2006
YEAR BOOK OF
VASCULAR SURGERY®

The 2006 Year Book Series

Year Book of Allergy, Asthma, and Clinical Immunology™: Drs Rosenwasser, Boguniewicz, Milgrom, Routes, and Weber

Year Book of Anesthesiology and Pain Management™: Drs Chestnut, Abram, Black, Gravlee, Lee, Mathru, and Roizen

Year Book of Cardiology®: Drs Gersh, Cheitlin, Elliott, Graham, Sundt, and Waldo

Year Book of Critical Care Medicine®: Drs Dellinger, Parrillo, Balk, Bekes, Dorman, and Dries

Year Book of Dentistry®: Drs McIntyre, Belvedere, Buhite, Davis, Henderson, Johnson, Jureyda, Ohrbach, Olin, Scott, Spencer, and Zakariasen

Year Book of Dermatology and Dermatologic Surgery™: Drs Thiers and Lang

Year Book of Diagnostic Radiology®: Drs Osborn, Birdwell, Dalinka, Gardiner, Levy, Maynard, Oestreich, and Rosado de Christenson

Year Book of Emergency Medicine®: Drs Burdick, Hamilton, Handly, Quintana, and Werner

Year Book of Endocrinology®: Drs Mazzaferri, Bessesen, Clarke, Howard, Kennedy, Leahy, Meikle, Molitch, Rogol, and Schteingart

Year Book of Family Practice®: Drs Bowman, Apgar, Dexter, Miser, Neill, and Scherger

Year Book of Gastroenterology™: Drs Lichtenstein, Burke, Campbell, Dempsey, Drebin, Ginsberg, Katzka, Kochman, Morris, Rombeau, Shah, and Stein

Year Book of Hand and Upper Limb Surgery®: Drs Chang and Steinmann

Year Book of Medicine®: Drs Barkin, Frishman, Loehrer, Garrick, Phillips, Pillinger, and Snydman

Year Book of Neonatal and Perinatal Medicine®: Drs Fanaroff, Maisels, and Stevenson

Year Book of Neurology and Neurosurgery®: Drs Gibbs and Verma

Year Book of Nuclear Medicine®: Drs Coleman, Blaufox, Royal, Strauss, and Zubal

Year Book of Obstetrics, Gynecology, and Women's Health®: Dr Shulman

Year Book of Oncology®: Drs Loehrer, Arceci, Glatstein, Gordon, Hanna, Morrow, and Thigpen

Year Book of Ophthalmology®: Drs Rapuano, Cohen, Eagle, Flanders, Hammersmith, Myers, Nelson, Penne, Sergott, Shields, Tipperman, and Vander

Year Book of Orthopedics®: Drs Morrey, Beauchamp, Peterson, Swiontkowski, Trigg, and Yaszemski

Year Book of Otolaryngology-Head and Neck Surgery®: Drs Paparella, Gapany, and Keefe

Year Book of Pathology and Laboratory Medicine®: Drs Raab, Parwani, Bejarano, and Bissell

Year Book of Pediatrics®: Dr Stockman

Year Book of Plastic and Aesthetic Surgery™: Drs Miller, Bartlett, Garner, McKinney, Ruberg, Salisbury, and Smith

Year Book of Psychiatry and Applied Mental Health®: Drs Talbott, Ballenger, Buckley, Frances, Jensen, and Markowitz

Year Book of Pulmonary Disease®: Drs Phillips, Barker, Lewis, Maurer, Tanoue, and Willsie

Year Book of Rheumatology, Arthritis, and Musculoskeletal Disease™: Drs Panush, Furst, Hadler, Hochberg, Lahita, and Paget

Year Book of Sports Medicine®: Drs Shephard, Alexander, Cantu, Feldman, McCrory, Nieman, Rowland, Sanborn, and Shrier

Year Book of Surgery®: Drs Copeland, Bland, Cerfolio, Daly, Eberlein, Fahey, Mozingo, Pruett, and Seeger

Year Book of Urology®: Drs Andriole and Coplen

Year Book of Vascular Surgery®: Dr Moneta

2006

The Year Book of VASCULAR SURGERY®

Editor-in-Chief

Gregory L. Moneta, MD

Professor and Chief of Vascular Surgery, Oregon Health and Science University; and Chief of Vascular Surgery, Oregon Health and Science University Hospital and Portland VA Hospital, Portland, Oregon

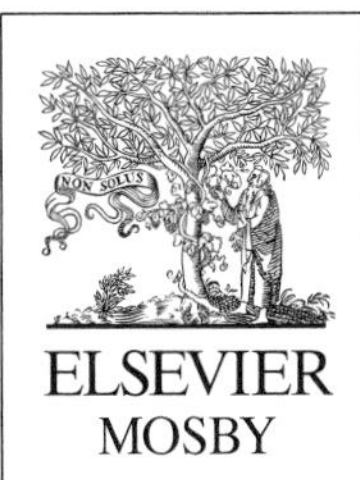

ELSEVIER
MOSBY

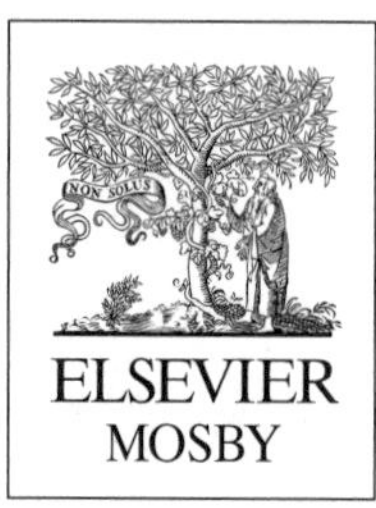

Vice President, Continuity Publishing: Andrea Stingelin
Publishing Director, Continuity: J. Heather Cullen
Developmental Editor: Ruth Malwitz
Senior Manager, Continuity Production: Idelle L. Winer
Senior Issue Manager: Pat Costigan
Illustrations and Permissions Coordinator: Dawn Vohsen

2006 EDITION

Printed in the United States of America
Composition by Thomas Technology Solutions, Inc.
Printing/binding by Sheridan Books, Inc

Editorial Office:
Elsevier
Suite 1800
1600 John F. Kennedy Blvd
Philadelphia, PA 19103-2899

International Standard Serial Number: 0749-4041
International Standard Book Number: 1-4160-3298-3
978-1-4160-3298-4

Contributors

James M. Edwards, MD

Associate Professor of Surgery, Oregon Health and Science University; and Chief of Surgery, Portland VA Hospital, Portland, Oregon

W. Anthony Lee, MD

Assistant Progessor of Surgery and Radiology, Division of Vascular Surgery and Endovascular Therapy, University of Florida, Gainesville, Florida

Fedor Lurie, MD, PhD

Clinical Assistant Professor of Surgery, University of Hawaii; and Vascular Surgeon, Kistner Vein Clinic, Honolulu, Hawaii

Amy B. Reed, MD

Assistant Professor of Surgery; Program Director, Vascular Surgery Fellowship, University of Cincinnati, Cincinnati, Ohio

Table of Contents

Journals Represented

Journals represented in this YEAR BOOK are listed below.

Acta Neurologica Scandinavica
American Journal of Kidney Diseases
American Journal of Medicine
American Journal of Neuroradiology
American Journal of Physiology Heart and Circulation Physiology
American Journal of Roentgenology
American Journal of Surgery
Anesthesiology
Annals of Internal Medicine
Annals of Otology, Rhinology and Laryngology
Annals of Rheumatic Diseases
Annals of Surgery
Annals of Vascular Surgery
Archives of Surgery
British Journal of Cancer
British Journal of General Practice
British Journal of Surgery
British Medical Journal
Canadian Medical Association Journal
Chest
Circulation
Clinical Radiology
Dermatologic Surgery
Diabetes Care
European Heart Journal
European Journal of Internal Medicine
European Journal of Vascular and Endovascular Surgery
Hypertension
Journal of Bone and Joint Surgery (American Volume)
Journal of Cardiothoracic and Vascular Anesthesia
Journal of Clinical Endocrinology and Metabolism
Journal of Immunology
Journal of Pediatric Surgery
Journal of Rheumatology
Journal of Surgical Research
Journal of Ultrasound in Medicine
Journal of Vascular Surgery
Journal of the American Academy of Dermatology
Journal of the American College of Cardiology
Journal of the American College of Surgeons
Journal of the American Geriatrics Society
Journal of the American Medical Association
Kidney International
Lancet
Metabolism: Clinical and Experimental
Microsurgery
Nephrology, Dialysis, Transplantation
Neurology
New England Journal of Medicine

Phlebology
Proceedings of the National Academy of Sciences
Radiology
Spine Journal
Stroke
Surgery
Thrombosis Research
Vascular and Endovascular Surgery
World Journal of Surgery

STANDARD ABBREVIATIONS

The following terms are abbreviated in this edition: acquired immunodeficiency syndrome (AIDS), cardiopulmonary resuscitation (CPR), central nervous system (CNS), cerebrospinal fluid (CSF), computed tomography (CT), deoxyribonucleic acid (DNA), electrocardiography (ECG), health maintenance organization (HMO), human immunodeficiency virus (HIV), intensive care unit (ICU), intramuscular (IM), intravenous (IV), magnetic resonance (MR) imaging (MRI), ribonucleic acid (RNA), and ultrasound (US).

NOTE

The YEAR BOOK OF VASCULAR SURGERY® is a literature survey service providing abstracts of articles published in the professional literature. Every effort is made to assure the accuracy of the information presented in these pages. Neither the editors nor the publisher of the YEAR BOOK OF VASCULAR SURGERY® can be responsible for errors in the original materials. The editors' comments are their own opinions. Mention of specific products within this publication does not constitute endorsement.

To facilitate the use of the YEAR BOOK OF VASCULAR SURGERY® as a reference tool, all illustrations and tables included in this publication are now identified as they appear in the original article. This change is meant to help the reader recognize that any illustration or table appearing in the YEAR BOOK OF VASCULAR SURGERY® may be only one of many in the original article. For this reason, figure and table numbers will often appear to be out of sequence within the YEAR BOOK OF VASCULAR SURGERY®.

Introduction

The introduction to the YEAR BOOK OF VASCULAR SURGERY stands at the beginning of the each year's volume. The introduction is, however, in reality the last thing that is prepared for each edition of the YEAR BOOK. These few pages can be used in any way the editor feels is appropriate. Elsevier is a great publisher to work with; there are no restrictions placed on the contents of the YEAR BOOK, the commentaries that accompany the abstracts, or on the editor's introductory comments. It would, of course, be a bit silly not to highlight in the Introduction some of the pivitol papers and topics of interest and controversy that appear in this volume. Below I will point out what are, in my opinion, particularly interesting or controversial papers. I will also provide a few comments on our field as it moves further into the endovascular era.

Over the last year, catheter-based therapies of the carotid artery and the superficial femoral artery have dominated the thoughts of many vascular surgeons. Such papers are featured frequently in this edition of the YEAR BOOK (Chapters 10 and 12 of the YEAR BOOK).

Carotid artery angioplasty and stenting (CAS) will be a viable alternative to carotid endarterectomy (CEA) for selected patients and under selected conditions. Exactly who those patients are and under what conditions CAS may be preferred over endarterectomy remains to be determined. It may even be CAS will be preferred over CEA for most patients with appropriate indications for carotid intervention. However, at the moment, there are lots of procedures being performed and little real science getting accomplished. The SAPHIERE trial was an abomination and everyone, except perhaps reviewers for *The New England Journal of Medicine*, know it.

It is actually relatively sad what is happening with CAS. The field now appears largely driven by zealots with agendas and is also driven by industry connections. Turf wars are waging between societies and in individual hospitals. There seems to be more concern regarding who will do CAS rather than to whom should CAS be offered. More than anything else in recent memory, CAS is illustrating just how petty, self-absorbed, and self-interested physicians can be. Eventually it will get sorted out, but in doing so a lot of money is going to be spent unnecessarily, a lot of patients are going to be subjected to unnecessary treatment, and many friendships will be destroyed. Of course, all of this will be under the guise of patient care and safety. The dirty little secrets of stock options, physician power, prestige and income will be glossed over. Nevertheless, those elephants are still in the room regardless of whether anyone is willing to acknowledge them. Suddenly, used car salesmen don't seem nearly as slimy as often portrayed.

The situation is similar but not quite as egregious with respect to catheter-based treatments of superficial femoral artery occlusive disease. This is a field also dominated and driven by industry. That is not all bad. Industry provides innovation and innovation eventually leads to progress. Nevertheless, I grow weary of the constant onslaught of industry representatives armed with 6-month data they really don't understand trying to tell me what is best for my patients, all the while knowing their next car payment may depend on whether I am really as stupid as they must think I am. At the moment, you can burn, scrape, freeze, cut out, radiate, dilate, and stent superficial femoral artery (SFA) lesions. The results are really not substantially different at the moment. Intimal hyperplasia roars back at about 18 months postprocedure. Technology is changing, but biology is still winning.

Similar to CAS, catheter-based treatments of the SFA will clearly have a role in the treatment of patients with lower-extremity ischemia. It is somewhat a matter of philosophy. When is a procedure with predictably limited patency acceptable? It seems to me that a nonhealing ulcer in an otherwise fairly well-perfused lower extremity may be an indication for a catheter based SFA procedure. In such cases, the SFA may have a reasonable chance of staying patent long enough to result in healing of the ulcer. However, when the patient is otherwise as healthy as a critical limb ischemia patient can be, and the indication for treatment is spontaneous gangrene or ischemic rest pain, a more durable procedure should be considered and is probably preferred. I don't think a catheter-based treatment is indicated simply because it is unlikely to hurt and may help. That is an irresponsible use of resources, tax dollars, insurance premiums, etc; a matter more of philosophy than science.

Catheter-based treatment of claudication is even more controversial. Careful assessment of comorbidities is required. Many claudicants have other medical conditions that impede their ambulation. In addition, survival is considerably better than in patients with critical limb ischemia. How many repeat procedures can be justified in the name of increased walking distance? I submit we don't even know how many claudication patients get a repeat catheter-based treatment when the initial treatment fails. The overall impact of catheter-based and bypass procedures on patient quality of life and their function is not known.

It is really no longer acceptable to evaluate any invasive treatment of limb ischemia, whether it be for critical limb ischemia or claudication, with only patency rates. Patients really only care if their graft or angioplasty is patent if the patency or lack of patency affects their quality of life and functional status. It may be acceptable for a SFA angioplasty to fail in a patient with exercise-induced leg pain if that patient's ambulation, once limited by claudication, is now more limited by arthritis or chronic obstructive pulmonary disease than by claudication. In the modern world, any phase III study of any form of treatment for limb ischemia must include assessment of quality of life as an end point. The importance of functional outcomes and quality of life evaluation in the assessment of peripheral arterial disease is highlighted in Chapter 10 of the YEAR BOOK.

Genetics is assuming an increasingly important role in basic vascular surgical research. Much of this research is, at the moment, best described as exploratory. Microarray DNA studies allow for study of thousands of genes whose expression may be up-regulated or down-regulated under specific conditions. These types of studies are being applied to aortic aneurysm, peripheral artery occlusive disease, as well as carotid disease (Chapters 1, 5, 9, 10, and 12). Currently, we are learning what genes are up-regulated and down-regulated in various disease states and respond to various treatments. We still have no idea of the timing of the changes in gene regulation, which genes are actually important in producing a clinically important effect, or which ones are potentially modifiable by therapy or risk factor reduction.

As always, I have tried to highlight in the YEAR BOOK major randomized clinical trials. With respect to aortic endografting, the British EVAR and Dutch DREAM trials have both found that endografting reduces perioperative mortality compared with open surgery. However, long-term mortality is not affected by endografting and after 1 year, health-related quality of life is no different in patients treated with open versus endovascular repair of their infrarenal aortic aneurysm (Chapter 6). An interesting trial conducted in patients after acute deep venous thrombosis (DVT) found the postthrombotic syndrome seems to be improved, or even eliminated, by early treatment of patients with acute DVT with elastic compression stockings (Chapter 15).

Papers with regard to perioperative management of vascular surgical patients are in Chapter 3 of the YEAR BOOK. In recent years, there has been a trend away from routine cardiac investigation of patients asymptomatic for cardiac symptoms about to undergo a vascular surgical procedure. A large muticenter Department of Veteran's Affairs trial should add to this movement in that it found no benefit of prophylactic cardiac revascularization in reducing mortality in patients with vascular disease undergoing a peripheral vascular procedure. There are more and more papers suggesting pleotropic effects of statins in vascular surgical patients in not only reducing progression of vascular disease, but also in reducing perioperative mortality in patients undergoing open carotid and aortic reconstructions as well as bypass procedures for lower extremity occlusive disease (Chapters 3, 5, 10, and 12).

In this year's YEAR BOOK, there are also a number of papers focusing on limiting contrast-induced nephropathy. N-acetylcysteine and fenoldopam mesylate appear less effective than previously thought, while simple infusions of sodium bicarbonate in conjunction with hydration appear quite effective in lowering contrast-induced nephropathy.

Screening for aortic aneurysm and for vascular disease in general has become a hot topic. Identifying patients with peripheral artery occlusive disease as a means of predicting cardiac mortality is now widely accepted but still not widely practiced. The US Preventative Task Force and the Society for Vascular Surgery along with the Society for Vascular Medicine and Biology have published separate recommendations on screening for aortic aneurysmal disease (Chapter 5).

Traditional vascular surgical topics and operations are continuing to undergo evaluation. Femoral vein as a conduit for primary reconstruction of aortoiliac disease in younger patients has been proposed (Chapter 7) and the traditional exclusion technique for popliteal aneurysm questioned (Chapter 10). Bypass to inframalleolar vessels results in better limb salvage than many may have thought (Chapter10), while transposed basilic vein as dialysis access is probably not as good an access as first thought (Chapter 11).

Iatrogentic vascular trauma is rapidly replacing street violence as the predominant source of vascular injury in many hospitals. Evaluation of possible popliteal artery injury associated with knee dislocation does not require routine angiography (Chapter 13). Repeat operation for a failed mesenteric bypass is both practical and effective (Chapter 8).

Acute and chronic venous disorders (Chapters 15 and 16) again constitute an important focus for the YEAR BOOK. The role of determining D-dimer levels as an aid to diagnosis of DVT and limiting the need for venous ultrasound studies continues to be explored. Over the last several years, the safety and efficacy of limiting venous ultrasound in the diagnosis of DVT has become more accepted. The literature by and large supports this approach. Development of an artificial venous valve is frustratingly slow but continues to inch forward in Portland (Chapter 16). We continue to be presented with new data verifying the endovenous approach to controlling reflux in the greater and lesser saphenous veins; at the same time, new sclerotherapy techniques are being developed and tested (Chapter 16).

Finally, I wish to thank all who work so hard on this project each year. I am very grateful to those who serve as associate editors. It is important that perspectives other than those of the editor be included in the YEAR BOOK. I put the associate editors in a difficult position by asking them to review articles that I choose for them. The fact they do their jobs so well greatly enhances the overall quality of the YEAR BOOK. I also express my appreciation to the YEAR BOOK staff at Elsevier and give special thanks to Jenna Bowker for her invaluable assistance in organizing the enormous amount of material required for production of the YEAR BOOK OF VASCULAR SURGERY. Jenna has provided a great service to the vascular community over the last 4 years by serving as the YEAR BOOK'S organizational focal point. She has recently been accepted to nursing school. We all wish her well in her career.

Gregory L. Moneta, MD

1 Basic Considerations

Effects of an Inhibitor of Cholesteryl Ester Transfer Protein on HDL Cholesterol

Brousseau ME, Schaefer EJ, Wolfe ML, et al (Tufts Univ, Boston; Univ of Pennsylvania, Philadelphia; Pfizer, Groton, Conn)

N Engl J Med 350:1505-1515, 2004 1–1

Background.—Decreased high-density lipoprotein (HDL) cholesterol levels constitute a major risk factor for coronary heart disease; however, there are no therapies that substantially raise HDL cholesterol levels. Inhibition of cholesteryl ester transfer protein (CETP) has been proposed as a strategy to raise HDL cholesterol levels.

Methods.—We conducted a single-blind, placebo-controlled study to examine the effects of torcetrapib, a potent inhibitor of CETP, on plasma lipoprotein levels in 19 subjects with low levels of HDL cholesterol (<40 mg per deciliter [1.0 mmol per liter]), 9 of whom were also treated with 20 mg of atorvastatin daily. All the subjects received placebo for four weeks and then received 120 mg of torcetrapib daily for the following four weeks. Six of the subjects who did not receive atorvastatin also participated in a third phase, in which they received 120 mg of torcetrapib twice daily for four weeks.

Results.—Treatment with 120 mg of torcetrapib daily increased plasma concentrations of HDL cholesterol by 61 percent (P<0.001) and 46 percent (P=0.001) in the atorvastatin and non-atorvastatin cohorts, respectively, and treatment with 120 mg twice daily increased HDL cholesterol by 106 percent (P<0.001). Torcetrapib also reduced low-density lipoprotein (LDL) cholesterol levels by 17 percent in the atorvastatin cohort (P=0.02). Finally, torcetrapib significantly altered the distribution of cholesterol among HDL and LDL subclasses, resulting in increases in the mean particle size of HDL and LDL in each cohort.

Conclusions.—In subjects with low HDL cholesterol levels, CETP inhibition with torcetrapib markedly increased HDL cholesterol levels and also decreased LDL cholesterol levels, both when administered as monotherapy and when administered in combination with a statin.

► This is a small study, but the results are dramatic. Torcetrapib was highly effective in increasing HDL cholesterol levels. Clinical studies have suggested that increased HDL levels are associated with decreased risk of coronary heart disease. A necessary subsequent step in the evaluation of torcetrapib will be to determine reduction in cardiovascular risk after raising HDL levels in patients with initially low HDL levels.

G. L. Moneta, MD

Clinical Pharmacology of Platelet, Monocyte, and Vascular Cyclooxygenase Inhibition by Naproxen and Low-Dose Aspirin in Healthy Subjects

Capone ML, Tacconnelli S, Sciulli MG, et al (G d'Annunzio Univ, Chieti, Italy; Univ of Rome; Univ of Verona, Italy)

Circulation 109:1468-1471, 2004 1–2

Background.—The current controversy on the potential cardioprotective effect of naproxen prompted us to evaluate the extent and duration of platelet, monocyte, and vascular cyclooxygenase (COX) inhibition by naproxen compared with low-dose aspirin.

Method and Results.—We performed a crossover, open-label study of low-dose aspirin (100 mg/d) or naproxen (500 mg BID) administered to 9 healthy subjects for 6 days. The effects on thromboxane (TX) and prostacyclin biosynthesis were assessed up to 24 hours after oral dosing. Serum TXB_2, plasma prostaglandin (PG) E_2, and urinary 11-dehydro-TXB_2 and 2,3-dinor-6-keto-$PGF_{1\alpha}$ were measured by previously validated radioimmunoassays. The administration of naproxen or aspirin caused a similar suppression of whole-blood TXB_2 production, an index of platelet COX-1 activity ex vivo, by 94±3% and 99±0.3% (mean±SD), respectively, and of the urinary excretion of 11-dehydro-TXB_2, an index of systemic biosynthesis of TXA_2 in vivo, by 85±8% and 78±7%, respectively, that persisted throughout the dosing interval. Naproxen, in contrast to aspirin, significantly reduced systemic prostacyclin biosynthesis by 77±19%, consistent with differential inhibition of monocyte COX-2 activity measured ex vivo.

Conclusions.—The regular administration of naproxen 500 mg BID can mimic the antiplatelet COX-1 effect of low-dose aspirin. Naproxen, unlike aspirin, decreased prostacyclin biosynthesis in vivo.

▶ The authors have shown that a nonsteroidal anti-inflammatory drug (NSAID) can virtually completely suppress COX-1–associated inhibition of TXA_2, the platelet inhibition thought to be responsible for the cardioprotective effect of aspirin. This suggests NSAIDs may serve as "aspirin substitutes" in patients at risk for cardiovascular disease and requiring NSAID therapy. The potential cardiac protective effect of naproxen in this study, however, only was present for 24 hours after dosing. This indicates compliance could be a problem using NSAIDs as cardioprotective drugs.

G. L. Moneta, MD

Strain-dependent Vascular Remodeling: The "Glagov Phenomenon" Is Genetically Determined

Korshunov VA, Berk BC (Univ of Rochester, NY)
Circulation 110:220-226, 2004 1–3

Background.—Atherosclerosis of the carotid artery, called intima-media thickening (IMT), is a form of vascular remodeling that is an important predictor for cardiovascular events and has a strong genetic component.

Method and Results.—Recently, we established a mouse model of vascular remodeling based on partial ligation of the carotid, which is relevant to the "Glagov phenomenon." We hypothesized that there would be genetically determined differences in outward remodeling and IMT induced by carotid flow alterations. We compared vascular remodeling among 5 inbred strains of mice. Despite similar changes in flow among the strains in the left carotid artery (LCA), we observed dramatic differences in remodeling of the partially ligated LCA relative to control. The smallest IMT volume (26±3 μm^3) was found in C3H/HeJ mice, and the largest were in SJL/J (59±10 μm^3) and FVB/NJ (81±6 μm^3). Shear stress did not differ after ligation among strains. Lumen area decreased only when stenosis was ≥55%. IMT correlated significantly with outward remodeling among inbred strains (except C3H). There were significant strain-dependent differences in remodeling index (measured as vessel area/IMT), which suggest fundamental alterations in sensing or transducing hemodynamic signals among strains. Among hemodynamic factors, low shear stress and high heart rate were predictive for IMT. Specifically, heart rate (bpm: C3H, 592±6; SJL, 649±6; FVB, 683±7) but not systolic blood pressure (mm Hg: C3H, 116±2; SJL, 119±1; FVB, 136±1) was predictive.

Conclusions.—The present study indicates that performing a genetic cross of these strains and total genome scan should identify genes that mediate vascular remodeling.

▶ The "Glagov phenomenon," that arteries enlarge during the early stages of atherosclerosis, is well known and well accepted. Recent advances in gene-specific research now promise to discern the underlying mechanisms of vascular remodeling. This research that links genetic differences to the phenotypic effects of shear stress is the beginning of the link between genetics, hemodynamics, and vascular remodeling in the development of atherosclerosis.

G. L. Moneta, MD

Arterial Enlargement, Tortuosity, and Intimal Thickening in Response to Sequential Exposure to High and Low Wall Shear Stress

Sho E, Nanjo H, Sho M, et al (Akita Univ, Japan; Stanford Univ, Calif)

J Vasc Surg 39:601-612, 2004 1–4

Introduction.—We investigated the effects of sequential and prolonged exposure to high and low wall shear stress on arterial remodeling using a rabbit arteriovenous fistula (AVF) model. Blood flow was increased by approximately 17-fold to 20-fold when the AVF was open, and returned to normal when the AVF was occluded. Repeated opening and closing of the AVF resulted in sequential exposure of the artery to high and low wall shear stress. High flow and high wall shear stress induced arterial dilatation, elongation, and tortuosity, without intimal thickening. The common carotid artery was elongated 37% after 4 weeks of high flow, and was shortened 10% after 6 weeks of normal flow. Subsequent cycles of high flow induced less elongation, with less shortening after return to normal flow. Enlargement of the distal segment was more dramatic than in the proximal segment, despite exposure to the same volume of flow and the same initial high wall shear stress after creation of the AVF. The distal carotid segment enlarged more than did the proximal segment during each exposure to high flow. In segments of carotid artery exposed to low wall shear stress (<5 dynes/cm^2) intimal thickening developed. These changes were maximal in the distal carotid segment, just before the AVF. Each cycle of low wall shear stress induced intimal thickening accompanied by medial hyperplasia. Intimal thickening was inhibited during periods of high flow when wall shear stress was high. Three cycles of flow alteration induced three layers of intimal thickening in the distal arterial segment, two layers of intimal thickening in the middle segment, and one layer of intimal thickening in the proximal segment. Long-term exposure to low wall shear stress induced severe intimal thickening and medial hyperplasia in different segments. Thus the response of the carotid artery afferent to an AVF varies along the length of the artery, with maximum enlargement, elongation, and tortuosity in the distal segment, just proximal to the AVF. Similarly, intimal thickening in response to low wall shear stress is maximal in the distal carotid artery. It appears that intimal thickening is related to local levels of low wall shear stress, and occurs when wall shear stress chronically falls to less than 5 dynes/cm^2.

► Low shear stress is known to be associated with the development of atherosclerosis. The authors' AVF model is obviously not directly analogous to atherogenesis. From clinical observations we know that arterial changes induced by AVFs do not generally resemble atherosclerotic arteries. Nevertheless, the idea that there is a threshold level of shear stress below which intimal medial thickness occurs is intriguing and seems to further link hemodynamics and the atherosclerotic process. The mediators of that link are likely genetically determined (see Abstract 1–3).

G. L. Moneta, MD

Deletion of p66^{shc} Gene Protects Against Age-Related Endothelial Dysfunction

Francia P, delli Gatti C, Bachschmid M, et al (Inst of Physiology, Zürich, Switzerland; Univ Hosp, Zürich, Switzerland; Univ "La Sapienza," Rome, et al)
Circulation 110:2889-2895, 2004 1–5

Background.—Enhanced production of reactive oxygen species (ROS) has been recognized as the major determinant of age-related endothelial dysfunction. The p66^{shc} protein controls cellular responses to oxidative stress. Mice lacking p66^{shc} (p66$^{shc-/-}$) have increased resistance to ROS and a 30% prolonged life span. The present study investigates age-dependent changes of endothelial function in this model.

Method and Results.—Aortic rings from young and old p66$^{shc-/-}$ or wild-type (WT) mice were suspended for isometric tension recording. Nitric oxide (NO) release was measured by a porphyrinic microsensor. Expression of endothelial NO synthase (eNOS), inducible NOS (iNOS), superoxide dismutase, and nitrotyrosine-containing proteins was assessed by Western blotting. Nitrotyrosine residues were also identified by immunohistochemistry. Superoxide (O_2^-) production was determined by coelenterazine-enhanced chemiluminescence. Endothelium-dependent relaxation in response to acetylcholine was age-dependently impaired in WT mice but not in p66$^{shc-/-}$ mice. Accordingly, an age-related decline of NO release was found in WT but not in p66$^{shc-/-}$ mice. The expression of eNOS and manganese superoxide dismutase was not affected by aging either in WT or in p66$^{shc-/-}$ mice, whereas iNOS was upregulated only in old WT mice. It is interesting that old WT mice displayed a significant increase of O_2^- production as well as of nitrotyrosine expression compared with young animals. Such age-dependent changes were not found in p66$^{shc-/-}$ mice.

Conclusions.—We report that inactivation of the p66^{shc} gene protects against age-dependent, ROS-mediated endothelial dysfunction. These findings suggest that the p66^{shc} is part of a signal transduction pathway also relevant to endothelial integrity and may represent a novel target to prevent vascular aging.

► As I get older, I get more interested in what makes me get older. Age-dependent endothelial dysfunction may be related to inactivation of particular gene products. This study has identified a gene that, when inactivated, seems to be protective against vascular aging. Maintaining bioavailability of NO is important for cardiovascular health. Deletion of the gene identified in this study leads to decreased vascular wall O_2^- production, which leads to decreased NO breakdown and therefore, theoretically, decreased vascular wall aging. And you thought you just had to live right!

G. L. Moneta, MD

Direct Effect of Ethanol on Human Vascular Function

Tawakol A, Omland T, Creager MA (Massachusetts Gen Hosp, Boston; Brigham and Women's Hosp, Boston; Akershus Univ, Nordbyhagen, Norway)

Am J Physiol Heart Circ Physiol 286:H2468-H2473, 2004 1–6

Introduction.—Epidemiological studies indicate that moderate ethanol consumption reduces cardiovascular mortality. Cellular and animal data suggest that ethanol confers beneficial effects on the vascular endothelium and increases the bioavailability of nitric oxide. The purpose of this study was to assess the effect of ethanol on endothelium-dependent, nitric oxide–mediated vasodilation in healthy human subjects. Forearm blood flow (FBF) was determined by venous occlusion plethysmography in healthy human subjects during intra-arterial infusions of either methacholine (0.3, 1.0, 3.0, and 10.0 mcg/min, $n = 9$), nitroprusside (0.3, 1.0, 3.0, and 10.0 mcg/min, $n = 9$), or verapamil (10, 30, 100, and 300 mcg/min, $n = 8$) before and during the concomitant intra-arterial infusions of ethanol (10% ethanol in 5% dextrose). Additionally, a time control experiment was conducted, during which the methacholine dose-response curve was measured twice during vehicle infusions ($n = 5$). During ethanol infusion, mean forearm and systemic alcohol levels were 227 ± 30 and 6 ± 0 mg/dl, respectively. Ethanol infusion alone reduced FBF (2.5 ± 0.1 to 1.9 ± 0.1 $ml \cdot dl^{-1} \cdot min^{-1}$, $P < 0.05$). Despite initial vasoconstriction, ethanol augmented the FBF dose-response curves to methacholine, nitroprusside, and verapamil ($P < 0.01$ by ANOVA for each). To determine whether this augmented FBF response was related to shear-stress-induced release of nitric oxide, FBF was measured during the co-infusion of ethanol and N^G-nitro-L-arginine (L-NAME; $n = 8$) at rest and during verapamil-induced vasodilation. The addition of L-NAME did not block the ability of ethanol to augment verapamil-induced vasodilation. Ethanol has complex direct vascular effects, which include basal vasoconstriction as well as potentiation of both endothelium-dependent and -independent vasodilation. None of these effects appear to be mediated by an increase in nitric oxide bioavailability, thus disputing findings from preclinical models.

▶ There are apparently mechanisms other than those mediated by nitric oxide (see also Abstract 1–5) that mediate endothelial-dependent vasoconstriction and vasodilatation. Alcohol, since it seems to act independent of nitric oxide, and clearly has vasoactive effects, may be a compound that someday will provide a clue to other methods of modifying vascular function and aging.

G. L. Moneta, MD

Preclinical Changes in the Mechanical Properties of Abdominal Aorta in Obese Children

Iannuzzi A, Licenziati MR, Acampora C, et al (Ospedale S Maria dell'Olmo e Costa d'Amalfi, Cava de' Tirreni, Italy; Ospedale A Cardarelli, Naples, Italy; Universita' di Napoli Federico II, Naples, Italy)

Metabolism 53:1243-1246, 2004 1–7

Introduction.—Obesity in childhood has been associated with the development of early cardiovascular abnormalities. The aim of the present study was to investigate whether preclinical functional changes are detectable in the abdominal aorta of obese children. One hundred consecutively seen obese children and 50 healthy controls were studied. The groups were matched in terms of age and gender. The pulsatile wall-motion of the abdominal aorta was determined using a B-mode ultrasound technique. The following mechanical property parameters were measured or computed: lumen diastolic and systolic diameters, relative aortic strain, elastic modulus, and stiffness. Compared to controls, obese children had higher blood pressure values and higher concentrations of total cholesterol, triglycerides, insulin, and C-reactive protein. Homeostasis model assessment (HOMA) score, a parameter of insulin resistance, was significantly higher in obese children than in controls (3.2 ± 1.9 *v* 1.4 ± 0.5, $P < .001$). Aortic mechanical parameters were significantly different in obese children as compared to controls: stiffness was higher (3.00 ± 1.45 *v* 2.22 ± 0.87, $P < .001$) as was elastic modulus (0.38 ± 0.18 *v* 0.24 ± 0.10 N/m^2, $P < .001$). Obese girls with insulin resistance (ie, in the highest tertile of HOMA, >3.7) had increased aortic stiffness (3.79 ± 2.25) compared to obese girls in the lowest tertiles of HOMA (2.67 ± 1.09, $P = .045$), even after adjustment for traditional cardiovascular risk factors ($P = .031$). The present findings suggest that preclinical changes in the aortic elastic properties are detectable in obese children. Insulin resistance seems to play an important role in the increased rigidity of the aortic wall in obese girls.

▶ It is not surprising there are changes in the mechanical properties of blood vessels in obese children. Childhood obesity is associated with early development of vascular abnormalities, and such abnormalities may well mediate or be mediated by mechanical changes. The differential effects of insulin resistance on aortic stiffness in male versus female children suggests a possible sex-linked determinant of atherosclerosis at an early age.

G. L. Moneta, MD

Weight Change Is Associated With Change in Arterial Stiffness Among Healthy Young Adults

Wildman RP, Farhat GN, Patel AS, et al (Tulane Univ, New Orleans, La; Univ of Pittsburgh, Pa)

Hypertension 45:187-192, 2005 1–8

Introduction.—Risk factors for arterial stiffness progression have not been well characterized. We examined the relationship between arterial stiffness progression and body weight and weight gain in a group of healthy young adults. Aortic pulse-wave velocity was assessed at 2 time points approximately 2 years apart in 152 white and black adults aged 20 to 40 years, and was standardized by the time between visits to obtain annualized pulse-wave velocity changes. Blacks had 15.5 cm/s per year larger annual pulse-wave velocity increases compared with whites (P=0.02), even after multivariable adjustment for weight and blood pressure changes. Larger annual pulse-wave velocity increases were also associated with larger baseline body weight (P=0.02), waist girth (P=0.003), and body mass index (P<0.001), and greater annual weight gain (P=0.02), after adjustment for baseline pulse-wave velocity. After multivariable adjustment that included blood pressure changes, larger baseline waist girth (P=0.009), baseline body mass index (P=0.001), body mass index increase (P=0.037), and weight gain (P=0.017) remained significantly associated with larger annual pulse-wave velocity progression. Weight change showed a direct relationship with pulse-wave velocity change; mean annual pulse-wave velocity changes were −29.9 cm/s per year (regression) for those with ≥4.5 kg annual weight loss and 18.2 cm/s per year (progression) for those with ≥4.5 kg annual weight gain. These data show strong associations between weight gain and arterial stiffness progression, as well as between weight loss and arterial stiffness regression. These data greatly underscore the vascular benefit of weight loss. Successful weight loss programs in young adults, particularly blacks, are needed.

► If atherosclerosis is in part mediated by arterial stiffness and, as shown by this and the previous abstract (Abstract 1–7), increased weight leads to increased arterial stiffness, then one would hope losing weight would lead to a decrease in arterial stiffness. Apparently, this is the case. Perhaps it is possible to reverse some of the early determinants of the atherosclerotic process. That would be good thing.

G. L. Moneta, MD

The Metabolic Syndrome Is Associated With Advanced Vascular Damage in Patients With Coronary Heart Disease, Stroke, Peripheral Arterial Disease or Abdominal Aortic Aneurysm

Olijhoek JK, for the SMART Study Group (UMC Utrecht, The Netherlands)

Eur Heart J 25:342-348, 2004 1–9

Aims.—The metabolic syndrome is associated with an increased risk of cardiovascular disease in patients without a cardiovascular history. We investigated whether the metabolic syndrome is related to the extent of vascular damage in patients with various manifestations of vascular disease.

Method and Results.—The study population of this cross-sectional survey consisted of 502 patients recently diagnosed with coronary heart disease (CHD), 236 with stroke, 218 with peripheral arterial disease (PAD) and 89 with abdominal aortic aneurysm (AAA). Metabolic syndrome was diagnosed according to Adult Treatment Panel III criteria. Carotid Intima Media Thickness (IMT), Ankle Brachial Pressure Index (ABPI) and albuminuria were used as non-invasive markers of vascular damage and adjusted for age and sex if appropriate.

The prevalence of the metabolic syndrome in the study population was 45%. In PAD patients this was 57%; in CHD patients 40%, in stroke patients 43% and in AAA patients 45%. Patients with the metabolic syndrome had an increased mean IMT (0.98 vs 0.92 mm, *P*-value <0.01), more often a decreased ABPI (14% vs 10%, *P*-value 0.06) and increased prevalence of albuminuria (20% vs 15%, *P*-value 0.03) compared to patients without this syndrome. An increase in the number of components of the metabolic syndrome was associated with an increase in mean IMT (*P*-value for trend <0.001), lower ABPI (*P*-value for trend <0.01) and higher prevalence albuminuria (*P*-value for trend <0.01).

Conclusion.—In patients with manifest vascular disease the presence of the metabolic syndrome is associated with advanced vascular damage.

▶ The data indicate that the metabolic syndrome is not only a marker for increased risk of cardiovascular disease but also a marker for worse cardiovascular disease in patients with a manifestation of peripheral atherosclerosis. This is another bit of evidence indicating the profound adverse health affects of obesity. Obesity is not only a risk factor for atherosclerosis but is also a risk factor for more severe atherosclerosis.

G. L. Moneta, MD

Lifestyle, Diabetes, and Cardiovascular Risk Factors 10 Years After Bariatric Surgery

Sjöström L, for the Swedish Obese Subjects Study (Sahlgrenska Univ, Göteborg, Sweden; et al)

N Engl J Med 351:2683-2693, 2004 1–10

Background.—Weight loss is associated with short-term amelioration and prevention of metabolic and cardiovascular risk, but whether these benefits persist over time is unknown.

Methods.—The prospective, controlled Swedish Obese Subjects Study involved obese subjects who underwent gastric surgery and contemporaneously matched, conventionally treated obese control subjects. We now report follow-up data for subjects (mean age, 48 years; mean body-mass index, 41) who had been enrolled for at least 2 years (4047 subjects) or 10 years (1703 subjects) before the analysis (January 1, 2004). The follow-up rate for laboratory examinations was 86.6 percent at 2 years and 74.5 percent at 10 years.

Results.—After two years, the weight had increased by 0.1 percent in the control group and had decreased by 23.4 percent in the surgery group ($P<0.001$). After 10 years, the weight had increased by 1.6 percent and decreased by 16.1 percent, respectively ($P<0.001$). Energy intake was lower and the proportion of physically active subjects higher in the surgery group than in the control group throughout the observation period. Two- and 10-year rates of recovery from diabetes, hypertriglyceridemia, low levels of high-density lipoprotein cholesterol, hypertension, and hyperuricemia were more favorable in the surgery group than in the control group, whereas recovery from hypercholesterolemia did not differ between the groups. The surgery group had lower 2- and 10-year incidence rates of diabetes, hypertriglyceridemia, and hyperuricemia than the control group; differences between the groups in the incidence of hypercholesterolemia and hypertension were undetectable.

Conclusions.—As compared with conventional therapy, bariatric surgery appears to be a viable option for the treatment of severe obesity, resulting in long-term weight loss, improved lifestyle, and, except for hypercholesterolemia, amelioration in risk factors that were elevated at baseline (Figs 3 and 4).

▶ This was not a randomized study. The data, however, strongly implicate bariatric surgery as an effective means of improving cardiovascular risk factors in the morbidly obese. The study does not tell us whether progression of established vascular disease in the morbidly obese can be slowed by bariatric surgery. We certainly are not at the point at which we can recommend bariatric surgery as a treatment to slow progression of peripheral vascular disease. However, in patients with established cardiovascular risk factors who are morbidly obese, bariatric surgery can be recommended to diminish these risk factors and improve lifestyle.

G. L. Moneta, MD

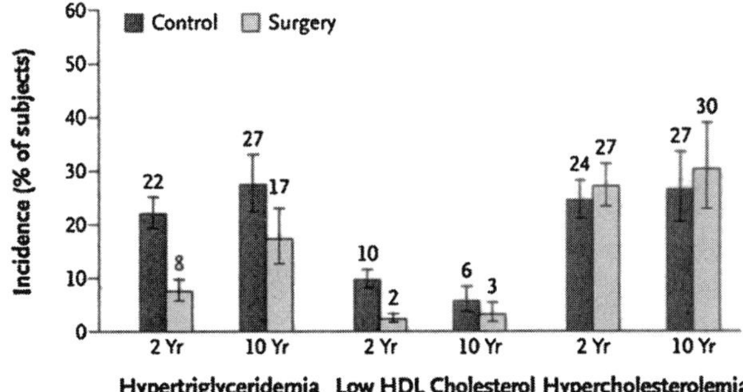

No. of subjects						
Control	801	281	1174	440	596	188
Surgery	731	225	1293	431	504	135
Odds ratio	0.29	0.61	0.21	0.57	1.27	1.16
95% CI	0.21–0.41	0.39–0.95	0.14–0.32	0.29–1.15	0.95–1.69	0.69–1.95
P value	<0.001	0.03	<0.001	0.12	0.11	0.57

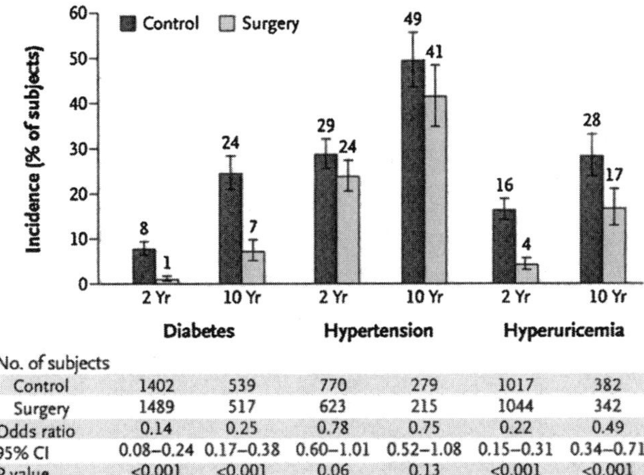

No. of subjects						
Control	1402	539	770	279	1017	382
Surgery	1489	517	623	215	1044	342
Odds ratio	0.14	0.25	0.78	0.75	0.22	0.49
95% CI	0.08–0.24	0.17–0.38	0.60–1.01	0.52–1.08	0.15–0.31	0.34–0.71
P value	<0.001	<0.001	0.06	0.13	<0.001	<0.001

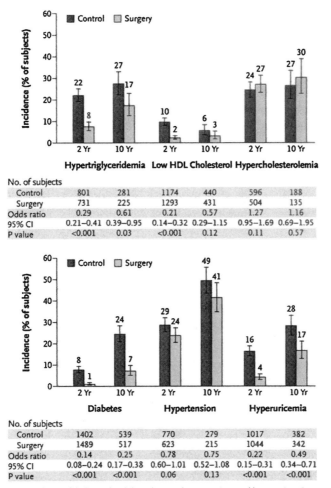

FIGURE 3.—Incidence of diabetes, lipid disturbances, hypertension, and hyperuricemia among subjects in the SOS Study over 2- and 10-year periods. Data are for subjects who completed 2 years and 10 years of the study. The *bars* and the values above the bars indicate unadjusted incidence rates; *I bars* represent the corresponding 95 percent confidence intervals (CIs). The odds ratios, 95 percent CIs for the odds ratios, and P values have been adjusted for sex, age, and body-mass index at the time of inclusion in the intervention study. (Reprinted by permission of *The New England Journal of Medicine* from Sjöström L, for the Swedish Obese Subjects Study Scientific Group: Lifestyle, diabetes, and cardiovascular risk factors 10 years after bariatric surgery. *N Engl J Med* 351:2683-2693, 2004.)

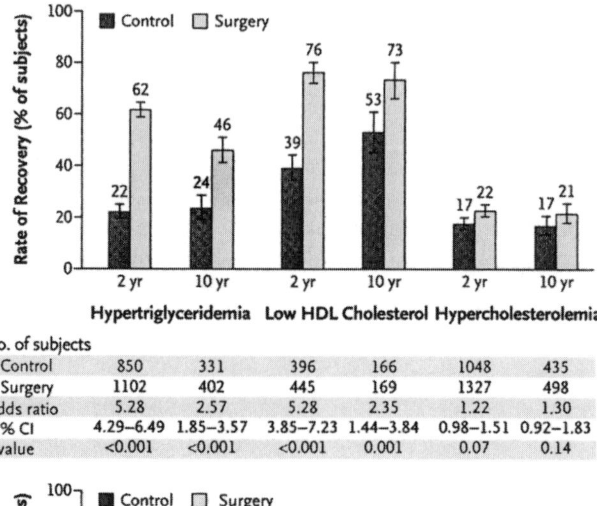

No. of subjects	Hypertriglyceridemia 2 yr	Hypertriglyceridemia 10 yr	Low HDL Cholesterol 2 yr	Low HDL Cholesterol 10 yr	Hypercholesterolemia 2 yr	Hypercholesterolemia 10 yr
Control	850	331	396	166	1048	435
Surgery	1102	402	445	169	1327	498
Odds ratio	5.28	2.57	5.28	2.35	1.22	1.30
95% CI	4.29–6.49	1.85–3.57	3.85–7.23	1.44–3.84	0.98–1.51	0.92–1.83
P value	<0.001	<0.001	<0.001	0.001	0.07	0.14

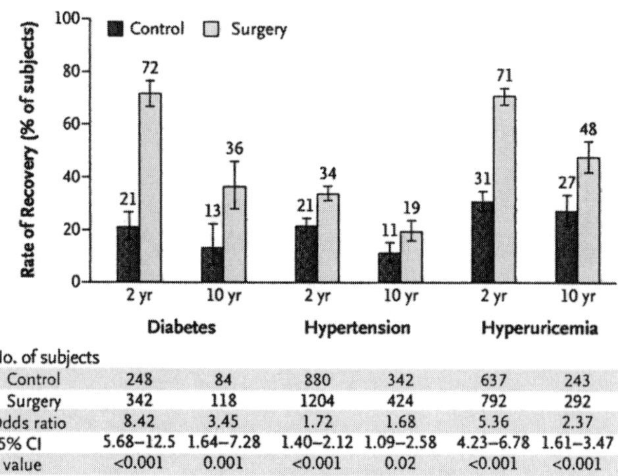

No. of subjects	Diabetes 2 yr	Diabetes 10 yr	Hypertension 2 yr	Hypertension 10 yr	Hyperuricemia 2 yr	Hyperuricemia 10 yr
Control	248	84	880	342	637	243
Surgery	342	118	1204	424	792	292
Odds ratio	8.42	3.45	1.72	1.68	5.36	2.37
95% CI	5.68–12.5	1.64–7.28	1.40–2.12	1.09–2.58	4.23–6.78	1.61–3.47
P value	<0.001	0.001	<0.001	0.02	<0.001	<0.001

FIGURE 4.—Recovery from diabetes, lipid disturbances, hypertension, and hyperuricemia over 2 and 10 years in surgically treated subjects and their obese controls. Data are for subjects who completed 2 years and 10 years of the study. The *bars* and the values above the bars indicate unadjusted rates of recovery; *I bars* represent the corresponding 95 percent confidence intervals (CIs). The odds ratios, 95 percent CIs for the odds ratios, and P values have been adjusted for sex, age, and body-mass index at the time of inclusion in the intervention study. (Reprinted by permission of *The New England Journal of Medicine* from Sjöström L, for the Swedish Obese Subjects Study Scientific Group: Lifestyle, diabetes, and cardiovascular risk factors 10 years after bariatric surgery. *N Engl J Med* 351:2683-2693, 2004.)

Arterial Neovascularization and Inflammation in Vulnerable Patients: Early and Late Signs of Symptomatic Atherosclerosis

Fleiner M, Kummer M, Mirlacher M, et al (Univ Hosp Bruderholz, Switzerland; Univ Hosp Basel, Switzerland; Univ of Basel, Switzerland; et al)

Circulation 110:2843-2850, 2004 1–11

Background.—Atherosclerosis is complicated by cardiovascular events such as myocardial infarction, stroke, or peripheral arterial occlusive disease. Inflammation and pathological neovascularization are thought to precipitate plaque rupture or erosion, both causes of arterial thrombosis and cardiovascular events. We tested the hypothesis that arterial inflammation and angiogenic events are increased throughout the arterial tree in vulnerable patients, ie, in patients who suffered from cardiovascular events, compared with patients who never suffered from complications of atherosclerosis.

Method and Results.—In a postmortem study, we quantified the inflammatory infiltrate and microvascular network in the arterial wall of iliac, carotid, and renal arteries. Tissue microarray technology was adapted to investigate full-thickness arterial sectors. We compared 22 patients with symptomatic atherosclerosis with 27 patients who never had suffered from any cardiovascular event. The absolute intimal macrophage content was 2- to 4-fold higher in vulnerable patients at all 3 arterial sites analyzed ($P<0.05$). Patients with symptomatic atherosclerosis had a denser network of vasa vasorum than patients with asymptomatic disease (33±2 versus 25±2 adventitial microvessels per 1 mm^2; $P=0.008$). Hyperplasia of vasa vasorum was an early and macrophage infiltration was a late sign of symptomatic atherosclerosis.

Conclusions.—High intimal macrophage content and a hyperplastic network of vasa vasorum characterize vulnerable patients suffering from symptomatic atherosclerosis. These changes are uniformly present in different arterial beds and support the concept of symptomatic atherosclerosis as a panarterial disease.

▶ Clearly, patients with symptomatic atherosclerosis generally have diffuse disease, but patients with diffuse disease may also be asymptomatic. In this study, the symptomatic patients had more plaque burden than the asymptomatic patients. The observation of increased neovascularization with greater burden of disease indicates a link between plaque burden and neovascularization. Whether these factors parallel each other or are caused by one or the other remains to be determined. (See also Abstracts 1–12 and 1–13.)

G. L. Moneta, MD

Loss of Collagen XVIII Enhances Neovascularization and Vascular Permeability in Atherosclerosis

Moulton KS, Olsen BR, Sonn S, et al (Children's Hosp, Boston; Brigham and Women's Hosp, Boston; Harvard Med School, Boston)

Circulation 110:1330-1336, 2004 1–12

Background.—Plaque neovascularization is thought to promote atherosclerosis; however, the mechanisms of its regulation are not understood. Collagen XVIII and its proteolytically released endostatin fragment are abundant proteoglycans in vascular basement membranes and the walls of major blood vessels. We hypothesized that collagen XVIII in the aortic wall inhibits the proliferation and intimal extension of vasa vasorum.

Method and Results.—To test our hypothesis, we bred collagen XVIII-knockout (*Col18a1*$^{-/-}$) mice into the atherosclerosis-prone apolipoprotein E–deficient (*ApoE*$^{-/-}$) strain. After 6 months on a cholesterol diet, aortas from *ApoE*$^{-/-}$; *Col18a1*$^{-/-}$ and *ApoE*$^{-/-}$; *Col18a1*$^{+/-}$ heterozygote mice showed increased atheroma coverage and enhanced lipid accumulation compared with wild-type littermates. We observed more extensive vasa vasorum and intimal neovascularization in knockout but not heterozygote aortas. Endothelial cells sprouting from *Col18a1*$^{-/-}$ aortas were increased compared with heterozygote and wild-type aortas. In contrast, vascular permeability of large and small blood vessels was enhanced with even heterozygous loss of collagen XVIII but was not suppressed by increasing serum endostatin to wild-type levels.

Conclusions.—Our results identify a previously unrecognized function for collagen XVIII that maintains vascular permeability. Loss of this basement membrane proteoglycan enhances angiogenesis and vascular permeability during atherosclerosis by distinct gene-dose–dependent mechanisms.

► The study highlights the potential downsides of angiogenesis in vascular disease. Whereas investigators are attempting to stimulate large-vessel angiogenesis in patients with limb ischemia, plaque neovascularization is essentially a localized form of angiogenesis that is thought to promote atherosclerosis by increasing entry of inflammatory cells into the arterial wall. Studies like this may lead to mechanisms to control plaque neovascularization and the adverse effects of local angiogenesis on the atherosclerotic plaque.

G. L. Moneta, MD

Plaque Neovascularization Is Increased in Ruptured Atherosclerotic Lesions of Human Aorta: Implications for Plaque Vulnerability

Moreno PR, Purushothaman KR, Fuster V, et al (Mount Sinai School of Medicine, New York; Univ of Kentucky, Lexington)

Circulation 110:2032-2038, 2004 1–13

Background.—Growth of atherosclerotic plaques is accompanied by neovascularization from vasa vasorum microvessels extending through the tunica media into the base of the plaque and by lumen-derived microvessels through the fibrous cap. Microvessels are associated with plaque hemorrhage and may play a role in plaque rupture. Accordingly, we tested this hypothesis by investigating whether microvessels in the tunica media, the base of the plaque, and the fibrous cap are increased in ruptured atherosclerotic plaques in human aorta.

Method and Results.—Microvessels, defined as CD34-positive tubuloluminal capillaries recognized in cross-sectional and longitudinal profiles, were quantified in 269 advanced human plaques by bicolor immunohistochemistry. Macrophages/T lymphocytes and smooth muscle cells were defined as CD68/CD3-positive and α-actin–positive cells. Total microvessel density was increased in ruptured plaques when compared with nonruptured plaques (P=0.0001). Furthermore, microvessel density was increased in lesions with severe macrophage infiltration at the fibrous cap (P=0.0001) and at the shoulders of the plaque (P=0.0001). In addition, microvessel density was also increased in lesions with intraplaque hemorrhage (P=0.04) and in thin-cap fibroatheromas (P=0.038). Logistic regression analysis identified plaque base microvessel density (P=0.003) as an independent correlate to plaque rupture.

Conclusions.—Thus, neovascularization as manifested by the localized appearance of microvessels is increased in ruptured plaques in the human aorta. Furthermore, microvessel density is increased in lesions with inflammation, with intraplaque hemorrhage, and in thin-cap fibroatheromas. Microvessels at the base of the plaque are independently correlated with plaque rupture, suggesting a contributory role for neovascularization in the process of plaque rupture.

► Another bit of information linking local plaque angiogenesis (ie, neovascularization) with adverse plaque events and potentially adverse clinical outcomes. (See also Abstracts 1–11 and 1–12.)

G. L. Moneta, MD

Unstable Carotid Plaques Exhibit Raised Matrix Metalloproteinase-8 Activity

Molloy KJ, Thompson MM, Jones JL, et al (Univ of Leicester, England; St George's Hosp, London)

Circulation 110:337-343, 2004 1–14

Background.—The fibrous cap of atherosclerotic plaques is composed predominantly of type I and III collagen. Unstable carotid plaques are characterized by rupture of their cap, leading to thromboembolism and stroke. The proteolytic mechanisms causing plaque disruption are undefined, but the collagenolytic matrix metalloproteinase (MMP)-1, -8, and -13 may be implicated. The aim of this study was to quantify the concentrations of these collagenases in carotid plaques and to determine their relationship to markers of plaque instability.

Method and Results.—Atherosclerotic plaques were collected from 159 patients undergoing carotid endarterectomy. The presence and timing of carotid territory symptoms were ascertained. Preoperative embolization was recorded by transcranial Doppler. Each plaque was assessed for histological features of instability. Plaque MMP concentrations were quantified with ELISA. Significantly higher concentrations of active MMP-8 were observed in the plaques of symptomatic patients (20.5 versus 11.4 ng/g; P=0.0002), in plaques of emboli-positive patients (22.7 versus 13.5 ng/g; P=0.0037), and in those plaques showing histological evidence of rupture (20.8 versus 14.7 ng/g; P=0.0036). No differences were seen in the levels of MMP-1 and MMP-13. Immunohistochemistry, in situ hybridization, and colocalization studies confirmed the presence of MMP-8 protein and mRNA within the plaque, which colocalized with macrophages.

Conclusions.—These data suggest that the active form of MMP-8 may be partly responsible for degradation of the collagen cap of atherosclerotic plaques. This enzyme represents an attractive target for drug therapy aimed at stabilizing vulnerable plaques.

▶ Disruption of the fibrous cap of an atherosclerotic plaque may lead to distal embolization or local thrombosis. Something local in the plaque must lead to disruption of the plaque, or at least contribute to it. This article suggests that MMP-8 may play a role in degeneration of the collagen content of the fibrous plaque. Previously, MMP-9 has been implicated in unstable plaques, but MMP-9 does not affect the type 1 and 3 collagens that are the principal collagen types of the fibrous cap. It is unlikely there will be only one "bad" enzyme that leads to plaque rupture. I suspect MMP-8 will be among a number of factors contributing to plaque rupture. If, however, it turns out MMP-8 is required for plaque rupture, then it will be an attractive target for drug therapy in patients at risk for atherosclerotic events.

G. L. Moneta, MD

Regulator of G Protein Signaling 5 Marks Peripheral Arterial Smooth Muscle Cells and Is Downregulated in Atherosclerotic Plaque

Li J, Adams LD, Wang X, et al (Wake Forest Univ, Winston-Salem, NC; Univ of Washington, Seattle)

J Vasc Surg 40:519-528, 2004 1–15

Objective.—Regulator of G protein signaling 5 (RGS5), an inhibitor of Gα(q) and Gα(i) activation, was recently identified among genes highly expressed in smooth muscle cells (SMCs) of aorta but not vena cava. This finding prompted the hypothesis that RGS5 provides long-term G protein inhibition specific to normal arterial SMC populations and that loss of expression may in turn contribute to arterial disease.

Methods.—To test this hypothesis we characterized RGS5 gene expression throughout the vasculature of nonhuman primates to determine whether RGS5 was restricted to arteries in other vascular beds and whether expression was altered in arterial disease.

Results.—In situ hybridization localized RGS5 message to medial SMCs of peripheral arteries, including carotid, iliac, mammary, and renal arteries, but not accompanying veins. SMCs of many small arteries and arterioles also expressed RGS5, including glomerular afferent arterioles critical to blood pressure regulation. Differential expression persisted in culture, inasmuch as RGS5 message was significantly higher in SMCs derived from arteries than from veins at real-time polymerase chain reaction. It was remarkable that the only major arterial bed lacking RGS5 was the coronary circulation. In atherosclerotic peripheral arteries RGS5 was expressed in medial SMCs, but was sharply downregulated in plaque SMCs.

Conclusion.—These data identify RGS5 as a new member of a short list of genes uniquely expressed in peripheral arteries but not coronary arteries. Persistence of an arterial pattern of RGS5 expression in culture and lack of expression in coronary arteries support a unique SMC phenotype fixed by distinct lineage or differentiation pathways. The association between loss of expression and arterial wall disease has prompted the new hypothesis that prolonged inhibition by RGS5 of vasoactive or trophic G protein signaling is critical to normal peripheral artery function.

▶ Atherosclerosis is both a diffuse disease and a site-specific disease. Varying levels of shear stress is one thing that may contribute to disease developing in a specific site. This article, along with Abstracts 1–4 and 1–11, suggests site-specific disease may also be determined by varying levels of expression of genes that act independently or dependently with other atherosclerotic risk factors to promote atherosclerotic plaque at specific locations. A long-term implication is the development of therapies both specific to generalized atherosclerosis and site-specific accumulation of atheroma.

G. L. Moneta, MD

Rates and Determinants of Site-Specific Progression of Carotid Artery Intima-Media Thickness: The Carotid Atherosclerosis Progression Study

Mackinnon AD, Jerrard-Dunne P, Sitzer M, et al (St George's Hosp, London; Johann Wolfgang Goethe Univ, Frankfurt am Main, Germany)

Stroke 35:2150-2154, 2004 1–16

Background and Purpose.—Carotid intima-media thickness (IMT) progression rates are increasingly used as an intermediate outcome for vascular risk. The carotid bifurcation (BIF) and internal carotid artery (ICA) are predilection sites for atherosclerosis. IMT measures from these sites may be a better estimate of atherosclerosis than common carotid artery (CCA) IMT. The study aim was to evaluate site-specific IMT progression rates and their relationships to vascular risk factors compared with baseline IMT measurements.

Methods.—In a community population (n=3383), ICA-IMT, BIF-IMT, CCA-IMT, and vascular risk factors were evaluated at baseline and at 3-year follow-up.

Results.—Mean (SD) IMT progression was significantly greater at the ICA (0.032 [0.109] mm/year) compared with the BIF (0.023 [0.108] mm/year) and the CCA (0.001 [0.040] mm/year) (P<0.001). Only ICA-IMT progression significantly correlated with baseline vascular risk factors (age, male gender, hypertension, diabetes, and smoking). Change in risk factor profile over follow-up, estimated using the Framingham risk score, was a predictor of IMT progression only. For all arterial sites, correlations were stronger, by a factor of 2 to 3, for associations with baseline IMT compared with IMT progression.

Conclusions.—Progression rates at the ICA rather than the CCA yield greater absolute changes in IMT and better correlations with vascular risk factors. Vascular risk factors correlate more strongly with baseline IMT than with IMT progression. Prospective data on IMT progression and incident vascular events are required to establish the true value of progression data as a surrogate measure of vascular risk.

► If something is a problem, and increases in IMT seem to be a problem, it would make sense to study where the problem is potentially the greatest problem! The CCA has traditionally been a classic site for studying IMT. However, the current data combined with improved ultrasound imaging capabilities, suggest that site-specific studies of IMT may be a future direction for this type of research.

G. L. Moneta, MD

Blockade of the Angiotensin II Type 1 Receptor Stabilizes Atherosclerotic Plaques in Humans by Inhibiting Prostaglandin E_2–Dependent Matrix Metalloproteinase Activity

Cipollone F, Fazia M, Iezzi A, et al ("G d'Annunzio" Univ of Chieti, Italy; Univ of Rome Tor Vergata)

Circulation 109:1482-1488, 2004 1–17

Background.—Clinical trials have demonstrated that agents that inhibit the angiotensin II pathway confer benefit beyond the reduction of blood pressure alone. However, the molecular mechanism underlying this effect has yet to be investigated. Recently, we have demonstrated enhanced expression of inducible cyclooxygenase (COX) and prostaglandin (PG)E_2-dependent synthase (COX-2/mPGES-1) in human symptomatic plaques and provided evidence that it is associated with metalloproteinase (MMP)-induced plaque rupture. Thus, the aim of this study was to characterize the effect of the angiotensin II type 1 (AT_1) receptor antagonist irbesartan on the inflammatory infiltration and expression of COX-2/mPGES-1 and MMPs in human carotid plaques.

Method and Results.—Seventy patients with symptomatic carotid artery stenosis were randomized to irbesartan (300 mg/d) or chlorthalidone (50 mg/d) for 4 months before endarterectomy. Plaques were subjected to analysis of COX-1, COX-2, mPGES-1, MMP-2, and MMP-9, angiotensin II, AT_1, AT_2, and collagen content by immunocytochemistry, Western blot, and reverse-transcriptase polymerase chain reaction, whereas zymography was used to detect MMP activity. Immunohistochemistry was also used to identify CD68+ macrophages, CD3+ T lymphocytes, smooth muscle cells (SMCs), and HLA-DR+ inflammatory cells. Plaques from the irbesartan group had fewer (P<0.0001) macrophages, T lymphocytes, and HLA-DR+ cells; less (P<0.0001) immunoreactivity for COX-2/mPGES-1 and MMPs; reduced (P<0.0001) gelatinolytic activity; and increased (P<0.0001) collagen content. It is worth noting that COX-2/mPGES-1 inhibition was observed after incubation in vitro with irbesartan but not with the selective AT_2 blockade PD123,319.

Conclusions.—This study demonstrates that irbesartan decreases inflammation and inhibits COX-2/mPGES-1 expression in plaque macrophages, and this effect may in turn contribute to plaque stabilization by inhibition of MMP-induced plaque rupture.

► MMPs may be crucial to fibrous cap rupture (see also Abstract 1–14). In most biologic systems, there are both promoting and opposing factors. The key is controlling the balance between the two. The promoting and opposing systems can be quite complex. However, identification of both ends of the system potentially allows control of the outcome at the end point by targeting multiple mechanisms.

G. L. Moneta, MD

Simvastatin Induces Heme Oxygenase-1: A Novel Mechanism of Vessel Protection

Lee T-S, Chang C-C, Zhu Y, et al (Univ of Californa, Riverside)

Circulation 110:1296-1302, 2004 1–18

Background.—Evidence from experimental and clinical studies indicates that statins can protect the vessel wall through cholesterol-independent mechanisms. The "pleiotropic" effects include the prevention of inflammation and proliferation of vascular cells. Here, we studied whether heme oxygenase-1 (HO-1), an important cytoprotective molecule, is induced by simvastatin and the role of HO-1 in the pleiotropic effects of simvastatin.

Method and Results.—Human and rat aortic smooth muscle cells treated with simvastatin showed an elevated level of HO-1 for up to 24 hours. The induction of HO-1 by simvastatin was not found in cultured endothelial cells and macrophages. Injecting C57BL/6J mice intraperitoneally with simvastatin increased the level of HO-1 in vascular SMCs (VSMCs) in the tunica media. Treating VSMCs with zinc protoporphyrin, an HO-1 inhibitor, or HO-1 small interfering RNA (siRNA) blocked the antiinflammatory effect of simvastatin, including the inhibition of nuclear factor-κB activation and nitric oxide production. Blockade of HO-1 also abolished the simvastatin-induced $p21^{Waf1}$ and the associated antiproliferative effect. Simvastatin activated p38 and Akt in VSMCs, and the respective inhibitor of p38 and phosphoinositide 3-kinase (PI3K) greatly reduced the level of simvastatin-induced HO-1, which suggests the involvement of p38 and the PI3K-Akt pathway in HO-1 induction.

Conclusions.—Simvastatin activates HO-1 in VSMCs in vitro and in vivo. The antiinflammatory and antiproliferative effects of simvastatin occur largely through the induced HO-1.

▶ In addition to lowering cholesterol levels, statins have so-called favorable "pleiotropic" anti-inflammatory and immunosuppressive effects limiting atherosclerosis. This may be a pivotal article in understanding the pleiotropic antiatherogenic effects of statins in that it suggests that many pleiotropic effects of statins may be mediated by an inducible gene. If so, dissecting the statin drugs to determine what leads to induction of the HO-1 gene may provide a new target for antiatherogenic drugs.

G. L. Moneta, MD

Prevalence of and Risk Factors for Peripheral Arterial Disease in the United States: Results From the National Health and Nutrition Examination Survey, 1999-2000

Selvin E, Erlinger TP (Johns Hopkins Univ, Baltimore, Md)

Circulation 110:738-743, 2004 1–19

Background.—Peripheral arterial disease (PAD) is associated with significant morbidity and mortality and is an important marker of subclinical coronary heart disease. However, estimates of PAD prevalence in the general US population have varied widely.

Method and Results.—We analyzed data from 2174 participants aged 40 years and older from the 1999-2000 National Health and Nutrition Examination Survey. PAD was defined as an ankle-brachial index <0.90 in either leg. The prevalence of PAD among adults aged 40 years and over in the United States was 4.3% (95% CI 3.1% to 5.5%), which corresponds to ≈ 5 million individuals (95% CI 4 to 7 million). Among those aged 70 years or over, the prevalence was 14.5% (95% CI 10.8% to 18.2%). In age- and gender-adjusted logistic regression analyses, black race/ethnicity (OR 2.83, 95% CI 1.48 to 5.42) current smoking (OR 4.46, 95% CI 2.25 to 8.84), diabetes (OR 2.71, 95% CI 1.03 to 7.12), hypertension (OR 1.75, 95% CI 0.97 to 3.13), hypercholesterolemia (OR 1.68, 95% CI 1.09 to 2.57), and low kidney function (OR 2.00, 95% CI 1.08 to 3.70) were positively associated with prevalent PAD. More than 95% of persons with PAD had 1 or more cardiovascular disease risk factors. Elevated fibrinogen and C-reactive protein levels were also associated with PAD.

Conclusions.—This study provides nationally representative prevalence estimates of PAD in the United States, revealing that PAD affects more than 5 million adults. PAD prevalence increases dramatically with age and disproportionately affects blacks. The vast majority of individuals with PAD have 1 or more cardiovascular disease risk factors that should be targeted for therapy.

► If anything, this study likely underestimates the prevalence of PAD. Patients with severe risk factors or severe chronic disease may have been less likely to participate in the survey.

G. L. Moneta, MD

Aortic Calcification and the Risk of Osteoporosis and Fractures

Schulz E, Arfai K, Liu X, et al (Loma Linda Univ, Calif; Univ of Southern California, Los Angeles; Univ of California, Los Angeles)

J Clin Endocrinol Metab 89:4246-4253, 2004 1–20

Introduction.—We investigated the relation between computed tomography measures of aortic calcification and values for bone density and the number of fragility fractures in 2348 healthy, postmenopausal women. To determine whether increases in vascular calcification and bone loss progress in parallel, baseline values were compared with measurements obtained 9 months to 8 yr later in a subgroup of 228 women. Of the 2348 subjects studied, 70% had osteoporosis, 30% had at least one vertebral fracture, and 9% had at least one hip fracture. Aortic calcifications were inversely related to bone density and directly related to fractures. After adjusting for age and potential confounders, measures for aortic calcification predicted 26.1% of the variance in bone density ($P < 0.001$). Compared with women without calcification, the odds ratios for vertebral and hip fractures in those with calcification were estimated to be 4.8 (95% confidence interval, 3.6-6.5) and 2.9 (95% confidence interval, 1.8-4.8), respectively. The subgroup analysis of 228 women longitudinally studied showed that the percentage of yearly increase in aortic calcification accounted for 47% of the variance in the percentage rate of bone loss ($P < 0.001$). Moreover, a strong graded association was observed between the progression of vascular calcification and bone loss for each quartile. Women in the highest quartile for gains in aortic calcification had four times greater yearly bone loss (5.3 *vs.*1.3% yearly; $P < 0.001$) than women of similar age in the lowest quartile. Smaller, but highly significant differences were also found between all other quartiles. We conclude that aortic calcifications are a strong predictor for low bone density and fragility fractures (Fig 6).

► Aortic calcification is a risk factor for cardiovascular disease. Previous studies have suggested women with osteoporosis are at increased risk of mortality due to stroke or coronary disease.[1] This study suggests a relationship between atherosclerosis and osteoporosis and implies a at least partially shared mech-

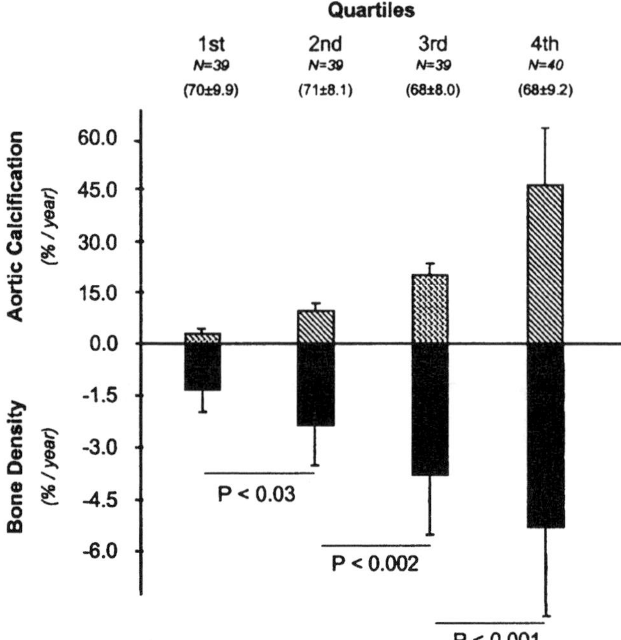

FIGURE 6.—Yearly percentage gains in aortic calcification and bone loss in the 157 women longitudinally studied with vascular calcifications at baseline. Subjects were divided into quartiles based on rates of change in aortic calcification. The different scales represent the range of yearly gains or losses for aortic calcification and bone density, respectively. *Numbers in parentheses* represent the age in years. Values are mean ± SD. (Courtesy of Schulz E, Arfai K, Liu X, et al: Aortic calcification and the risk of osteoporosis and fractures. *J Clin Endocrinol Metab* 89:4246-4253, 2004. Copyright 2004, The Endocrine Society.)

anism for mineral deposition in connective tissue. Effective treatment strategies for either osteoporosis or atherosclerosis may modify the risk of both of these common conditions.

G. L. Moneta, MD

Reference

1. von der Recke P, Hansen MA, Hassager C: The association between low bone mass at the menopause and cardiovascular mortality. *Am J Med* 106:273-278, 1999.

Noninvasive Phenotypes of Atherosclerosis: Similar Windows but Different Views

Spence JD, Hegele RA (Robarts Research Inst, London, Ont, Canada)
Stroke 35:649-653, 2004 1–21

Background and Purpose.—Noninvasive measures of atherosclerosis, such as carotid intima-media thickness, total carotid plaque area, and carotid stenosis, probably represent different phenotypes with distinct determinants. For instance, total carotid plaque area may reflect atherosclerotic lesion size more closely than carotid stenosis, which instead may reflect hemodynamic compromise within the arterial lumen.

Methods.—In 1821 patients from a Premature Atherosclerosis Clinic, we studied determinants of total carotid plaque area and carotid stenosis as measured by ultrasound using multivariate regression analysis with traditional risk factors and some emerging risk factors.

Results.—Regression modeling showed that (1) traditional atherosclerosis risk factors were more strongly associated with total carotid plaque area than with carotid stenosis (R=0.53 and 0.13, respectively), and (2) individual risk factors had different relationships with total carotid plaque area and carotid stenosis. For instance, age accounted for 53% and 26% of the explained variance of total carotid plaque area and carotid stenosis, respectively. Female sex was inversely associated with total carotid plaque area but positively associated with carotid stenosis. Nontraditional risk variables such as plasma homocysteine had different associations with the 2 analytes.

Conclusions.—Total carotid plaque area and carotid stenosis had different associations with specific atherosclerosis risk factors. Thus, for future studies of the determinants of atherosclerosis, it is important to distinguish between different phenotypes and to appreciate that they will not necessarily have the same determinants.

▶ Some of the authors' findings do not surprise me. Stenosis would be expected to correlate with plaque area only if atherosclerotic lesions were concentric. Clearly they are not concentric. The smaller arteries of females makes an association of female sex with stenosis seem likely. What is perhaps more interesting in this study is that plaque area rather than stenosis was more strongly associated with atherosclerotic risk factors. Stenosis has never correlated all that well with risk factors in the carotid artery and certainly correlates only poorly with symptoms. Perhaps plaque area will prove to be a better marker of future neurologic symptoms than stenosis.

G. L. Moneta, MD

Relationship of High and Low Ankle Brachial Index to All-Cause and Cardiovascular Disease Mortality: The Strong Heart Study

Resnick HE, Lindsay RS, McDermott MM, et al (MedStar Research Inst, Hyattsville, Md; Northwestern Univ, Chicago; Cornell Univ, New York; et al)
Circulation 109:733-739, 2004 1–22

Background.—The associations of low (<0.90) and high (>1.40) ankle brachial index (ABI) with risk of all-cause and cardiovascular disease (CVD) mortality have not been examined in a population-based setting.

Method and Results.—We examined all-cause and CVD mortality in relation to low and high ABI in 4393 American Indians in the Strong Heart Study. Participants had bilateral ABI measurements at baseline and were followed up for 8.32.2 years (36 589 person-years). Cox regression was used to quantify mortality rates among participants with high and low ABI relative to those with normal ABI (0.90 ≤ABI ≤1.40). Death from all causes occurred in 1022 participants (23.3%; 27.9 deaths per 1000 person-years), and of these, 272 (26.6%; 7.4 deaths per 1000 person-years) were attributable to CVD. Low ABI was present in 216 participants (4.9%), and high ABI occurred in 404 (9.2%). Diabetes, albuminuria, and hypertension occurred with greater frequency among persons with low (60.2%, 44.4%, and 50.1%) and high (67.8%, 49.9%, and 45.1%) ABI compared with those with normal ABI (44.4%, 26.9%, and 36.5%), respectively ($P<0.0001$). Adjusted risk estimates for all-cause mortality were 1.69 (1.34 to 2.14) for low and 1.77 (1.48 to 2.13) for high ABI, and estimates for CVD mortality were 2.52 (1.74 to 3.64) for low and 2.09 (1.49 to 2.94) for high ABI.

Conclusions.—The association between high ABI and mortality was similar to that of low ABI and mortality, highlighting a U-shaped association between this noninvasive measure of peripheral arterial disease and mortality risk. Our data suggest that the upper limit of normal ABI should not exceed 1.40.

▶ It doesn't take a genius to recognize that incompressible vessels (ie, ABIs > 1.4) indicate significant atherosclerotic disease. The new bit of information here is that high ABIs portend an equally bad prognosis as low ABIs.

G. L. Moneta, MD

Prevalence of Lower-Extremity Disease in the US Adult Population ≥40 Years of Age With and Without Diabetes: 1999-2000 National Health and Nutrition Examination Survey

Gregg EW, Wolz M, Sorlie P, et al (Ctrs for Disease Control and Prevention, Atlanta, Ga; NIH, Bethesda, Md; Ctrs for Disease Control and Prevention, Hyattsville, Md)

Diabetes Care 27:1591-1597, 2004 1–23

Objective.—Although lower-extremity disease (LED), which includes lower-extremity peripheral arterial disease (PAD) and peripheral neuropathy (PN), is disabling and costly, no nationally representative estimates of its prevalence exist. The aim of this study was to examine the prevalence of lower-extremity PAD, PN, and overall LED in the overall U.S. population and among those with and without diagnosed diabetes.

Research Design and Methods.—The analysis consisted of data for 2873 men and women aged ≥40 years, including 419 with diagnosed diabetes, from the 1999-2000 National Health and Nutrition Examination Survey. The main outcome measures consisted of the prevalence of lower-extremity PAD (defined as ankle-brachial index <0.9), PN (defined as ≥1 insensate area based on monofilament testing), and of any LED (defined as either PAD, PN, or history of foot ulcer or lower-extremity amputations).

Results.—Of the U.S. population aged ≥40 years, 4.5% (95% CI 3.4-5.6) have lower-extremity PAD, 14.8% (12.8-16.8) have PN, and 18.7% (15.9-

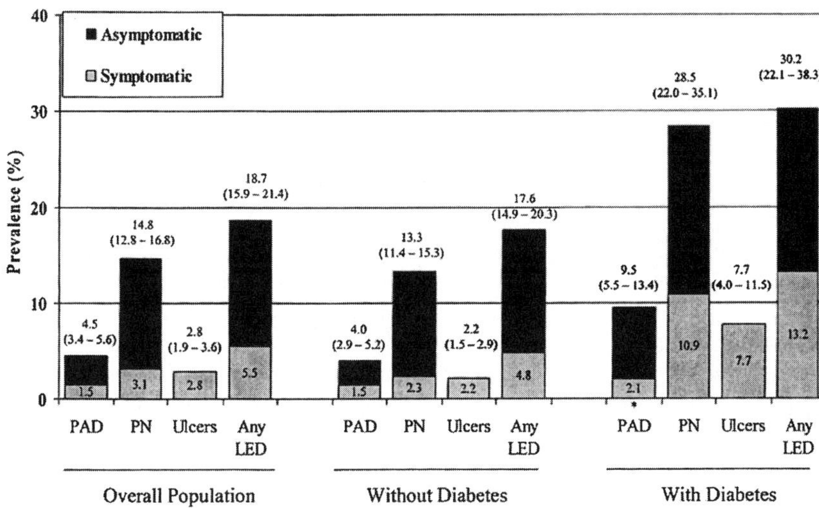

FIGURE 1.—Prevalence of LED among the overall, nondiabetic population, and diabetic population aged ≥40 years in the U.S., 1999-2000. *Does not meet standard of statistical reliability and precision (relative SE >30%). (Courtesy of Gregg EW, Wolz M, Sorlie P, et al: Prevalence of lower-extremity disease in the US adult population ≥40 years of age with and without diabetes: 1999-2000 National Health And Nutrition Examination Survey. *Diabetes Care* 27;1591-1597, 2004. Copyright 2004, with permission from The American Diabetes Association.)

21.4) have any LED. Prevalence of PAD, PN, and overall LED increases steeply with age and is higher ($P < 0.05$) in non-Hispanic blacks and Mexican Americans than non-Hispanic whites. The prevalence of LEDs is approximately twice as high for individuals with diagnosed diabetes (PAD 9.5% [5.5-13.4]; PN 28.5% [22.0-35.1]; any LED 30.2% [22.1-38.3]) as the overall population.

Conclusions.—LED is common in the U.S. and twice as high among individuals with diagnosed diabetes. These conditions disproportionately affect the elderly, non-Hispanic blacks, and Mexican Americans (Fig 1).

▶ The high incidence of peripheral neuropathy is alarming. The detection of PAD identifies cardiac risk. I wonder if limb loss risk would be better assessed by detection of neuopathy? This type of information, while admittedly boring, is very important for those trying to anticipate future national health care needs. Of course, this assumes that those anticipating future health care needs, the policy makers, actually think beyond the next election. I am sure there is no paper suggesting that assumption has been proven.

G. L. Moneta, MD

Effect of Type 2 Diabetes and Its Duration on the Risk of Peripheral Arterial Disease Among Men

Al-Delaimy WK, Merchant AT, Rimm EB, et al (Harvard School of Public Health, Boston; Harvard Med School, Boston)
Am J Med 116:236-240, 2004 1–24

Purpose.—To assess the relation between the duration of diabetes and the risk of peripheral arterial disease among men.

Methods.—A total of 48,607 men in the Health Professionals Follow-up Study who returned a questionnaire in 1986 were followed for 12 years. Peripheral arterial disease (intermittent claudication or surgery for peripheral arterial diseases in the lower extremities) was ascertained by biennial questionnaire and confirmed by medical record review. Diabetes status and other cardiovascular risk factors were also ascertained by biennial questionnaire.

Results.—During follow-up (534,588 person-years), we documented 387 cases of peripheral arterial disease. After adjusting for cardiovascular risk factors, the relative risk of developing peripheral arterial disease among men with diabetes compared with men without diabetes was 2.61 (95% confidence interval [CI]: 1.98 to 3.45). Compared with men without diabetes, the relative risk of peripheral arterial disease among men with diabetes increased with duration of disease, even after adjusting for cardiovascular risk factors: 1.39 (95% CI: 0.82 to 2.36) for 1 to 5 years of diabetes, 3.63 (95% CI: 2.23 to 5.88) for 6 to 10 years, 2.55 (95% CI: 1.50 to 4.32) for 11 to 25 years, and 4.53 (95% CI: 2.39 to 8.58) for >25 years of diabetes (*P* for trend ≤0.0001).

Conclusion.—These results indicate that duration of type 2 diabetes is associated strongly with the risk of developing peripheral arterial disease.

► The Health Professionals Follow-up Study is a long-running study of primarily dentists, veterinarians, pharmacists, and optometrists (95% of participants). Data from the study are widely quoted but of little use in determining overall behavior of disease. Health professionals are hardly a true cross section of the population. However, people are people, and the relationship between the risk of diabetes and development of peripheral arterial disease is likely real. It is important to remember that most patients with diabetes likely had the disease long before they had an official diagnosis. The true lag time for development of peripheral arterial disease in diabetics, I think, is still unknown.

G. L. Moneta, MD

Regression of Carotid Atherosclerosis by Control of Postprandial Hyperglycemia in Type 2 Diabetes Mellitus

Esposito K, for the Campanian Postprandial Hyperglycemia Study Group (Univ of Naples, Italy)

Circulation 110:214-219, 2004 1–25

Background.—Postprandial hyperglycemia may be a risk factor for cardiovascular disease. We compared the effects of two insulin secretagogues, repaglinide and glyburide, known to have different efficacy on postprandial hyperglycemia, on carotid intima-media thickness (CIMT) and markers of systemic vascular inflammation in type 2 diabetic patients.

Method and Results.—We performed a randomized, single-blind trial on 175 drug-naive patients with type 2 diabetes mellitus (93 men and 82 women), 35 to 70 years of age, selected from a population of 401 patients who participated in an epidemiological analysis assessing the relation of postprandial hyperglycemia to surrogate measures of atherosclerosis. Eighty-eight patients were randomly assigned to receive repaglinide and 87 patients to glyburide, with a titration period of 6 to 8 weeks for optimization of drug dosage and a subsequent 12-month treatment period. The effects of repaglinide (1.5 to 12 mg/d) and glyburide (5 to 20 mg/d) on CIMT were compared by using blinded, serial assessments of the far wall. After 12 months, postprandial glucose peak was 148±28 mg/dL in the repaglinide group and 180±32 mg/dL in the glyburide group ($P<0.01$). HbA_{1c} showed a similar decrease in both groups (−0.9%). CIMT regression, defined as a decrease of >0.020 mm, was observed in 52% of diabetics receiving repaglinide and in 18% of those receiving glyburide ($P<0.01$). Interleukin-6 ($P=0.04$) and C-reactive protein ($P=0.02$) decreased more in the repaglinide group than in the glyburide group. The reduction in CIMT was associated with changes in postprandial but not fasting hyperglycemia.

Conclusions.—Reduction of postprandial hyperglycemia in type 2 diabetic patients is associated with CIMT regression.

► This article suggests a possible new strategy for glucose control. The authors found that a suppression of postprandial glucose increases reduced CIMT more effectively than lowering fasting hyperglycemia in patients with the same levels of hemoglobin A_{1c}. The results indicate that excessive excursions of postprandial plasma glucose levels promote atherogenesis. Promoting minimal excursions of glucose beyond baseline may be a treatment strategy or preventive strategy for atherosclerosis in patients with diabetes.

G. L. Moneta, MD

Vascular Effects of Improving Metabolic Control With Metformin or Rosiglitazone in Type 2 Diabetes

Natali A, Barbaro D, Baldeweg S, et al (Univ of Pisa, Italy; Univ College, London; "Federico II" Univ, Naples, Italy; et al)

Diabetes Care 27:1349-1357, 2004 1–26

Objective.—The aim of this study was to test whether vascular reactivity is modified by improving metabolic control and peripheral insulin resistance in type 2 diabetes.

Research Design and Methods.—In a randomized, double-blind design, we assigned 74 type 2 diabetic patients to rosiglitazone (8 mg/day), metformin (1,500 mg/day), or placebo treatment for 16 weeks and measured insulin sensitivity (euglycemic insulin clamp), ambulatory blood pressure, and forearm blood flow response to *1*) intra-arterial acetylcholine (ACh), *2*) intra-arterial nitroprusside, *3*) the clamp, and *4*) blockade of nitric oxide (NO) synthase.

Results.—Compared with 25 nondiabetic subjects, patients had reduced insulin sensitivity (30 ± 1 vs. 41 ± 3 μmol · min^{-1} · kg fat-free mass^{-1}; $P <$ 0.001) and reduced maximal response to ACh (586 ± 42 vs. 883 ± 81%; $P <$ 0.001). Relative to placebo, 16 weeks of rosiglitazone and metformin similarly reduced fasting glucose (−2.3 ± 0.5 and −2.3 ± 0.5 mmol/l) and HbA_{1c} (−1.2 ± 0.3 and −1.6 ± 0.3%). Insulin sensitivity increased with rosiglitazone (+6 ± 3 μmol · min^{-1} · kg fat-free mass^{-1}; $P < 0.01$) but not with metformin or placebo. Ambulatory diastolic blood pressure fell consistently (−2 ± 1 mmHg; $P < 0.05$) only in the rosiglitazone group. Nitroprusside dose response, clamp-induced vasodilatation, and NO blockade were not affected by either treatment. In contrast, the slope of the ACh dose response improved with rosiglitazone (+40% versus baseline, $P < 0.05$, +70% versus placebo, $P < 0.005$) but did not change with either metformin or placebo. This improvement in endothelium-dependent vasodilatation was accompanied by decrements in circulating levels of free fatty acids and tumor necrosis factor-α.

Conclusions.—At equivalent glycemic control, rosiglitazone, but not metformin, improves endothelium dependent vasodilatation and insulin sensitivity in type 2 diabetes.

► Apparently, achieving glucose control in itself is not enough to prevent or mollify the proatherogenic effects of diabetes (see Abstract 1–25). How glucose control is achieved may also be important. The obvious implication of this data is that diabetes may, at least in part, promote atherosclerosis in ways that are not directly linked to glucose control.

G. L. Moneta, MD

Association Between High Serum Ferritin Levels and Carotid Atherosclerosis in the Study of Health in Pomerania (SHIP)

Wolff B, Völzke H, Lüdemann J, et al (Universität Greifswald, Germany)

Stroke 35:453-457, 2004 1–27

Background and Purpose.—Several studies have provided evidence for a relationship between body iron load and cardiovascular disease. We analyzed the association of serum ferritin levels with carotid atherosclerosis.

Methods.—We assessed intima-media thickness and plaque prevalence in the carotid arteries by high-resolution ultrasound among 2443 participants (1200 women; age, 45 to 79 years) in the Study of Health in Pomerania (SHIP), a population-based study in northeast Germany.

Results.—In multivariate analysis, serum ferritin levels were not independently associated with carotid intima-media thickness among women or men. In contrast, the relationship between serum ferritin levels and carotid plaque prevalence was significant among men (odds ratio per 1-SD increase of serum ferritin levels, 1.33; 95% confidence interval, 1.08 to 1.44) yet not among women (odds ratio, 1.29; 95% confidence interval, 0.98 to 1.75). However, both men and women showed a dose-response relation between serum ferritin levels and carotid atherosclerosis in which higher serum ferritin levels were associated with greater odds ratios for carotid plaque prevalence. Additionally, there was an interaction of serum ferritin levels with low-density lipoprotein (LDL) cholesterol ($P=0.039$) among men in which the association of serum ferritin levels with carotid plaque prevalence became stronger with increasing LDL cholesterol levels.

Conclusions.—Our study identified a relationship between serum ferritin levels and carotid atherosclerosis that was potentiated by LDL cholesterol. This relationship adds support to the hypothesis of a link between iron and cardiovascular disease.

▶ The study demonstrates a synergistic relationship where the magnitude of association between serum ferritin levels and carotid atherosclerosis becomes greater with higher LDL cholesterol levels. This suggests some mechanism whereby iron interferes with lipid metabolism. While there is a certain level of biologic plausibility to such an interaction, the overall data supporting a relationship between serum ferritin levels and atherosclerosis still seem weak. Any relationship is likely to be overwhelmed by the effects of more traditional risk factors such as hypercholesterolemia, smoking, and diabetes.

G. L. Moneta, MD

Serum Total 8-Iso-Prostaglandin $F_{2\alpha}$: A New and Independent Predictor of Peripheral Arterial Disease

Mueller T, Dieplinger B, Gegenhuber A, et al (Konventhospital Barmherzige Brueder, Linz, Austria; Univ of Linz, Austria)

J Vasc Surg 40:768-773, 2004 1–28

Objective.—Circulating 8-iso-prostaglandin $F_{2\alpha}$ (8-iso-$PGF_{2\alpha}$) has been proposed as new indicator of oxidative stress, which is involved in the pathophysiologic changes of atherosclerosis. We proposed to test the hypothesis that 8-iso-$PGF_{2\alpha}$ is an independent predictor of symptomatic peripheral arterial disease (PAD).

Methods.—A case-control study in 100 patients with symptomatic PAD and 100 control subjects matched for age, sex, and diabetes mellitus was conducted. Smokers and subjects using lipid-lowering drugs were excluded. Serum total 8-iso-$PGF_{2\alpha}$ was quantified with an enzyme immunoassay.

Results.—Median 8-iso-$PGF_{2\alpha}$ was higher in patients with PAD than in control subjects (63 vs 42 pg/mL; $P = .001$). Logistic regression with hypertension, body mass index, and creatinine, low-density lipoprotein (LDL) cholesterol, triglyceride, high-sensitivity C-reactive protein (hs-CRP), 8-iso-$PGF_{2\alpha}$, and total homocysteine concentrations as independent variables and case-control status as dependent variable revealed significant odds ratios (OR) for hypertension (OR, 3.74; 95% confidence interval [CI], 1.85-7.53), low-density lipoprotein cholesterol (OR, 1.16, for an increment of 10 mg/dL; 95% CI, 1.07-1.27), high-sensitivity C-reactive protein (OR, 1.02, for an increment of 1 mg/L; 95% CI, 1.00-1.03), and 8-iso-$PGF_{2\alpha}$ (OR, 1.11, for an increment of 10 pg/mL; 95% CI, 1.03-1.20).

Conclusions.—Serum total 8-iso-$PGF_{2\alpha}$ was an independent predictor of PAD in the population studied. This finding supports the hypothesis that 8-iso-$PGF_{2\alpha}$ is a risk marker for PAD. Our results indicate increased systemic oxidative stress in patients with PAD.

▶ There are so may "predictors" of atherosclerosis that one needs a Ouija board to keep track of them all and a crystal ball to try and figure out which ones are truly important. I bet you this one will generate articles and grants but will be of little practical importance in comparison to tried-and-true clinical risk factors such as smoking, hypertension, and diabetes.

G. L. Moneta, MD

Dietary Folate and Vitamin B6 Are Independent Predictors of Peripheral Arterial Occlusive Disease

Wilmink ABM, Welch AA, Quick CRG, et al (Univ of Birmingham, England; Univ of Cambridge, England)

J Vasc Surg 39:513-516, 2004 1–29

Background.—It has been suggested that hyperhomocysteinemia (HHcy) is an independent risk factor for peripheral arterial occlusive disease

(PAOD). However, the relationship between dietary folate and vitamin B6, cofactors in the metabolism of homocysteine (Hcy), and PAOD is unclear.

Aims.—To study the relationship between dietary folate and B6 and PAOD.

Methods.—Case-control population based study of 392 men older than 50 years living in Huntingdon, United Kingdom. PAOD, defined as an ankle-brachial pressure index (ABPI) < 0.9, was present in 86 (22%) of subjects. Folate, vitamin B6, and vitamin B12 intakes were calculated by means of the EPIC (European Prospective Investigation into Cancer) food frequency questionnaire.

Results.—Daily folate intake was significantly lower in case subjects (mean, 288; 95% confidence interval [CI], 266-309 µg) than in control subjects (324; 95% CI, 313-335 µg). Daily vitamin B6 intake was also lower in case subjects (2.05; 95% CI, 1.92-2.19 mg versus 2.26; 95% CI, 2.19-2.33 mg). Daily folate and vitamin B6 intakes were independent predictors of PAOD after adjusting for age, blood pressure, cholesterol levels, diabetes, and smoking status in a logistic regression model. This model suggests that increasing daily folate intake by 1 standard deviation decreased the risk of PAOD by 46%. A similar increase in daily vitamin B6 intake decreased the risk of PAOD by 29%.

Conclusion.—In men older than 50 years, dietary folate and B6 intakes are independent predictors of PAOD. Longitudinal studies are required to determine whether dietary modification can reduce the incidence of PAOD in the population.

▶ This study is well done. It is, however, based on results of a questionnaire purporting to accurately identify food intake of 130 items over one year with no specific validation of its ability to reflect folate and B12 intake. I am sorry, but I can't even remember what I had for lunch yesterday, much less six months ago. I will wait for a study using blood samples, not questionnaires.

G. L. Moneta, MD

Safety Evaluation of Clinical Gene Theapy Using Hepatocyte Growth Factor to Treat Peripheral Arterial Disease

Morishita R, Aoki M, Hashiya N, et al (Osaka Univ, Japan)

Hypertension 44:203-209, 2004 1–30

Introduction.—Therapeutic angiogenesis using angiogenic growth factors is expected to be a new treatment for patients with critical limb ischemia (CLI). Because hepatocyte growth factor (HGF) has potent angiogenic activity, we investigated the safety and efficiency of HGF plasmid DNA in patients with CLI as a prospective open-labeled clinical trial. Intramuscular injection of naked HGF plasmid DNA was performed in ischemic limbs of 6 CLI patients with arteriosclerosis obliterans (n=3) or Buerger disease (n=3) graded as Fontaine III or IV. The primary end points were safety and improvement of ischemic symptoms at 12 weeks after transfection. Severe complications and adverse effects caused by gene transfer were not detected in any patients. Of particular importance, no apparent edema was observed in any patient throughout the trial. In addition, serum HGF concentration was not changed throughout the therapy period in all patients. In contrast, a reduction of pain scale of more than 1 cm in visual analog pain scale was observed in 5 of 6 patients. Increase in ankle pressure index more than 0.1 was observed in 5 of 5 patients. The long diameter of 8 of 11 ischemic ulcers in 4 patients was reduced >25%. Intramuscular injection of naked HGF plasmid is safe, feasible, and can achieve successful improvement of ischemic limbs. Although the present data are conducted to demonstrate the safety as phase I/early phase IIa, the initial clinical outcome with HGF gene transfer seems to indicate usefulness as sole therapy for CLI.

▶ Patients with CLI have a poor prognosis. In that regard, the outcome of this initial study is encouraging. However, it is known that there is a large placebo effect in drug treatment of patients with CLI. This study should be regarded as preliminary data suggesting safety of the procedure. It has far too few patients to suggest efficacy or provide conclusive data about safety.

G. L. Moneta, MD

Improved Vascular Gene Transfer With a Helper-Dependent Adenoviral Vector

Wen S, Graf S, Massey PG, et al (Univ of Washington, Seattle)
Circulation 110:1484-1491, 2004 1–31

Background.—Adenoviral vectors are the most widely used agents for vascular gene transfer. However, the utility of adenoviral vectors for vascular gene transfer is limited by brevity of expression and by the induction of a significant host inflammatory response. Third-generation or "helper-dependent" adenoviral vectors have achieved prolonged recombinant gene expression in liver and muscle with minimal associated inflammation; however, they have never been tested for vascular gene transfer.

Method and Results.—We constructed a helper-dependent adenoviral vector expressing rabbit urokinase plasminogen activator (HD-AduPA). HD-AduPA was compared, in a rabbit model of carotid gene transfer, with a first-generation adenovirus, also expressing rabbit uPA (FG-AduPA). uPA expression and vector DNA were measured in arteries harvested from 3 to 56 days after gene transfer. Vector-specific mRNA, vascular inflammation, and neointimal formation were assessed 14 days after gene transfer. uPA expression was lost, and vector DNA declined rapidly in arteries infused with FG-AduPA. In contrast, uPA expression and vector DNA persisted in HD-AduPA arteries for ≥56 days, with stable expression from 14 to 56 days. Increased uPA expression in HD-AduPA arteries was accompanied by high levels of vector-specific uPA mRNA. Moreover, HD-AduPA arteries had significantly less inflammation and neointimal formation than FG-AduPA arteries.

Conclusions.—Helper-dependent adenoviral vectors can stably express a therapeutic gene in the vascular wall for ≥8 weeks, with minimal associated inflammation. Helper-dependent adenoviral vectors will be useful agents for vascular gene transfer and gene therapy.

► The Holy Grail of gene therapy is to transfer a therapeutic gene to an individual requiring the gene product with subsequent stable expression of the gene product and minimal adverse reaction of the host. Research such as this is crucial to making gene therapy a therapeutic reality.

G. L. Moneta, MD

Endograft Technology: A Delivery Vehicle for Intravascular Gene Therapy

Eton D, Yu H, Wang Y, et al (Univ of Miami, Fla)

J Vasc Surg 39:1066-1073, 2004 1–32

Purpose.—The purpose of this study was to determine whether vascular smooth muscle cells (SMCs) suffused into a bilayered stent graft retain and express a retrovirally transduced gene for 7 months in vivo.

Methods.—SMCs harvested from dog jugular vein were retrovirally transduced to introduce genes for tissue plasminogen activator (t-PA) and β-galactosidase. These cells were then suffused into a novel dual-layered Dacron graft and cultured for 36 to 48 hours. The grafts were mounted on a Palmaz stent and balloon- expanded in the infrarenal aorta of the SMC donor dogs (n = 6). Grafts were recovered at 1, 2, 3, 4, 5, and 7 months. A control endograft suffused with SMCs transduced with only the β-galactosidase gene was placed in the dogs with grafts recovered at 2, 3, and 4 months. t-PA antigen concentration and expression were analyzed with an enzyme-linked immunosorbent assay.

Results.—Retained engineered SMCs (blue nuclei) were identified in the explanted grafts, neointima, and underlying aorta with X-gal staining. The t-PA antigen concentration and t-PA activity from the SMCs recovered from the grafts remained elevated for the duration of the experiment (7 months) at levels significantly higher (3.7 ± 0.2 ng/mL per 10^5 cells per 24 hours and 1.4 ± 0.1 IU/mL per 10^5 cells per 24 hours) than in control endografts (0.5 ± 0.03 ng/mL per 10^5 cells per 24 hours and 0.07 ± 0.00 IU/mL per 10^5 cells per 24 hours; P <.001). No graft stenosis was observed.

Conclusion.—Retrovirally engineered vascular SMCs survived the implantation trauma, repopulated each graft, migrated into the underlying aorta, and expressed the transduced genes for the 7-month duration of the experiment. This bilayered Dacron endograft model provides a platform to study direct intravascular gene therapy.

► This is interesting technology. It may prove to be a major advantage to delivering genes for gene therapy in that adenoviral delivery mechanisms and their toxicity are avoided. The cart may be a bit before the horse. So far, gene therapy, while theoretically having great promise, has not provided much in the way of practical application.

G. L. Moneta, MD

Temporal Gene Expression Following Prosthetic Arterial Grafting

Willis DJ, Kalish JA, Li C, et al (Beth Israel Deaconess Med Ctr, Boston; Children's Hosp, Boston; Harvard Med School, Boston)

J Surg Res 120:27-36, 2004 1–33

Background.—Following prosthetic arterial grafting, cytokines and growth factors released within the perianastomotic tissues stimulate smooth muscle cell proliferation and matrix production. While much in vitro work has characterized this response, little understanding exists regarding the sequential up- and down-regulation of genes following prosthetic arterial grafting. This study evaluates temporal gene expression at the distal anastomosis of prosthetic arterial grafts using microarray analysis.

Methods.—Expanded polytetrafluoroethylene (ePTFE) carotid interposition grafts ($n = 12$) were surgically implanted into mongrel dogs. Distal anastomotic segments were harvested at 7, 14, 30, or 60 days. Contralateral carotid artery served as control. Total RNA was isolated from the anastomotic tissue and paired controls. Samples were probed with oligonucleotide microarrays consisting of approximately 10,000 human genes to analyze differential gene expression at each time point.

Results.—Forty-nine genes were found to be up-regulated and 37 genes were found to be down-regulated at various time points. Six genes were found to be consistently up-regulated at all time intervals, including collagen type 1 α-1 and α-2, 80K-L protein (MARCKS), and osteopontin. Six genes were found to be consistently down-regulated, including smoothelin and tropomyosin 2. RT-PCR and immunohistochemistry confirmed the microarray data.

Conclusions.—This study uses microarray analysis to identify genes that were temporally up- and down-regulated after prosthetic arterial grafting. Genes with similar patterns of expression have been identified, providing insights into related cellular pathways that may result in the formation of anastomotic intimal hyperplasia.

► There is no consensus regarding the most appropriate method for analyzing gene expression using microarrays. Studies such as this are basically "shotgun approaches" that seek to identify gene expression associated with a biologic process. They do, however, provide a useful starting point and likely will ultimately lead to further studies specifically linking gene expression with biologic function.

G. L. Moneta, MD

Interleukin-6 Promoter Genotype and Restenosis After Femoropopliteal Balloon Angioplasty: Initial Observations

Exner M, Schillinger M, Minar E, et al (Univ of Vienna)

Radiology 231:839-844, 2004 1–34

Purpose.—To investigate whether there is an association between a functional polymorphism in the interleukin (IL)-6 gene promoter (−174)G/C and restenosis after percutaneous transluminal angioplasty (PTA) of the femoropopliteal artery.

Materials and Methods.—A total of 281 patients underwent PTA of the femoropopliteal artery during the study period; 23 (8%) patients had to be excluded due to missing genetic data. We studied 258 patients with intermittent claudication (n = 174) or critical limb ischemia (n = 84). The IL-6 promoter genotype was determined from venous blood samples before intervention by using a mutagenically separated polymerase chain reaction, and patients were followed up for 6 months with duplex ultrasonography for the occurrence of restenosis (≥=50%) after angioplasty. Multivariate Cox proportional hazards analysis was performed to assess the association between the IL-6 promoter genotype and restenosis, with adjustment for possible confounders such as atherosclerotic risk factors and angiographic covariates.

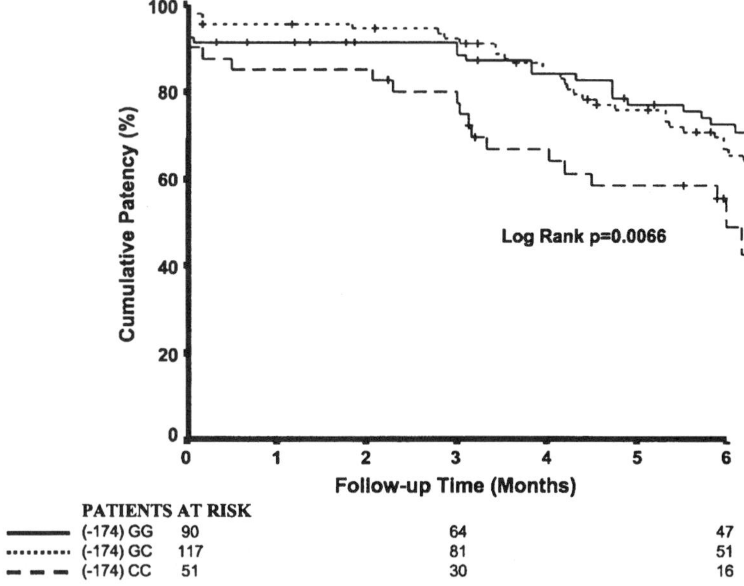

FIGURE.—Graph shows cumulative patency in 258 patients after PTA of the femoropopliteal artery according to IL-6 genotype. Homozygous carriers of (−174)C allele exhibited an increased rate of restenosis within 6 months after PTA (log-rank text, P = .0066). (Courtesy of Exner M, Schillinger M, Minar E, et al: Interleukin-6 promoter genotype and restenosis after femoropopliteal balloon angioplasty: Initial observations. *Radiology* 231:839-844, 2004. Radiological Society of North America.)

Results.—The 6-month restenosis rate was 26% (23 of 90) in patients with the (−174)GG genotype, 28% (33 of 117) with the (−174)GC genotype, and 43% (22 of 51) with the (−174)CC genotype (P =.044). Homozygous carriers of the (−174)C allele ([−174]CC) exhibited a 2.42-fold increased adjusted risk for restenosis (95% CI: 1.28, 4.58; P =.007) compared with homozygous (−174)G allele carriers ([−174]GG). Heterozygous carriers ([−174]GC) had no significantly increased restenosis risk (hazard ratio, 1.37; 95% CI: 0.84, 2.22; P =.21).

Conclusion.—The IL-6 promoter polymorphism (−174)G/C seems to influence the occurrence of restenosis after PTA. Homozygous carriers of the (−174)C allele have an increased rate of intermediate-term restenosis (Figure).

▶ Vascular injury is characterized, in part, by inflammation, and IL-6 is likely involved in the regulation of the inflammatory response secondary to injury following balloon angioplasty, with this inflammatory response resulting in restenosis. The study suggests that IL-6 polymorphism may influence restenosis, but the study is far from conclusive. Venous samples, not samples directly from the artery treated, were used to sample for IL-6. In addition, there were differences in blood pressure and lipid levels between the IL-6 subtypes. Other studies have also failed to confirm the observations of this study.[1] Nevertheless, a genetic basis is likely to contribute to differential molecular responses to injury. Further work in the genetics of restenosis is eagerly awaited.

G. L. Moneta, MD

Reference

1. Nauck M, Winkelmann BR, Hoffmann MM, et al: The interleukin-6 G(−174)C promoter polymorphism in the LURIC cohort: No association with plasma interleukin-6, coronary artery disease, and myocardial infarction. *J Mol Med* 80:507-513, 2002.

Comparison of Turbidimetric Aggregation and In Vitro Bleeding Time (PFA-100) for Monitoring the Platelet Inhibitory Profile of Antiplatelet Agents in Patients Undergoing Stent Implantation

Van der Planken MG, Claeys MJ, Vertessen FJ, et al (Univ Hosp Antwerp, Edegem, Belgium; Antwerp Univ, Belgium)

Thromb Res 111:159-164, 2003 1–35

Introduction.—The present study compared classical ADP-induced platelet aggregation vs. PFA-100 closure times using collagen/ADP membrane cartridges to monitor the degree of platelet-inhibiting effect of three drug regimens: ticlopidin, abciximab/ticlopidin and loading dose clopidogrel, each on top of aspirin (acetylsalicylic acid, ASA) during and after elective stent placement (intervention) in a total of 31 patients with acute coronary syndrome. Ticlopidin was started directly after stent implantation, abciximab was started before coronary intervention and given intravenously for 12 h, and a clopidogrel loading dose was given before intervention. The 10 patients treated with ticlopidin (500 mg daily) showed no significant prolongation of PFA closure times and a slight increase of ADP-induced platelet aggregation shortly after intervention (Fig 1). In 11 patients treated with abciximab/ticlopidin, the PFA closure times were significantly prolonged, and ADP-induced platelet aggregation was reduced by more than 80% during the 12-h abciximab infusion after intervention. The 10 patients pretreated with loading dose clopidogrel (450 mg followed by 75 mg daily)

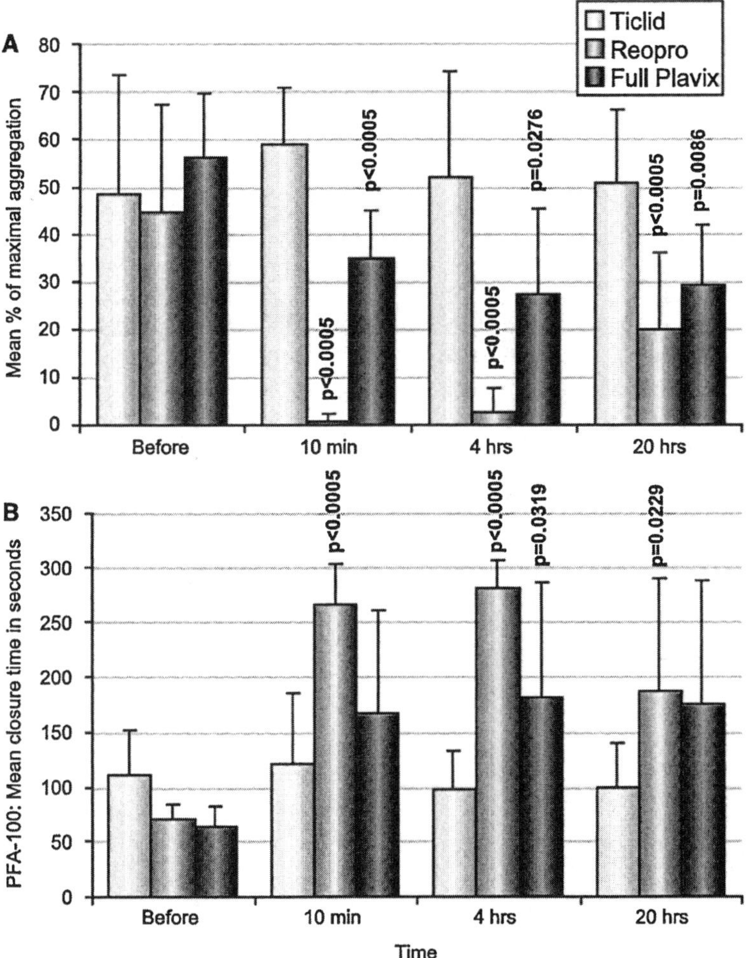

FIGURE 1.—A, Mean percentage of maximal aggregation. B, Mean closure time in seconds. (Reprinted from Van der Planken MG, Claeys MJ, Vertessen FJ, et al: Comparison of turbidimetric aggregation and in vitro bleeding time (PFA-100) for monitoring the platelet inhibitory profile of antiplatelet agents in patients undergoing stent implantation. *Thromb Res* 111:159-164, 2003. Copyright 2003, with kind permission from Elsevier Science Ltd, The Boulevard, Langford Lane, Kidlington OX5 1GB, UK.)

showed an intermediate but significant prolongation of PFA closure times and reduction of ADP-induced platelet aggregation at levels between the ticlopidin/aspirin- and the abciximab/ticlopidin/aspirin-treated groups. At 20 h after intervention, a similar degree of PFA closure time prolongation and inhibition of ADP-induced aggregation was observed in the abciximab/ticlopidin/aspirin- and the clopidogrel/aspirin-treated patient groups. Both measurement of PFA-100 closure times and inhibition of ADP-induced platelet aggregation showed a similar degree of platelet inhibition, but had rather broad SD ranges, which limit their precision for the follow-up of individual patients. In conclusion, abciximab on top of ticlopidin/aspirin showed a stronger antiplatelet effect for only less than 20 h, as compared to loading dose clopidogrel/aspirin in acute coronary syndrome patients undergoing stent implantation. Whether such a short-term superiority of abciximab, as compared to loading dose clopidogrel, translates into an overall clinical benefit of thombotic and bleeding complications remains to be established in a randomized clinical trial.

▶ Thienopyridines (clopidogrel and ticlopidin) along with aspirin have synergistic effects on platelet inhibition in that they inhibit arachidonic acid and ADP-mediated platelet activation and reduce collagen- and thrombin-induced activation. This study indicates that the addition of the IIb/IIIa inhibitor abciximab to a thienopyridine/aspirin combination gives more rapid platelet inhibition. One worries that it will also result in more bleeding at the angio access site and, therefore, potential increased complications of angioplasty and stenting. While this was a study of coronary stent patients, the principles likely apply to peripheral arterial disease patients as well.

G. L. Moneta, MD

Folate Therapy and In-Stent Restenosis After Coronary Stenting

Lange H, Suryapranata H, De Luca G, et al (Heart Ctr, Bremen, Germany; Hosp De Weezenlanden, Zwolle, The Netherlands; Diagram, Zwolle, the Netherlands)

N Engl J Med 350:2673-2681, 2004 1–36

Background.—Vitamin therapy to lower homocysteine levels has recently been recommended for the prevention of restenosis after coronary angioplasty. We tested the effect of a combination of folic acid, vitamin B_6, and vitamin B_{12} (referred to as folate therapy) on the risk of angiographic restenosis after coronary-stent placement in a double-blind, multicenter trial.

Methods.—A total of 636 patients who had undergone successful coronary stenting were randomly assigned to receive 1 mg of folic acid, 5 mg of vitamin B_6, and 1 mg of vitamin B_{12} intravenously, followed by daily oral doses of 1.2 mg of folic acid, 48 mg of vitamin B_6, and 60 μg of vitamin B_{12} for six months, or to receive placebo. The angiographic end points (minimal luminal diameter, late loss, and restenosis rate) were assessed at six months by means of quantitative coronary angiography.

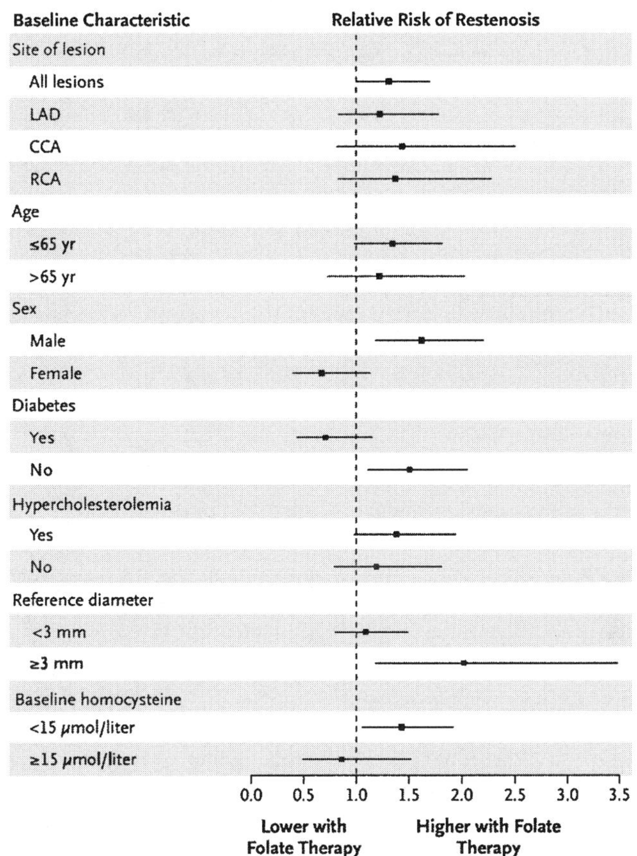

FIGURE 2.—Relative risk of restonsis with folate therapy, according to baseline characteristics.*Squares* indicate means, and *horizontal lines* 95 percent confidence intervals. Folate therapy did not uniformly increase the risk of restenosis. Women (P for heterogeneity = 0.002), patients with diabetes (P for heterogeneity = 0.02), and patients with high baseline homocysteine levels tended to have a lower risk of restenosis with folate therapy. *Abbreviations: LAD*, Left anterior descending coronary artery; *CCA*, circumflex coronary artery; *RCA*, right coronary artery. (Reprinted by permission of *The New England Journal of Medicine* from Lange H, Suryapranata H, De Luca G, et al: Folate therapy and in-stent restenosis after coronary stenting. *N Engl J Med* 350:2673-2681, 2004. Copyright 2004, Massachusetts Medical Society. All rights reserved.)

Results.—At follow-up, the mean (±SD) minimal luminal diameter was significantly smaller in the folate group than in the placebo group (1.59±0.62 mm vs. 1.74±0.64 mm, P=0.008), and the extent of late luminal loss was greater (0.90±0.55 mm vs. 0.76±0.58 mm, P=0.004). The restenosis rate was higher in the folate group than in the placebo group (34.5 percent vs. 26.5 percent, P=0.05), and a higher percentage of patients in the folate group required repeated target-vessel revascularization (15.8 percent vs. 10.6 percent, P=0.05). Folate therapy had adverse effects on the risk of restenosis in all subgroups except for women, patients with diabetes, and patients with markedly elevated homocysteine levels (15 μmol per liter or more) at baseline.

Conclusions.—Contrary to previous findings, the administration of folate, vitamin B_6, and vitamin B_{12} after coronary stenting may increase the risk of in-stent restenosis and the need for target-vessel revascularization (Fig 2).

▶ The role of homocysteine in predicting restenosis after angioplasty is controversial. Some studies have suggested it facilitates restenosis, whereas others have not. The results of this study clearly do not indicate a role of homocysteine in restenosis following coronary angioplasty. The data, however, do not indicate that folate therapy is harmful. The folate-treated patients did not have increased incidence of death or myocardial infarction. Based on this study, it may be reasonable to limit folate therapy in patients with hyperhomocysteinemia around the time of stent placement. The results, however, do not argue for discontinuation of chronic folate therapy in patients with hyperhomocysteinemia.

G. L. Moneta, MD

Effect of Stent Coating Alone on In Vitro Vascular Smooth Muscle Cell Proliferation and Apoptosis

Curcio A, Torella D, Cuda G, et al (Magna Graecia Univ, Catanzaro, Italy; Federico II Univ, Naples, Italy; Genecor Found, Naples, Italy)

Am J Physiol Heart Circ Physiol 286:H902-H908, 2004 1–37

Introduction.—Synthetic polymers, like methacrylate (MA) compounds, have been clinically introduced as inert coatings to locally deliver drugs that inhibit restenosis after stent. The aim of the present study was to evaluate the effects of MA coating alone on vascular smooth muscle cell (VSMC) growth in vitro. Stainless steel stents were coated with MA at the following doses: 0.3, 1.5, and 3 ml. Uncoated/bare metal stents were used as controls. VSMCs were cultured in dishes, and a MA-coated stent or an uncoated bare metal stent was gently added to each well. VSMC proliferation was assessed by bromodeoxyuridine (BrdU) incorporation. Apoptosis was analyzed by three distinct approaches: *1*) annexin V/propidium iodide fluorescence detection; *2*) DNA laddering; and *3*) caspase-3 activation and PARP cleavage. MA-coated stents induced a significant decrease of BrdU incorporation compared with uncoated stents at both the low and high concentrations. In VSMCs incubated with MA-coated stents, annexin V/propidium iodide fluorescence detection showed a significant increase in apoptotic cells, which was corroborated by the typical DNA laddering. Apoptosis of VSMCs after incubation with MA-coated stents was characterized by caspase-3 activation and PARP cleavage. The MA-coated stent induced VSMC growth arrest by inducing apoptosis in a dose-dependent manner. Thus MA is not an inert platform for eluting drugs because it is biologically active per se. This effect should be taken in account when evaluating an association of this coating with antiproliferative agents for in-stent restenosis prevention.

▶ Huge efforts are under way to determine the best drug for a drug-eluting stent. The current study indicates the polymers used to deliver the drugs may also have biologic activity. Biocompatibility between delivery polymers and drugs must therefore be considered in the design of drug-eluting stents. The overall success of drug-eluting stents may be dependent not only on the drug, but also on the polymer component of the delivery system.

G. L. Moneta, MD

Specific Binding to Intracellular Proteins Determines Arterial Transport Properties for Rapamycin and Paclitaxel

Levin AD, Vukmirovic N, Hwang C-W, et al (Harvard-MIT, Cambridge, Mass; Harvard Med School, Boston)

Proc Natl Acad Sci U S A 101:9463-9467, 2004 1–38

Introduction.—Endovascular drug-eluting stents have changed the practice of medicine, and yet it is unclear how they so dramatically reduce restenosis and how to distinguish between the different formulations available. Biological drug potency is not the sole determinant of biological effect. Physicochemical drug properties also play important roles. Historically, two classes of therapeutic compounds emerged: hydrophobic drugs, which are retained within tissue and have dramatic effects, and hydrophilic drugs, which are rapidly cleared and ineffective. Researchers are now questioning whether individual properties of different drugs beyond lipid avidity can further distinguish arterial transport and distribution. In bovine internal carotid segments, tissue-loading profiles for hydrophobic paclitaxel and rapamycin are indistinguishable, reaching load steady state after 2 days. Hydrophilic dextran reaches equilibrium in several hours at levels no higher than surrounding solution concentrations. Both paclitaxel and rapamycin bind to the artery at 30-40 times bulk concentration. Competitive binding assays confirm binding to specific tissue elements. Most importantly, transmural drug distribution profiles are markedly different for the two compounds, reflecting, perhaps, different modes of binding. Rapamycin, which binds specifically to FKBP12 binding protein, distributes evenly through the artery, whereas paclitaxel, which binds specifically to microtubules, remains primarily in the subintimal space. The data demonstrate that binding of rapamycin and paclitaxel to specific intracellular proteins plays an essential role in determining arterial transport and distribution and in distinguishing one compound from another. These results offer further insight into the mechanism of local drug delivery and the specific use of existing drug-eluting stent formulations.

▶ Recent data suggest rapamycin and paclitaxel drug-eluting stents may have different clinical efficacies, with paclitaxel stents being perhaps slightly more effective. This may be explained by the more specific affinity of paclitaxel for the subintimal space. Delineation of the precise targets of the drugs coating drug-eluting stents may allow development of even more efficacious drug-eluting stents and a better understanding of the intimal hyperplastic process.

G. L. Moneta, MD

Genome Scan for Familial Abdominal Aortic Aneurysm Using Sex and Family History as Covariates Suggests Genetic Heterogeneity and Identifies Linkage to Chromosome 19q13

Shibamura H, Olson JM, van Vlijmen-van Keulen C, et al (Wayne State Univ, Detroit; Case Western Reserve Univ, Cleveland, Ohio; Free Univ, Amsterdam; et al)

Circulation 109:2103-2108, 2004 1–39

Background.—Abdominal aortic aneurysm (AAA) is a relatively common disease, with 1% to 2% of the population harboring aneurysms. Genetic risk factors are likely to contribute to the development of AAAs, although no such risk factors have been identified.

Method and Results.—We performed a whole-genome scan of AAA using affected-relative-pair (ARP) linkage analysis that includes covariates to allow for genetic heterogeneity. We found strong evidence of linkage (logarithm of odds [LOD] score=4.64) to a region near marker *D19S433* at 51.88 centimorgans (cM) on chromosome 19 with 36 families (75 ARPs) when including sex and the number of affected first-degree relatives of the proband (N_{aff}) as covariates. We then genotyped 83 additional families for the same markers and typed additional markers for all families and obtained a LOD score of 4.75 (P=0.00014) with sex, N_{aff}, and their interaction as covariates near marker *D19S416* (58.69 cM). We also identified a region on chromosome 4 with a LOD score of 3.73 (P=0.0012) near marker *D4S1644* using the same covariate model as for chromosome 19.

Conclusions.—Our results provide evidence for genetic heterogeneity and the presence of susceptibility loci for AAA on chromosomes 19q13 and 4q31.

▶ The authors linkage mode for demonstration of a genetic basis for AAA depends on including sex and family history as covariants in the model. This makes sense, as AAA is unlikely to be solely a genetically determined disease, but rather a disease in which genetics interact with additional patient and environmental factors to produce an aneurysm. By determining the presence of "susceptible" genes, it may be possible to more precisely identify patients at an early age who are at risk for AAA. Clinicians can then potentially provide more effective counseling regarding modification of specific risk factors linked to genetic susceptibility to AAA.

G. L. Moneta, MD

Accelerated Enlargement of Experimental Abdominal Aortic Aneurysms in a Mouse Model of Chronic Cigarette Smoke Exposure

Buckley C, Wyble CW, Borhani M, et al (Washington Univ, St Louis)

J Am Coll Surg 199:896-903, 2004 1–40

Background.—Cigarette smoking and pulmonary emphysema are strongly associated with abdominal aortic aneurysms (AAAs), but the biologic mechanisms linking these conditions are undefined.

Study Design.—To determine if exposure to cigarette smoke influences formation and growth of experimental AAAs, 129/SvEv mice were acclimated to daily cigarette smoke exposure for 2 weeks followed by transient elastase perfusion of the abdominal aorta to induce aneurysmal degeneration. Smoking was continued for intervals of either 2 or 12 weeks (8 mice per group). Nonsmoking 129/SvEv controls (n = 29) underwent elastase perfusion and followup evaluation at the same time intervals. In all animals, abdominal aortic diameter (AD) was measured to determine interval increases in AD (ΔAD), with AAAs defined as a ΔAD > 100%.

Results.—Preperfusion and immediate postperfusion ADs were not significantly different between experimental groups. Aneurysmal dilatation was present 2 weeks after elastase perfusion in both smoking mice and non-

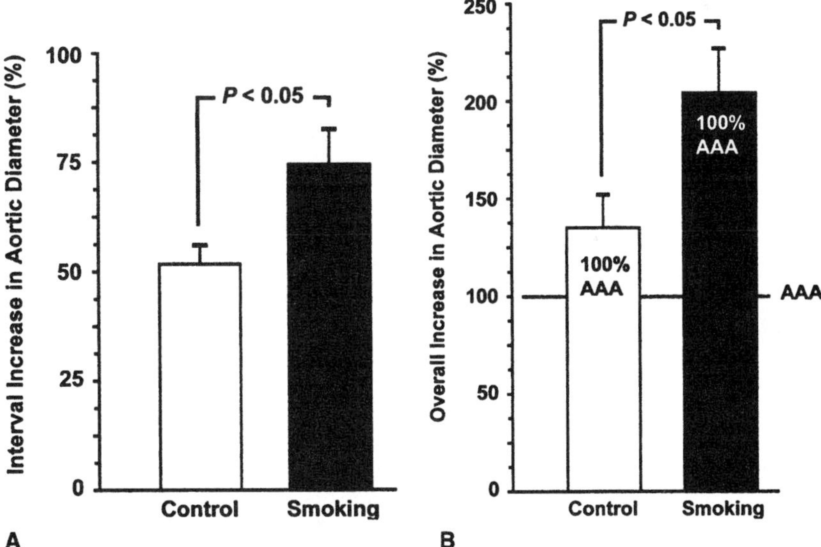

FIGURE 3.—Extent of aortic dilation in smoking and nonsmoking mice 12 weeks after elastase perfusion. Smoking and nonsmoking C57B1/6 wild-type mice were examined 12 weeks after elastase perfusion to induce development of abdominal aortic aneurysms (AAAs). Data shown represent the mean ± SEM for the (A) interval and (B) overall extent of aortic dilation, with *solid bars* indicating smoking mice and *open bars* indicating nonsmoking controls. The incidence of AAAs is indicated for each group, with aneurysmal dilation defined as an overall increase in aortic diameter >100% (indicated by the *horizontal line*). (Reprinted from Buckley C, Wyble CW, Borhani M, et al: Accelerated enlargement of experimental abdominal aortic aneurysms in a mouse model of chronic cigarette smoke exposure. *J Am Coll Surg* 199:896-903, 2004. Copyright 2004, with permission from American College of Surgeons.)

smoking controls, with no significant difference in final AD (mean ± SEM: smoking, 1.23 ± 0.11 mm versus nonsmoking, 1.22 ± 0.05 mm). There were also no differences in the overall extent of aortic dilatation (ΔAD smoking, 136 ± 24% versus nonsmoking, 138 ± 10%), or the incidence of AAAs (smoking, 75% versus nonsmoking, 79%). Although all animals had developed AAAs by 12 weeks after elastase perfusion, the overall extent of aortic dilatation was 50% greater in smoking mice compared with nonsmoking controls (ΔAD smoking, 204 ± 23% versus nonsmoking, 135 ± 17%; $p < 0.05$).

Conclusions.—Short-term exposure to cigarette smoke did not alter initial development of experimental AAAs, but chronic smoke exposure was associated with a substantial increase in the late progression of aneurysmal dilatation. This novel combination of in vivo experimental models offers a new approach to investigate mechanisms by which cigarette smoking promotes aneurysmal degeneration (Fig 3).

▶ This study serves as a first step toward determining how cigarette smoking may influence the development of aneurysms. It represents a combination of 2 well-characterized experimental models, an elastase-induced model of AAAs combined with a model of cigarette smoke–induced pulmonary emphysema. This study indicates that it is feasible to combine the 2 models in a single model. It may eventually yield clues as to the mechanism of tobacco-induced aortic degeneration.

G. L. Moneta, MD

Vascular Surgery Training in the United States, 1994 to 2003

Cronenwett JL (Dartmouth-Hitchcock Med Ctr, Lebanon, NH)

J Vasc Surg 40:660-669, 2004 1–41

Objective.—The purpose of this study was to analyze the use of operative training resources for vascular surgery residents (VSRs) and general surgery residents (GSRs) over the past 10 years in the United States, to address questions concerning adequate endovascular versus open surgical training and the potential to expand the number of VSRs to meet future workforce needs.

Methods.—National operative data from the Residency Review Committee for Surgery (RRC) were analyzed for all vascular surgery (VS) and general surgery (GS) training programs from 1994 to 2003. GSR experience in programs with and without associated VS programs was also compared.

Results.—Mean total VS volume per VSR increased from 220 operations in 1994 to 368 in 2003, owing to the addition of 140 endovascular procedures by 2003. GSR volume was more stable, with 117 mean total VS operations in 1994 and 122 in 2003. This volume was distributed as approximately 50% major open VS operations for both VSR and GSR. In addition, 39% of VSR experience was endovascular, whereas 32% of GSR experience was vascular access. The average VSR performed 2.7 times more major open VS operations than each GSR, but because of the 10-fold greater number of

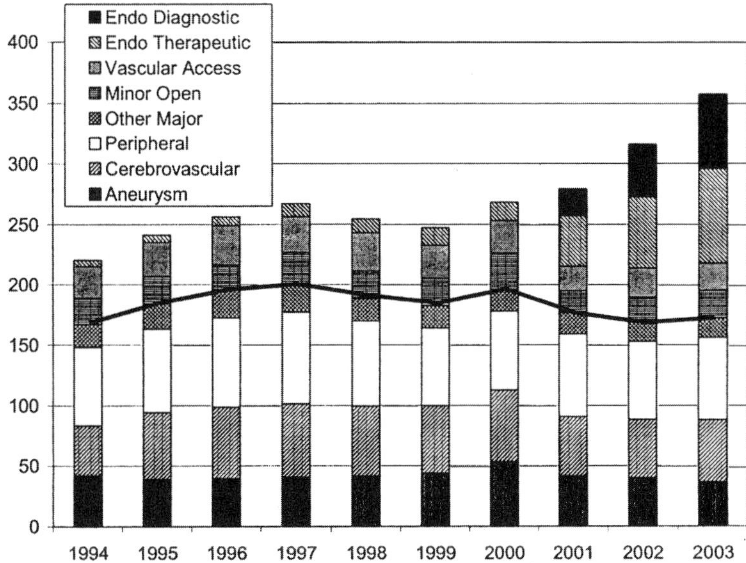

FIGURE 1.—Mean volume of total vascular operations per vascular surgery resident completing training from 1994 to 2003. *Black line* indicates total major open operations. Only primary operations are included. (Reprinted by permission of the publisher from Cronenwett JL: Vascular surgery training in the United States, 1994 to 2003. *J Vasc Surg* 40:660-669, 2004. Copyright 2004 by Elsevier.)

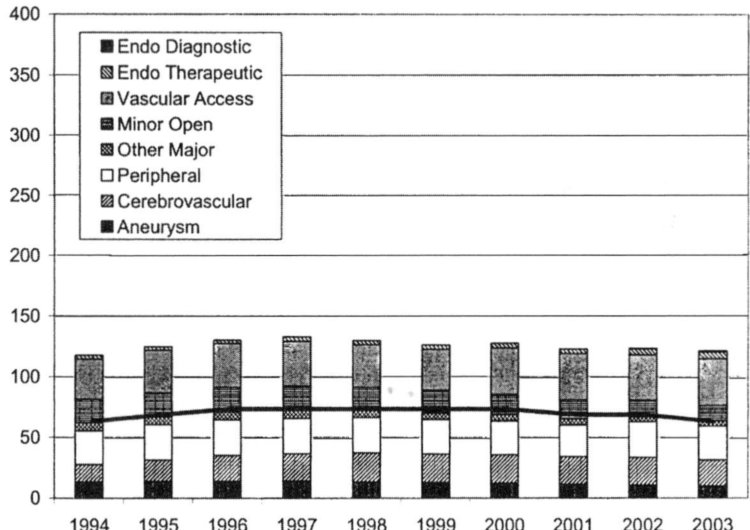

FIGURE 2.—Mean volume of total vascular operations per general surgery resident completing training from 1994 to 2003. *Black line* indicates total major open operations. Only primary operations are included. (Reprinted by permission of the publisher from Cronenwett JL: Vascular surgery training in the United States, 1994 to 2003. *J Vasc Surg* 40:660-669, 2004. Copyright 2004 by Elsevier.)

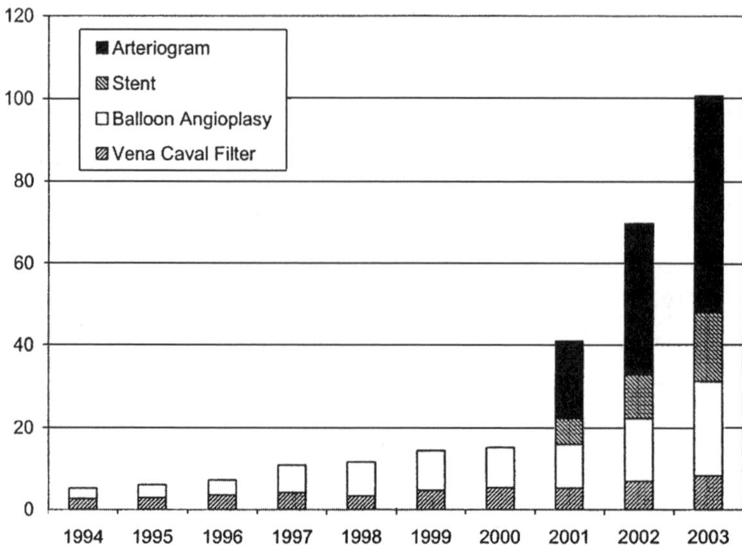

FIGURE 4.—Mean volume of interventional procedures by category per vascular surgery residents completing training from 1994 to 2003. Only primary procedures are included. (Reprinted by permission of the publisher from Cronenwett JL: Vascular surgery training in the United States, 1994 to 2003. *J Vasc Surg* 40:660-669, 2004. Copyright 2004 by Elsevier.)

GSRs, VSRs performed only 20% of the total major operations available for VS training. Selective procedures, such as renal revascularization and open infrarenal abdominal aortic aneurysm repair decreased over time, while endovascular abdominal aortic aneurysm repair increased dramatically, accounting for 46% of aortic aneurysm repairs per VSR in 2003. The mean volume of total interventional procedures per VSR in 2003 was 152 diagnostic and 213 therapeutic. GSRs in programs with and without an associated VS program had very similar operative volumes.

Conclusions.—Interventional procedures have increased VSR operative volume by 50% in recent years, with only a 12% decrease in major open operations. Nearly all VSRs currently meet RRC minimum requirements for open and endovascular procedures. Mean GSR operative volume has been stable, and far exceeds RRC minimum requirements. Based on the number of major open vascular operations available for training in 2003, the current number of VSR positions could be increased by 50% if GSR operative volume was decreased by 15%. However, increased interventional volume would also be required, for which there is competition with other specialties (Figs 1, 2, and 4).

► Vascular residents are busier than ever but doing different things than they were 5 years ago. I think the current worries about vascular residents having enough open cases is a bit overblown. The data suggest that for the next 5 to 10 years vascular residents will have sufficient open experience. The exception may be programs with an endovascular agenda.

G. L. Moneta, MD

Postmenopausal Hormone Therapy Is Associated With Atherosclerosis Progression in Women With Abnormal Glucose Tolerance

Howard BV, Hsia J, Ouyang P, et al (MedStar Research Inst, Hyattsville, Md)

Circulation 110:201-206, 2004 1–42

Background.—Abnormal glucose tolerance (AGT; diabetes or impaired glucose tolerance) is associated with increased risk of cardiovascular disease, especially in women. Cardiovascular disease rates in women increase after menopause. The Women's Health Initiative found that postmenopausal hormone therapy (PHT) increased the risk of cardiovascular disease and that effects in diabetic women did not differ from those in women without diabetes. In this study, we hypothesized that PHT would have a worse effect on disease among women with AGT.

Method and Results.—We randomly assigned 423 postmenopausal women with angiographically defined atherosclerosis (321 women had exit angiograms) with (n=140) or without (n=181) AGT to receive estrogen, estrogen plus progestin, or a placebo for 2.8±0.9 years. LDL was lower and HDL and triglycerides were higher after PHT in non-AGT and AGT women, but more adverse changes occurred in C-reactive protein and fibrinogen in women with AGT (P=0.11 and P=0.02 for interactions). PHT had no effect on fasting glucose or insulin concentrations in women without AGT, but in women with AGT, fasting glucose levels, insulin concentration, and insulin resistance as assessed by the HOMA (homeostasis model) calculation decreased slightly (P=0.28, P=0.25, P=0.14 for interaction, respectively). Atherosclerotic progression was greater in women with AGT. Atherosclerotic progression in previously nondiseased segments was enhanced by PHT to a greater extent in women with AGT (P=0.11 for interaction).

Conclusions.—PHT is associated with a worsening of coronary atherosclerosis and exacerbation of the profile of inflammatory markers in women with AGT. Therefore, PHT is not warranted for use in diabetic women. Further study is needed to explore the improvement in insulin resistance and glycemia that appears to occur with PHT in women with AGT.

▶ Diabetes promotes atherosclerosis in women as well as men. This is not new news. The fact that PHT is even worse for women with diabetes than for those without is yet another blow to the concept of the use of estrogen replacement in the postmenopausal woman. The follow-up of this study is short, and additional and possibly adverse effects of PHT are therefore likely to become evident over time.

G. L. Moneta, MD

2 Vascular Laboratory and Imaging

Integrating Surgery and Radiology in One Suite: A Multicenter Study

ten Cate G, Fosse E, Hol PK, et al (Rikshospitalet Univ, Oslo, Norway; Mission Hosps, Asheville, NC; Univ of Chicago; et al)

J Vasc Surg 40:494-499, 2004 2–1

Purpose.—The study was performed to evaluate the performance of digital fixed-mounted angiographic C-arm systems in the operating room as used by surgeons, cardiologists, and interventional radiologists (Fig 2).

Methods.—An observational study in the operating room was performed, along with a structured questionnaire and semi-structured interviews. Twenty interventions were observed at 5 sites. Workflow was analyzed.

Results.—Integration of high-end angiographic imaging equipment in the operating room enables image-guided surgery with high-quality images, on-table quality assessment of surgical procedures, and "one-stop shopping" procedures. Integrated suites were run by surgery as well as radiology departments, and are used for a variety of procedures, including vascular, car-

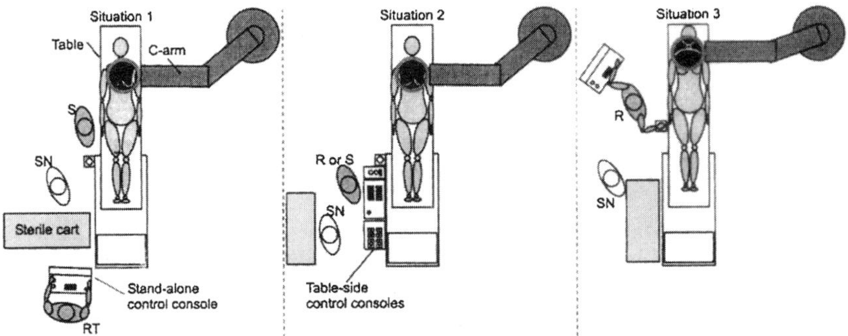

FIGURE 2.—Overview system operation. The following arrangements were observed: a vascular surgeon, together with a technician, who controlled the system from behind the table with a stand-alone control console (*Situation 1*); a radiologist or surgeon operating the table and system alone with control consoles attached to the table (*Situation 2*); and a radiologist controlling the table and system alone with a stand-alone control console positioned behind his back (*Situation 3*). (Reprinted by permission of the publisher from ten Cate G, Fosse E, Hol PK, et al: Integrating surgery and radiology in one suite: A multicenter study. *J Vasc Surg* 40:494-499, 2004. Copyright 2004 by Elsevier.)

diothoracic, open surgical, percutaneous, and combined procedures. Operation of the angiographic system and its user interface design were not considered ideal for operating room use. Limited patient accessibility was observed, sometimes leading to uncomfortable positions for the operating physicians. Certain procedures, such as tibial artery surgery, were difficult to perform, owing to lack of accessories. Patient transfer was considered inadequate. Cleaning of the system was rated as poor. Operating room use puts an even higher demand on reliability of the system.

Conclusion.—Integration of digital angiographic systems into operating rooms has produced opportunities for new treatments and offers a superior solution for interdisciplinary work among surgeons, cardiologists, and radiologists. However, the context of use differs radically from that in the traditional radiologic examination room; the environment, users, and procedures are all different. Integration of imaging methods into the operating room can be more successful if special operating room conditions are taken into account by medical systems manufacturers.

▶ The integration of fixed imaging systems into the operating room is becoming more and more common. However, it appears the cart is a bit ahead of the horse in that manufacturers have not, and architects have not fully considered the ergonomic needs of the operating surgeon during long open procedures. This is not good news for those surgeons who already have neck or back discomfort during a long procedure.

G. L. Moneta, MD

Imaging of Carotid Arteries in Symptomatic Patients: Cost-effectiveness of Diagnostic Strategies

Buskens E, Nederkoorn PJ, Buijs-van der Woude T, et al (Univ Med Ctr Utrecht, The Netherlands; Erasmus MC, Rotterdam, The Netherlands; Harvard School of Public Health, Boston)

Radiology 233:101-112, 2004 2–2

Purpose.—To assess the cost-effectiveness of noninvasive imaging strategies in patients who have had a transient ischemic attack (TIA) or minor stroke and are suspected of having significant carotid artery stenosis.

Materials and Methods.—From 1997 through 2000, 350 patients were included in a multicenter blinded consecutive cohort study. The sensitivities and specificities of duplex ultrasonography (US), magnetic resonance (MR) angiography, and these two examinations combined were estimated by using digital subtraction angiography (DSA) as the reference standard. The actual costs (from a societal perspective) of performing imaging and endarterectomy were estimated. The survival, quality of life, and costs associated with stroke were based on data reported in the literature. Markov modeling was used to predict long-term outcomes. Subsequently, a decision model was used to calculate costs, quality-adjusted life-years (QALYs), and incremental costs per QALY gained for 62 examination-treatment strategies. Extensive sensitivity analyses were performed.

Results.—Duplex US had 88% sensitivity and 76% specificity with use of conventional cutoff criteria. MR angiography had comparable values: 92% sensitivity and 76% specificity. Combined concordant duplex US and MR angiography had superior diagnostic performance: 96% sensitivity and 80% specificity. Duplex US alone was the most efficient strategy. Adding MR angiography led to a marginal increase in QALYs gained but at prohibitive costs (cost-effectiveness ratio > €1,500,000 per QALY gained). Performing DSA owing to discordant duplex US and MR angiographic findings and to confirm duplex US and MR angiographic findings led to extra costs and QALY loss owing to complications. Sensitivity analyses revealed that duplex US as a stand-alone examination remained the preferred strategy while estimates and assumptions were varied across plausible ranges.

Conclusion.—Duplex US performed without additional imaging is cost-effective in the selection of symptomatic patients suitable for endarterectomy. Adding MR angiography increases effectiveness slightly at disproportionately high costs, whereas DSA is inferior because of associated complications.

► I have always felt that adding a confirming MR angiographic examination to a technically adequate duplex study in the evaluation of carotid stenosis was unnecessary and needlessly expensive. This study confirms that impression. All advantages of the duplex-alone strategy will be lost if the test is poorly performed or interpreted. Ongoing quality assurance in the vascular laboratory is essential.

G. L. Moneta, MD

Ocular Findings as Predictors of Carotid Artery Occlusive Disease: Is Carotid Imaging Justified?

McCullough HK, Reinert CG, Hynan LS, et al (Univ of Texas, Dallas; Veterans Affairs North Texas Health Care System, Dallas)

J Vasc Surg 40:279-286, 2004 2–3

Objectives.—Hemispheric neurologic symptoms, amaurosis fugax, and Hollenhorst plaques at eye examination are standard indications for carotid imaging to identify carotid artery occlusive disease (CAOD). Previous reports have suggested that other ocular findings, such as retinal artery occlusion and anterior ischemic optic neuropathy, are associated with CAOD. However, the predictive value of ocular findings for the presence of CAOD is controversial. The purpose of this study was to define the predictive value of ocular symptoms and ophthalmologic examination in identifying significant CAOD.

Methods.—Over 3 years 145 patients were referred for carotid imaging on the basis of ocular indications in 160 eyes. Forty patients were excluded because of concurrent non-ocular indications for carotid imaging, leaving

105 patients referred exclusively for ocular indications to evaluate. Ophthalmologic history and eye examination were correlated with carotid duplex ultrasound findings.

Results.—Amaurosis fugax was associated with a positive scan in 20.0% of carotid arteries (P =.022). Hollenhorst plaques at fundoscopic examination were associated with a positive scan in 18.2% of carotid arteries (P =.02). Ocular findings exclusive of Hollenhorst plaques were particularly poor predictors of CAOD, inasmuch as only 1 of 64 arteries (1.6%) had significant ipsilateral internal carotid artery stenosis (P =.022). Venous stasis retinopathy was the only ocular finding other than Hollenhorst plaques with any predictive value (1 of 5 scans positive; positive predictive value, 20.0%).

Conclusions.—Ocular symptoms and findings are poor predictors of CAOD. Amaurosis fugax, Hollenhorst plaques, and venous stasis retinopathy demonstrated moderate predictive value, whereas all other ocular findings demonstrated no predictive value in identifying CAOD.

► The results of this study need to be disseminated to primary care physicians and ophthalmologists. A 20% yield of greater than 50% carotid stenosis when evaluating for amaurosis fugax or Hollenhorst plaques is not all that bad when one compares the cost of duplex to that of a stroke. Clearly, other ocular "indications" for carotid duplex provide too low of a yield to ever be cost-effective.

G. L. Moneta, MD

Quantification of Internal Carotid Artery Stenosis With Duplex US: Comparative Analysis of Different Flow Velocity Criteria

Sabeti S, Schillinger M, Mlekusch W, et al (Vienna Gen Hosp)

Radiology 232:431-439, 2004 2–4

Purpose.—To compare 13 previously published sets of duplex ultrasonographic (US) criteria with the US criteria used at the authors' institution in terms of agreement with carotid artery angiographic results.

Materials and Methods.—The authors studied 1,006 carotid arteries in 503 patients at duplex US and angiography. The degree of stenosis was determined by using duplex flow US velocities and applying 13 previously published sets of criteria and the criteria used at the authors' institution. Two independent observers evaluated the angiograms according to North American Symptomatic Carotid Endarterectomy Trial (NASCET) criteria. κ statistics, sensitivities, specificities, positive predictive values (PPVs), negative predictive values (NPVs), and generalized linear mixed regression models were used to assess agreement between duplex US and angiographic findings.

Results.—Stenoses of 0%-29%, 30%-49%, 50%-69%, 70%-99%, and 100% could be differentiated with 73% overall agreement between duplex US and angiographic findings according to flow velocity criteria (κ = 0.57; 95% confidence interval [CI]: 0.54, 0.60); however, with duplex US, the an-

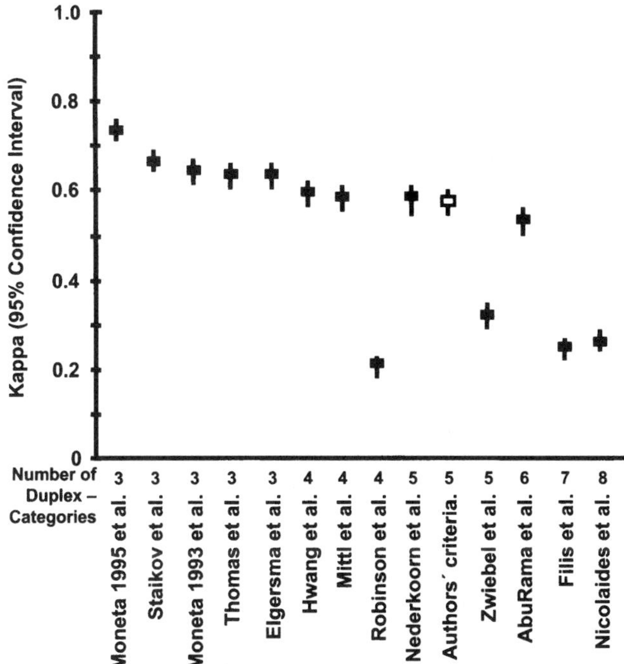

FIGURE 3.—Graph illustrates agreement between duplex US stenosis grade and angiographic stenosis grade. Angiographic findings for 1,006 carotid arteries in 503 patients were compared with those obtained by using 13 previously published sets of duplex US criteria (*solid rectangles*, listed in Fig 1) and the duplex US criteria used at the authors' institution (*open rectangles*). With increasing specificity of duplex US owing to increasing numbers of stenosis degree ranges, agreement between US and angiographic findings decreased. (Courtesy of Sabeti S, Schillinger M, Mlekusch W, et al: Quantification of internal carotid artery stenosis with duplex US: Comparative analysis of different flow velocity criteria. *Radiology* 232:431-439, 2004. Copyright 2004, Radiological Society of North America.)

giographic degree of stenosis tended to be overestimated. In the differentiation of stenoses of less than 70%, only 45% agreement ($\kappa = 0.26$; 95% CI: 0.23, 0.29) was observed, whereas in the differentiation of high-grade (≥70%) stenoses, 96% agreement was observed ($\kappa = 0.85$; 95% CI: 0.83, 0.87). The PPV and NPV for the identification of 70%-99% angiographic stenosis were 69% and 98%, respectively, with use of the most sensitive duplex US criteria.

Conclusion.—Duplex US is an excellent examination to screen for high-grade carotid artery stenosis; however, it tends to lead to an overestimation of the degree of stenosis. Exclusion of 70%-99% angiographic stenosis can be achieved with a sensitivity of up to 98% (Fig 3).

► The more categories into which one tries to subdivide duplex-determined carotid stenoses, the less will be the overall accuracy of the examination. Duplex works best for identifying whether or not a particular lesion exceeds a threshold level of stenosis. That the threshold concept works best for the higher levels of stenosis is not surprising, as minimal degrees of carotid stenosis do not produce reproducible changes in quantitative measures of velocity waveforms.

G. L. Moneta, MD

Three-Dimensional Assessment of Extracranial Doppler Sonography in Carotid Artery Stenosis Compared With Digital Subtraction Angiography

Wessels T, Harrer JU, Stetter S, et al (Justus-Liebig-Univ Giessen, Germany; Aachen Univ, Germany; Kliniken Schmieder Allensbach/Singen, Germany)
Stroke 35:1847-1851, 2004 2–5

Background and Purpose.—Difficulties in data presentation, data storage, and a high interobserver variability may influence color-coded Duplex sonography assessment of internal carotid artery stenosis (ICAS). The aim of our study was to evaluate the between-method agreement of ICAS using 3D color Doppler sonography (CDS) compared with digital subtraction angiography (DSA).

Methods.—Forty-nine patients with 64 ICASs (age 64±9 years) were involved. The patients were investigated with a color-coded duplex system using the power mode. The 3D system consists of an electromagnet that induces a low-intensity magnetic field near the patient's head. A magnetic position sensor is attached to the probe and transmits the spatial orientation to a personal computer.

Results.—A total of 62 ICASs were reconstructed successfully with 3D CDS in 47 of 49 patients. High agreement for 2 independent observers was found in 3D CDS (weighted κ coefficient of 0.88). Three-dimensional CDS slightly underestimated the mean stenotic degree (mean 3D CDS 68.47±10.5 versus DSA 71.3±10.0). The intermethod agreement comparing DSA with 3D CDS was analyzed with the Bland and Altman test, which showed good agreement. Mean sensitivity of 3D CDS was 93%, mean specificity 82.5%, mean positive predictive value 82%, and mean negative predictive value 98%.

Conclusions.—The 3D CDS findings demonstrated good agreement compared with the gold standard, DSA, yielding higher accuracy than CDS alone. Compared with angiography or magnetic resonance angiography, 3D CDS can be performed easily on critically ill patients in stroke or intensive care units and may therefore provide a useful tool for patients unable to undergo more invasive imaging techniques.

▶ Previous reports of 3D US reconstruction of the carotid bifurcation have utilized techniques that were time-consuming, required personal computers, and produced low-quality reconstructive pictures. The current technique seems much more efficient, with reconstruction times for the images averaging 7.1 mintues. A serious drawback to 3D US in this study was frequent underestimation of high-grade ICAS. The technique in its present form, therefore, should not be used as a stand alone test, but rather as a study to confirm findings of standard color duplex examination. Clearly, if both by 3D color duplex scanning and standard color duplex scanning the patient has a high grade ICAS, it is very likely that the patient does have critical carotid stenosis.

G. L. Moneta, MD

Characterization of Carotid Artery Plaques Using Real-time Compound B-mode Ultrasound

Kern R, Szabo K, Hennerici M, et al (Univ of Heidelberg, Mannheim, Germany)

Stroke 35:870-875, 2004 2–6

Background and Purpose.—Real-time compound ultrasound imaging is a new technique for improving the image quality of B-mode scanning. We investigated the value of this method for the characterization of atherosclerotic plaques in the internal carotid artery.

Methods.—Thirty-two patients (22 men, 10 women; mean age, 75 years) with plaques of the internal carotid artery as identified by high-resolution B-mode scanning were investigated with real-time compound ultrasound imaging with the use of a 5- to 12-MHz dynamic range linear transducer on a duplex scanner. Two independent observers rated plaque morphology according to a standardized protocol.

Results.—The majority of plaques was classified as predominantly echogenic and as plaques of irregular surface, whereas ulcerated plaques were rarely observed. The interobserver agreement for plaque surface characterization was good for both compound ultrasound (κ=0.72) and conventional B-mode (κ=0.65). For the determination of plaque echogenicity, the reproducibility of compound ultrasound (κ_w=0.83) was even higher than that of conventional B-mode ultrasound (κ_w=0.74). According to a semiquantitative analysis, real-time compound ultrasound was rated superior in the categories plaque texture resolution, plaque surface definition, and vessel wall demarcation. Furthermore, there was a significant reduction of acoustic shadowing and reverberations.

Conclusions.—Real-time compound ultrasound is a suitable technique for the characterization of atherosclerotic plaques, showing good general agreement with high-resolution B-mode imaging. This advanced technique allows reduction of ultrasound artifacts and improves the assessment of plaque texture and surface for enhanced evaluation of carotid plaque morphology.

▶ One of many examples in medicine of technology in search of an application. US characterization of plaques continues to generate great interest. So far, however, it has been of little practical value. Reliable criteria for identifying dangerous plaques have yet to be developed. Compounding US images result in a reduction of US artifact and "speckling" by averaging images from different perspectives. Image quality is improved but is unlikely to provide sufficiently increased information to identify the asymptomatic plaque that will eventually result in a neurologic deficit. In my opinion, identification of the truly dangerous plaque with sufficient predictive value to be clinically useful is going to require quantitative assessment of plaque histologic or biochemical features.

G. L. Moneta, MD

Measurement of Carotid Plaque Volume by 3-Dimensional Ultrasound

Landry A, Spence JD, Fenster A (Robarts Research Inst, London, Ont, Canada)
Stroke 35:864-869, 2004 2–7

Background and Purpose.—Measurement of carotid plaque volume and its progression are important tools for research and patient management. In this study, we investigate the observer variability in the measurement of plaque volume as determined by 3-dimensional (3D) ultrasound (US). We also investigate the effect of interslice distances (ISD) and repeated 3D US scans on measurement variability.

Materials and Methods.—Forty 3D US patient images of plaques (range, 37.43 to 604.1 mm^3) were measured by manual planimetry. We applied ANOVA to determine plaque volume measurement variability and reliability. Plaque volumes were measured with 9 ISDs to determine the effect of ISD on measurement variability. Additional plaque volumes were also measured from multiple 3D US scans to investigate repeated scan acquisition variability.

Results.—Intraobserver and interobserver measurement reliabilities were 94% and 93.2%, respectively. Plaque volume measurement variability decreased with increasing plaque volume (range, 27.1% to 2.2%). Measurement precision was constant for ISDs between 1.0 and 3.0 mm, whereas plaque volume measurement variability increased with ISD. Repeated 3D US scan measurements were not different from single-scan measurements ($P=0.867$).

Conclusions.—The coefficient of variation in the measurement of plaque volume decreased with plaque size. The volumetric change that must be observed to establish with 95% confidence that a plaque has undergone change is ≈20% to 35% for plaques <100 mm^3 and ≈10% to 20% for plaques >100 mm^3. Measurement precision was unchanged for ISDs <3.0 mm, whereas measurement variability increased with ISD. Repeated 3D US scans did not affect plaque volume measurement variability.

► Another example of technology in search of an application (see previous article [Abstract 2–6]). Measurement of plaque volume, however, may be a useful application. Potentially, intimal medial thickness can be used to follow minimal carotid disease and plaque response to experimental pharmacologic therapies. Intimal medial thickness is not as useful for larger plaques of more immediate clinical interest. 3D US measurement of plaque volume may eventually be sufficiently accurate and reproducible to assess subtle effects of pharmacologic therapy on plaques of sufficient size to be clinically important.

G. L. Moneta, MD

Vertebral Artery Occlusion in Duplex Color-Coded Ultrasonography

Saito K, Kimura K, Nagatsuka K, et al (Natl Cardiovascular Ctr, Japan; Nara Med Univ, Japan)

Stroke 35:1068-1072, 2004 2–8

Background and Purpose.—To establish the diagnostic criteria for the site of occlusion in the vertebral arteries (VAs) using duplex color-coded ultrasonography.

Methods.—In 128 consecutive patients who underwent conventional cerebral angiography, we prospectively measured the diameter, mean flow velocity (MV), peak systolic flow velocity, and end-diastolic flow velocity of both VAs. The diameter-ratio (diameter of contralateral VA divided by that of target VA) and MV-ratio (MV of contralateral VA divided by that of target VA) were determined. Based on the angiographic findings, we classified the VAs into 4 types (5 groups) as follows: (1) the origin of VA occlusion (Origin group: n=9); (2) VA occlusion before branching into the posterior inferior cerebellar artery (PICA) (Before group: n=10); (3A) symptomatic VA occlusion after branching into the PICA (After group: n=12); (3B) asymptomatic or hypoplastic occlusive VA after branching into the PICA (PICA end group: n=15); and (4) no significant occlusive lesions in the VA (Control group: n=194).

Results.—No flow signals in the VAs apparently indicated the Origin group. Preserved peak systolic flow velocity but end-diastolic flow velocity of zero cm/s indicated the Before group. MV <18 cm/s and MV-ratio ≥1.4 indicated the PICA end group or After group. Furthermore, these groups could be distinguished as follows: a diameter-ratio <1.4 indicated the After group. A diameter-ratio ≥1.4 indicated the PICA end group. Either MV ≥18 cm/s or MV <18 cm/s in combination with MV-ratio <1.4 indicated the Control group.

Conclusions.—Duplex color-coded ultrasonography can accurately diagnose the site of VA occlusion.

▶ This is an excellent systematic analysis of VA duplex findings with respect to angiography. The data may allow differentiation of resistive VA waveforms (those with flow to 0 in diastole or very low peak systolic velocities) with respect to the specific site of upstream stenosis or occlusion. The days of interpreting VA waveforms as only antegrade or retrograde will likely disappear over the next few years.

G. L. Moneta, MD

The Role of Color Duplex Sonography in the Diagnosis of Giant Cell Arteritis

Romera-Villegas A, Vila-Coll R, Poca-Dias V, et al (Hosp Universitari de Bellvitge, Barcelona)

J Ultrasound Med 23:1493-1498, 2004 2–9

Objective.—To determine the clinical usefulness of color duplex sonography in the diagnosis of giant cell arteritis as an alternative to temporal artery biopsy.

Methods.—From May 1998 to November 2002, 68 consecutive patients seen in our hospital with a clinical suggestion of active temporal arteritis were included. Forty-eight patients were female and 20 were male, with a mean age of 77 years. Color duplex sonography with a linear array transducer (5-10 MHz) was used to assess temporal artery morphologic characteristics before a biopsy was performed. The main sonographic criterion for a positive diagnosis was visualization of a hypoechoic halo around the temporal artery. These data were compared with pathologic findings. The κ statistic was used to determine the level of agreement. Sensitivity, specificity, positive and negative predictive values, and accuracy of duplex sonography as a diagnostic test were assessed.

Results.—The color duplex sonographic findings were positive in 25 of 68 patients with a clinical suggestion of giant cell arteritis. The diagnosis was confirmed by biopsy in 22 patients; there were 4 false-positive results and 1 false-negative result by duplex sonography. The κ value was 0.84. Sensitivity, specificity, positive and negative predictive values, and accuracy for duplex sonography were 95.4%, 91.3%, 84%, 97.6%, and 92.6%, respectively.

Conclusions.—The use of high-resolution color duplex sonography may replace biopsy in the diagnosis of giant cell arteritis.

▶ It must be remembered that the American College of Rheumatology diagnostic criteria for temporal arteritis allow the diagnosis of temporal arteritis to be based on the clinical picture alone. Temporal artery biopsy is not required.[1] Since temporal arteritis can be diagnosed on clinical features alone, the current study suggests that duplex sonography can substitute for temporal artery biopsy to confirm the clinical diagnosis of temporal arteritis. Additional studies will be required before duplex can be accepted as an alternative to biopsy that will permit withholding treatment in patients with possible temporal arteritis.

G. L. Moneta, MD

Reference

1. Hunder GG, Bloch DA, Beat AM: The American College of Rheumatology 1990 criteria for the classification of giant cell arteritis. *Arthritis Rheum* 33:1122-1228, 1990.

Measuring Carotid Stenosis on Contrast-Enhanced Magnetic Resonance Angiography: Diagnostic Performance and Reproducibility of 3 Different Methods

U-King-Im JMKS, Trivedi RA, Cross JJ, et al (Addenbrooke's Hosp, Cambridge, England)

Stroke 35:2083-2088, 2004 2–10

Background and Purpose.—The aim of this study was to compare diagnostic performance and reproducibility of 3 different methods of quantifying stenosis on contrast-enhanced magnetic resonance angiography (CEMRA), with intra-arterial digital subtraction angiography (DSA) as the reference standard.

Methods.—167 symptomatic patients scheduled for DSA, after screening Doppler ultrasound, were prospectively recruited to undergo CEMRA. Severity of stenosis was measured according to the North American Symptomatic Trial Collaborators (NASCET), European Carotid Surgery Trial (ECST), and the common carotid (CC) methods. Measurements for each method were made for 284 vessels (142 included patients) on both CEMRA and DSA in a blinded and randomized manner by 3 independent attending neuroradiologists.

Results.—Significant differences in prevalence of severe stenosis were seen with the 3 methods on both DSA and CEMRA, with ECST yielding the least and NASCET the most cases of severe stenosis. Overall, all 3 methods performed similarly well in terms of intermodality correlation and agreement. No significant differences in interobserver agreement were found on either modality. With CEMRA, however, we found a significantly lower sensitivity for detection of severe stenosis with ECST (79.8%) compared with NASCET (93.0%), with DSA as reference standard.

Conclusions.—Uniformity of carotid stenosis measurement methods is desirable because patient management may otherwise differ substantially. All 3 methods are adequate for use with DSA. With CEMRA, however, this study supports use of the NASCET method because of improved sensitivity for detecting severe stenosis.

▶ The NASCET method should be used for comparing noninvasive methods of assessing internal carotid artery stenosis to angiography. It is the most clinically relevant comparison and, apparently, the most sensitive for MR angiographic assessment of high-grade internal carotid artery stenosis.

G. L. Moneta, MD

Determination of Carotid Artery Atherosclerotic Lesion Type and Distribution in Hypercholesterolemic Patients With Moderate Carotid Stenosis Using Noninvasive Magnetic Resonance Imaging

Chu B, Hatsukami TS, Polissar NL, et al (Univ of Washington, Seattle; Mountain-Whisper-Light Statistical Consulting, Seattle; Univ of Utah, Salt Lake City; et al)

Stroke 35:2444-2448, 2004 2–11

Purpose.—The aims of this study were to noninvasively determine carotid atherosclerotic lesion type and distribution and to evaluate the reproducibility of determining lesion types in asymptomatic patients with moderate hypercholesterolemia and moderate carotid artery (CA) stenosis using MRI.

Methods.—Forty-two asymptomatic patients with moderate CA stenosis underwent bilateral carotid MRI in a 1.5-T scanner using a protocol that generated 4 contrast weightings (T1, T2, proton density, and 3D time of flight). MRI-modified American Heart Association criteria were used to evaluate lesion types at 3 locations (common and internal CA [CCA and ICA, respectively] and CA bifurcation) and at the minimum lumen area. Two identical MR scans were conducted to evaluate reproducibility of lesion types.

Results.—Lesion types were obtained from 230 locations. Type III (39%) occurred most commonly, followed by types IV-V (25%), I-II (20%), VI (12%), and VII (4%). Type III was more commonly distributed in the CCA (n=35, 39%) and ICA (n=32, 36%). Type IV-V was more commonly distributed in the CCA (n=24, 41%) and at the bifurcation (n=21, 36%). Forty-two lesions were available at the site of minimum lumen area: type III (33%), IV-V (33%), VI (29%), and VII (5%). There was good agreement of lesion types between both MRI scans (Cohen's κ=0.73; 95% CI: 0.65 to 0.81).

Conclusions.—MRI can determine lesion types reproducibly as well as the distribution of lesions in hypercholesterolemic patients with moderate CA stenosis. A wide range of lesion types, including advanced lesions, were found in these patients.

► Attempts to characterize atherosclerotic plaque composition and morphology are not limited to US (see Abstract 3–6). This study and many before it show that MRI techniques also provide reproducible information about plaque composition. However, I think it is unlikely that MR assessment of plaque composition will be used clinically in the intermediate future. It is likely to remain primarily a research tool at a limited number of centers. I disagree with the authors that "operator dependence" of US limits its potential utility in the study of plaque composition. They should take the time to actually read the US literature. US imaging has also improved dramatically over the last 5 years, and quantitative, nearly operator-independent methods of plaque assessment are being rapidly developed.

G. L. Moneta, MD

Histological Correlates of Carotid Plaque Surface Morphology on Lumen Contrast Imaging

Lovett JK, Gallagher PJ, Hands LJ, et al (Radcliffe Infirmary, Oxford, England; Southampton Gen Hosp, England; John Radcliffe Hosp, Oxford, England)

Circulation 110:2190-2197, 2004 2–12

Background.—Carotid angiographic plaque surface morphology is a powerful risk factor for stroke and systemic vascular risk. However, the underlying pathology is unclear, and a better understanding is required both to evaluate other forms of carotid imaging and to develop new treatments. Previous studies comparing angiographic plaque surface morphology with pathology have been small and unblinded, and the vast majority assessed only the crude macroscopic appearance of the plaque. We performed the first large study comparing angiographic surface morphology with detailed histology.

Method and Results.—Carotid plaque surface morphology was classified as ulcerated, irregular, or smooth on 128 conventional selective carotid artery angiograms from consecutive patients undergoing endarterectomy for severe symptomatic stenosis. Blinded angiographic assessments were compared with 10 histological features recorded on detailed microscopy of the plaque using reproducible semiquantitative scales. Angiographic ulceration was associated with plaque rupture ($P=0.001$), intraplaque hemorrhage ($P=0.001$), large lipid core ($P=0.005$), less fibrous tissue ($P=0.003$), and increased instability overall ($P=0.001$). For example, angiographically ulcerated plaques were much more likely than smooth plaques to be ruptured (OR=15.4, 95% CI=2.7 to 87.3, $P<0.001$), show a large lipid core (OR=26.7, 95% CI=2.6 to 270, $P<0.001$) or a large hemorrhage (OR=17.0, 95% CI=2.0 to 147, $P=0.02$). The equivalent odds ratios for angiographically irregular versus smooth plaque were 6.3 (1.3 to 31, $P=0.02$), 6.7 (1.5 to 30, $P=0.008$), and 9.2 (1.1 to 77, $P=0.02$), respectively.

Conclusions.—In contrast to previous studies based on macroscopic assessment, we found very strong associations between detailed histology and carotid angiographic plaque surface morphology. Plaque surface morphology on carotid angiography is a highly sensitive marker of plaque instability. Studies of the predictive value of MR- and CT-based lumen contrast plaque surface imaging are required.

► We used to think surface ulceration was a marker of potential plaque virulence because the ulcer could serve as a site for platelet aggregates or thrombus accumulation. This study, however, raises the question that perhaps it is not the presence of the ulcer that increases plaque virulence. The ulcer may reflect the fact the plaque has additional histologic features, such as high lipid content and hemorrhage, that are associated with plaque rupture and neurologic symptoms. The sequence of cart and horse has not been established with respect to plaque ulcers.

G. L. Moneta, MD

Segmental Waveform Analysis in the Diagnosis of Peripheral Arterial Occlusive Diseases

de Morais Filho D, Miranda F Jr, del Carmen Janeiro Peres M, et al (Universidade Estadual de Londrina, Paraná, Brazil; Universidade Federal de São Paulo, Brazil; Jobst Vascular Ctr, Toledo, Ohio)

Ann Vasc Surg 18:714-724, 2004 2–13

Introduction.—The duplex exam is widely used in the diagnosis of peripheral arterial occlusive disease. It presents some drawbacks, however, such as calcified plaques, sequential stenosis, and time-consuming examinations. A type of waveform analysis, referred to in this study as segmental analysis, was conducted to try to find solutions to these problems. Parameters of waveform analysis (peak systolic velocity, acceleration time, pulsatility, and resistance indices) taken at the common femoral and popliteal arteries in 177 arterial segments (aortoiliac and femoropopliteal) were compared to angiography results in a prospective manner. The statistical analysis showed an accuracy rate above 95% for all parameters in defining hemodynamic-significant (stenosis and occlusions) lesions in both segments. Also, a combination of measurements (parallel tests) was used to differentiate between hemodynamic-significant stenosis and occlusions, showing sensitivity and specificity rates between 84.8% and 94.8%. Findings from this study show that the hemodynamics of an arterial segment can be evaluated by segmental waveform analysis. It can also be used as a screening test for peripheral arterial occlusive diseases alone or combined with the standard duplex color exam.

► Segmental waveform analysis has been used for over 30 years to distinguish hemodynamically significant from hemodynamically insignificant lesions in peripheral arteries. The authors also found that peak systolic velocity to pulsatility index ratios and pulsatility to resistive index ratios for the aortoiliac and femoral-popliteal segments, respectively, can also reasonably well distinguish hemodynamically significant stenosis from occlusion. This ability to distinguish stenosis from occlusion is a new attribute for waveform analysis. However, it is not good enough. To screen for application of catheter-based procedures it is also useful, in most cases, to know the length of the stenotic or occlusive lesion.

G. L. Moneta, MD

Speed Rather Than Distance: A Novel Graded Treadmill Test to Assess Claudication

Manfredini F, Conconi F, Malagoni AM, et al (Univ of Ferrara, Italy)

Eur J Vasc Endovasc Surg 28:303-309, 2004 2–14

Objective.—To evaluate a new treadmill test, determining pain threshold speed (PTS) for use in assessment and measuring rehabilitation of patients with intermittent claudication.

Methods and Design.—Twenty-nine patients with claudication were evaluated, and the ankle-brachial index (ABI) was assessed. PTS was determined with a treadmill protocol based on level walking, low starting speed, and progressive increments at a predetermined distance up to the onset of pain. Repeatability and equivalence with a time-based protocol were verified. PTS was compared to pain-free walking distance, 6-minute walking distance, and ABI.

Results.—PTS was measured in all patients (3.6 ± 1.1 km/h). Repeatability and equivalence between established tests were demonstrated. PTS showed a significant correlation with pain-free walking distance ($r = 0.833$; $P = 0.0001$), with 6-minute walking distance ($r = 0.724$; $P = 0.005$), and with ABI in the more ischemic limb ($r = 0.641$; $P = 0.0001$).

Conclusions.—PTS is a reliable parameter that correlates well with other established measures. It is useful for determining the degree of functional handicap and for designing and guiding rehabilitation protocols.

▶ After more than 3 decades of widespread use, we cannot agree on the most reliable testing protocol and measurement parameters to quantify the arterial component of exercised-induced lower extremity pain. Absolute claudication distance, initial claudication distance, ABI decrease, measurement of ischemic "windows," graded testing and maximum walking distance under varying inclines and, now, PTS as a parameter for treadmill testing have all been suggested. With so many variables, it is unlikely any of them are actually all that good. Maybe treadmill testing is not all that good?

G. L. Moneta, MD

Contrast-Enhanced Duplex Scanning of Crural Arteries by Means of Continuous Infusion of Levovist

Coffi SB, Ubbink DT, Zwiers I, et al (Academic Med Ctr, Amsterdam)

J Vasc Surg 39:517-522, 2004 2–15

Objectives.—To estimate the dosage needed for continuous infusion and to investigate whether continuous infusion of the ultrasound contrast-enhancing agent Levovist (SH U 508A) can improve duplex scanning of crural arteries in patients with peripheral arterial obstructive disease (PAOD) eligible for distal bypass graft surgery.

Design, Patients, and Methods.—The study design consisted of two parts. Part 1 investigated the color and spectral Doppler scan enhancement of three different Levovist dosages (200, 300, and 400 mg/mL) in one arterial segment of a patent lumen of a crural artery in seven patients with PAOD. Part 2 investigated the value of the optimum Levovist dosage in the assessment of 10 crural arteries in 10 consecutive patients with PAOD. Angiography was the reference standard.

Results.—Part 1: Levovist significantly enhanced color and spectral Doppler scan as compared with baseline ultrasound scan, but no differences were found between the Levovist dosages. Thus, the lowest Levovist dosage sufficed for application in part 2, because of its infusion volume and prolonged enhancement time. Part 2: The agreement between contrast-enhanced duplex scanning and angiography was moderate (κ = 0.50; 95% confidence interval [CI], 0.03-0.97). Five (50%) of 10 crural arteries that could not adequately be visualized with routine duplex scanning could be visualized with contrast-enhanced duplex scanning.

Conclusion.—Contrast-enhanced duplex scanning by means of continuous infusion of Levovist in patients with PAOD improves the ultrasound scan investigation of crural arteries in case routine duplex scanning is inconclusive and might reduce the need for angiography.

► I have yet to find much utility for use of US contrast agents. They are expensive, and their use is limited by only short periods of enhancement when administered as a bolus infusion. Continuous infusion may increase the period of enhancement, but the overall improvement in data acquisition appears to be inadequate for routine use. If you are on a limited budget, and who isn't, better to invest in training of your technologists than US contrast agents.

G. L. Moneta, MD

Duplex Arteriography Prior to Femoral-Popliteal Reconstruction in Claudicants: A Proposal for a New Shortened Protocol

Ascher E, Markevich N, Schutzer RW, et al (Maimonides Med Ctr, Brooklyn, NY)

Ann Vasc Surg 18:544-551, 2004 2–16

Introduction.—The standard preoperative duplex arteriography (DA) from the aorta to the pedal vessels is time consuming and may be unnecessary in patients presenting with calf claudication alone. The feasibility of a shortened protocol was evaluated. Of 286 femoral-popliteal reconstruction based on DA during the last 4 years, 79 (28%) were primary operations for calf claudication. Eliminating the aortoiliac portion of the test except for the distal external iliac artery and limiting the scanning of the infrapopliteal vessels to one or two arteries in the leg would significantly shorten the exam. To confirm the adequacy of the inflow tract, we relied on the common femoral artery Doppler waveform analysis and the intraoperative graft pressure upon completion of the bypass. Of the 79 primary femoral-popliteal bypasses, 53 (67%) had triphasic common femoral artery waveform and the remaining 26 had monophasic or biphasic waveforms. Three (6%) of the 53 femoral-popliteal bypasses in the former group had significant pressure gradients measured intraoperatively and were treated with iliac angioplasties and stents for unsuspected stenoses in 2 cases and a covered stent for a common iliac aneurysm in 1 case. Three, two, and one infrapopliteal vessel runoff was observed in 24 (45%), 16 (30%), and 9 (17%) extremities, respectively. Four patients (8%) had significant stenoses (>50%) or occlusion of all three infrapopliteal arteries. Eighty-one percent of the patients would have completed the short protocol had we scanned the peroneal artery initially.

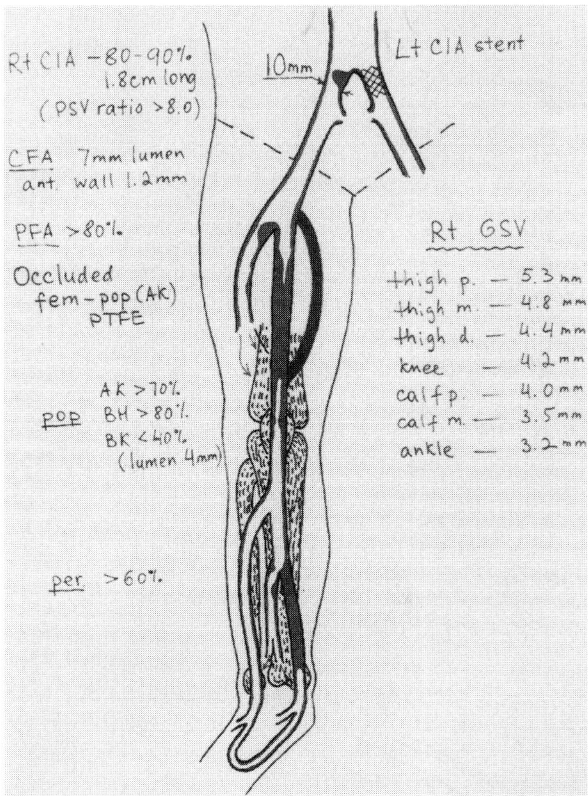

FIGURE 1.—Diagram depicting color-coded arterial mapping from the aorta to the pedal vessels. (Courtesy of Ascher E, Markevich N, Schutzer RW, et al: Duplex arteriography prior to femoral-popliteal reconstruction in claudicants: A proposal for a new shortened protocol. *Ann Vasc Surg* 18[5]:544-551, 2004.)

An additional 8% would have required scanning of a second vessel (anterior tibial) and only 11%, scanning of all three infrapopliteal vessels. The time interval for completion of short-protocol DA was significantly less than the time for the standard DA (16.2 ± 5.2 min vs. 35.1 ± 10.6 min) ($p < 0.01$). We believe that the proposed short DA protocol combined with intraoperative graft pressure measurements can be used in 94% of the patients who have a patent popliteal artery (≥7 cm). It is a totally noninvasive approach that is particularly suitable for vascular technologists and surgeons who wish to start utilizing DA instead of contrast arteriography prior to infrainguinal reconstructions. However, the short protocol does not avert the need for completion arteriography of the inflow arteries and readiness to perform endovascular procedures to correct lesions not suspected by common femoral artery waveform analysis (Fig 1).

▶ We also, but only on occasion, perform infrainguinal arterial reconstructions based only on duplex scanning using a protocol very similar to that described. However, I am not sure about the overall gain described in this article.

Everyone appears to get an angiogram anyway, and there are some nasty surprises, which I hate in the operating room, regarding unexpected inflow and outflow lesions. In addition, you need to have a very good imaging person available at all times. I suppose if you don't have access to the angio suite in your hospital, this approach does have the advantage of shifting revenue from the radiologist to the surgeon.

G. L. Moneta, MD

Infrarenal Aortic and Lower-Extremity Arterial Disease: Diagnostic Performance of Multi–Detector Row CT Angiography

Catalano C, Fraioli F, Laghi A, et al (Univ of Rome)

Radiology 231:555-563, 2004 2–17

Purpose.—To compare multi–detector row spiral computed tomographic (CT) angiography with digital subtraction angiography (DSA) in evaluation of the infrarenal aorta and lower-extremity arterial system.

Materials and Methods.—Fifty patients with peripheral arterial occlusive disease were evaluated with multi–detector row CT angiography and DSA. Arteries depicted at CT angiography and DSA were graded separately for degree of stenosis as 23 anatomic segments (infrarenal aorta, right and left common iliac artery, internal iliac artery, external iliac artery, common femoral artery, superficial femoral artery, deep femoral artery, popliteal artery, anterior tibial artery, tibioperoneal trunk, posterior tibial artery, and peroneal artery). Grades included the following: 1, normal patency; 2, moderate (≤50%) stenosis; 3, focal severe (>50%) stenosis; 4, multiple severe stenoses; and 5, occlusion. Three readers independently interpreted the images, and statistical analysis was performed. The results of image interpretation were evaluated for strength of agreement by using Cohen κ statistics. On the basis of consensus readings, sensitivity, specificity, and accuracy for detection of stenotic lesions were calculated, with findings at DSA used as the reference standard.

Results.—Substantial to almost perfect interobserver agreement was achieved in all cases. At DSA, 349 diseased segments were found among the 1,137 segments evaluated (Fig 4). Sensitivity, specificity, and accuracy, based on a consensus reading of multi–detector row CT angiograms, were 96%, 93%, and 94%, respectively. A statistically significant difference ($P < .05$) between DSA and multi–detector row CT angiography was present only in arteries graded 1 or 2. Interobserver agreement was almost perfect among the three readers for treatment recommendations based on findings at CT angiography and DSA.

Conclusion.—Multi–detector row CT angiography appears consistent and accurate in the assessment of patients with peripheral arterial occlusive disease.

► CT angiography obtained with multi-detector scanners promises to be better than traditional CT angiography; although I doubt it will be applicable to all

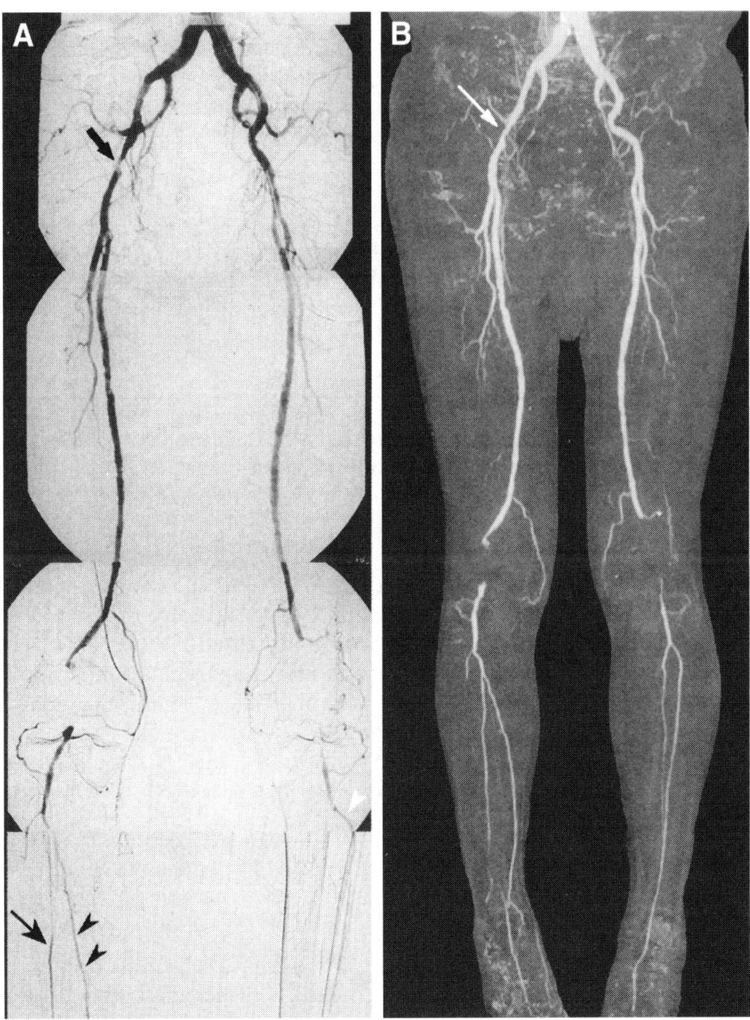

FIGURE 4.—Rutherford and Becker grade II (category 3) disease in a 48-year-old man. (**a**) Composite digital subtraction angiography (DSA) image obtained with multiple injections of contrast agent depicts a focal severe (>50%) stenosis in the proximal right common femoral artery (*thick arrow*) and bilateral occlusion of the popliteal artery. In the right calf, the patency of the peroneal (*thin arrow*) and posterior tibial (*black arrowheads*) arteries is evident; in the left calf, although arterial enhancement is poor, the patency of the anterior tibial artery (*white arrowhead*) is demonstrated. (**b**) Coronal MIP image from multi–detector row CT angiography with bone segmentation correlates well with the DSA image and depicts the right femoral stenosis (*arrow*) and bilateral popliteal occlusion with excellent distal enhancement. (Courtesy of Catalano C, Fraioli F, Laghi A, et al: Infrarenal aortic and lower-extremity arterial disease: Diagnostic performance of multi–detector row CT angiography. *Radiology* 231:555-563, 2004. Copyright 2004, Radiological Society of North America.)

patients requiring arterial reconstruction. Patients with significant calcification of distal arteries where calcium can be confused with contrast, and those with renal insufficiency are obvious examples. In addition, while the radiologists agreed about treatment decisions based on the CT angiograms, I find those data unconvincing. Treatment decisions were simplistic and based only on image interpretation without consideration of available vein, patient condition, or patient functional status. In addition, only patients without previous arterial intervention were subjects for this study. These are increasingly rare patients in many practices.

G. L. Moneta, MD

Whole-Body 3D MR Angiography of Patients With Peripheral Arterial Occlusive Disease

Herborn CU, Goyen M, Quick HH, et al (Univ Hosp Essen, Germany; Catholic Hosps Essen-Nord, Germany)

AJR 182:1427-1434, 2004 2–18

Objective.—We assessed the diagnostic performance of whole-body 3D contrast-enhanced MR angiography in comparison with digital subtraction angiography (DSA) of the lower extremities in patients with peripheral arterial occlusive disease.

Subjects and Methods.—Fifty-one patients with clinically documented peripheral arterial occlusive disease referred for DSA of the lower extremity arterial system underwent whole-body MR angiography on a 1.5-T MR scanner. Paramagnetic gadobutrol was administered and five contiguous stations were acquired with 3D T1-weighted gradient-echo sequences in a total scanning time of 72 sec. DSA was available as a reference standard for the peripheral vasculature in all patients. Separate blinded data analyses were performed by two radiologists. Additional vascular disease detected by whole-body MR angiography was subsequently assessed on sonography, dedicated MR angiography, or both.

Results.—All whole-body MR angiography examinations were feasible and well tolerated. AngioSURF-based whole-body MR angiography had overall sensitivities of 92.3% and 93.1% (both 95% confidence intervals [CIs], 78-100%) with specificities of 89.2% and 87.6% (both CIs, 84-98%) and excellent interobserver agreement ($\kappa = 0.82$) for the detection of high-grade stenoses. Additional vascular disease was detected in 12 patients (23%) (Fig 2).

Conclusion.—Whole-body MR angiography permits a rapid, noninvasive, and accurate evaluation of the lower peripheral arterial system in patients with peripheral arterial occlusive disease, and it may allow identification of additional relevant vascular disease that was previously undetected.

► This is the radiology equivalent of the cardiology "drive-by" carotid and renal arteriogram.

G. L. Moneta, MD

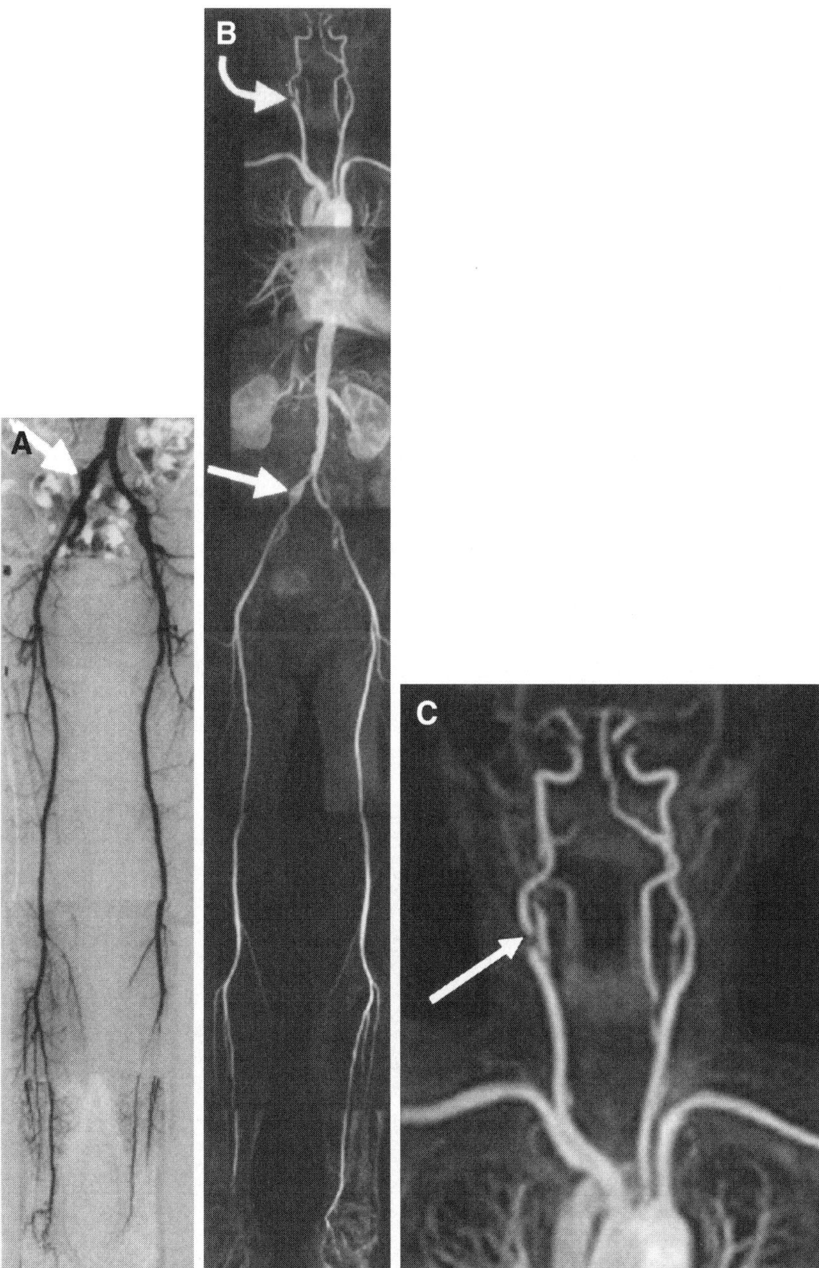

FIGURE 2.—68-year-old woman with history of peripheral vascular disease and pain-free walking distance of more than 200 m. **A,** Intra-arterial digital subtraction angiogram shows sacciform aneurysm (*arrow*) of right common iliac artery. **B,** Coronal maximum intensity projection of 3D whole-body MR angiogram using moving table shows aneurysm of right common iliac artery (*straight arrow*) and additional high-grade stenosis of right internal carotid artery (*curved arrow*). **C,** Magnification of coronal maximum intensity projection of 3D whole-body MR angiogram shows lesion of right internal carotid artery (*arrow*). Stenosis was initially unsuspected and verified on duplex sonography (not shown). (Courtesy of Herborn CU, Goyen M, Quick HH, et al: Whole-body 3D MR angiography of patients with peripheral arterial occlusive disease. *AJR* 182:1427-1434, 2004. Reprinted with permission from the *American Journal of Roentgenology.*)

Abdominal Aortic Aneurysm: Contrast-Enhanced US for Missed Endoleaks After Endoluminal Repair

Napoli V, Bargellini I, Sardella SG, et al (Univ of Pisa, Italy)

Radiology 233:217-225, 2004 2–19

Purpose.—To evaluate contrast material-enhanced ultrasonography (US) for depiction of endoleaks after endovascular abdominal aortic aneurysm repair (or endovascular aneurysm repair [EVAR]) in patients with aneurysm enlargement and no evidence of endoleak.

Materials and Methods.—From November 1998 to February 2003, 112 patients underwent EVAR. At follow-up, duplex US and biphasic multi–detector row computed tomographic (CT) angiography were performed. In 10 patients (group A), evident aneurysm enlargement was observed, with no evidence of complications, at both CT angiography and duplex US. Group A patients, 10 men (mean age, 69.6 years ± 10 [standard deviation]), underwent US after intravenous bolus injection of a second-generation contrast agent, with continuous low-mechanical index (0.01-0.04) real-time tissue harmonic imaging. Group B patients, 10 men (mean age, 71.3 years ± 8.2) with aneurysm shrinkage and no evidence of complications, and group C patients, 10 men (mean age, 73.2 years ± 6) with CT angiographic evidence of endoleak, underwent contrast-enhanced US. Digital subtraction angiography (DSA) was performed in groups A and C. Endoleak detection and characterization were assessed with imaging modalities used in groups A–C; at

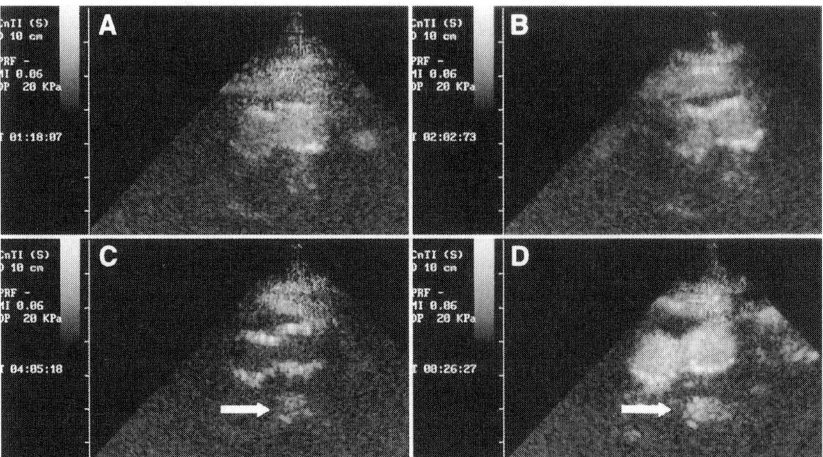

FIGURE 1.—Transverse contrast-enhanced US scans obtained with anterior approach in patient 6 with enlarging abdominal aortic aneurysm. Endoleak or other complications were not visualized at duplex US and CT angiography. **A-C,** Images obtained after administration of an initial bolus of 2.4 mL of second-generation contrast agent show enhancement and slight contrast agent uptake 4 minutes after contrast agent administration. **A,** Image obtained in arterial phase. **B,** Image obtained in venous phase. **C,** Image shows contrast agent uptake posterior to iliac branches (*arrow*). **D,** Image obtained after administration of second bolus of 2.4 mL of contrast agent better depicts endoleak (*arrow*). (Courtesy of Napoli V, Bargellini I, Sardella SG, et al: Abdominal aortic aneurysm: Contrast-enhanced US for missed endoleaks after endoluminal repair. *Radiology* 233:217-225, 2004. Copyright 2004, Radiological Society of North America.)

contrast-enhanced US, time of detection of endoleak, persistence of sac enhancement, and morphology of enhancement were evaluated.

Results.—In group A, contrast-enhanced US depicted one type I, six type II, one type III, and two undefined endoleaks that were not detected at CT angiography. All leakages were characterized by slow and delayed echo enhancement detected at longer than 150 seconds after contrast agent administration (Fig 1). DSA results confirmed findings in all patients; percutaneous treatment was performed. In group B, contrast-enhanced US did not show echo enhancement; in group C, results with this modality confirmed findings at CT angiography and DSA.

Conclusion.—Contrast-enhanced US depicts endoleaks after EVAR, particularly when depiction fails with other imaging modalities.

▶ The article addresses the problem of why some patients after EVAR have expansion of their abdominal aortic aneurysms without detectable endoleak. Turns out, some actually have an endoleak that may be detected by use of contrast-enhanced duplex techniques. I still would not omit follow-up CT, but if the CT shows an increase in aneurysm sac diameter and no endoleak is detected, then a contrast-enhanced US may demonstrate that leak. The situation is more complicated if the patient has one of the old Gore exluder grafts where abdominal aortic aneurysm expansion may occur without endoleak secondary to perigraft seroma.

G. L. Moneta, MD

Is Ultrasound More Accurate Than Axial Computed Tomography for Determination of Maximal Abdominal Aortic Aneurysm Diameter?

Sprouse LR II, Meier GH III, Parent FN, et al (Eastern Virginia Med School, Norfolk)

Eur J Vasc Endovasc Surg 28:28-35, 2004 2–20

Objective(s).—Clinical assessment of maximal abdominal aortic aneurysm (AAA) diameter assumes clinical equivalency between ultrasound (US) and axial computed tomography (CT). Three-dimensional (3D) CT reconstruction allows for the assessment of AAA in the orthogonal plane and avoids oblique cuts due to AAA angulation. This study was undertaken to compare maximal AAA diameter by US, axial CT, and orthogonal CT, and to assess the effect that AAA angulation has on each measurement.

Methods.—Maximal AAA diameter by US (US^{max}), axial CT ($axial^{max}$), and orthogonal CT ($orthogonal^{max}$) along with aortic angulation and minor axis diameters were measured prospectively. Spiral CT data was processed by Medical Media Systems (West Lebanon, NH) to produce computerized axial CT and reformatted orthogonal CT images. The US technologists were blinded to all CT results and vice versa.

Results.—Thirty-eight patients were analyzed. Mean $axial^{max}$ (58.0 mm) was significantly larger ($P < 0.05$) than US^{max} (53.9 mm) or $orthogonal^{max}$ (54.7 mm). The difference between US^{max} and $orthogonal^{max}$ (0.8 mm) was insignificant ($P > 0.05$). When aortic angulation was ≤25°, axial^{max} (55.3 mm), US^{max} (54.3 mm), and orthogonal^{max} (54.1 mm) were similar ($P > 0.05$); however, when aortic angulation was >25°, axial^{max} (60.1 mm) was significantly larger ($P < 0.001$) than US^{max} (53.8 mm) and orthogonal^{max} (55.0 mm). The limits of agreement (LOA) between axial^{max} and both US^{max} and orthogonal^{max} were poor and exceeded clinical acceptability (±5 mm). The variation between US^{max} and orthogonal^{max} was minimal with an acceptable LOA of −2.7 to 4.5 mm.

Conclusion.—Compared to axial CT, US is a better approximation of true perpendicular AAA diameter as determined by orthogonal CT. When aortic angulation is greater than 25° axial CT becomes unreliable. However, US measurements are not affected by angulation and agree strongly with orthogonal CT measurements.

► The problem is not that US or CT is inaccurate in measuring AAA diameter. Both are accurate when performed properly with the measurement taken perpendicular to the axis of the aneurysm. This issue, I believe, is rapidly becoming moot as routine spiral CT scanning replaces standard axial-only views.

G. L. Moneta, MD

Diagnosis of Deep Venous Thrombosis and Alternative Diseases in Symptomatic Outpatients

Blättler W, Martinez I, Blättler IK (Ctr for Vascular Diseases, Zürich, Switzerland)

Eur J Intern Med 15:305-311, 2004 2–21

Background.—The management of patients with suspected deep vein thrombosis (DVT) is controversial. Recent studies have suggested that anticoagulant treatment can safely be withheld if the clinical probability is low and the D-dimer concentration in blood is normal. We examined a diagnostic algorithm comparing a score-based, explicit assessment model with our empirical, implicit approach, which was designed to be more sensitive for distal DVT. We further investigated what information would be lost by not performing a routine ultrasound examination in each patient.

Methods.—Consecutive patients with suspected DVT first received a D-dimer estimation, then an examination to assess the clinical probability, and ultimately objective testing for DVT or alternative diseases. Ultrasound was used in all patients; venography and other tests were performed as indicated. The implicit assessment of clinical probability was compared with the explicit scoring system of Wells et al, and the value of ultrasound was assessed retrospectively.

Results.—In 57 of 206 patients (28%), DVT was confirmed. A high clinical probability was attributed to all pelvic and femoral DVT (except one), but popliteal and crural DVT were missed in 78% by the explicit approach and in 34% by the implicit approach. The negative predictive values for any DVT were 83% for the explicit assessment and 92% for the implicit assess-

TABLE 3.—Preultrasound Probability of Isolated Crural DVT

Implicit Clinical Probability + SimpliRED Test	Isolated DVT Present	Absent
Low + negative	1	82
Not low + negative	18	67

N = 168 (149 patients without DVT, 19 with isolated calf DVT).
Sensitivity = 95% (95% CI 75-99).
Negative predictive value = 99% (95% CI 93-100).
Abbreviations: DVT, Deep vein thrombosis; *CI*, confidence interval.
(Courtesy of Blättler W, Martinez I, Blättler IK: Diagnosis of deep venous thrombosis and alternative diseases in symptomatic outpatients. *Eur J Intern Med* 15:305-311, 2004.)

ment, 95% for the D-dimer estimation, and 98% (95% CI 92-99) for the combination of low implicit clinical probability and a negative D-dimer test. This combination yielded the same NPV for isolated crural DVT and was found in 41% of all suspected cases. An alternative organic diagnosis was established in 100 patients (48%) and no organic diagnosis was made in 49 (24%). In half of all suspected cases, irrespective of whether DVT was present or not, concomitant or alternative venous pathologies were observed. Ultrasound was found useful in 91% of cases.

Conclusions.—Proximal as well as distal DVT can reliably be excluded when both a sensitive assessment of clinical probability and a bedside D-dimer assay are negative. Nevertheless, ultrasound is helpful in establishing alternative diagnoses. Strategies to reduce the number of ultrasound investigations appear to lack comprehensiveness (Tables 3 and 6).

▶ When a patient comes to the doctor with a complaint of leg pain, it is important to tell the patient what is wrong. A negative D-dimer may exclude DVT, but it doesn't tell you what is causing the leg pain. The negative D-dimer at 2 AM may save a 2 AM US examination, but it does not release the physician of the responsibility of determining the etiology of the lower extremity pain. This

TABLE 6.—Relative Prevalence of Concomitant Venous Diseases and Malignancies in Patients With Cruro-Popliteal Versus Proximal DVT

	Number of Patients	Concomitant Venous Diseases	Malignancy or Severe Systemic Diseases
Cruro-popliteal DVT	32	19 (59%)	0
Proximal DVT	25	7 (28%)	8 (32%)

Two-sided $\chi^2 = 13.25$; Fisher's exact test, $P < .001$.
Abbreviation: DVT, Deep vein thrombosis.
(Courtesy of Blättler W, Martinez I, Blättler IK: Diagnosis of deep venous thrombosis and alternative diseases in symptomatic outpatients. *Eur J Intern Med* 15:305-311, 2004.)

study suggests that in spite of negative D-dimer studies, US will still be useful in helping answer the etiology of the patient's complaints.

G. L. Moneta, MD

The Effect of Helical Computed Tomography on Diagnostic and Treatment Strategies in Patients With Suspected Pulmonary Embolism

Trowbridge RL, Araoz PA, Gotway MB, et al (Univ of California, San Francisco)
Am J Med 116:84-90, 2004 2–22

Background.—Helical computed tomography (CT) has been proposed as a first-line test for the diagnosis of pulmonary embolism. How the test affects the diagnostic evaluation of patients with suspected pulmonary embolism is unknown.

Methods.—We examined a cohort of 360 patients evaluated for pulmonary embolism at a teaching hospital in the 4 years following the introduction of the helical CT scan. We collected patient demographic and clinical data to calculate the pretest likelihood of pulmonary embolism; we then read the test results and determined rates of further testing and treatment for pulmonary embolism.

Results.—After the helical CT scan became available, the number of patients referred for pulmonary embolism testing increased markedly from 170 to 624 total evaluations during 1997 to 2000 ($P < 0.01$). This rise was due to increased use of the helical CT scan (9% to 83% of evaluations, $P < 0.01$) as the use of ventilation-perfusion scanning (79% to 17%, $P = 0.03$)

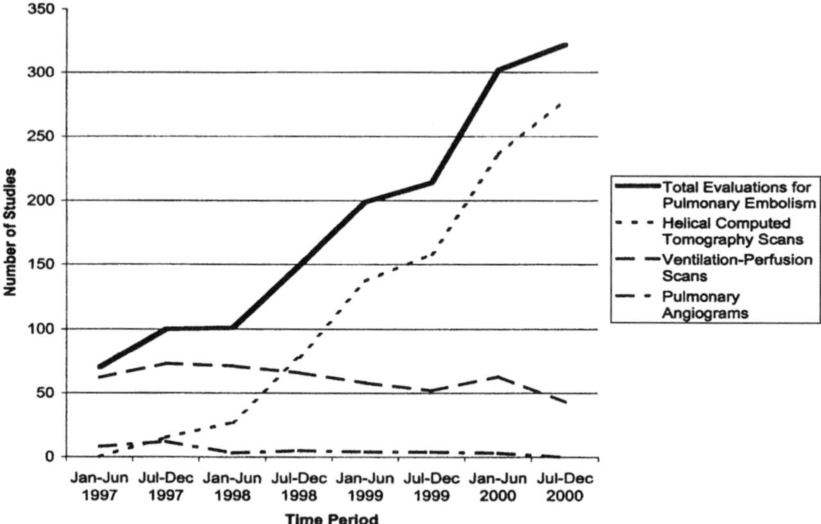

FIGURE.—Trends in testing for pulmonary embolism, 1997 to 2000. (Courtesy of Trowbridge RL, Araoz PA, Gotway MB, et al: The effect of helical computed tomography on diagnostic and treatment strategies in patients with suspected pulmonary embolism. *Am J Med* 116:84-90, 2004. Copyright 2004, with permission from Excerpta Medica Inc.)

and pulmonary angiography (12% to <1%, $P < 0.01$) fell (Figure). There was no change in the pre-test likelihood of disease over time, but the percentage of scans that were positive for pulmonary embolism rose (14% to 32%, $P = 0.02$). Clinicians treated all patients who had a positive CT scan, but became less likely over time to order further testing for patients who had a negative scan (30% to 12%, $P = 0.02$).

Conclusion.—At this academic medical center, introduction of the helical CT scan had a profound effect on the evaluation of pulmonary embolism, resulting in more frequent use of the CT scan, and more frequent diagnosis and treatment of pulmonary embolism, despite no change in the pretest probability of disease. Future studies should confirm our findings and determine whether increased detection of pulmonary emboli results in improved outcomes.

▶ It is almost as easy to get a CT scan as a glass of water. The study shows that when a test is readily available, accurate, and directly answers the clinical question, it will be rapidly accepted. Given that only half of patients with proven pulmonary embolism have deep venous thrombosis detected in the legs, I hope studies such as this are harbingers of the end of "shortness of breath" as an indication for venous duplex scans (see also Abstract 2–23).

G. L. Moneta, MD

Risk of Pulmonary Embolism After Negative MDCT Pulmonary Angiography Findings

Kavanagh EC, O'Hare A, Hargaden G, et al (Mater Misericordiae Hosp, Dublin)
AJR 182:499-504, 2004 2–23

Objective.—The purpose of our study was to determine the risk of pulmonary embolism in patients who have negative MDCT pulmonary angiography findings.

Subjects and Methods.—In this prospective study, one hundred two consecutive patients with suspected pulmonary embolism underwent MDCT pulmonary angiography. Scans were reviewed jointly by two observers and findings recorded by consensus. Observers noted whether pulmonary embolism or other disease was present. No pulmonary embolism was seen in 85 patients (52 men and 33 women; age range, 20-94 years; mean age, 60 years) who were followed up for a mean of 9 months (range, 4-13 months) for evidence of subsequent pulmonary embolism.

Results.—One patient had a diagnosis of pulmonary embolism made within 3 weeks of undergoing CT pulmonary angiography. MDCT pulmonary angiography showed additional potentially significant findings in 76% of patients; 47% of these findings were not suspected on chest radiography.

Conclusion.—The risk of pulmonary embolism at a mean of 9 months after negative MDCT pulmonary angiography findings is 1%. In our study of patients without pulmonary embolism, MDCT pulmonary angiography revealed other causes for individual patients' signs or symptoms in most cases.

► CT pulmonary angiography has already replaced ventilation-perfusion scanning as the noninvasive test of choice for the diagnosis of pulmonary embolism. It has, or has in most cases, also replaced catheter-based pulmonary angiography as well. Ventilation-perfusion scanning and catheter-based pulmonary angiography are rapidly following the path of the whaler and buffalo hunter. They will not be needed and few will miss them.

G. L. Moneta, MD

Lower Extremity Deep Venous Thrombosis: Vascular Laboratory Quality Assurance Without Correlation Between Ultrasound and Venography

Salles-Cunha SX, Ascher E, Hingorani A, et al (Vascular Inst of New York, Brooklyn)

Vasc Endovasc Surg 38:443-447, 2004 2–24

Introduction.—Venography is rarely available for comparison with ultrasonography (US) as a means for quality assurance (QA) in the detection of lower extremity venous thrombosis. New QA methods must be implemented. We compared results of multiple serial studies performed in the same extremity as a QA indicator. From a 3-year sample of close to 9,000 venous tests, we obtained a subset of 44 patients who had 331 tests in 71 lower extremities throughout the years. A positive or negative study preceded or followed by another positive or negative study was considered as a confirmed study. A negative or positive study not preceded or followed by a negative or positive study was considered as unconfirmed. Explanations were then sought to explain unconfirmed results. There were 169 (51%) and 124 (37%) confirmed positive and negative studies, respectively, and 13 (4%) and 25 (8%) unconfirmed positive and negative studies, respectively. Of the 13 unconfirmed positive tests, 2 were preceded by negative tests, 3 were preceded and followed by negative tests, and 8 were followed by negative tests. Of these 13 tests, 4 documented extensive venous thrombosis. Of the 25 unconfirmed negative tests, 11 followed treatment for venous thrombosis, 6 had recurrent thrombosis with intermittent lysis, and 8 were followed by positive tests. Considering the low probability of extensive thrombosis being a false-positive test, positive predictive value was 95% (173/182). Excluding 11 negative tests following treatment for venous thrombosis, negative predictive value was 90% (124/138) and accuracy was 93% (297/320). US versus US and literature US versus venography comparisons of these statistics were similar.

► Validating venous duplex studies via the traditional method of comparison with contrast studies is not possible. The use of serial examinations is one approach to this problem. However, this is basically a retrospective study design. A better approach would be to perform blinded examinations by 2 different technologists on the same day and to prospectively track the data. Another method is to follow patients with negative exams and make sure they do not develop symptoms of venous thromboembolism or have a positive venous duplex study within 30 days of the initial study. Either approach should be acceptable to vascular laboratory accrediting agencies.

G. L. Moneta, MD

Hemodynamic and Clinical Impact of Ultrasound-Derived Venous Reflux Parameters

Neglén P, Eggert JF III, Olivier J, et al (River Oaks Hosp, Flowood, Miss; Univ of Mississippi, Jackson)

J Vasc Surg 40:303-310, 2004 2–25

Purpose.—This study was undertaken to assess which ultrasound-derived parameter was superior for measuring venous reflux quantitatively and to evaluate the importance of popliteal vein valve reflux.

Patients and Methods.—A retrospective analysis was performed of 244 refluxive limbs in 182 patients who underwent ultrasound scanning, venous pressure measurement, air plethysmography, and clinical classification of severity according to the CEAP score. Reflux time (RT, s), peak reflux velocity (PRV, m/s), time of average rate of reflux (TAF, mL/min), absolute displaced volume retrogradely (ADV, mL) were compared to clinical class, ambulatory venous pressure (% drop), venous filling time (s), and venous filling index (mL/s) using nonparametric statistical tests. A *P* value of <.05 was considered significant. Limbs were divided into 3 groups: (A) axial great saphenous vein reflux only (n = 68); (B) axial deep reflux including popliteal vein incompetence with or without concomitant gastrocnemius or great or small saphenous vein reflux (all ultrasound reflux parameters of each refluxive vein added at the knee level) (n = 79); and (C) all limbs with popliteal vein reflux (the ultrasound data of the refluxive popliteal vein exclusively was used in comparison regardless of concomitant associated reflux) (n = 103). Limbs were also stratified into limbs with skin changes and ulcer (C-class 4-6) and those without (C-class 1-3) and subsequently compared.

Results.—No meaningful significant correlation was found between RT and the clinical and hemodynamic results in groups A and B. The PRV and TAF correlated significantly with the hemodynamic parameters. The PRV and TAF and clinical severity trended towards correlation in group A (*P* = .0554 and *P* = .0998, respectively), but was significantly correlated in group B. The poor hemodynamic condition in the subset of C-class 4-6 limbs in groups A and B was reflected in a greater PRV, TAF, and ADV in this subset as compared with the limbs in C-class 1-3. RT was not significantly different in the subsets of limbs, further suggesting that RT is not related to hemodynamic or clinical state of the limbs. No meaningful correlations were found in group C. Although the hemodynamic data were significantly poorer in the subset of limbs with C-class 4-6 than in C-class 1-3, the ultrasound-derived parameters were not significantly different.

Conclusion.—The duration of valve reflux time (or valve closure time) cannot be used to quantify severity of reflux and is purely a qualitative measurement. The PRV and the rate of reflux appeared to better reflect the magnitude of venous incompetence. In the presence of axial reflux, it appeared logical and physiologically correct to sum up these reflux parameters for each venous segment crossing the knee. The popliteal valve reflux (the "gatekeeper" function) was not in itself an important determinant of venous hemodynamics and clinical severity. Additional reflux in other venous segments must be taken into account.

▶ This is a complicated article with complicated results and therefore is not very useful. It reflects the difficulties of trying to correlate noninvasive vascular laboratory testing with the clinical severity of chronic venous insufficiency. This difficulty makes it almost impossible to objectively assess the impact of venous procedures on venous hemodynamics in the individual patient. I am convinced the reliability of venous testing and reproducibility of venous testing for chronic venous insufficiency will also be affected by the severity of the underlying disease, with results in more advanced disease likely to be less reproducible. We have a long way to go to objectively evaluate the hemodynamic results of venous procedures.

G. L. Moneta, MD

Laser Doppler Skin Perfusion Pressure in the Assessment of Raynaud's Phenomenon

Kanetaka T, Komiyama T, Onozuka A, et al (Univ of Tokyo)

Eur J Vasc Endovasc Surg 27:414-416, 2004 2–26

Objectives.—In the assessment of Raynaud's phenomenon, objective evaluation of digital microcirculatory flow is important, and so we investigated whether the measurement of laser Doppler skin perfusion pressure could be of use.

Materials and Methods.—Ten fingers of five patients with secondary Raynaud's phenomenon due to systemic sclerosis, 22 fingers of 11 patients with primary Raynaud's phenomenon and 10 fingers of five control patients were examined. Skin perfusion pressure was measured on the third finger of both hands at rest, and then again 3 min after local cold exposure.

Results.—Laser Doppler skin perfusion pressure at rest in patients with secondary Raynaud's phenomenon was significantly lower than that in patients with primary Raynaud's phenomenon and the control patients ($p < 0.05$). Skin perfusion pressure decreased significantly in both patient groups upon local cold exposure ($p = 0.005$). There were significant differences in perfusion pressure after cold exposure among both groups ($p < 0.05$).

Conclusions.—The low skin perfusion pressure at rest in patients with secondary Raynaud's phenomenon suggested the presence of obstructive arterial lesions. The marked pressure decrease in all Raynaud's patients after local cold exposure might be due to vasospasm of the microvasculature in the digits. These results indicate that the measurement of laser Doppler skin perfusion pressure is valuable in the diagnosis of Raynaud's phenomenon.

▶ The results suggest laser Doppler measurements of skin perfusion pressure may be able to detect and quantify the hypersensitivity of digital vasospasm to cold in patients with Raynaud's syndrome. With the exception of the digital hyperthermic challenge test utilized in selected centers, there are no validated quantitative noninvasive assessments of the severity of Raynaud's syndrome. Perhaps this test will offer quantitative assessment of cold-induced vasospasm; if so, it will be a valuable addition, especially in evaluation of cold-associated workers' compensation claims.

G. L. Moneta, MD

3 Perioperative Considerations

Coronary-Artery Revascularization Before Elective Major Vascular Surgery

McFalls EO, Ward HB, Moritz TE, et al (Univ of Minnesota, Minneapolis; VA Med Ctr, Hines, Ill; Univ of Arizona, Tucson; et al)

N Engl J Med 351:2795-2804, 2004 3–1

Background.—The benefit of coronary-artery revascularization before elective major vascular surgery is unclear.

Methods.—We randomly assigned patients at increased risk for perioperative cardiac complications and clinically significant coronary artery disease to undergo either revascularization or no revascularization before elective major vascular surgery. The primary end point was long-term mortality.

Results.—Of 5859 patients scheduled for vascular operations at 18 Veterans Affairs medical centers, 510 (9 percent) were eligible for the study and were randomly assigned to either coronary-artery revascularization before surgery or no revascularization before surgery. The indications for a vascular operation were an expanding abdominal aortic aneurysm (33 percent) or arterial occlusive disease of the legs (67 percent). Among the patients assigned to preoperative coronary-artery revascularization, percutaneous coronary intervention was performed in 59 percent, and bypass surgery was performed in 41 percent. The median time from randomization to vascular surgery was 54 days in the revascularization group and 18 days in the group not undergoing revascularization ($P<0.001$). At 2.7 years after randomization, mortality in the revascularization group was 22 percent and in the no-revascularization group 23 percent (relative risk, 0.98; 95 percent confidence interval, 0.70 to 1.37; $P=0.92$). Within 30 days after the vascular operation, a postoperative myocardial infarction, defined by elevated troponin levels, occurred in 12 percent of the revascularization group and 14 percent of the no-revascularization group ($P=0.37$).

Conclusions.—Coronary-artery revascularization before elective vascular surgery does not significantly alter the long-term outcome. On the basis of these data, a strategy of coronary-artery revascularization before elective vascular surgery among patients with stable cardiac symptoms cannot be recommended.

▶ This study, as with all studies, must be interpreted with respect to the patients studied and the study conditions. Patients were carefully screened for unstable cardiac disease. Such patients were excluded. In addition, approximately 85% of the patients in the coronary and no coronary revascularization group were treated with perioperative β-blockers, 77% of the patients in the revascularization group were treated with aspirin, and 70% in the no revascularization group were treated with aspirin. The overall results therefore indicate that patients treated with aggressive medical management who are carefully screened for unstable coronary disease will not benefit from coronary revascularization before major vascular surgery. In patients with stable cardiac symptoms, a strategy of coronary artery revascularization cannot be recommended before elective vascular surgery.

G. L. Moneta, MD

Preoperative Cardiac Evaluation Does Not Improve or Predict Perioperative or Late Survival in Asymptomatic Diabetic Patients Undergoing Elective Infrainguinal Arterial Reconstruction

Monahan TS, Shrikhande GV, Pomposelli FB Jr, et al (Beth Israel Deaconess Med Ctr, Boston)

J Vasc Surg 41:38-45, 2005 3–2

Objective.—Patients undergoing infrainguinal arterial reconstruction frequently have increased cardiac risk factors. Diabetic patients are often asymptomatic despite advanced cardiac disease. This study investigates whether preoperative cardiac testing improves the outcome in diabetic patients at risk for cardiac disease.

Methods.—We retrospectively reviewed all patients undergoing lower-extremity arterial reconstructions in a 32-month period from July 1999 to February 2002. Of the 433 patients identified undergoing 539 procedures, 295 had diabetes mellitus and considered in this study. The patients were stratified into two groups according to the present American College of Cardiology, American Heart Association (ACC/AHA) algorithm. We identified 140 patients with two or more of ACC (Eagle) criteria who met the inclusion criteria for a preoperative cardiac evaluation. These patients were separated into two groups: those undergoing a cardiac work-up (WU) according to the ACC/AHA algorithm and those not undergoing the recommended work-up (NWU). Outcomes included perioperative mortality, postoperative myocardial infarction, congestive heart failure, arrhythmia, and length of hospitalization. Significance of association was assessed by the Fisher exact test. Length of hospitalization was compared using the Kruskal-Wallis rank sum test. Survival data was analyzed with the Kaplan-Meier method (Fig 2).

Results.—One hundred forty patients met the criteria for moderate risk. There were 61 patients in the NWU group and 79 in the WU group. Ten pa-

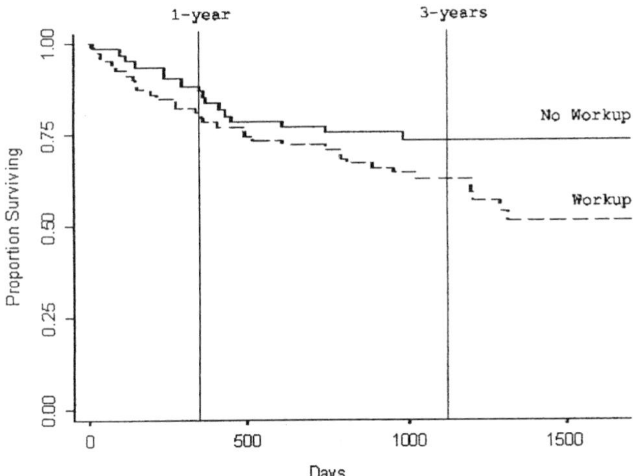

FIGURE 2.—Kaplan-Meier analysis for patients with and without a preoperative cardiac evaluation. The *dashed line* represents the cohort that had a cardiac evaluation, the *solid line* represents the cohort that did not. (Reprinted by permission of the publisher from Monahan TS, Shrikhande GV, Pomposelli FB Jr, et al: Preoperative cardiac evaluation does not improve or predict perioperative or late survival in asymptomatic diabetic patients undergoing elective infrainguinal arterial reconstruction. *J Vasc Surg* 41:38-45, 2005. Copyright 2005 by Elsevier.)

tients in the WU group underwent preoperative coronary revascularization (6 had percutaneous transluminal coronary angioplasty, 4 underwent coronary artery bypass grafting). There was no difference between perioperative mortality (WU, 1%; NWU, 2%; P = 1.00) or in postoperative cardiac morbidity, including myocardial infarction, congestive heart failure, and arrhythmia requiring treatment (WU, 5%; NWU, 6%; P = .71). There were no perioperative deaths and one episode of congestive heart failure in the group that had preoperative coronary revascularization. Median length of hospitalization was 10 days in the WU group and 8 days in the NWU group (P = .11). Patient survival at 12 months for the NWU, WU, and revascularized groups was 85.3%, 78.5%, and 80.0%, respectively; 36-month survival was 73.6%, 62.9%, and 80.0%, respectively. The three survival curves did not differ significantly (P = .209).

Conclusions.—Preoperative cardiac evaluation, as defined by the ACC/AHA algorithm, does not predict or improve postoperative morbidity, mortality, or 36-month survival in asymptomatic, diabetic patients undergoing elective lower-extremity arterial reconstruction. These data do not support the current ACC/AHA recommendations as a standard of care for diabetic patients with an intermediate clinical predictor who undergo peripheral arterial reconstruction, a high-risk surgical procedure.

► Our group has long espoused the view that all patients with peripheral arterial disease should be assumed to have coronary artery disease and treated with β-blockers and antiplatelet agents perioperatively, with close postoperative monitoring and control of blood pressure and heart rate. Only patients with changing cardiac symptoms or a history of severe congestive heart failure or refractory angina are selected for more detailed perioperative cardiac evaluation. The era of routine perioperative cardiac workup for peripheral arterial disease patients hopefully has passed. Such workups are inefficient, expensive, and have positive predictive values that are too low to be useful.

G. L. Moneta, MD

Long-term Survival After Vascular Surgery: Specific Influence of Cardiac Factors and Implications for Preoperative Evaluation

Back MR, Leo F, Cuthbertson D, et al (Univ of South Florida, Tampa)
J Vasc Surg 40:752-760, 2004 3–3

Objective.—We sought to identify specific determinants of long-term cardiac events and survival in patients undergoing major arterial operations after preoperative cardiac risk stratification by American College of Cardiology/American Heart Association guidelines. A secondary goal was to define the potential long-term protective effect of previous coronary revascularization (coronary artery bypass grafting [CABG] or percutaneous coronary intervention [PCI]) in patients with vascular disease.

Methods.—Four hundred fifty-nine patients underwent risk stratification (high, intermediate, low) before 534 consecutive elective or urgent (<24 hours after presentation) open cerebrovascular, aortic, or lower limb reconstruction procedures between August 1996 and January 2000. Long-term follow-up (mean, 56 ± 14 months) was possible in 97% of patients. The Kaplan-Meier method was used for survival data. Long-term prognostic variables were identified with the multivariate Cox proportional hazards

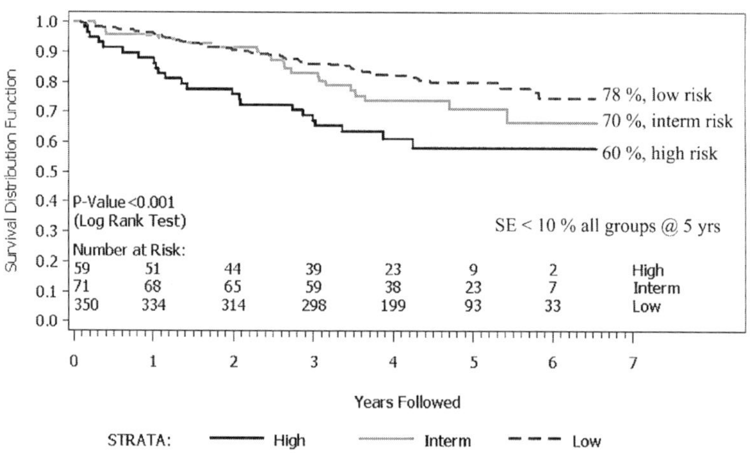

FIGURE 2.—Significant differences in 5-year survival between preoperatively determined cardiac risk stratification levels favoring low risk populations. *SE,* Standard error. (Reprinted by permission of the publisher from Back MR, Leo F, Cuthbertson D, et al: Long-term survival after vascular surgery: Specific influence of cardiac factors and implications for preoperative evaluation. *J Vasc Surg* 40:752-760, 2004. Copyright 2004 by Elsevier.)

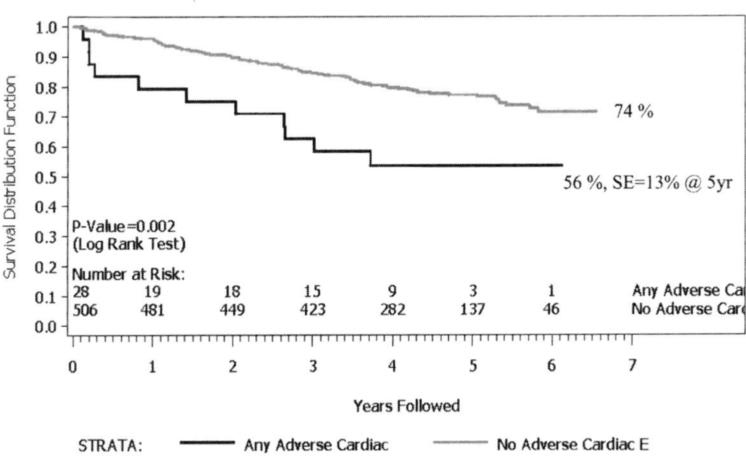

FIGURE 4.—Significantly reduced 5-year survival in patients with early adverse cardiac events (myocardial infarction, congestive heart failure, ventricular arrhythmias) after vascular operations, even with censoring of perioperative deaths. Standard error less than 10% in group without complications. (Reprinted by permission of the publisher from Back MR, Leo F, Cuthbertson D, et al: Long-term survival after vascular surgery: Specific influence of cardiac factors and implications for preoperative evaluation. *J Vasc Surg* 40:752-760, 2004. Copyright 2004 by Elsevier.)

model and contingency table analysis censoring early (<30 days) perioperative deaths.

Results.—While 5-year survival was 72% for the overall cohort, cardiac causes accounted for only 24% of all deaths, and new cardiac events (myocardial infarction, congestive heart failure, arrhythmia, unstable angina, new coronary angiography, new CABG or PCI, cardiac death) affected only 4.6% of patients per year during follow-up (Figs 2 and 4). High cardiac risk stratification level (hazards ratio [HR], 2.2, 95% confidence interval [CI], 1.4-3.4), adverse perioperative cardiac events (myocardial infarction, congestive heart failure, ventricular arrhythmia; HR, 2.2; 95% CI, 1.2-4.1), and age (HR, 0.33; 95% CI, 0.2-0.6) were independently prognostic for late mortality. Preoperative cardiac risk levels also correlated with new cardiac event rates ($P < .01$) and late cardiac mortality ($P = .02$). Modestly improved survival in patients who had undergone CABG or PCI less than 5 years before vascular operations compared with those who had undergone revascularization 5 or more years previously and those at high risk without previous coronary intervention (73% vs 58% vs 62% 5-year survival; $P = .02$) could be demonstrated with univariate testing, but not with multivariate analysis. Type of operation, urgency, noncardiac complications, and presence of diabetes did not affect long-term survival.

Conclusion.—Despite cardiac events being a less common cause of late mortality after vascular surgery, perioperative cardiac factors (age, preoperative risk level, early cardiac complications) are the primary determinants of patient longevity. Patients undergoing more recent (<5 years) CABG or PCI before vascular surgery do not have an obvious survival advantage compared with patients at high cardiac risk without previous coronary interventions.

▶ Past studies have suggested that 40% of late deaths in patients who had undergone abdominal aortic aneurysm or peripheral vascular surgery were from cardiac causes. In the current study, this number is roughly half that (24%). I doubt this implies modern vascular surgical patients have less cardiac disease than those previously studied. I doubt there is something special about the water in Tampa. My guess is the care of patients with cardiac disease has improved over the last 10 to 15 years, and that the decreased late deaths from cardiac causes in patients with peripheral arterial disease merely reflects the decreased death rate from cardiac disease in the population as a whole.

G. L. Moneta, MD

Long-term Prognostic Value of Asymptomatic Cardiac Troponin T Elevations in Patients After Major Vascular Surgery

Kertai MD, Boersma E, Klein J, et al (Erasmus Med Ctr, Rotterdam, The Netherlands)

Eur J Vasc Endovasc Surg 28:59-66, 2004 3–4

Background.—Cardiac troponin T (cTnT) is a sensitive and specific marker for myocardial injury, but elevations of cTnT without clinical evidence of ischemia and persistent or new electrocardiographic (ECG) abnormalities are common in patients undergoing major vascular surgery. We explored the long-term prognostic value of cTnT levels in these patients.

Methods.—A follow-up study was conducted between 1996–2000 in 393 patients who underwent successful aortic or infrainguinal vascular surgery and routine sampling of cTnT. Patients were followed until May 2003 (median of 4 years [25th–75th percentile, 2.8–5.3 years]). Total creatine kinase (CK), CK-MB, and cTnT were routinely screened in all patients, and included sampling after surgery and the mornings of postoperative days 2, 3 and 7. Electrocardiograms were also routinely evaluated for sign of ischemia. An elevated cTnT was defined as serum concentrations $\geq$0.1 ng/ml in any of these samples. All-cause mortality was evaluated during long-term follow-up (Fig 1).

Results.—Eighty patients (20%) had late death. The incidence of all-cause mortality (41% vs. 17%; $p < 0.001$) was significantly higher in patients with an elevated cTnT level compared to patients with normal cTnT. After adjustment for baseline clinical characteristics, the association between an elevated cTnT level and increased incidence of all-cause mortality (adjusted hazard ratio, 1.9; 95% CI, 1.1–3.1) persisted. Elevated cTnT had significant prognostic value in patients with and without renal dysfunction, abnormal levels of CK-MB, and in patients with transient ECG abnormalities.

Conclusions.—Elevated cTnT levels are associated with an increased incidence of all-cause mortality in patients undergoing major vascular surgery.

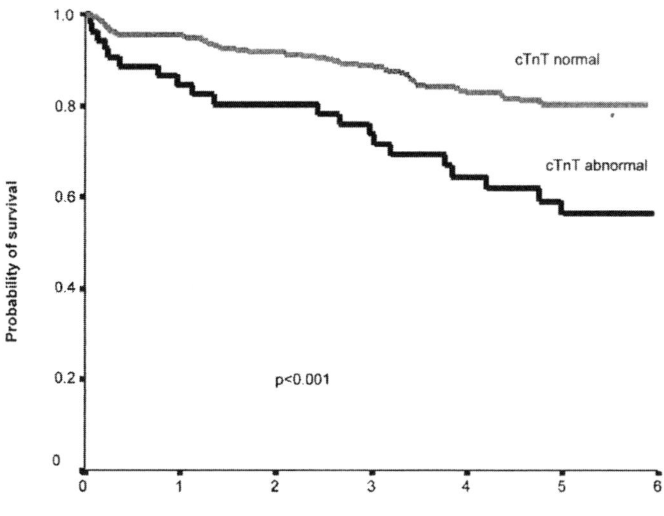

FIGURE 1.—Kaplan–Meier estimates of all-cause mortality according to normal and elevated levels of cardiac troponin T. (Reprinted from Kertai MD, Boersma E, Klein J, et al: Long-term prognostic value of asymptomatic cardiac troponin T elevations in patients after major vascular surgery. *Eur J Vasc Endovasc Surg* 28:59-66, 2004. By permission of the publisher.)

► It is difficult to know how to apply these data clinically. The adverse prognosis imparted by elevated cTnT levels does not become known until after the patient has undergone the surgical procedure. The findings are interesting but do not argue for routine screening for elevated cTnT levels in asymptomatic patients.

G. L. Moneta, MD

Risk of Acute Myocardial Infarction and Sudden Cardiac Death in Patients Treated With Cyclo-oxygenase 2 Selective and Non-selective Non-steroidal Anti-inflammatory Drugs: Nested Case-Control Study

Graham DJ, Campen D, Hui R, et al (Food and Drug Administration, Rockville, Md; Kaiser Permanente, Oakland, Calif; Vanderbilt Univ, Nashville, Tenn; et al)
Lancet 365:475-481, 2005 3–5

Background.—Controversy has surrounded the question about whether high-dose rofecoxib increases or naproxen decreases the risk of serious coronary heart disease. We sought to establish if risk was enhanced with rofecoxib at either high or standard doses compared with remote non-steroidal anti-inflammatory drug (NSAID) use or celecoxib use, because celecoxib was the most common alternative to rofecoxib.

Methods.—We used data from Kaiser Permanente in California to assemble a cohort of all patients age 18-84 years treated with a NSAID between Jan 1, 1999, and Dec 31, 2001, within which we did a nested case-control study. Cases of serious coronary heart disease (acute myocardial infarction and sudden cardiac death) were risk-set matched with four controls for age, sex, and health plan region. Current exposure to cyclooxygenase 2 selective and non-selective NSAIDs was compared with remote exposure to any NSAID, and rofecoxib was compared with celecoxib.

Findings.—During 2302029 person-years of follow-up, 8143 cases of serious coronary heart disease occurred, of which 2210 (27.1%) were fatal. Multivariate adjusted odds ratios versus celecoxib were: for rofecoxib (all doses), 1.59 (95% CI 1.10–2.32, p=0.015); for rofecoxib 25 mg/day or less, 1.47 (0.99–2.17, p=0.054); and for rofecoxib greater than 25 mg/day, 3.58 (1.27–10.11, p=0.016). For naproxen versus remote NSAID use the adjusted odds ratio was 1.14 (1.00–1.30, p=0.05).

Interpretation.—Rofecoxib use increases the risk of serious coronary heart disease compared with celecoxib use. Naproxen use does not protect against serious coronary heart disease.

▶ Parts of this article were first posted on the US Food and Drug Administration (FDA) Web site on November 2, 2004. At that point, the document was considered preliminary and was a source of great controversy within the FDA. It is important to recognize that the current document represents the opinion of the authors and not necessarily that of the FDA and that the FDA did not participate in the study design, data collection, analysis, or writing of this report. This study, however, obviously has enormous implications for the entire class of COX-2 inhibitors and the mechanisms of oversight used by the FDA.

G. L. Moneta, MD

Risk of Myocardial Infarction and Stroke After Acute Infection or Vaccination

Smeeth L, Thomas SL, Hall AJ, et al (London School of Hygiene and Tropical Medicine; Univ of Nottingham, England; Open Univ, Milton Keynes, England; et al)

N Engl J Med 351:2611-2618, 2004 3–6

Background.—There is evidence that chronic inflammation may promote atherosclerotic disease. We tested the hypothesis that acute infection and vaccination increase the short-term risk of vascular events.

Methods.—We undertook within-person comparisons, using the case-series method, to study the risks of myocardial infarction and stroke after common vaccinations and naturally occurring infections. The study was based on the United Kingdom General Practice Research Database, which contains computerized medical records of more than 5 million patients.

Results.—A total of 20,486 persons with a first myocardial infarction and 19,063 persons with a first stroke who received influenza vaccine were included in the analysis. There was no increase in the risk of myocardial infarction or stroke in the period after influenza, tetanus, or pneumococcal vaccination. However, the risks of both events were substantially higher after a diagnosis of systemic respiratory tract infection and were highest during the first three days (incidence ratio for myocardial infarction, 4.95; 95 percent confidence interval, 4.43 to 5.53; incidence ratio for stroke, 3.19; 95 percent confidence interval, 2.81 to 3.62). The risks then gradually fell during the following weeks. The risks were raised significantly but to a lesser degree after a diagnosis of urinary tract infection. The findings for recurrent myocardial infarctions and stroke were similar to those for first events.

Conclusions.—Our findings provide support for the concept that acute infections are associated with a transient increase in the risk of vascular events. By contrast, influenza, tetanus, and pneumococcal vaccinations do not produce a detectable increase in the risk of vascular events.

► This very large database supports a link between acute infection and vascular events. It now needs to be established whether the risk is from alterations in white cell activation, dehydration, or perhaps the institution of bed rest with the illness. The authors correctly point out that the associated increased risk of cardiovascular events with infection in 2 very different organ systems suggests the possibility of an underlying genetic basis for this increased risk.

G. L. Moneta, MD

Intensive Versus Moderate Lipid Lowering With Statins After Acute Coronary Syndromes

Cannon CP, for the Pravastatin or Atorvastatin Evaluation and Infection Therapy–Thrombolysis in Myocardial Infarction 22 Investigators (Harvard Med School, Boston; et al)

N Engl J Med 350:1495-1504, 2004 3–7

Background.—Lipid-lowering therapy with statins reduces the risk of cardiovascular events, but the optimal level of low-density lipoprotein (LDL) cholesterol is unclear.

Methods.—We enrolled 4162 patients who had been hospitalized for an acute coronary syndrome within the preceding 10 days and compared 40 mg of pravastatin daily (standard therapy) with 80 mg of atorvastatin daily (intensive therapy). The primary end point was a composite of death from any cause, myocardial infarction, documented unstable angina requiring rehospitalization, revascularization (performed at least 30 days after randomization), and stroke. The study was designed to establish the noninferiority of pravastatin as compared with atorvastatin with respect to the time to an end-point event. Follow-up lasted 18 to 36 months (mean, 24).

Results.—The median LDL cholesterol level achieved during treatment was 95 mg per deciliter (2.46 mmol per liter) in the standard-dose pravastatin group and 62 mg per deciliter (1.60 mmol per liter) in the high-dose atorvastatin group ($P<0.001$) (Fig 1). Kaplan–Meier estimates of the rates of the primary end point at two years were 26.3 percent in the pravastatin group and 22.4 percent in the atorvastatin group, reflecting a 16 percent reduction

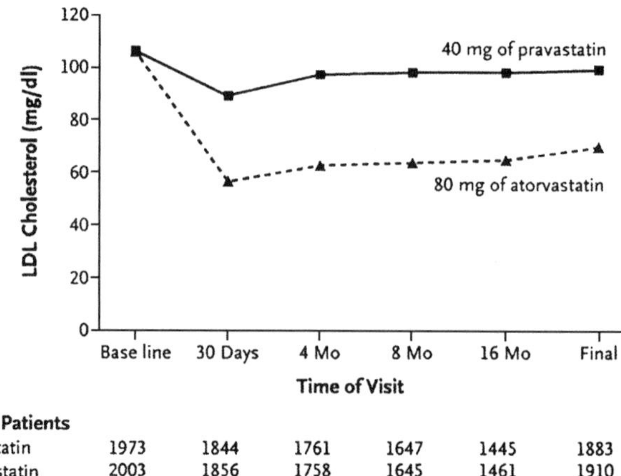

No. of Patients						
Pravastatin	1973	1844	1761	1647	1445	1883
Atorvastatin	2003	1856	1758	1645	1461	1910

FIGURE 1.—Median low-density lipoprotein (LDL) cholesterol levels during the study. *Note:* To convert values for LDL cholesterol to millimoles per liter, multiply by 0.02586. (Reprinted by permission of *The New England Journal of Medicine* from Cannon CP, for the Pravastatin or Atorvastatin Evaluation and Infection Therapy–Thrombolysis in Myocardial Infarction 22 Investigators: Intensive versus moderate lipid lowering with statins after acute coronary syndromes. *N Engl J Med* 350:1495-1504, 2004. Copyright 2004, Massachusetts Medical Society. All rights reserved.)

in the hazard ratio in favor of atorvastatin (P=0.005; 95 percent confidence interval, 5 to 26 percent) (Fig 2). The study did not meet the prespecified criterion for equivalence but did identify the superiority of the more intensive regimen.

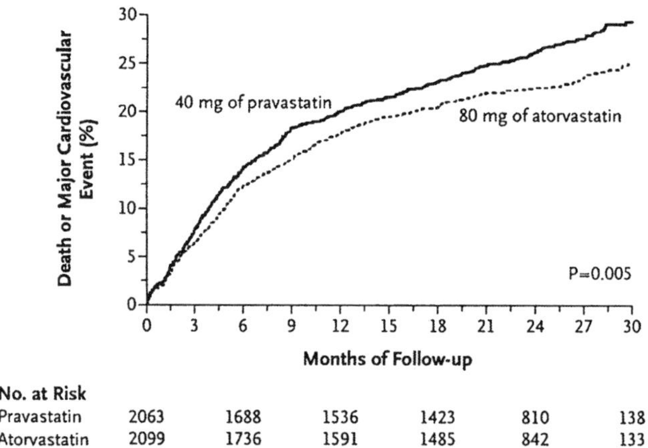

No. at Risk						
Pravastatin	2063	1688	1536	1423	810	138
Atorvastatin	2099	1736	1591	1485	842	133

FIGURE 2.—Kaplan-Meier estimates of the incidence of the primary end point of death from any cause or a major cardiovascular event. Intensive lipid lowering with the 80-mg dose of atorvastatin, as compared with moderate lipid lowering with the 40-mg dose of pravastatin, reduced the hazard ratio for death or a major cardiovascular event by 16 percent. (Reprinted by permission of *The New England Journal of Medicine* from Cannon CP, for the Pravastatin or Atorvastatin Evaluation and Infection Therapy–Thrombolysis in Myocardial Infarction 22 Investigators: Intensive versus moderate lipid lowering with statins after acute coronary syndromes. *N Engl J Med* 350:1495-1504, 2004. Copyright 2004, Massachusetts Medical Society. All rights reserved.)

Conclusions.—Among patients who have recently had an acute coronary syndrome, an intensive lipid-lowering statin regimen provides greater protection against death or major cardiovascular events than does a standard regimen. These findings indicate that such patients benefit from early and continued lowering of LDL cholesterol to levels substantially below current target levels.

▶ When it comes to lipids, there appear to be no "normal" levels. Currently, it appears the lower the LDL cholesterol level the better. It should be noted, and the authors point out, that the patients in this study generally had fewer coexisting conditions than might be expected in the usual population. Patients encountered in clinical practice may not be as tolerant of the high-dose statin regimen utilized in this study.

G. L. Moneta, MD

Statin Therapy, LDL Cholesterol, C-Reactive Protein, and Coronary Artery Disease

Nissen SE, for the Reversal of Atherosclerosis with Aggressive Lipid Lowering (REVERSAL) Investigators (Cleveland Clinic Found, Ohio; et al)

N Engl J Med 352:29-38, 2005 3–8

Background.—Recent trials have demonstrated better outcomes with intensive than with moderate statin treatment. Intensive treatment produced greater reductions in both low-density lipoprotein (LDL) cholesterol and C-reactive protein (CRP), suggesting a relationship between these two biomarkers and disease progression.

Methods.—We performed intravascular ultrasonography in 502 patients with angiographically documented coronary disease. Patients were randomly assigned to receive moderate treatment (40 mg of pravastatin orally per day) or intensive treatment (80 mg of atorvastatin orally per day). Ultrasonography was repeated after 18 months to measure the progression of atherosclerosis. Lipoprotein and CRP levels were measured at baseline and follow-up.

Results.—In the group as a whole, the mean LDL cholesterol level was reduced from 150.2 mg per deciliter (3.88 mmol per liter) at baseline to 94.5 mg per deciliter (2.44 mmol per liter) at 18 months ($P<0.001$), and the geometric mean CRP level decreased from 2.9 to 2.3 mg per liter ($P<0.001$) (Figs 1 and 2). The correlation between the reduction in LDL cholesterol levels and that in CRP levels was weak but significant in the group as a whole ($r=0.13$, $P=0.005$), but not in either treatment group alone. In univariate analyses, the percent change in the levels of LDL cholesterol, CRP, apolipoprotein B-100, and non-high-density lipoprotein cholesterol were related to the rate of progression of atherosclerosis. After adjustment for the reduction in these lipid levels, the decrease in CRP levels was independently and significantly correlated with the rate of progression. Patients with reductions in both LDL cholesterol and CRP that were greater than the median had signif-

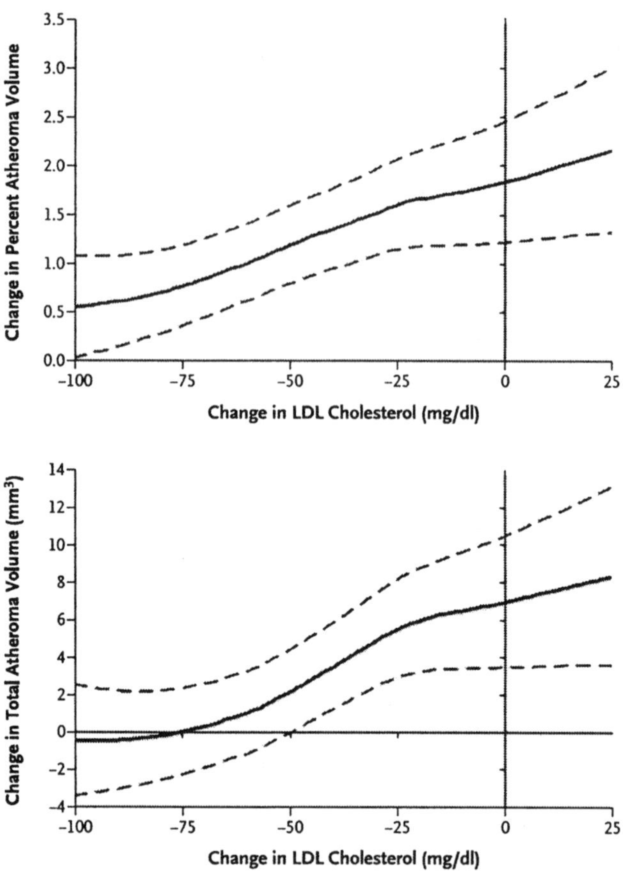

FIGURE 1.—Locally weighted smoothed scatterplots showing the relationship between the change in LDL cholesterol levels and the rate of progression of atherosclerosis in the entire group of 502 patients. In each plot, the solid line represents the point estimates and the upper and lower lines the 95 percent confidence intervals. To convert values for LDL cholesterol to millimoles per liter, multiply by 0.02586. (Reprinted by permission of *The New England Journal of Medicine* from Nissen SE, for the Reversal of Atherosclerosis with Aggressive Lipid Lowering (REVERSAL) Investigators: Statin therapy, LDL cholesterol, C-reactive protein, and coronary artery disease. *N Engl J Med* 352:29-38, 2005.)

icantly slower rates of progression than patients with reductions in both biomarkers that were less than the median (P=0.001).

Conclusions.—For patients with coronary artery disease, the reduced rate of progression of atherosclerosis associated with intensive statin treatment, as compared with moderate statin treatment, is significantly related to greater reductions in the levels of both atherogenic lipoproteins and CRP.

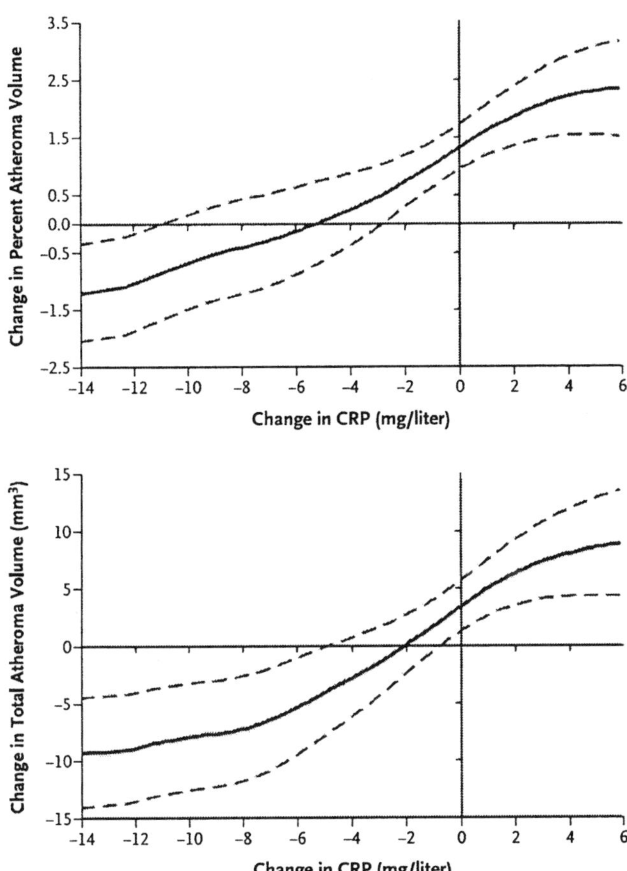

FIGURE 2.—Locally weighted smoothed scatterplots showing the relationship between the changes in CRP levels and the rate of progression of atherosclerosis in the entire group of 502 patients. In each plot, the solid line represents the point estimates and the upper and lower lines the 95 percent confidence intervals. (Reprinted by permission of *The New England Journal of Medicine* from Nissen SE, for the Reversal of Atherosclerosis with Aggressive Lipid Lowering (REVERSAL) Investigators: Statin therapy, LDL cholesterol, C-reactive protein, and coronary artery disease. *N Engl J Med* 352:29-38, 2005.

▶ This is another bit of evidence that statin-mediated reductions in LDL cholesterol and CRP are for the most part unrelated. Reductions in levels of atherogenic proteins in this study were not closely correlated with reductions in CRP levels. This study, along with a similar study in the same issue of *The New England Journal of Medicine* (Abstract 3–9), suggest both CRP and atherogenic protein levels in patients on statin therapy should be monitored.

G. L. Moneta, MD

C-Reactive Protein Levels and Outcomes After Statin Therapy

Ridker PM, for the Pravastatin or Atorvastatin Evaluation and Infection Therapy–Thrombolysis in Myocardial Infarction 22 (PROVE IT–TIMI 22) Investigators (Harvard Med School, Boston)

N Engl J Med 352:20-28, 2005 3–9

Background.—Statins lower the levels of low-density lipoprotein (LDL) cholesterol and C-reactive protein (CRP). Whether this latter property affects clinical outcomes is unknown.

Methods.—We evaluated relationships between the LDL cholesterol and CRP levels achieved after treatment with 80 mg of atorvastatin or 40 mg of pravastatin per day and the risk of recurrent myocardial infarction or death from coronary causes among 3745 patients with acute coronary syndromes.

Results.—Patients in whom statin therapy resulted in LDL cholesterol levels of less than 70 mg per deciliter (1.8 mmol per liter) had lower event rates than those with higher levels (2.7 vs. 4.0 events per 100 person-years, P=0.008). However, a virtually identical difference was observed between those who had CRP levels of less than 2 mg per liter after statin therapy and those who had higher levels (2.8 vs. 3.9 events per 100 person-years, P=0.006), an effect present at all levels of LDL cholesterol achieved. For patients with post-treatment LDL cholesterol levels of more than 70 mg per deciliter, the rates of recurrent events were 4.6 per 100 person-years among those with CRP levels of more than 2 mg per liter and 3.2 events per 100 person-years among those with CRP levels of less than 2 mg per liter; the respective rates among those with LDL cholesterol levels of less than 70 mg per deciliter were 3.1 and 2.4 events per 100 person-years (P<0.001). Although atorvastatin was more likely than pravastatin to result in low levels of LDL cholesterol and CRP, meeting these targets was more important in determining the outcomes than was the specific choice of therapy. Patients who had LDL cholesterol levels of less than 70 mg per deciliter and CRP levels of less than 1 mg per liter after statin therapy had the lowest rate of recurrent events (1.9 per 100 person-years).

Conclusions.—Patients who have low CRP levels after statin therapy have better clinical outcomes than those with higher CRP levels, regardless of the resultant level of LDL cholesterol. Strategies to lower cardiovascular risk with statins should include monitoring CRP as well as cholesterol.

▶ The data imply that therapies designed to reduce both inflammation and cholesterol levels may improve outcomes in patients with atherosclerotic disease. The current data obviously directly apply only to patients who have had acute coronary artery syndromes. Nevertheless, this is another suggestion that patients with diffuse atherosclerosis will benefit not only from cholesterol lowering, but also from control of inflammation.

G. L. Moneta, MD

Statins Decrease Perioperative Cardiac Complications in Patients Undergoing Noncardiac Vascular Surgery: The Statins for Risk Reduction in Surgery (StaRRS) Study

O'Neil-Callahan K, Katsimaglis G, Tepper MR, et al (Harvard Med School, Boston; Hygeia Hosp, Athens, Greece; Naval Hosp, Athens, Greece; et al)

J Am Coll Cardiol 45:336-342, 2005 3–10

Objectives.—We sought to assess whether statins may decrease cardiac complications in patients undergoing noncardiac vascular surgery.

Background.—Cardiovascular complications account for considerable morbidity in patients undergoing noncardiac surgery. Statins decrease cardiac morbidity and mortality in patients with coronary disease, and the beneficial treatment effect is seen early, before any measurable increase in coronary artery diameter.

Methods.—A retrospective study recorded patient characteristics, past medical history, and admission medications on all patients undergoing carotid endarterectomy, aortic surgery, or lower extremity revascularization over a two-year period (January 1999 to December 2000) at a tertiary referral center. Recorded perioperative complication outcomes included death, myocardial infarction, ischemia, congestive heart failure, and ventricular tachyarrhythmias occurring during the index hospitalization. Univariate and multivariate logistic regressions identified predictors of perioperative cardiac complications and medications that might confer a protective effect.

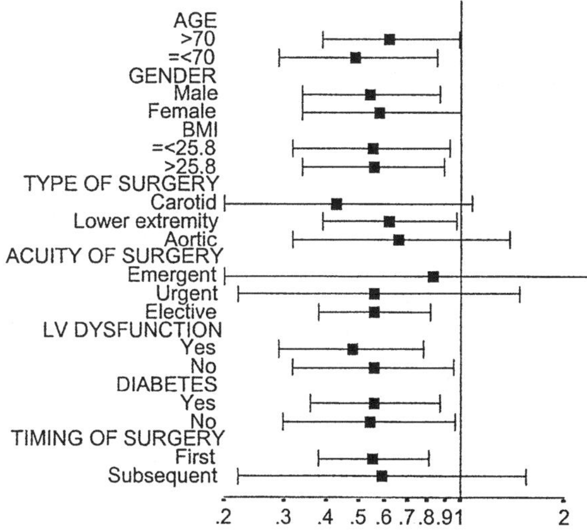

FIGURE 1.—The odds ratio and 95% confidence interval for complications in patients receiving versus those not receiving statins across subgroups defined by various parameters. BMI = body mass index; LV = left ventricular. (Courtesy of O'Neil-Callahan K, Katsimaglis G, Tepper MR, et al: Statins decrease perioperative cardiac complications in patients undergoing noncardiac vascular surgery: The Statins for Risk Reduction in Surgery (StaRRS) study. *J Am Coll Cardiol* 45:336-342, 2005. Reprinted with permission from the American College of Cardiology.)

Results.—Complications occurred in 157 of 1,163 eligible hospitalizations and were significantly fewer in patients receiving statins (9.9%) than in those not receiving statins (16.5%, $p = 0.001$) (Fig 1). The difference was mostly accounted by myocardial ischemia and congestive heart failure. After adjusting for other significant predictors of perioperative complications (age, gender, type of surgery, emergent surgery, left ventricular dysfunction, and diabetes mellitus), statins still conferred a highly significant protective effect (odds ratio 052, $p = 0.001$). The protective effect was similar across diverse patient subgroups and persisted after accounting for the likelihood of patients to have hypercholesterolemia by considering their propensity to use statins.

Conclusions.—Use of statins was highly protective against perioperative cardiac complications in patients undergoing vascular surgery in this retrospective study.

► It is now well appreciated that statins have significant pleiotropic effects in addition to lowering lipid levels. This report does not indicate when statins need to be started before an operation or how long they need to be continued after an operation. If vascular surgeons are going to prescribe statins to reduce perioperative complications, they must be prepared to monitor the potential side effects and complications. Alternatively, they must communicate with primary care physicians to ensure the medications are properly prescribed and the patients adequately monitored.

G. L. Moneta, MD

Reduction in Cardiovascular Events After Vascular Surgery With Atorvastatin: A Randomized Trial

Durazzo AES, Machado FS, Ikeoka DT, et al (Univ of São Paulo, Brazil)

J Vasc Surg 39:967-976, 2004 3–11

Objectives.—This prospective, randomized, placebo-controlled, double-blind clinical trial was performed to analyze the effect of atorvastatin compared with placebo on the occurrence of a 6-month composite of cardiovascular events after vascular surgery. Cardiovascular complications are the most important cause of perioperative morbidity and mortality among patients undergoing vascular surgery. Statin therapy may reduce perioperative cardiac events through stabilization of coronary plaques.

Methods.—One hundred patients were randomly assigned to receive 20 mg atorvastatin or placebo once a day for 45 days, irrespective of their serum cholesterol concentration. Vascular surgery was performed on average 30 days after randomization, and patients were prospectively followed up over 6 months. The cardiovascular events studied were death from cardiac cause, nonfatal myocardial infarction, unstable angina, and stroke.

Results.—Fifty patients received atorvastatin, and 50 received placebo. During the 6-month follow-up primary end points occurred in 17 patients, 4 in the atorvastatin group and 13 in the placebo group. The incidence of car-

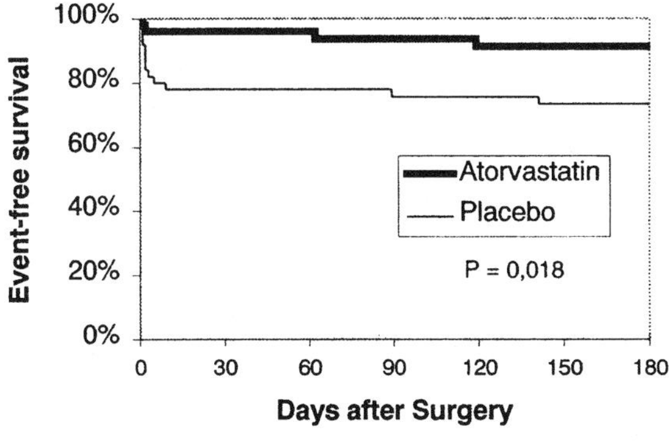

Atorvastatin	50	44	43	41	40	40	40
Placebo	50	38	36	35	34	33	33

FIGURE 2.—Event-free survival in the 6 months after vascular surgery according to study group. Outcome measures included death from cardiac causes, nonfatal acute myocardial infarction, ischemic stroke, and unstable angina. Rate of event-free survival at 6 months (180 days) was 91.4% in the atorvastatin group and 73.5% in the placebo group (*P* = .018). (Reprinted by permission of the publisher from Durazzo AES, Machado FS, Ikeoka DT, et al: Reduction in cardiovascular events after vascular surgery with atorvastatin: A randomized trial. *J Vasc Surg* 39:967-976, 2004. Copyright 2004 by Elsevier.)

diac events was more than three times higher with placebo (26.0%) compared with atorvastatin (8.0%; *P* = .031). The risk for an event was compared between the groups with the Kaplan-Meier method, as event-free survival after vascular surgery (Fig 2). Patients given atorvastatin exhibited a significant decrease in the rate of cardiac events, compared with the placebo group, within 6 months after vascular surgery (*P* = .018).

Conclusion.—Short-term treatment with atorvastatin significantly reduces the incidence of major adverse cardiovascular events after vascular surgery.

▶ This is part of a series of reports in this year's YEAR BOOK suggesting benefits of statins perioperatively in patients undergoing vascular surgery. The numbers of patients in this particular study are small and the groups not exactly the same. It is therefore important to keep in mind that while suggestive, this study does not conclusively prove perioperative benefit of statins. It is a little disappointing the statins were not continued beyond 6 months in many of patients in this series, as long-term benefits of statins in vascular patients seem reasonably well established regardless of cholesterol level.

G. L. Moneta, MD

Statin Therapy Improves Cardiovascular Outcome of Patients With Peripheral Artery Disease

Schillinger M, Exner M, Mlekusch W, et al (Vienna Gen Hosp)

Eur Heart J 25:742-748, 2004 3–12

Aims.—We sought to examine the interrelationship between statin use, inflammation, and outcome of high-risk patients with advanced atherosclerosis.

Methods and Results.—We prospectively studied 515 patients with severe peripheral artery disease (median age 70 years, 296 males). The cardiovascular risk profile and laboratory parameters of inflammation (high-sensitivity C-reactive protein [hs-CRP], serum amyloid A [SAA], fibrinogen, serum albumin, neutrophil counts) were obtained, and patients were followed for a median of 21 months (interquartile range 12–25) for the occurrence of myocardial infarction (MI) and death. We observed 19 MIs (5 fatal and 14 nonfatal) and 65 deaths. Cumulative survival and event-free survival rates (freedom from death and MI) at 6, 12, and 24 months were 97%, 95%, and 89%, and 96%, 93% and 87%, respectively (Fig 2). Patients receiving statin therapy ($n = 269$, 52%) had a lower level of inflammation (hs-CRP $p < 0.001$, SAA $p = 0.001$, fibrinogen $p = 0.007$, albumin $p < 0.001$, neutrophils $p = 0.049$) and better survival (adjusted hazard ratio [HR] 0.52, $p = 0.022$) and event-free survival rates (adjusted HR 0.48, $p = 0.004$) than patients not treated with statins. However, patients with low inflammatory activity (hs-CRP $\leq$0.42 mg/dl) had no significant benefit from statin therapy ($p = 0.74$ for survival; $p = 0.83$ for event-free survival), whereas in patients with high hs-CRP (>0.42 mg/dl) statin therapy was associated with a significantly re-

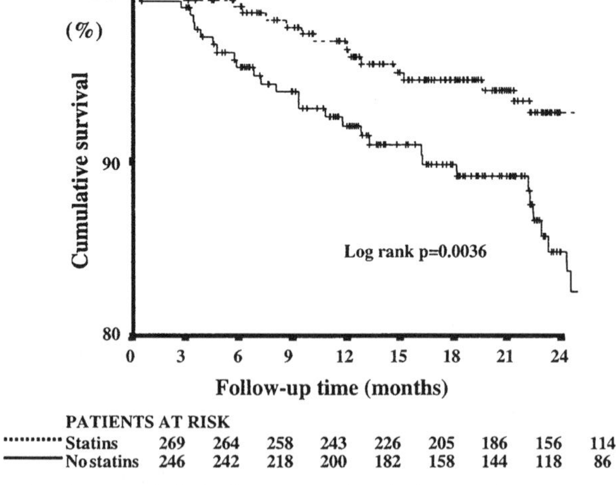

PATIENTS AT RISK

·········· Statins	269	264	258	243	226	205	186	156	114
——— No statins	246	242	218	200	182	158	144	118	86

FIGURE 2.—Cumulative survival of 515 patients with and without statin pretreatment. (Courtesy of Schillinger M, Exner M, Mlekusch W, et al: Statin Therapy improves cardiovascular outcome of patients with peripheral artery disease. *Eur Heart J* 25:742-748, 2004. Reprinted by permission of Oxford University Press.)

duced risk for mortality (adjusted HR 0.58, $p = 0.046$) and the composite of myocardial infarction and death (adjusted HR 0.46, $p = 0.016$).

Conclusion.—Statin therapy is associated with a substantially improved intermediate-term survival of patients with severe peripheral artery disease and a high inflammatory activity, whereas in patients with low hs-CRP no survival benefit was observed.

▶ It has become increasingly clear that statin therapy is associated with improved survival in patients with peripheral arterial disease. This study suggests CRP levels may be used to select patients with peripheral arterial disease who may most benefit from statins. These results are consistent with previously documented benefits of statin therapy on levels of inflammatory markers associated with cardiovascular disease and the association of elevated inflammatory markers for cardiovascular disease with decreased long-term survival.

G. L. Moneta, MD

A Combination of Statins and Beta-Blockers Is Independently Associated With a Reduction in the Incidence of Perioperative Mortality and Nonfatal Myocardial Infarction in Patients Undergoing Abdominal Aortic Aneurysm Surgery

Kertai MD, Boersma E, Westerhout CM, et al (Erasmus MC, Rotterdam, The Netherlands)

Eur J Vasc Endovasc Surg 28:343-352, 2004 3–13

Objective.—To investigate the combined beneficial effect of statin and beta-blocker use on perioperative mortality and myocardial infarction (MI) in patients undergoing abdominal aortic aneurysm surgery (AAA).

Background.—Patients undergoing elective AAA-surgery identified by clinical risk factors and dobutamine stress echocardiography (DSE) as being at high-risk often have considerable cardiac complication rate despite the use of beta-blockers.

Methods.—We studied 570 patients (mean age 69±9 years, 486 males) who underwent AAA-surgery between 1991 and 2001 at the Erasmus MC. Patients were evaluated for clinical risk factors (age>70 years, histories of MI, angina, diabetes mellitus, stroke, renal failure, heart failure and pulmonary disease), DSE, statin and beta-blocker use. The main outcome was a composite of perioperative mortality and MI within 30 days of surgery.

Results.—Perioperative mortality or MI occurred in 51 (8.9%) patients (Fig 1). The incidence of the composite endpoint was significantly lower in statin users compared to nonusers (3.7% vs. 11.0%; crude odds ratio (OR): 0.31, 95% confidence interval (CI): 0.13–0.74; p=0.01). After correcting for other covariates, the association between statin use and reduced incidence of the composite endpoint remained unchanged (OR: 0.24, 95% CI: 0.10–0.70; p=0.01). Beta-blocker use was also associated with a significant reduction in the composite endpoint (OR: 0.24, 95% CI: 0.11–0.54). Pa-

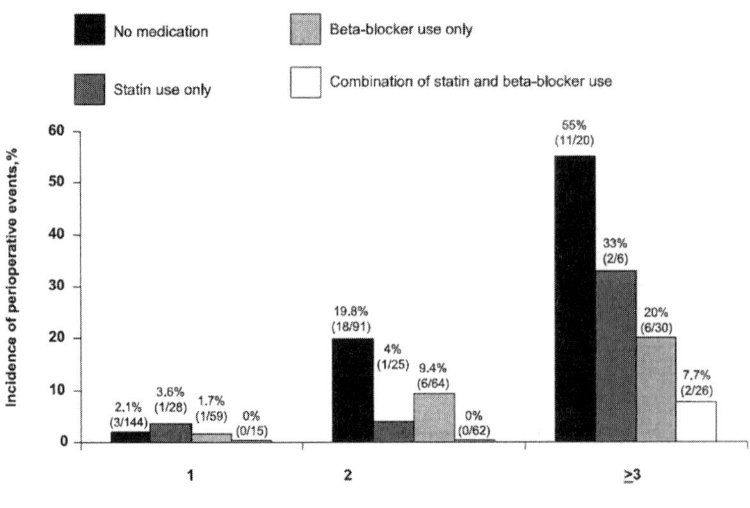

FIGURE 1.—Incidence of perioperative mortality and myocardial infarction. Results are based on the number of clinical risk factors by the revised cardiac risk index (ischemic heart disease, history of congestive heart failure, history of cerebrovascular disease, insulin therapy for diabetes, preoperative serum creatinine >2 mg/dl), statin and beta-blocker use. (Reprinted from Kertai MD, Boersma E, Westerhout CM, et al: A Combination of statins and beta-blockers is independently associated with a reduction in the incidence of perioperative mortality and nonfatal myocardial infarction in patients undergoing abdominal aortic aneurysm. *Eur J Vasc Endovasc Surg*28:343-352, 2004. By permission of the publisher.)

tients using a combination of statins and beta-blockers appeared to be at lower risk for the composite endpoint across multiple cardiac risk strata; particularly patients with 3 or more risk factors experienced significantly lower perioperative events.

Conclusions.—A combination of statin and beta-blocker use in patients with AAA-surgery is associated with a reduced incidence of perioperative mortality and nonfatal MI particularly in patients at the highest risk.

► It is now well recognized that β-blockers lower perioperative mortality rate and adverse cardiovascular events in patients undergoing peripheral vascular surgery. Statins also lower long-term mortality rate in patients with vascular disease. Emerging data such as this indicate statins may also have beneficial effects in the perioperative period as well. (See also Abstract 3–11.)

G. L. Moneta, MD

Early Post-operative Glucose Levels Are an Independent Risk Factor for Infection After Peripheral Vascular Surgery. A Retrospective Study

Vriesendorp TM, Morélis QJ, DeVries JH, et al (Academic Med Ctr, Amsterdam)

Eur J Vasc Endovasc Surg 28:520-525, 2004 3–14

Objective.—To evaluate whether hyperglycaemia in the first 48 h after infrainguinal vascular surgery is a risk factor for post-operative infection, independent from factors associated with insulin resistance and surgical stress.

Design.—Retrospective cohort study.

Patients and Methods.—Patients who underwent infrainguinal vascular surgery in our hospital between March 1998 and March 2003 were included. Glucose values until 48 h after surgery were retrieved from laboratory reports. Post-operative infections, treated with antibiotics, during hospital stay were scored until 30 days after surgery. Data were analysed with univariate and multivariate logistic regression analyses.

Results.—At least one post-operative glucose value was retrieved for 211/275 (77%) patients. The incidence of post-operative infections was 84/275 (31%). When corrected for factors associated with insulin resistance and surgical stress, post-operative glucose levels were found to be an independent risk factor for post-operative infections (odds ratio top quartile versus lowest quartile: 5.1; 95% confidence interval: 1.6-17.1; $P = 0.007$).

Conclusion.—Post-operative glucose levels appear to be an independent risk factor for infections after infrainguinal vascular surgery. This finding requires confirmation in a prospective study (Fig 1).

► Perioperative glucose control is currently under intense scrutiny. It appears strict glucose control improves morbidity and mortality rates in ICU patients.[1] Extrapolation of these data to wound healing and infection in vascular surgical

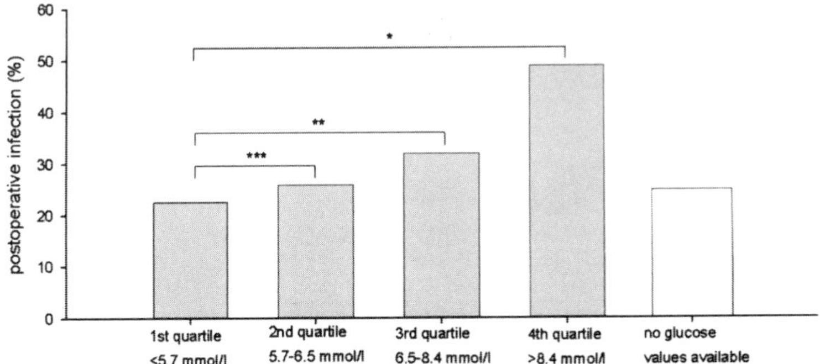

FIGURE 1.—Results of univariate analysis. Percentage of patients with at least one post-operative infection per post-operative glucose quartile. P for trend = 0.003; $^{*}P = 0.006$; $^{**}P = 0.28$; $^{***}P = 0.69$. (Reprinted from Vriesendorp TM, Morélis QJ, DeVries JH, et al: Early post-operative glucose levels are an independent risk factor for infection after peripheral vascular surgery. A retrospective study. *Eur J Vasc Endovasc Surg* 28:520-525, 2004. By permission of the publisher.)

patients is somewhat of a leap but does make some sense. The old days of tolerating high glucose levels in the perioperative period are over.

G. L. Moneta, MD

Reference

1. van de Berghe G, Wouters P, Weekers F, et al: Intensive insulin therapy in the critically ill patients. *N Engl J Med* 345:1359-1367, 2001.

A Comparison of Albumin and Saline for Fluid Resuscitation in the Intensive Care Unit

Finfer S, for the SAFE Study Investigators (ANZICS CTG, Carlton, Australia; et al)

N Engl J Med 350:2247-2256, 2004 3–15

Background.—It remains uncertain whether the choice of resuscitation fluid for patients in intensive care units (ICUs) affects survival. We conducted a multicenter, randomized, double-blind trial to compare the effect of fluid resuscitation with albumin or saline on mortality in a heterogeneous population of patients in the ICU.

Methods.—We randomly assigned patients who had been admitted to the ICU to receive either 4 percent albumin or normal saline for intravascular-fluid resuscitation during the next 28 days. The primary outcome measure was death from any cause during the 28-day period after randomization.

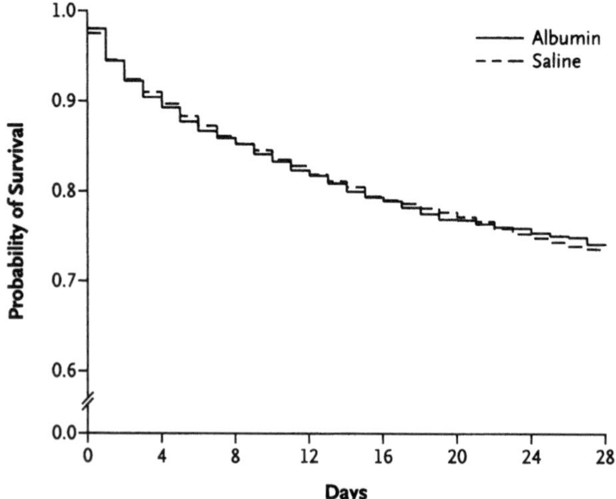

FIGURE 1.—Kaplan–Meier Estimates of the Probability of Survival. P=0.96 for the comparison between patients assigned to receive albumin and those assigned to receive saline. (Reprinted with permission from *The New England Journal of Medicine* from Finfer S, for the SAFE Study Investigators: A comparison of albumin and saline for fluid resuscitation in the intensive care unit. *N Engl J Med* 350:2247-2256, 2004.)

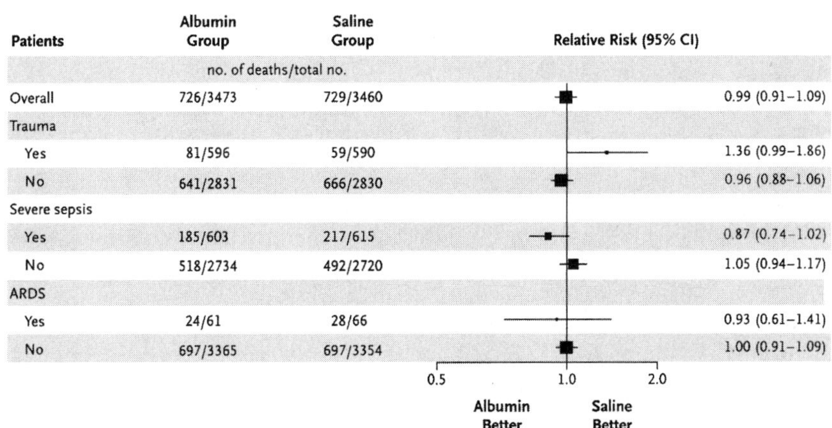

Patients
Albumin Group
Saline Group
Relative Risk (95% CI)
no. of deaths/total no.
Overall 726/3473 729/3460 0.99 (0.91–1.09)
Trauma
Yes 81/596 59/590 1.36 (0.99–1.86)
No 641/2831 666/2830 0.96 (0.88–1.06)
Severe sepsis
Yes 185/603 217/615 0.87 (0.74–1.02)
No 518/2734 492/2720 1.05 (0.94–1.17)
ARDS
Yes 24/61 28/66 0.93 (0.61–1.41)
No 697/3365 697/3354 1.00 (0.91–1.09)
0.5
1.0
2.0
Albumin Better
Saline Better

FIGURE 2.—Relative Risk of Death from Any Cause among All the Patients and among the Patients in the Six Predefined Subgroups. The size of each symbol indicates the relative number of events in the given group. The horizontal bars represent the confidence intervals (CI). ARDS denotes the acute respiratory distress syndrome. (Reprinted with permission from *The New England Journal of Medicine* from Finfer S, for the SAFE Study Investigators: A comparison of albumin and saline for fluid resuscitation in the intensive care unit. *N Engl J Med* 350:2247-2256, 2004. Copyright 2004, Massachusetts Medical Society. All rights reserved.)

Results.—Of the 6997 patients who underwent randomization, 3497 were assigned to receive albumin and 3500 to receive saline; the two groups had similar baseline characteristics. There were 726 deaths in the albumin group, as compared with 729 deaths in the saline group (relative risk of death, 0.99; 95 percent confidence interval, 0.91 to 1.09; P=0.87). The proportion of patients with new single-organ and multiple-organ failure was similar in the two groups (P=0.85). There were no significant differences between the groups in the mean (SD) numbers of days spent in the ICU (6.5±6.6 in the albumin group and 6.2±6.2 in the saline group, P=0.44), days spent in the hospital (15.3±9.6 and 15.6±9.6, respectively; P=0.30), days of mechanical ventilation (4.5±6.1 and 4.3±5.7, respectively; P=0.74), or days of renal-replacement therapy (0.5±2.3 and 0.4±2.0, respectively; P=0.41).

Conclusions.—In patients in the ICU, use of either 4 percent albumin or normal saline for fluid resuscitation results in similar outcomes at 28 days (Figs 1 and 2).

► Because it appeared in *The New England Journal of Medicine,* this article will likely be widely cited. The data, however, may not apply to surgical patients undergoing massive resuscitation or to vascular surgical patients. There is no breakdown of the number of patients undergoing elective or urgent aortic surgery or those who required massive amounts of fluid resuscitation. The study provides the results of an overview of ICU patients. It should not be used to justify therapies in specific subgroups of surgical patients, especially those who require massive resuscitation.

G. L. Moneta, MD

Haemodilutional Effect of Standard Fluid Management Limits the Effectiveness of Acute Normovolaemic Haemodilution in AAA Surgery—Results of a Pilot Trial

Wolowczyk L, Nevin M, Smith FCT, et al (Bristol Royal Infirmary, England)
Eur J Vasc Endovasc Surg 26:405-411, 2003 3–16

Objective.—To evaluate the impact of standard fluid management on the effectiveness of ANH as a blood conservation method in elective open AAA repair.

Design.—Prospective randomised controlled study.

Methods.—Thirty-four patients undergoing elective AAA repair were randomised to have ANH (16) or act as controls (18). Intra-operative cell salvage was permitted in both groups. Haemoglobin (Hb) concentrations were determined at variable intervals peri-operatively. Blood loss and the use of heterologous blood were recorded.

Results.—The pre- and post-operative Hb concentrations, surgical blood loss and the use of cell salvage were similar in both groups. Hb concentration (median, range) decreased significantly from pre-operative to aortic clamping (with blood loss <100 ml) in ANH patients from 8.8 (7.5–10.2) to 5.7 (4.2–6.6)mmol/l following ANH but also in controls from 8.6 (7.5–9.7) to 7.0 (4.5–9.0)mmol/l due to fluid infusion ($P < 0.01$ for every comparison). Bank blood requirements were similar: median 2 units in ANH and 2.5 units in control patients ($P = 0.68$).

Conclusions.—Large volumes of fluids infused during AAA repair already conserve blood by the mechanism of hypervolaemic haemodilution. When cell salvage is used with standard fluid management during AAA repair, additional ANH is ineffective in saving blood.

► I have never been convinced that ANH (acute normovolemic hemodilution) in patients undergoing aortic aneurysm surgery was of much value. This is especially so with the wide availability of cell savers in most operating rooms. There is no reason for ANH in vascular surgical patients.

G. L. Moneta, MD

Randomized Clinical Trial of Intraoperative Autotransfusion in Surgery for Abdominal Aortic Aneurysm

Mercer KG, Spark JI, Berridge DC, et al (St James's Univ, Leeds, England)
Br J Surg 91:1443-1448, 2004 3–17

Background.—Perioperative homologous blood transfusion (HBT) is associated with adverse reactions and risks transmission of infection. It has also been implicated as an immunosuppressive agent. Intraoperative autotransfusion (IAT) is a potential method of autologous transfusion.

Methods.—This was a single-centre randomized clinical trial of IAT in surgery for abdominal aortic aneurysm. Forty patients were randomized to IAT and 41 underwent surgery with HBT only. Patients in both groups received HBT to maintain haemoglobin levels above 8 g/dl. Transfusion requirements, and incidence of systemic inflammatory response syndrome (SIRS) and infection, were compared.

Results.—Significantly fewer patients in the IAT group required HBT (21 *versus* 31; $P = 0.038$) and the median blood requirement per patient was 2 units lower ($P = 0.012$). There was a higher incidence of chest infection (12 *versus* four patients; $P = 0.049$) and SIRS (20 *versus* nine patients; $P = 0.020$) in the HBT group. Risk of SIRS was related to aortic cross-clamp time in the IAT group only.

Conclusion.—Use of autotransfusion effectively reduced the need for HBT and was associated with a reduced incidence of postoperative SIRS and infective complications.

▶ The authors' findings that IAT is associated with reduced postoperative infection is consistent with observational studies linking a diminished immunologic response with HBT. The mechanism of this potential decrease in immunologic competence with HBT is unknown. The observation, however, provides another reason, in addition to conserving blood bank resources and diminishing direct bloodborne infections, to use IAT.

G. L. Moneta, MD

Genomic and Proteomic Determinants of Outcome in Patients Undergoing Thoracoabdominal Aortic Aneurysm Repair

Feezor RJ, Baker HV, Xiao W, et al (Univ of Florida, Gainesville; Stanford Genome Technology Ctr, Palo Alto, Calif; Zyomyx, Hayward, Calif)

J Immunol 172:7103-7109, 2004 3–18

Introduction.—Thoracoabdominal aortic aneurysm repair, with its requisite intraoperative mesenteric ischemia-reperfusion, often results in the development of systemic inflammatory response syndrome, multiorgan dysfunction syndrome (MODS), and death. In the present study, an adverse clinical outcome following thoracoabdominal aortic aneurysm repair was identified by blood leukocyte genomic and plasma proteomic responses. Time-dependent changes in the expression of 146 genes from blood leukocytes were observed ($p < 0.001$). Expression of 138 genes ($p < 0.001$) and the concentration of seven plasma proteins discriminated between patients who developed MODS and those who did not, and many of these differences were evident even before surgery. These findings suggest that changes in blood leukocyte gene expression and plasma protein concentrations can illuminate pathophysiological processes that are subsequently associated with the clinical sequelae of systemic inflammatory response syndrome and MODS. These changes in gene expression and plasma protein concentrations are often observed before surgery, consistent with either a genetic predisposition or pre-existing inflammatory state.

► Genetic array studies are producing some fascinating information. This study parallels previous studies suggesting activation of specific genes and gene products after vascular procedures. The current study, like those previously, is too much of a "shotgun" approach to be clinically useful. The idea that systemic inflammatory response syndrome or MODS can be predicted preoperatively does, however, have clear implications as to selection of patients for complex aortic surgery.

G. L. Moneta, MD

Activation of Fibrinolytic Pathways Is Associated With Duration of Supraceliac Aortic Cross-Clamping

Haithcock BE, Shepard AD, Raman SBK, et al (Henry Ford Hosp, Detroit)
J Vasc Surg 40:325-333, 2004 3–19

Purpose.—The cause of the coagulopathy seen with supraceliac aortic cross-clamping (SC AXC) is unclear. SC AXC for 30 minutes results in both clotting factor consumption and activation of fibrinolytic pathways. This study was undertaken to define the hemostatic alterations that occur with longer intervals of SC AXC.

Methods.—Seven pigs underwent SC AXC for 60 minutes. Five pigs that underwent infrarenal aortic cross-clamping (IR AXC) for 60 minutes and 11 pigs that underwent SC AXC for 30 minutes served as controls. No heparin was used. Blood samples were drawn at baseline, 5 minutes before release of the aortic clamp, and 5, 30, and 60 minutes after unclamping. Prothrombin time, partial thromboplastin time, platelet count, and fibrinogen concentration were measured as basic tests of hemostatic function. Thrombin-antithrombin complexes were used to detect the presence of intravascular thrombosis. Fibrinolytic pathway activation was assessed with levels of tissue plasminogen activator antigen and tissue plasminogen activator activity, plasminogen activator inhibitor-1 activity, and $\alpha2$-antiplasmin activity. Statistical analysis was performed with the Student *t* test and repeated measures of analysis of variance.

Results.—Prothrombin time, partial thromboplastin time, and platelet count did not differ between groups at any time. Fibrinogen concentration decreased 5 minutes ($P = .005$) and 30 minutes ($P = .006$) after unclamping in both SC AXC groups, but did not change in the IR AXC group. Thrombin-antithrombin complexes increased in both SC AXC groups, but were not significantly greater than in the IR AXC group. SC AXC for both 30 and 60 minutes produced a significant increase in tissue plasminogen activator antigen during clamping and 5 minutes after clamping. This increase persisted for 30 and 60 minutes after clamp release in the 60-minute SC AXC group. Tissue plasminogen activator activity, however, increased only in the 60-min SC AXC group during clamping ($P = .02$), and 5 minutes ($P = .05$)

and 30 minutes (P = .06) after unclamping, compared with both control groups.

Conclusions.—Thirty and 60 minutes of SC AXC results in similar degrees of intravascular thrombosis and fibrinogen depletion. Although SC AXC for both 30 and 60 minutes leads to activation of fibrinolytic pathways, only 60 minutes of SC AXC actually induces a fibrinolytic state. Fibrinolysis appears to be an important component of the coagulopathy associated with SC AXC, and is related to the duration of aortic clamping.

▶ I would predict that almost any human being who has his or her supraceliac aorta clamped for more than 1 hour is going to have problems. This study extends that impression to pigs as well. Studies in human beings are needed to confirm the hypothesis that specific types of coagulopathy can be induced by aortic clamping. If this is true, specific types of blood product replacement as the duration of ischemia increases may be advisable.

G. L. Moneta, MD

Prospective Decision Analysis Modeling Indicates That Clinical Decisions in Vascular Surgery Often Fail to Maximize Patient Expected Utility

Brothers TE, Cox MH, Robison JG, et al (Med Univ of South Carolina, Charleston)

J Surg Res 120:278-287, 2004 3–20

Background.—Applied prospectively to patients with peripheral arterial disease, individualized decision analysis has the potential to improve the surgeon's ability to optimize patient outcome.

Methods.—A prospective, randomized trial comparing Markov surgical decision analysis to standard decision-making was performed in 206 patients with symptomatic lower extremity arterial disease. Utility assessment and quality of life were determined from individual patients prior to treatment. Vascular surgeons provided estimates of probability of treatment outcome, intended and actual treatment plans, and assessment of comfort with the decision (PDPI). Treatment plans and PDPI evaluations were repeated after each surgeon was made aware of model predictions for half of the patients in a randomized manner.

Results.—Optimal treatments predicted by decision analysis differed significantly from the surgeon's initial plan and consisted of bypass for 30 *versus* 29%, respectively, angioplasty for 28 *versus* 11%, amputation for 31 *versus* 6%, and medical management for 34 *versus* 54% (agreement 50%, kappa 0.28). Surgeon awareness of the decision model results did not alter the verbalized final plan, but did trend toward less frequent use of bypass. Patients for whom the model agreed with the surgeon's initial plan were less likely to undergo bypass (13 *versus*30%, $P < 0.01$). Greater surgeon comfort was present when the initial plan and model agreed (PDPI score 47.5 *versus* 45.6, $P < 0.005$).

Conclusions.—Individualized application of a decision model to patients with peripheral arterial disease suggests that arterial bypass is frequently recommended even when it may not maximize patient expected utility.

► Anyone who has been in practice for more than 2 heartbeats does not need decision analysis to realize that a lot of surgery gets done that is not likely to truly help the patient. This study is basically quantifying the obvious.

G. L. Moneta, MD

Are Patients Receiving Maximal Medical Therapy Following Carotid Endarterectomy?

Betancourt M, Van Stavern RB, Share D, et al (Wayne State Univ, Detroit; Blue Cross and Blue Shield of Michigan Ctr for Health Care Quality & Evaluative Studies, Detroit)

Neurology 63:2011-2015, 2004 3–21

Background.—Most patients in the North American Symptomatic Carotid Endarterectomy Trial (NASCET) did not receive lipid-lowering treatment. As vascular event rates can be lowered with statins, antihypertensive agents, and newer antiplatelet agents, the authors conducted a study to determine the usage of these medications in patients following carotid endarterectomy (CE).

Methods.—Claims data from Blue Cross and Blue Shield Michigan were used to study non-Medicare members who underwent CE in the years 1999 to 2001 (n = 1,049). Prescription of pharmacotherapy and sustained use (>80% use of the follow-up period) were examined in the 365-day period following index CE.

Results.—Overall, 1,049 individuals underwent CE during the years 1999 to 2001. For the 1-year period following CE, the statin prescription rate was 70, 66, and 73% for the 3 study years. Sustained statin use was noted, on average, in 38%. The 3-year average was lower for sustained use of angiotensin-converting enzyme inhibitor (19%) and even lower for prescription antiplatelet agents (5%).

Conclusions.—Use of statins has increased following carotid endarterectomy (CE) compared with the North American Symptomatic Carotid Endarterectomy Trial era, but sustained treatment with statins remains at <40%. Recent studies have shown a decrease in vascular event rates with statins regardless of low-density lipoprotein level, suggesting that statin use should be routine following CE. Increased statin use as part of a multimodality intensive medical regimen following CE has the potential to improve long-term vascular event rates in this population.

► The answer to the question posed in the title of the paper appears to be no. We all need to do better.

G. L. Moneta, MD

Predictors of Complications After a Prospective Evaluation of Diagnostic and Therapeutic Endovascular Procedures

Danetz JS, McLafferty RB, Schmittling ZC, et al (Southern Illinois Univ, Springfield)

J Vasc Surg 40:1142-1148, 2004 3–22

Objective.—To prospectively evaluate complications after diagnostic and therapeutic endovascular procedures (DTEPs) and determine what factors are predictive.

Methods.—From December 2002 to December 2003, all patients undergoing DTEPs performed by university vascular surgeons in a catheterization laboratory were prospectively evaluated. Medical demographics, procedure-related details, and type and severity of complications were recorded at the time of the procedure, during the first 24 hours, and at 2 to 4 weeks. Complications were classified as local vascular (LV), local nonvascular (LNV), systemic remote (SR), and major, minor, and nonsignificant.

Results.—Three hundred-three DTEPs were performed (54.5% DEPs, 45.5% TEPs). At the time of DTEP, 28 complications occurred in 23 patients: 10 LV (3.3%), 15 LNV (5.0%), and 3 SR (1.0%). At 24 hours, 26 complications occurred in 25 patients: 5 LV (1.7%), 7 LNV (2.3%), and 14 SR (4.7%). At 2 to 4 weeks, 26 complications occurred 25 patients: 5 LV (1.7%), 7 LNV (2.3%), and 14 SR (4.7%). The combined major (7.3%) and minor (4.3%) complication rate attributed to DTEPs was 11.6%. Significant predictors ($P < .05$) by multivariate analysis included thrombolysis, prior stroke, an additional procedure during the study period, and diabetes mellitus (odds ratios: 9.1, 3.2, 2.7, and 2.4, respectively).

Conclusion.—According to newly applied reporting standards, the prospective evaluation of DTEPs reveals that complications are uniformly distributed by type and follow-up period. Just over 1 in 10 patients will suffer either a major or minor complication. Potential predictors have been identified that may assist in patient selection and treatment plans to lower complications resulting from DTEPs.

▶ This is a rare prospective assessment of complications of catheter-based DTEPs. The authors' use of strict reporting standards is to be commended. Vascular surgical units need to update their databases to track complications of endovascular as well as open vascular procedures, otherwise they are guilty of the same reporting standard offenses of interventional radiologies in the 1980s.

G. L. Moneta, MD

Biological Assessment of Aspirin Efficacy on Healthy Individuals: Heterogeneous Response or Aspirin Failure?

Gonzalez-Conejero R, Rivera J, Corral J, et al (Univ of Murcia, Spain)

Stroke 36:276-280, 2005 3–23

Background and Purpose.—The widespread use of aspirin requires clarification of the aspirin resistance phenomenon. Most studies on this field are focused on patients which may affect the action of aspirin.

Methods.—We evaluated the biological efficacy of aspirin in healthy subjects.

Results.—Agonist-induced platelet aggregation was fully abrogated by 100 mg of aspirin in all individuals. By contrast, with the platelet function analyzer-100 device, 33.3% of the subjects displayed no response. This failure was overcome by 500 mg or by in vitro treatment of blood with 30 μmol/L acetylsalicylic acid. Intake of 100 mg of aspirin efficiently reduced by 75% the level of 11-dehydro thromboxane B_2 (11-dTxB_2) in all cases. However, variability on the pre-aspirin level (range 72.4 to 625.9 ng/mmol creatinine) led to substantial differences in the residual amount of the metabolite between subjects treated with aspirin (range 12.9 to 118.0 ng/mmol creatinine). Finally, there was no influence of platelet glycoprotein IIb/IIIa (Pro33Leu), platelet glycoprotein Ia/IIa, (C807T), and FXIII (Val34Leu) polymorphisms on the efficacy of aspirin. However, the cyclooxygenase (Cox)-1 *50T* allele associated with higher level of 11-dTxB_2, both before and after aspirin. Moreover, the Cox-2 −765C variant displayed a slightly higher reduction in 11-dTxB_2 level on treatment with aspirin.

Conclusions.—Our findings suggest that full resistance of healthy subjects to aspirin is rather unlikely. However, differences in aspirin absorption, or pharmacokinetic, or other unrecognized factors may lead to lack of effect of low dose of aspirin in some subjects when using tests like platelet function analyzer-100. Whether Cox polymorphisms are thrombotic risk factor for patients under aspirin will require further research.

► Studies of the aspirin resistance phenomenon have reported conflicting results. The next 2 reports (Abstracts 3–24 and 3–25) examine issues surrounding aspirin resistance and possible clinical importance of this phenomenon. This study suggests so-called aspirin resistance may be multifactorial and include differences in bioavailability (ie, absorption) of aspirin as well as polymorphisms of the COX genes. Testing for true aspirin resistance is going to require more than one blood test.

G. L. Moneta, MD

Randomized Clinical Trial of the Antiplatelet Effects of Aspirin–Clopidogrel Combination Versus Aspirin Alone After Lower Limb Angioplasty

Cassar K, Ford I, Greaves M, et al (Univ of Aberdeen, United Kingdom; Aberdeen Royal Infirmary, United Kingdom)

Br J Surg 92:159-165, 2005 3–24

Background.—There is a high risk of reocclusion after successful lower limb angioplasty. Platelets play a central role in this process. The aim of this study was to investigate the antiplatelet effect of a combination of aspirin and clopidogrel compared with aspirin alone in patients with claudication undergoing endovascular revascularization.

Methods.—This was a double-blind randomized placebo-controlled trial Some 132 patients were randomized to clopidogrel and aspirin or placebo and aspirin, with a loading dose 12 h before endovascular intervention. Flow cytometric measurements of platelet fibrinogen binding and P-selectin expression were taken as measures of platelet function at baseline, 12 h after the loading dose, and 1 h, 24 h and 30 days after intervention.

Results.—Within 12 h of the loading dose, platelet activation in the clopidogrel group had decreased (P-selectin by 27.3 per cent, $P = 0.017$; fibrinogen binding by 34.7 per cent, $P = 0.024$; stimulated fibrinogen binding by 49.2 per cent, $P < 0.001$). No change was observed in the placebo group. Platelet function in the clopidogrel group was significantly suppressed compared with baseline at 1 h, 24 h and 30 days after endovascular intervention (stimulated fibrinogen binding by 53.9, 51.7 and 57.2 per cent respectively; all $P < 0.001$).

Conclusion.—A combination of clopidogrel and aspirin inhibited platelet function more than aspirin alone in patients with claudication before and after angioplasty.

► The data here show a much greater antiplatelet effect with clopidogrel and aspirin versus aspirin alone in patients undergoing lower limb angioplasty. Clinical efficacy was not examined. Perhaps someone needs another publication. It is certainly easier to study blood samples than patients.

G. L. Moneta, MD

Chronic Kidney Disease and the Risks of Death, Cardiovascular Events, and Hospitalization

Go AS, Chertow GM, Fan D, et al (Kaiser Permanente of Northern California, Oakland; Univ of California, San Francisco)

N Engl J Med 351:1296-1305, 2004 3–25

Background.—End-stage renal disease substantially increases the risks of death, cardiovascular disease, and use of specialized health care, but the effects of less severe kidney dysfunction on these outcomes are less well defined.

Methods.—We estimated the longitudinal glomerular filtration rate (GFR) among 1,120,295 adults within a large, integrated system of health care delivery in whom serum creatinine had been measured between 1996 and 2000 and who had not undergone dialysis or kidney transplantation. We examined the multivariable association between the estimated GFR and the risks of death, cardiovascular events, and hospitalization.

Results.—The median follow-up was 2.84 years, the mean age was 52 years, and 55 percent of the group were women. After adjustment, the risk of death increased as the GFR decreased below 60 ml per minute per 1.73 m^2 of body-surface area: the adjusted hazard ratio for death was 1.2 with an estimated GFR of 45 to 59 ml per minute per 1.73 m^2 (95 percent confidence interval, 1.1 to 1.2), 1.8 with an estimated GFR of 30 to 44 ml per minute per 1.73 m^2 (95 percent confidence interval, 1.7 to 1.9), 3.2 with an estimated GFR of 15 to 29 ml per minute per 1.73 m^2 (95 percent confidence interval, 3.1 to 3.4), and 5.9 with an estimated GFR of less than 15 ml per minute per 1.73 m^2 (95 percent confidence interval, 5.4 to 6.5). The adjusted hazard ratio for cardiovascular events also increased inversely with the estimated GFR: 1.4 (95 percent confidence interval, 1.4 to 1.5), 2.0 (95 percent confidence interval, 1.9 to 2.1), 2.8 (95 percent confidence interval, 2.6 to 2.9), and 3.4 (95 percent confidence interval, 3.1 to 3.8), respectively. The adjusted risk of hospitalization with a reduced estimated GFR followed a similar pattern.

Conclusions.—An independent, graded association was observed between a reduced estimated GFR and the risk of death, cardiovascular events, and hospitalization in a large, community-based population. These findings highlight the clinical and public health importance of chronic renal insufficiency.

► Chronic renal disease, even when it does not necessitate dialysis, has considerable adverse effects. While clearly the prevention of end-stage renal disease is important, more effective management of patients with milder levels of renal insufficiency is also needed to reduce the adverse health effects of lesser levels of impaired renal function.

G. L. Moneta, MD

Effect of *N*-Acetylcysteine for Prevention of Contrast Nephropathy in Patients With Moderate to Severe Renal Insufficiency: A Randomized Trial

Fung JWH, Szeto CC, Chan WWM, et al (Chinese Univ of Hong Kong)

Am J Kidney Dis 43:801-808, 2004 3–26

Background.—The effect of *N*-acetylcysteine (NAC) to prevent contrast nephropathy (CN) in patients with moderate to severe renal insufficiency undergoing coronary angiography or interventions is not clear.

Methods.—This is a prospective, open-label, randomized, controlled trial. Ninety-one consecutive patients with a serum creatinine level of 1.69 to 4.52 mg/dL (149 to 400 μmol/L) undergoing coronary procedures were recruited and randomly assigned to administration of either oral NAC, 400 mg, thrice daily the day before and day of the contrast procedure (the NAC group) or no drug (the control group). Serum creatinine was measured before and 48 hours after contrast exposure. The primary end point of this study was the development of CN, defined as an increase in serum creatinine concentration of 0.5 mg/dL or greater (≥44 μmol/L) or a reduction in estimated glomerular filtration rate (GFR) of 25% or greater of the baseline value 48 hours after the procedure.

Results.—There were no significant differences between the 2 groups (46 patients, NAC group; 45 patients, control group) in baseline characteristics or mean volume of contrast agent administered. Six patients (13.3%) in the control group and 8 patients (17.4%) in the NAC group developed CN (P = 0.8). Serum creatinine levels increased from 2.27 ± 0.54 to 2.45 ± 0.65 mg/dL (201 ± 48 to 217 ± 57 μmol/L; P = 0.003) in the NAC group and 2.37 ± 0.61 to 2.40 ± 0.70 mg/dL (210 ± 54 to 212 ± 62 μmol/L; P = 0.6) in the control group. The increase in serum creatinine levels between the 2 groups had no difference (P = 0.7). Estimated GFR decreased from 30.3 ± 8.4 to 28.1 ± 8.4 mL/min (P = 0.01) in the NAC group and 28.4 ± 8.6 to 27.5 ± 8.8 mL/min (P = 0.3) in the control group. The decline in estimated GFR between the 2 groups had no difference (P = 0.7).

Conclusion.—In the current study, oral NAC had no effect on the prevention of CN in patents with moderate to severe renal insufficiency undergoing coronary angiography or interventions. However, the sample size of our present study is small. Our findings highlight the need for a large-scale, randomized, controlled trial to determine the exact beneficial effect of NAC.

▶ This and the following 3 articles (Abstracts 3–27 to 3–29) examine the issue of venal protection at the time of contrast administration. In this article, the authors also summarized 15 previous reports evaluating the effect of NAC on prevention of CN in patients with renal insufficiency. Only 5 of the 15 reports indicated benefit for NAC to prevent CN. The largest trial evaluating NAC in the prevention of CN showed a positive result, but the patients in that study had relatively mild renal impairment. The potential benefit of NAC in preventing CN in patients with more significant degrees of renal impairment remains unproven. This study indicates administration of prophylactic NAC to prevent CN in patients with significant renal impairment is not effective.

G. L. Moneta, MD

Prevention of Contrast-Induced Nephropathy in Vascular Patients Undergoing Angiography: A Randomized Controlled Trial of Intravenous N-Acetylcysteine

Rashid ST, Salman M, Myint F, et al (Royal Free Hosp, London)

J Vasc Surg 40:1136-1141, 2004 3–27

Objectives.—Apart from proper hydration, only oral N-acetylcysteine (NAC) has shown efficacy in reducing radiographic contrast media (RCM)-

induced acute renal failure, though its benefit has been challenged. We investigated the effect of intravenous (i.v.) NAC on renal function in patients with vascular disease receiving RCM for angiography.

Methods.—Single-center, randomized, double-blind, placebo-controlled trial. Based on a previous study, a trial with 44 patients each in placebo and treatment arms would give at least 80% power to show a statistically significant difference at the 5% level. Vascular patients undergoing angiography were consented and segregated into those whose serum creatinine (SC) level was normal or raised (men >1.32 mg/dl; women >1.07 mg/dL). All patients received 500 mL i.v. normal saline 6 to 12 hours prior to and then after angiography. Groups with normal SC and raised SC were randomly assigned to either 1 g of NAC with normal saline before and after angiography or nothing (placebo). Main outcome measures were change in SC and creatinine clearance (CrCl) as measured 1, 2, and 7 days postangiography (with comparison between active and placebo groups using unpaired t test) and incidence of acute renal decline (>25% or 0.5 mg/dL rise in SC) at 48 hours (with comparison between active and placebo using the Fisher exact test).

Results.—Forty-six patients received NAC (29 normal SC, 17 raised SC), and 48 received placebo (27 normal SC, 21 raised SC). There was no significant difference in postangiography SC or CrCl at any of the time points measured between NAC and placebo in patients with either normal or raised SC. In the raised SC group, 3 patients from both the NAC and placebo groups suffered acute renal declines. Importantly, at 48 hours, the impaired SC group had a significant reduction in CrCl (−14% ± 41% vs +18% ± 58%: P = .0142) and a significant rise in SC (+7.0 ± 25% vs −1.6% ± 10%; P = .0246) when compared with the normal SC group.

Conclusions.—NAC (i.v. at 1 g) precontrast and postcontrast does not confer any benefit in preventing RCM-induced nephropathy in vascular patients. Patients with pre-existing raised SC have an increased risk of renal impairment as defined by a fall in CrCl and a rise in SC post-RCM when compared with patients with normal SC who appear to benefit from hydration.

► Similar results as in the previous abstract (Abstract 3–26), only this time in vascular patients with varying levels of renal function. There should be decreasing interest in the use of *N*-acetylcystine in vascular surgical patients.

G. L. Moneta, MD

N-Acetylcysteine Versus Fenoldopam Mesylate to Prevent Contrast Agent-associated Nephrotoxicity

Briguori C, Colombo A, Airoldi F, et al (Clinica Mediterranea, Naples, Italy; "Vita e Salute" Univ, Milan, Italy)

J Am Coll Cardiol 44:762-765, 2004 3–28

Objectives.—We performed a study to assess the efficacy of fenoldopam mesylate (a specific agonist of the dopamine-1 receptor) as compared with

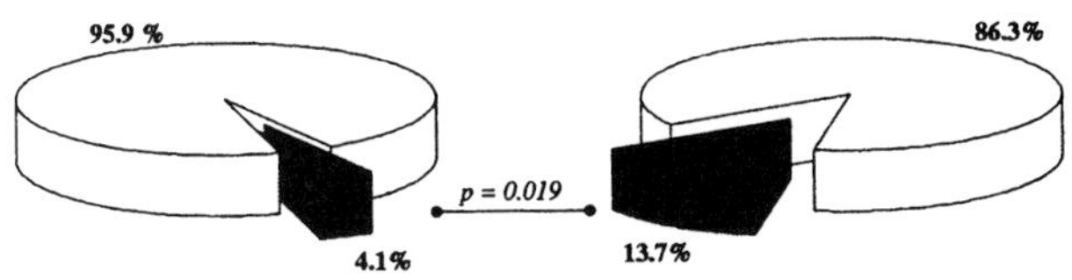

NAC Group **Fenoldopam Group**

FIGURE 1.—Schematic representation of the distribution of the occurrence of contrast agent–associated nephrotoxicity in patients with the N-acetylcysteine (NAC group) and with fenoldopam mesylate (fenoldopam group). *Filled areas* = cases with event; *open areas* = cases without event. (Courtesy of Brigouri C, Colombo A, Airoldi F, et al: N-acetylcysteine versus fenoldopam mesylate to prevent contrast agent-associated nephrotoxicity. *J Am Coll Cardiol* 44:762-765, 2004. Reprinted with permission from the American College of Cardiology.)

N-acetylcysteine (NAC) in preventing contrast agent-associated nephrotoxicity (CAN).

Background.—Prophylactic administration of NAC, along with hydration, prevents CAN in patients with chronic renal insufficiency who are undergoing contrast media administration. Preliminary data support the hypothesis that fenoldopam might be as effective as NAC.

Methods.—One hundred ninety-two consecutive patients with chronic renal insufficiency, referred to our institution for coronary and/or peripheral procedures, were assigned randomly to receive 0.45% saline intravenously and NAC (1,200 mg orally twice daily; NAC group; n = 97) or fenoldopam (0.10 µg/kg/min; fenoldopam group; n = 95) before and after a nonionic, iso-osmolality contrast dye administration.

Results.—Baseline creatinine levels were similar in the two groups: NAC group = 1.72 mg/dl (interquartile range, 1.55 to 1.90 mg/dl) and fenoldopam group = 1.75 mg/dl (interquartile range, 1.62 to 2.01 mg/dl) (p = 0.17). An increase of at least 0.5 mg/dl of the creatinine concentration 48 h after the procedure occurred in 4 of 97 patients (4.1%) in the NAC group and in 13 of 95 patients (13.7%) in the fenoldopam group (p = 0.019; odds ratio 0.27; 95% confidence interval 0.08 to 0.85) (Fig 1). The amount of contrast media administration was similar in the two groups (NAC group = 160 ± 82 ml; fenoldopam group = 168 ± 104 ml; p = 0.54).

Conclusions.—N-acetylcysteine seems to be more effective than fenoldopam in preventing CAN.

► Fenoldopam is thought to potentially selectively increase blood flow to the renal medulla. The findings in this study, however, indicate fenoldopam is ineffective in preventing further renal function deterioration in patients with chronic renal insufficiency receiving an iodated contrast agent. Based on these data and considering the high cost of fenoldopam, the strategy of hydration plus fenoldopam should not be used as a prophylactic measure to prevent contrast nephropathy. The study is difficult to interpret given the results of the previous 2 abstracts (Abstracts 3–26 and 3–27). Could fenoldopam actually make things worse?

G. L. Moneta, MD

Prevention of Contrast-Induced Nephropathy With Sodium Bicarbonate: A Randomized Controlled Trial

Merten GJ, Burgess WP, Gray LV, et al (Carolinas Med Ctr, Charlotte, NC)
JAMA 291:2328-2334, 2004 3–29

Context.—Contrast-induced nephropathy remains a common complication of radiographic procedures. Pretreatment with sodium bicarbonate is more protective than sodium chloride in animal models of acute ischemic renal failure. Acute renal failure from both ischemia and contrast are postulated to occur from free-radical injury. However, no studies in humans or animals have evaluated the efficacy of sodium bicarbonate for prophylaxis against contrast-induced nephropathy.

Objective.—To examine the efficacy of sodium bicarbonate compared with sodium chloride for preventive hydration before and after radiographic contrast.

Design, Setting, and Patients.—A prospective, single-center, randomized trial conducted from September 16, 2002, to June 17, 2003, of 119 patients with stable serum creatinine levels of at least 1.1 mg/dL (≥97.2 µmol/L) who were randomized to receive a 154-mEq/L infusion of either sodium chloride (n = 59) or sodium bicarbonate (n = 60) before and after iopamidol administration (370 mg iodine/mL). Serum creatinine levels were measured at baseline and 1 and 2 days after contrast.

Interventions.—Patients received 154 mEq/L of either sodium chloride or sodium bicarbonate, as a bolus of 3 mL/kg per hour for 1 hour before iopamidol contrast, followed by an infusion of 1 mL/kg per hour for 6 hours after the procedure.

Main Outcome Measure.—Contrast-induced nephropathy, defined as an increase of 25% or more in serum creatinine within 2 days of contrast.

Results.—There were no significant group differences in age, sex, incidence of diabetes mellitus, ethnicity, or contrast volume. Baseline serum creatinine was slightly higher but not statistically different in patients receiving sodium bicarbonate treatment (mean [SD], 1.71 [0.42] mg/dL [151.2 [37.1] µmol/L] for sodium chloride and 1.89 [0.69] mg/dL [167.1 [61.0] µmol/L] for sodium bicarbonate; P=.09). The primary end point of contrast-induced nephropathy occurred in 8 patients (13.6%) infused with sodium chloride but in only 1 (1.7%) of those receiving sodium bicarbonate (mean difference, 11.9%; 95% confidence interval [CI], 2.6%-21.2%; P=.02). A follow-up registry of 191 consecutive patients receiving prophylactic sodium bicarbonate and meeting the same inclusion criteria as the study resulted in 3 cases of contrast-induced nephropathy (1.6%; 95% CI, 0%-3.4%).

Conclusion.—Hydration with sodium bicarbonate before contrast exposure is more effective than hydration with sodium chloride for prophylaxis of contrast-induced renal failure.

▶ The success of sodium bicarbonate in reducing contrast-induced nephropathy in this study is consistent with the hypothesis that contrast injury is induced by free radicals. This is an excellent study with well-analyzed data. It presents persuasive data that sodium bicarbonate, rather than sodium chloride, should be used to provide preprocedure and postprocedure hydration in patients undergoing contrast administration. We have adopted the protocol for administration of sodium bicarbonate in conjunction with contrast angiography in our vascular surgery patients.

G. L. Moneta, MD

Vascular Risk Factors and Diabetic Neuropathy

Tesfaye S, for the EURODIAB Prospective Complications Study Group (Royal Hallamshire Hosp, Sheffield, England; et al)
N Engl J Med 352:341-350, 2005 3–30

Background.—Other than glycemic control, there are no treatments for diabetic neuropathy. Thus, identifying potentially modifiable risk factors for neuropathy is crucial. We studied risk factors for the development of distal symmetric neuropathy in 1172 patients with type 1 diabetes mellitus from 31 centers participating in the European Diabetes (EURODIAB) Prospective Complications Study.

Methods.—Neuropathy was assessed at baseline (1989 to 1991) and at follow-up (1997 to 1999), with a mean (±SD) follow-up of 7.3±0.6 years. A standardized protocol included clinical evaluation, quantitative sensory testing, and autonomic-function tests. Serum lipids and lipoproteins, glycosylated hemoglobin, and the urinary albumin excretion rate were measured in a central laboratory.

Results.—At follow-up, neuropathy had developed in 276 of 1172 patients without neuropathy at baseline (23.5 percent). The cumulative incidence of neuropathy was related to the glycosylated hemoglobin value and the duration of diabetes. After adjustment for these factors, we found that higher levels of total and low-density lipoprotein cholesterol and triglycerides, a higher body-mass index, higher von Willebrand factor levels and urinary albumin excretion rate, hypertension, and smoking were all significantly associated with the cumulative incidence of neuropathy. After adjustment for other risk factors and diabetic complications, we found that duration of diabetes, current glycosylated hemoglobin value, change in glycosylated hemoglobin value during the follow-up period, body-mass index, and smoking remained independently associated with the incidence of neuropathy. Cardiovascular disease at baseline was associated with double the risk of neuropathy, independent of cardiovascular risk factors.

Conclusions.—This prospective study indicates that, apart from glycemic control, the incidence of neuropathy is associated with potentially modifiable cardiovascular risk factors, including a raised triglyceride level, body-mass index, smoking, and hypertension.

▶ Glycemic control is the only method to treat diabetic neuropathy. The authors have identified potentially modifiable risk factors for diabetic neuropathy in patients with type 1 diabetes. The obvious hope is that by identification of such risk factors, treatment may lower the incidence of diabetic neuropathy and subsequent amputations resulting from complications of neuropathy.

G. L. Moneta, MD

Effect of Low Molecular Weight Heparin (Dalteparin) and Fondaparinux (Arixtra) on Human Osteoblasts In Vitro

Handschin AE, Trentz OA, Hoerstrup SP, et al (Univ Hosp of Zurich, Switzerland; Univ of Heidelberg, Germany)

Br J Surg 92:177-183, 2005 3–31

Background.—The prolonged administration of heparin for prevention and treatment of venous thromboembolism has been associated with a risk of heparin-induced osteoporosis. Fondaparinux is a new antithrombotic drug that specifically inhibits factor Xa. Because of the known interactions of other antithrombotic agents with bone remodelling, the effects of fondaparinux on human osteoblasts were analysed in vitro.

Methods.—Primary human osteoblast cell cultures were incubated with either the low molecular weight heparin dalteparin at concentrations of 30, 300 and 900 µg/ml or with fondaparinux at concentrations of 25, 50, 100, 150, 200 and 250 µg/ml. Cellular proliferation rate and protein synthesis were measured. Expression of genes encoding osteocalcin, collagen type I and alkaline phosphatase was examined by reverse transcriptase–polymerase chain reaction.

Results.—Incubation with dalteparin led to a significant, dose-dependent inhibition of osteoblast proliferation, inhibition of protein synthesis, and inhibited expression of phenotype markers (*osteocalcin* and *alkaline phosphatase* genes) after 3 and 7 days. No inhibitory effects were observed in the fondaparinux-treated cells.

Conclusion.—Fondaparinux did not inhibit osteoblast proliferation in vitro and may reduce the risk of heparin-induced osteoporosis associated with long-term heparin administration.

▶ Heparin-induced osteoporosis occurs after prolonged use of high doses of heparin. This study suggests fondaparinux may have less or no osteoporotic effects when administered at comparable high doses. This is obviously a laboratory investigation, but it appears to have been well conducted with analysis of reasonable surrogates for osteoblastic function. There is probably enough here, given the other advantages of fondaparinux compared with heparin, to recommend fondaparinux for patients requiring long-term anticoagulation and who are not candidates for warfarin therapy.

G. L. Moneta, MD

Variable Ventilation Improves Perioperative Lung Function in Patients Undergoing Abdominal Aortic Aneurysmectomy

Boker A, Haberman CJ, Girling L, et al (Abdulaziz Univ, Jeddah, Kingdom of Saudi Arabia; Univ of Manitoba, Winnipeg, Canada)

Anesthesiology 100:608-616, 2004 3–32

Background.—Optimizing perioperative mechanical ventilation remains a significant clinical challenge. Experimental models indicate that "noisy" or variable ventilation (VV)—return of physiologic variability to respiratory rate and tidal volume—improves lung function compared with monotonous control mode ventilation (CV). VV was compared with CV in patients undergoing abdominal aortic aneurysmectomy, a patient group known to be at risk of deteriorating lung function perioperatively.

Methods.—After baseline measurements under general anesthesia (CV with a tidal volume of 10 ml/kg and a respiratory rate of 10 breaths/min), patients were randomized to continue CV or switch to VV (computer control of the ventilator at the same minute ventilation but with 376 combinations of respiratory rate and tidal volume). Lung function was measured hourly for the next 6 h during surgery and recovery.

Results.—Forty-one patients for aneurysmectomy were studied. The characteristics of the patients in the two groups were similar. Repeated-measures analysis of variance (group $\times$ time interaction) revealed greater arterial oxygen partial pressure ($P = 0.011$), lower arterial carbon dioxide partial pressure ($P = 0.012$), lower dead space ventilation ($P = 0.011$), increased compliance ($P = 0.049$), and lower mean peak inspiratory pressure ($P = 0.013$) with VV.

Conclusions.—The VV mode of ventilation significantly improved lung function over CV in patients undergoing abdominal aortic aneurysmectomy.

▶ Normal ventilation is characterized by variability. In fact, most, if not all, physiologic parameters manifest some variability. Other data suggest variability of physiologic function is associated with health, and loss of variability may indicate deterioration.[1] The authors' findings are therefore compatible with the old adage "variety is the spice of life."

G. L. Moneta, MD

Reference

1. Goldberger AL: Heartbeats, hormones, and health: Is variability the spice of life? *Am J Crit Care Med* 163:1289-1296, 2001.

4 Grafts and Graft Complications

A Randomized Comparison of Radial-Artery and Saphenous-Vein Coronary Bypass Grafts

Desai ND, for the Radial Artery Patency Study Investigators (Univ of Toronto)

N Engl J Med 351:2302-2309, 2004 4–1

Background.—In the past decade, the radial artery has frequently been used for coronary bypass surgery despite concern regarding the possibility of graft spasm. Graft patency is a key predictor of long-term survival. We therefore sought to determine the relative patency rate of radial-artery and saphenous-vein grafts in a randomized trial in which we controlled for bias in the selection of patients and vessels.

Methods.—We enrolled 561 patients at 13 centers. The left internal thoracic artery was used to bypass the anterior circulation. The radial-artery graft was randomly assigned to bypass the major vessel in either the inferior (right coronary) territory or the lateral (circumflex) territory, with the saphenous-vein graft used for the opposing territory (control). The primary end point was graft occlusion, determined by angiography 8 to 12 months postoperatively.

Results.—Angiography was performed at one year in 440 patients: 8.2 percent of radial-artery grafts and 13.6 percent of saphenous-vein grafts were completely occluded (P=0.009). Diffuse narrowing of the graft (the angiographic "string sign") was present in 7.0 percent of radial-artery grafts and only 0.9 percent of saphenous-vein grafts (P=0.001). The absence of severe native-vessel stenosis was associated with an increased risk of occlusion of the radial-artery graft and diffuse narrowing of the graft. Harvesting of the radial artery was well tolerated.

Conclusions.—Radial-artery grafts are associated with a lower rate of graft occlusion at one year than are saphenous-vein grafts. Because the patency of radial-artery grafts depends on the severity of native-vessel stenosis, such grafts should preferentially be used for target vessels with high-grade lesions.

► This is the best study available evaluating the relative efficacy of radial artery and saphenous vein grafts in coronary revascularization. Despite good overall performance of radial artery grafts, there was a decrement in their performance when they were used to bypass less severe coronary stenoses. Radial artery grafts are, however, superior to saphenous vein grafts for coronary artery revascularization of target vessels with high-grade stenosis.

G. L. Moneta, MD

Radial Artery Bypass Grafts Have an Increased Occurrence of Angiographically Severe Stenosis and Occlusion Compared With Left Internal Mammary Arteries and Saphenous Vein Grafts

Khot UN, Friedman DT, Pettersson G, et al (Cleveland Clinic Found, Ohio)

Circulation 109:2086-2091, 2004 4–2

Background.—The radial artery has been increasingly used in CABG. However, angiographic outcome data have been limited.

Method and Results.—We reviewed all coronary angiography procedures from February 1996 to October 2001 and selected patients with a radial artery bypass graft. Angiographic outcomes were divided into groups as (1) occluded, (2) severe disease (≥70% stenosis, or string sign), or (3) patent (<70% stenosis). Multivariable analyses determined predictors of severe disease or occlusion. A total of 310 patients had a radial artery graft. Mean follow-up after coronary artery bypass grafting was 565±511 days. Radial artery grafts had a patency rate of 51.3%, which was significantly lower than that for left internal mammary arteries (90.3%, $P<0.0001$) or saphenous vein grafts (64.0%, $P=0.0016$). Radial artery grafts had an occlusion rate of 33.7%, compared with 4.8% for left internal mammary arteries ($P<0.0001$), and had a severe stenosis rate of 15.1%, compared with 5.9% for saphenous vein grafts ($P=0.0003$) and 4.8% for left internal mammary arteries ($P<0.0001$). Women had a worse overall radial artery patency rate than men (38.9% versus 56.1%, $P=0.025$). A radial artery graft was the most powerful multivariable predictor of severe stenosis or occlusion ($\chi^2=28.87$, $P<0.0001$). Because of diseased radial artery grafts, 58 patients required subsequent percutaneous intervention, and 26 patients required repeat CABG.

Conclusions.—In patients predominantly presenting with signs and symptoms of myocardial ischemia after CABG, radial artery grafts have lower patency rates than left internal mammary artery and saphenous vein grafts. Selective use of the radial artery is warranted, particularly in women.

► It is hard to reconcile this article with the previous one (Abstract 4–1). The results appear in contrast with the widespread belief that radial artery grafts have a high rate of patency in coronary artery bypass grafting. These data may suggest improvements in harvesting techniques, and postoperative administration of calcium channel blockers delays, rather than prevents, the previously documented poor outcome of radial artery grafts in the coronary circulation. The results in this study are certainly different from the previous abstract (Abstract 4–1). The previous study used more rigorous methods in that it was prospective, while in this study angiography was obtained for clinical suspicion of recurrent cardiac ischemia.

G. L. Moneta, MD

Temporal Genomics of Vein Bypass Grafting Through Oligonucleotide Microarray Analysis

Kalish JA, Willis DJ, Li C, et al (Beth Israel Deaconess Med Ctr, Boston; Harvard School of Public Health, Boston)

J Vasc Surg 39:645-654, 2004 4–3

Objective.—Autologous vein is the conduit of choice for small artery reconstruction. Despite excellent patency, these conduits undergo remodeling over time. The purpose of this study was to identify temporal gene expression in vein grafts versus control veins through microarray analysis.

Method.—Cephalic vein grafts (n = 12) were used to bypass femoral arteries in canines. Vein grafts were harvested after 1, 7, 14, and 30 days. Normal contralateral cephalic vein served as control. Total RNA was isolated; its quantity and quality were confirmed with spectrophotometry and gel electrophoresis. Affymetrix U133A GeneChips, comprising approximately 15,000 genes, were used to analyze differential gene expression at each time point. Statistical analysis was performed with Affymetrix and dChip software to identify consistently upregulated and downregulated genes. Real-time, quantitative reverse transcriptase polymerase chain reaction (qRT-PCR) and immunohistochemistry were used to validate microarray data.

Results.—Statistical analysis revealed that 49 genes were consistently upregulated and 31 genes were consistently downregulated in all three animals at various time points. qRT-PCR to quantitatively assess messenger RNA expression was performed on specific genes to validate the microarray data. Immunohistochemistry to qualitatively assess protein expression was used for further validation. Hierarchical clustering with dChip identified additional genes with similar temporal or functional expression patterns.

Conclusions.—This is the first study to use microarray analysis with confirmatory qRT-PCR to identify altered genes after vein bypass grafting. Oligonucleotide microarrays and hierarchical clustering are powerful tools to generate hypotheses as the basis for additional research on gene expression in vein graft remodeling. Ultimately, identification of a temporal sequence of differential gene expression may provide insights not preferred into the molecular mechanisms of vein graft remodeling, but also into the pathways leading to intimal hyperplasia.

► As pointed out elsewhere in the YEAR BOOK, genetic microarrays are being utilized to examine upregulation and downregulation of genes that accompany many vascular conditions. This research will not have immediate practical impact. It merely identifies differing gene expression but offers no insight into how or why the genes upregulate or downregulate, what gene products are involved, and the sequence or magnitude of gene expression. Studies such as this may eventually suggest more targeted research projects, but I bet it will be awhile.

G. L. Moneta, MD

Endothelium Properties of a Tissue-Engineered Blood Vessel for Small-Diameter Vascular Reconstruction

Rémy-Zolghadri M, Laganière J, Oligny J-F, et al (Saint-Sacrement Hosp, Sainte-Foy, Québec, Canada; Laval Univ, Québec, Canada)

J Vasc Surg 39:613-620, 2004 4–4

Purpose.—A tissue-engineered blood vessel (TEBV) produced in vitro by the self-assembly method was developed in our laboratory for the replacement of small-diameter blood vessels. The interior of this vessel is covered by an endothelium. The aim of the present study was to evaluate whether the endothelial layer would make a favorable contribution at the time of implantation of the TEBV by investigating in vitro the hemocompatible properties of the endothelial cells covering its interior.

Methods.—The secretion of the von Willebrand factor (vWF) and expression of thrombomodulin by the endothelium were assessed, and the adhesive molecules E-selectin and intercellular adhesion molecule-1 (ICAM-1) were quantified as a function of maturation time. To evaluate the functional response of the endothelium on injury, the cellular response to physiological stimulatory factors (thrombin and lipopolysaccharide [LPS]) was analyzed.

Results.—The endothelial cells formed a confluent monolayer displaying favorable hemocompatible properties (78% ± 10% of cells expressing thrombomodulin with only 12 ± 3 mU/10^6 cells of vWF secreted over a 2-hour period), which acquired their full expression after a culture period of 4 days. Moreover, pro-adhesive properties toward inflammatory cells were not observed. The cells were also able to respond to physiological-stimulating agents (thrombin and LPS) and demonstrated a statistically significant overexpression of the corresponding molecules under the conditions tested.

Conclusions.—These results indicate that the endothelium of the tissue-engineered blood vessel produced by the self-assembly approach displays advantageous qualities with regard to the vessel's future implantation as a small-diameter vascular prosthesis.

► For a small-caliber arterial substitute to be successful, it is critical the luminal surface be hemocompatible. The authors have utilized well-established surrogate markers of endothelial function to establish the hemocompatibility of their arterial substitute. Of course, there are probably many more endothelial cell functions critical to maintaining patency of an arterial substitute that were not studied in this in vitro model. We await future patency and implantibility studies of this graft.

G. L. Moneta, MD

Decellularized Vein as a Potential Scaffold for Vascular Tissue Engineering

Schaner PJ, Martin ND, Tulenko TN, et al (Thomas Jefferson Univ, Philadelphia)

J Vasc Surg 40:146-153, 2004 4–5

Purpose.—Current strategies to create small-diameter vascular grafts involve seeding biocompatible, compliant scaffolds with autologous vascular cells. Our purpose was to study the composition and strength of decellularized vein to determine its potential as a vascular tissue-engineering scaffold.

Methods.—Intact human greater saphenous vein specimens were decellularized by using sodium dodecyl sulfate (SDS). Residual cellular and extracellular matrix composition was studied with light and electron microscopy as well as immunohistochemistry. Burst and suture-holding strength was measured in vitro by insufflation and pull-through techniques. To assess initial handling and durability of decellularized vein in vivo, a canine model was developed wherein decellularized canine jugular veins were implanted as carotid interposition grafts in recipient animals. After two weeks of arterial perfusion, these grafts were studied with duplex imaging and histologic methods.

Results.—Human saphenous vein decellularized by using SDS was devoid of endothelial cells and >94% of the cells resident within the vein wall (Fig 2). Collagen morphology appeared unchanged, and elastin staining decreased only slightly. Basement membrane collagen type IV remained intact. Compared with fresh vein, decellularized vein had similar in vitro burst (2480 ± 460 mm Hg vs 2380 ± 620 mm Hg; $P > .05$) and suture-holding (185 ± 30 gm vs 178 ± 66 gm; $P > .05$) strength. Decellularized canine vein func-

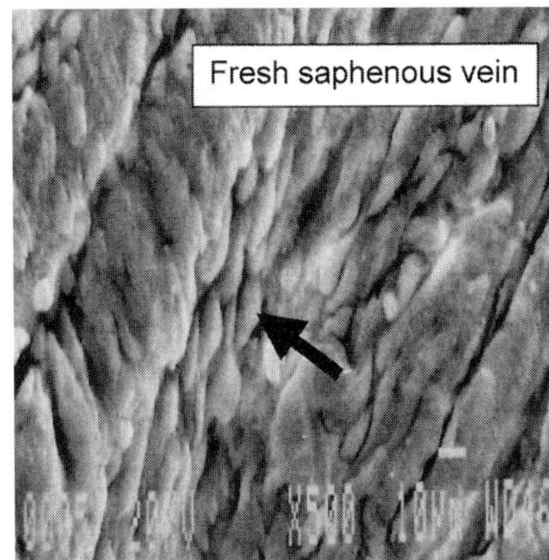

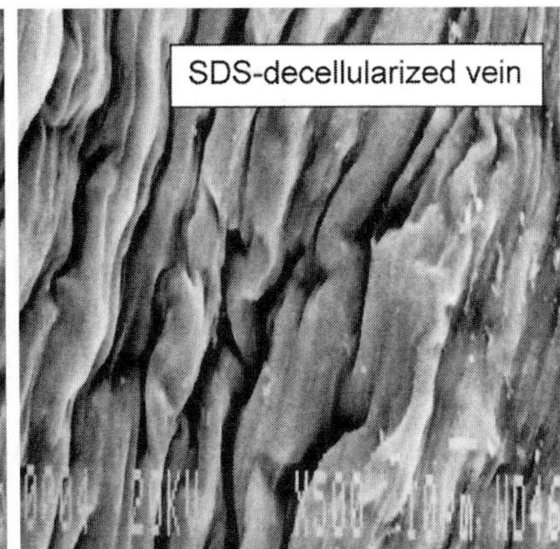

FIGURE 2.—Scanning electron micrograph of luminal surface of human greater saphenous vein before (**left**) and after (**right**) treatment with 0.075% sodium dodecyl sulfate (*SDS*) (500×). Endothelial cells seen on the **left** *arrow* are completely absent on the **right**, where only basement membrane is seen. (Reprinted by permission of the publisher from Schaner PJ, Martin ND, Tulenko TN, et al: Decellularized vein as a potential scaffold for vascular tissue engineering. *J Vasc Surg* 40:146-153, 2004. Copyright 2004 by Elsevier.)

tioned well in vivo without dilation, anastomotic complication, or rupture over 2 weeks of arterial perfusion.

Conclusions.—Vein rendered acellular with SDS has well-preserved extracellular matrix, basement membrane structure, and strength sufficient for vascular grafting. These properties suggest proof of concept for its use as a scaffold for further vascular tissue engineering.

► These guys are attempting to build a small-caliber arterial substitute from "the outside in." I think they have it backward. Success or failure will depend upon achieving reliable coverage of the luminal surface with functioning endothelial cells. This has been the Achilles' heel of small caliber arterial substitutes thus far. Perhaps the authors of this study should talk to the authors of the previous abstract (Abstract 4–4)! I think the luminal surface of a small-caliber graft will be much more important to the success or failure of that graft than the surrounding scaffold.

G. L. Moneta, MD

Allograft Replacement for Infrarenal Aortic Graft Infection: Early and Late Results in 179 Patients

Kieffer E, Gomes D, Chiche L, et al (Pitié-Salpêtrière Univ Hosp, Paris)

J Vasc Surg 39:1009-1017, 2004 4–6

Objectives.—We evaluated early and late results of allograft replacement to treat infrarenal aortic graft infection in a large number of patients and compared the results in patients who received fresh allografts versus patients who received cryopreserved allografts.

Methods.—From 1988 to 2002 we operated on 179 consecutive patients (mean age, 64.6 ± 9.0 years; 88.8% men). One hundred twenty-five patients (69.8%) had primary graft infections, and 54 patients (30.2%) had secondary aortoenteric fistulas (AEFs). Fresh allografts were used in 111 patients (62.0%) until 1996, and cryopreserved allografts were used in 68 patients (38.0%) thereafter.

Results.—Early postoperative mortality was 20.1% (36 patients), including four (2.2%) allograft-related deaths from rupture of the allograft (recurrent AEF, n = 3), all in patients with fresh allografts. Thirty-two deaths were not allograft related. Significant risk factors for early mortality were septic shock ($P < .001$), presence of AEF ($P = .04$), emergency operation ($P = .003$), emergency allograft replacement ($P = .0075$), surgical complication ($P = .003$) or medical complication ($P < .0001$), and need for repeat operation ($P = .04$). There were five (2.8%) nonlethal allograft complications (rupture, n = 2; thromboses, which were successfully treated at repeat operation, n = 2; and amputation, n = 1), all in patients with fresh allografts. Four patients (2.2%) were lost to follow-up. Mean follow-up was 46.0 ± 42.1 months (range, 1-148 months). Late mortality was 25.9% (37 patients). There were three (2.1%) allograft-related late deaths from rupture of the allograft, at 9, 10, and 27 months, respectively, all in patients with fresh

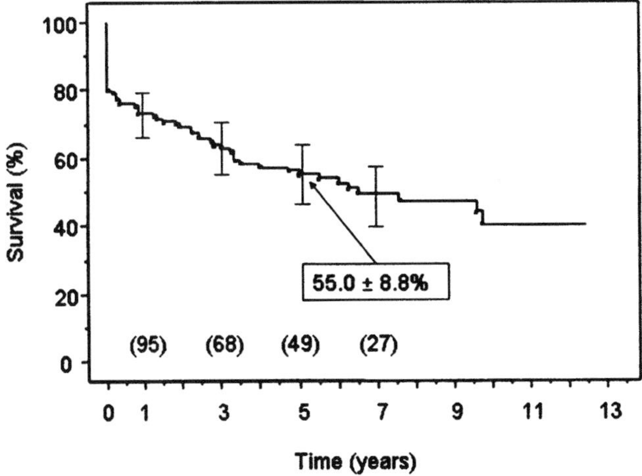

FIGURE 2.—Cumulative Kaplan-Meier curve shows early and late survival in 179 patients after allograft replacement to treat infrarenal aortic graft infection. (Reprinted by permission of the publisher from Kieffer E, Gomes D, Chiche L, et al: Allograft replacement for infrarenal aortic graft infection: Early and late results in 179 patients. *J Vasc Surg* 39:1009-1017, 2004. Copyright 2004 by Elsevier.)

allografts. Actuarial survival was 73.2% ± 6.8% at 1 year, 55.0% ± 8.8% at 5 years, and 49.4% ± 9.6% at 7 years (Fig 2). Late nonlethal aortic events occurred in 10 patients (7.2%; occlusion, n = 4; dilatation < 4 cm, n = 5; aneurysm, n = 1), at a mean of 28.3 ± 28.2 months, all but two in patients with fresh allografts. The only significant risk factor for late aortic events was use of an allograft obtained from the descending thoracic aorta (*P* = .03). Actuarial freedom from late aortic events was 96.6% ± 3.4% at 1 year,

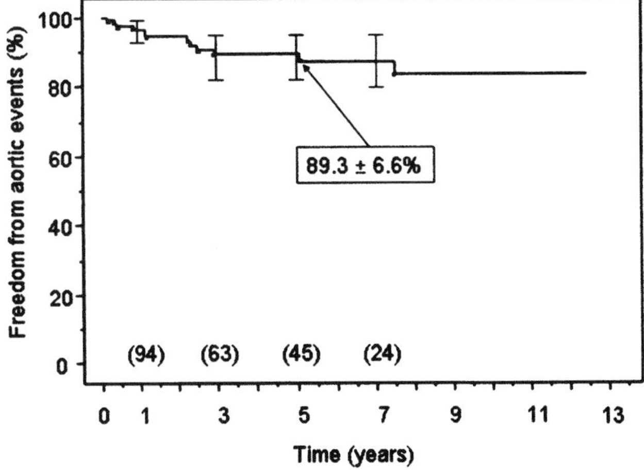

FIGURE 4.—Cumulative Kaplan-Meier curve shows freedom from aortic events after allograft replacement to treat infrarenal aortic graft infection. (Reprinted by permission of the publisher from Kieffer E, Gomes D, Chiche L, et al: Allograft replacement for infrarenal aortic graft infection: Early and late results in 179 patients. *J Vasc Surg* 39:1009-1017, 2004. Copyright 2004 by Elsevier.)

89.3% ± 6.6% at 3 years, and 89.3% ± 6.6% at 5 years (Fig 4). There were 63 late, mostly occlusive, iliofemoral events, which occurred at a mean of 34.9 ± 33.7 months in 38 patients (26.6%), 28 of whom (73.7%) had received fresh allografts. The only significant risk factor for late iliofemoral events was use of fresh allografts versus cryopreserved allografts (P = .03). Actuarial freedom from late iliofemoral events was 84.6% ± 7.0% at 1 year, 72.5% ± 9.0% at 3 years, and 66.4% ± 10.2% at 5 years.

Conclusions.—Early and long-term results of allograft replacement are at least similar to those of other methods to manage infrarenal aortic graft infections. Rare specific complications include early or late allograft rupture and late aortic dilatation. The more frequent late iliofemoral complications may be easily managed through the groin. These complications are significantly reduced by using cryopreserved allografts rather than fresh allografts and by not using allografts obtained from the descending thoracic aorta.

▶ These are reasonable results by excellent, experienced surgeons. It should be noted that, basically, the allografts used in this series were locally obtained and prepared. Durability of allografts may relate to their processing. The authors' results with regard to graft durability may not directly reflect those that would be obtained with commercially available allografts in the United States. Don't discount surgical experience. I doubt the guy who tries 1 graft infection every 2 years will achieve similar results.

G. L. Moneta, MD

Cryopreserved Arterial Allografts for In Situ Reconstruction of Infected Arterial Vessels

Teebken OE, Pichlmaier MA, Brand S, et al (Hannover Med School, Germany)

Eur J Vasc Endovasc Surg 27:597-602, 2004 4–7

Objective.—To review our experience of using cryopreserved allografts for in situ reconstruction in the presence of infection involving the aorta, iliac or femoral arteries.

Design.—Retrospective clinical study.

Methods.—From 3/2000 to 8/2003 all patients with mycotic aneurysms or secondary infection following earlier prosthetic replacement were treated with cryopreserved human allografts (Fig 1). Forty-two patients, 39 (93%) with a prosthetic graft infection and 3 (7%) with a mycotic aneurysm of the abdominal aorta were treated. Six (14%) had aorto-enteric fistulas, 5 (12%) had ruptured aneurysms, and 2 also had vertebral destruction. The median follow-up time was 20 months (range 1-42 months).

Results.—Thirty-day mortality was 14%. Three patients died due to multi-organ failure, two patients died from hypovolaemic shock due to allograft rupture and one from rupture of the native aorta. The overall mortality was 24% (four additional patients). Graft patency was 100% at 30 days and 97% at follow up in the survivors. The mean actuarial survival time was 32 months (95% CI = 27-37 months).

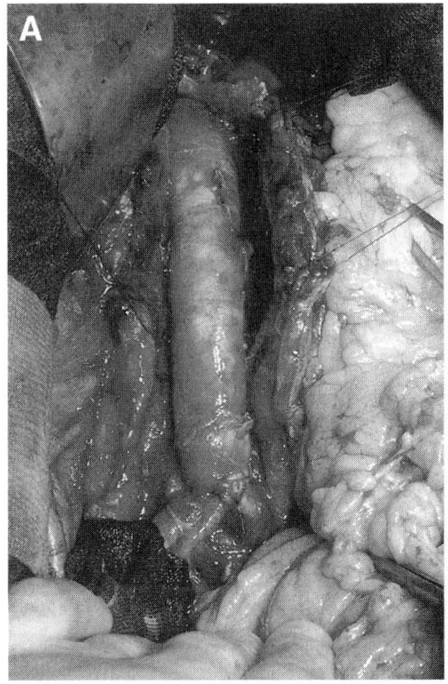

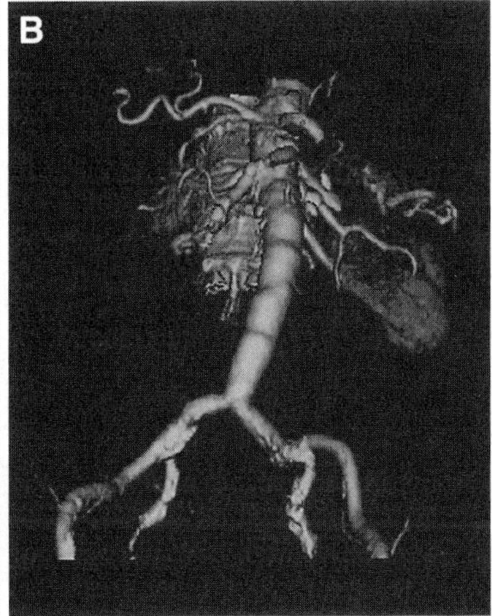

FIGURE 1.—Intraoperative view (**a**) and computed tomography scan reconstruction (**b**) after aorto-bi-iliac in situ replacement with a cryopreserved homograft made from an infrarenal aortic segment and 2 iliac arteries. (Reprinted from Teebken OE, Pichlmaier MA, Brand S, et al: Cryopreserved arterial allografts for in situ reconstruction of infected arterial vessels. *Eur J Vasc Endovasc Surg* 27:597-602, 2004. Copyright 2004 by permission of the publisher.)

Conclusions.—Cryopreserved allografts for the in situ reconstruction of infected arteries or grafts have acceptable intermediate results.

▶ A smaller series than that of Dr Kieffer (Abstract 4–6) but with basically similar results.

G. L. Moneta, MD

Cryopreserved Arterial Allografts in the Treatment of Prosthetic Graft Infections

Gabriel M, Pukacki F, Dzieciuchowicz L, et al (Med Univ, Poznań, Poland)
Eur J Vasc Endovasc Surg 27:590-596, 2004 4–8

Aim.—The purpose of this study was to evaluate the effectiveness of cryopreserved arterial allografts in the management of prosthetic graft infection.

Material and Methods.—Over a 5-year period 45 patients with infection of prosthetic vascular grafts were treated. There were 39 intra-abdominal infected grafts (group I) and six extra-abdominal infected grafts (group II). Treatment consisted of total graft removal and in situ or extra-anatomic implantation of cryopreserved arterial allografts. Six patients were operated on as an emergency. Four patients presented with aorto-enteric fistula. Follow-up ranged from 30 to 78 months.

Results.—There were six in-hospital deaths and two additional patient deaths during follow-up, yielding an overall mortality rate of 18%. Six patients died due to complications directly related to infection or insertion of an allograft. Combined short and long-term mortality rate was much higher in patients operated on as an emergency (67%) compared to elective cases (11%). Patients with aorto-enteric fistula had the highest mortality rate (75%). Primary and secondary 3-year allograft patency rates for group I were 84 and 94%, respectively and for group II were 60 and 80%, respectively.

Conclusions.—Aortic allografts are useful in the treatment of infection of major vascular prosthetic grafts, except for patients with aorto-enteric fistula. Patients with infection of the prosthetic graft should be promptly assessed for graft removal, since results of elective surgery are much better than results of emergency procedures.

► Another European series of allografts to treat prosthetic graft infection (see previous 2 articles [Abstracts 4–6 and 4–7]). These 3 articles outline the expected complications and mortality with allograft replacement for prosthetic graft infection. Compared with axillofemoral grafting for aortic graft infection, use of allografts for inline reconstruction has reasonable patency and fewer graft-related infections, but will be associated with some graft-related deaths. I have observed that more patients survive infected axillofemoral grafts than survive death.

G. L. Moneta, MD

Multicenter Randomized Prospective Trial Comparing a Pre-cuffed Polytetrafluoroethylene Graft to a Vein Cuffed Polytetrafluoroethylene Graft for Infragenicular Arterial Bypass

Panneton JM, Hollier LH, Hofer JM (Mayo Clinic, Rochester, Minn; Mount Sinai Med Ctr, New York)

Ann Vasc Surg 18:199-206, 2004 4–9

Introduction.—Poor patency of synthetic grafts for infragenicular revascularization has led to use of distal vein patches or cuffs. The aim of this study was to compare the distally widened Distaflo PTFE graft, which mimics a vein cuff, with a PTFE graft with distal vein modification. In this prospective, randomized, multicenter trial we compared use of a precuffed PTFE graft with that of PTFE grafts with distal vein modification for infragenicular revascularization in patients with critical limb ischemia without saphenous vein. Study end points were primary and secondary patency and limb salvage rates at 2 years. From January 28, 1999 to November 1, 2000, 104 patients were enrolled in 10 North American centers. Thirteen were excluded for protocol violation. Ninety-one bypasses were performed in 89 patients with a mean age of 73 years (range 47-90). By randomization,

47 bypasses were done with the precuffed graft and 44 with PTFE graft with vein cuff. Both groups were comparable for comorbidities and operative variables, except for a higher incidence of acute ischemia in the precuffed group (19% vs. 4.5%, $p = 0.03$). Bypass was a redo procedure in 53% and was performed at the infrapopliteal vessels in 79%. Operative mortality was 2.2% (2/91). Mean follow-up was 14 months (range 1-30). At 1 and 2 years, primary patency was 52% and 49% for the precuffed group and 62% and 44% for the vein cuffed group, respectively ($p = 0.53$). At 1 year and 2 years, the limb salvage rate was 72% and 65% for the precuffed group and 75% and 62% in the vein cuffed group ($p = 0.88$). Although numbers are small and follow-up short, this midterm analysis shows similar results for the Distaflo precuffed grafts and PTFE grafts with vein cuff. A precuffed graft is a reasonable alternative conduit for infragenicular reconstruction in the absence of saphenous vein and provides favorable limb salvage.

▶ The Distaflo graft is slowly gaining popularity. Results are obviously inferior to what would be expected with autogenous grafting with single-segment saphenous veins. However, if there is no need for a distal vein cuff for those cases where infrainguinal prosthetic grafting truly is required, the Distaflo graft is an advance.

G. L. Moneta, MD

Silyl-Heparin Bonding Improves the Patency and In Vivo Thromboresistance of Carbon-Coated Polytetrafluoroethylene Vascular Grafts

Laredo J, Xue L, Husak VA, et al (Loyola Univ, Maywood, Ill; Edward Hines VA Hosp, Ill; Biosurface Engineering Technologies, College Park, Md)

J Vasc Surg 39:1059-1065, 2004 4–10

Objectives.—Our purpose was to improve the performance of carbon-coated expanded polytetrafluoroethylene vascular grafts by bonding the grafts with silyl-heparin, a biologically active heparin analog, using polyethylene glycol as a cross-linking agent.

Material and Method.—Silyl-heparin-bonded carbon-coated expanded polytetrafluoroethylene vascular grafts (Bard Peripheral Vascular, Tempe, Ariz), were evaluated for patency and platelet deposition 2 hours, 7 days, and 30 days after graft implantation in a canine bilateral aortoiliac artery model. Platelet deposition was determined by injection of autologous, (111) Indium-radiolabeled platelets, followed by a 2-hour circulation period prior to graft explantation. Histologic studies were performed on a 2-mm longitudinal strip of each graft (7-day and 30-day groups). Heparin activity of the explanted silyl-heparin grafts was determined by using an antithrombin-III based thrombin binding assay.

Results.—Overall chronic graft patency (7-day and 30-day groups) was 100% for the silyl-heparin bonded (16/16) grafts versus 68.75% for control (11/16) grafts ($P = .043$). Acute 2-hour graft patency was 100% for the silyl-heparin bonded (6/6) grafts versus 83.3% for control (5/6) grafts. Radiola-

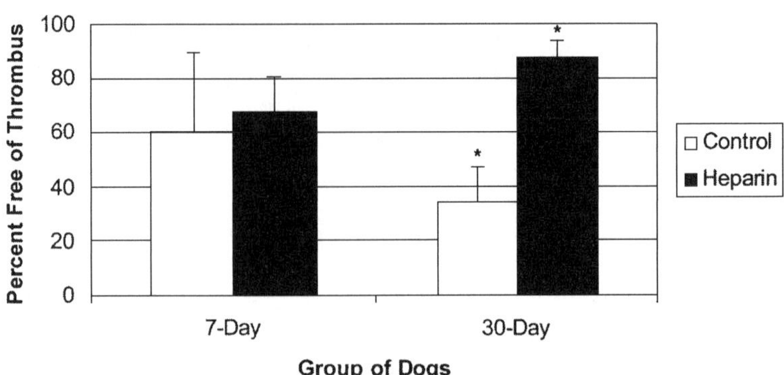

FIGURE 2.—The percentage of silyl-heparin and control graft length free of thrombus is shown for both 7-day and 30-day groups of dogs (n = 5, mean ± SD, P = .0451 by Wilcoxon rank sum test). (Reprinted by permission of the publisher from Laredo J, Xue L, Husak VA, et al: Silyl-heparin bonding improves the patency and in vivo thromboresistance of carbon-coated polytetrafluoroethylene vascular grafts. *J Vasc Surg* 39:1059-1065, 2004. Copyright 2004 by Elsevier.)

beled platelet deposition studies revealed a significantly lower amount of platelets deposited on the silyl-heparin grafts as compared with control grafts in the 30-day group (13.8 ± 7.18 vs 28.4 ± 9.73, CPM per cm^2 per million platelets, mean ± SD, P = .0451, Wilcoxon rank sum test). In the 2-hour group of dogs, a trend towards a lower deposition of platelets on the silyl-heparin grafts was observed. There was no significant difference in platelet deposition between the two grafts in the 7-day group. Histologic studies revealed a significant reduction in intraluminal graft thrombus present on the silyl-heparin grafts as compared with control grafts in the 30-day group of animals (Fig 2). In contrast, there was no difference in amount of graft thrombus present on both graft types in the 7-day group of dogs. Preimplant heparin activity on the silyl-heparin bonded grafts was 2.0 IU/cm^2 (international units[IU]/cm^2). Heparin activity remained present on the silyl-heparin grafts after explantation at all 3 time points (2 hours: above upper limit of assay, upper limit = 0.57, n = 6; 7 days: 0.106 ± 0.015, n = 5; 30 days: 0.007 ± 0.001, n = 5; mean ± SD, IU/cm^2).

Conclusion.—Silyl-heparin bonding onto carbon-coated expanded polytetrafluoroethylene vascular grafts resulted in (1) improved graft patency, (2) increased in vivo graft thromboresistance, and (3) a significant reduction in intraluminal graft thrombus. This graft may prove to be useful in the clinical setting.

► I have seen many animal studies expounding the virtues of various luminal modifications of polytetrafluoroethylene grafts. Here is another one. My advice is to wait for the human data.

G. L. Moneta, MD

Early Results With Use of Gracilis Muscle Flap Coverage of Infected Groin Wounds After Vascular Surgery

Morasch MD, Sam AD II, Kibbe MR, et al (Northwestern Univ, Chicago)

J Vasc Surg 39:1277-1283, 2004 4–11

Introduction.—Management of a nonhealing femoral wound after vascular surgery can pose a challenging problem, particularly when there is prosthetic material involved. We prefer to use pedicled gracilis muscle flaps (PGMFs) to cover problematic groin wounds when more conventional management is not possible.

Methods.—We describe the technique for using PGMFs to provide groin coverage (Figs 2 and 3), report a summary of our short-term and long-term results, and describe why we prefer this reconstructive technique.

Results.—Twenty PGMFs were placed in 18 patients to treat nonhealing and infected groin wounds. Exposed prosthetic vascular reconstructions were covered with the PGMF in 14 wounds, and in situ autogenous vascular reconstructions were covered in four. Seven wound infections were polymicrobial, 10 had a single gram-positive organism, and one had a single gram-negative organism. *Pseudomonas* cultured out in four wounds, and *Candida* in one wound. Two patients had a virulent combination of methicillin-resistant *Staphylococcus aureus* and vancomycin-resistant enterococcus. Complete healing was initially achieved in all wounds, and no patient died within 30 days of surgery. Two PGMFs failed, at 2 weeks and 2 months, re-

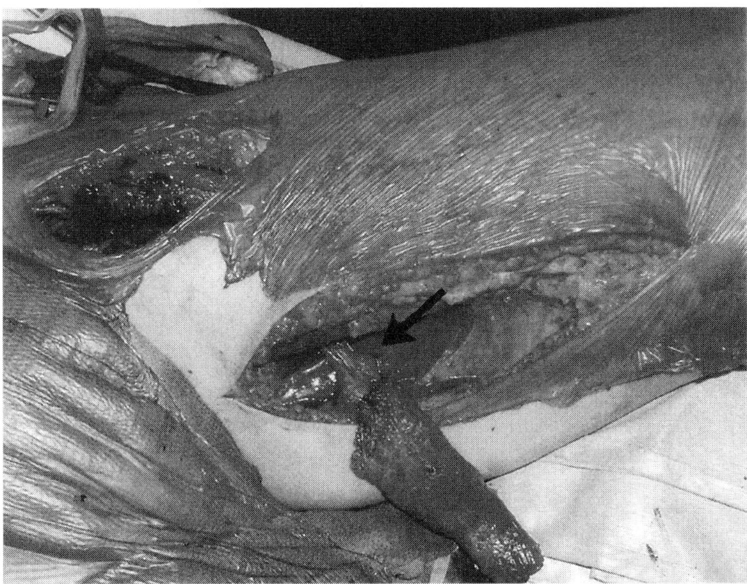

FIGURE 2.—Harvested gracilis muscle on single profunda-based pedicle (*arrow*). (Reprinted by permission of the publisher from Morasch MD, Sam AD II, Kibbe MR, et al: Early results with use of gracilis muscle flap coverage of infected groin wounds after vascular surgery. *J Vasc Surg* 39:1277-1283, 2004. Copyright 2004 by Elsevier.)

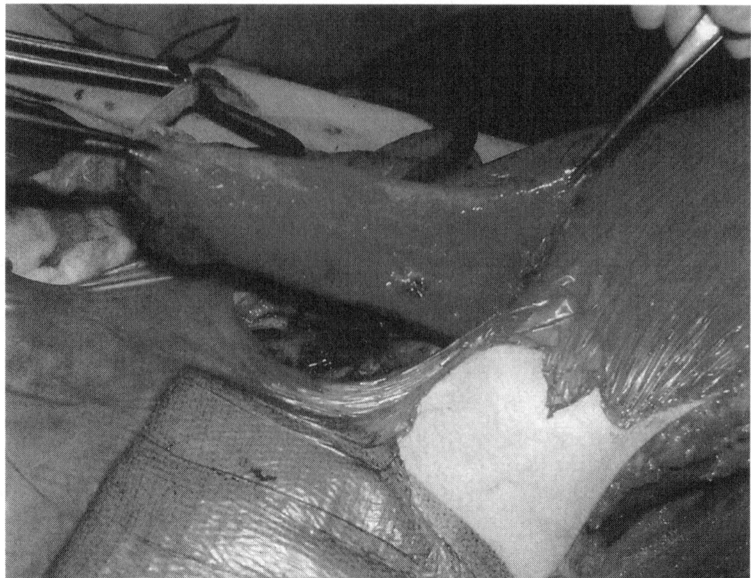

FIGURE 3.—Gracilis flap mobilized and tunneled up to groin wound. (Reprinted by permission of the publisher from Morasch MD, Sam AD II, Kibbe MR, et al: Early results with use of gracilis muscle flap coverage of infected groin wounds after vascular surgery. *J Vasc Surg* 39:1277-1283, 2004. Copyright 2004 by Elsevier.)

spectively, one from tension on the flap pedicle and one from acute inflow occlusion. Underlying prosthetic reconstruction was salvaged in 12 of 14 wounds; the remaining wounds with autogenous reconstructions or exposed femoral vessels all closed successfully. At a mean follow-up of 40 ± 10 months there were no recurrent groin infections. Seven patients died, at 2.5, 3, 8, 12, 14, 22, and 28 months, respectively.

Conclusion.—PGMF transposition is an effective option to cover infected or exposed femoral vessels or salvage prosthetic graft material in the groin. In appropriately selected patients, when complete graft removal and extra-anatomic bypass is not an acceptable option, gracilis muscle flap coverage is a viable alternative. The technique is relatively simple, and morbidity from PGMF harvest is minimal.

► Another muscle flap procedure to deal with groin wound complications. This one looks simple enough that I wonder if a plastic surgeon is really needed. (See also Abstract 17–7.)

G. L. Moneta, MD

5 Aortic Aneurysm

Screening for Abdominal Aortic Aneurysm: A Best-Evidence Systematic Review for the U.S. Preventive Services Task Force

Fleming C, Whitlock EP, Beil TL, et al (Kaiser Permanente, Portland, Ore; Veterans Affairs Med Ctr, Minneapolis)

Ann Intern Med 142:203-211, 2005 5–1

Background.—While the prognosis for abdominal aortic aneurysm (AAA) rupture is poor, ultrasound imaging is an accurate and reliable test for detecting AAAs before rupture.

Purpose.—To examine the benefits and harms of population-based AAA screening.

Data Sources.—MEDLINE (1994 to July 2004) supplemented by the Cochrane Library, a reference list of retrieved articles, and expert suggestions.

Study Selection.—Randomized trials of AAA population screening, population studies of AAA risk factors, and data on adverse screening and treatment events from randomized trials and cohort studies.

Data Extraction.—All studies were reviewed, abstracted, and rated for quality by using predefined criteria.

Data Synthesis.—The authors identified 4 population-based randomized, controlled trials of AAA screening in men 65 years of age and older. On the basis of meta-analysis, an invitation to attend screening was associated with a significant reduction in AAA-related mortality (odds ratio, 0.57 [95% CI, 0.45 to 0.74]). A meta-analysis of 3 trials revealed no significant difference in all-cause mortality (odds ratio, 0.98 [CI, 0.95 to 1.02]). No significant reduction in AAA-related mortality was found in 1 study of AAA screening in women. Screening does not appear to be associated with significant physical or psychological harms. Major treatment harms include an operative mortality rate of 2% to 6% and significant risk for major complications.

Limitations.—The population screening studies focused on men and provided no information on racial or ethnic groups. No information was available on uninvited control group characteristics, so the importance of risk factors such as tobacco use or family history could not be assessed. Since all trials were conducted in countries other than the United States, generalizability to the U.S. population is uncertain.

Conclusion.—For men age 65 to 75 years, an invitation to attend AAA screening reduces AAA-related mortality.

► This is the most comprehensive analysis of potential effectiveness for AAA screening that has been published. It is more conservative and restrictive than that suggested by the Society for Vascular Surgery (SVS) and Society for Vascular Medicine and Biology (SVMB). The SVS/SVMB screening recommendations for AAA screening are for all men aged 60 to 85 years, women aged 60 to 85 years with cardiovascular risk factors, and men and women 50 years or older with a family history of AAA.[1] Recommendations in the current article are derived from a more stringent analysis than the recommendations of the SVS/SVMB. As such, the recommendations of the US Preventive Service Task Force are likely to have more influence with Medicare and other insurance payers than the SVS/SVMB recommendations.

G. L. Moneta, MD

Reference

1. Kent KC, Zwolak RM, Jaff MR, et al: Screening for abdominal aortic aneurysm: A consensus statement. *J Vasc Surg* 39:267-269, 2004.

Population Based Randomised Controlled Trial on Impact of Screening on Mortality From Abdominal Aortic Aneurysm

Norman PE, Jamrozik K, Lawrence-Brown MM, et al (Univ of Western Australia, Fremantle; Univ of Queensland, Herston, Australia; Mount Med Centre, Perth, Australia; et al)

BMJ 329:1259-1262, 2004 5–2

Objective.—To assess whether screening for abdominal aortic aneurysms in men reduces mortality.

Design.—Population based randomised controlled trial of ultrasound screening, with intention to treat analysis of age standardised mortality.

Setting.—Community based screening programme in Western Australia.

Participants.—41,000 men aged 65-83 years randomised to intervention and control groups.

Intervention.—Invitation to ultrasound screening.

Main Outcome Measure.—Deaths from abdominal aortic aneurysm in the five years after the start of screening.

Results.—The corrected response to invitation to screening was 70%. The crude prevalence was 7.2% for aortic diameter ≥30 mm and 0.5% for diameter ≥55 mm. Twice as many men in the intervention group than in the control group underwent elective surgery for abdominal aortic aneurysm (107 *v* 54, $P = 0.002$, χ^2 test). Between scheduled screening and the end of follow up 18 men in the intervention group and 25 in the control group died from abdominal aortic aneurysm, yielding a mortality ratio of 0.61 (95% confidence interval 0.33 to 1.11). Any benefit was almost entirely in men aged between 65 and 75 years, where the ratio was reduced to 0.19 (0.04 to 0.89).

Conclusions.—At a whole population level screening for abdominal aortic aneurysms was not effective in men aged 65-83 years and did not reduce overall death rates. The success of screening depends on choice of target age group and the exclusion of ineligible men. It is also important to assess the current rate of elective surgery for abdominal aortic aneurysm as in some communities this may already approach a level that reduces the potential benefit of population based screening.

▶ This is one of the articles that the US Preventive Service Task Force based its recommendations upon (Abstract 5–1). The finding here that is most important is that the benefit of screening in reducing aneurysm-related mortality was confined almost entirely to men aged 65 to 75 years. Screening programs providing a reasonable yield will require careful targeting of appropriate aged patients.

G. L. Moneta, MD

Low Quality of Life Prior to Screening for Abdominal Aortic Aneurysm: A Possible Risk Factor for Negative Mental Effects

Wanhainen A, Rosén C, Rutegård J, et al (Uppsala Univ, Sweden; Örnsköldsvik County Hosp, Sweden; Örebro Univ, Örebro, Sweden)

Ann Vasc Surg 18:287-293, 2004 5–3

Introduction.—The objective of this study was to evaluate the effect on quality of life (QOL) of screening for abdominal aortic aneurysm (AAA) in a population-based AAA screening program. Twenty-four patients with screening-detected AAA and 45 controls with normal aortic diameter were studied in a prospective, controlled, population-based study. Prior to and 12 months after the ultrasonography examination, all participants completed Short-Form 36 and at 12 months, 10 AAA-specific questions were added. Comparisons were made between the two groups (AAA patients and controls), within each group, and between the groups and norms for the general Swedish population in the same age interval. Our results showed that screening for AAA results in impairment of QOL among those who have the disease and who suffered a low QOL prior to screening. Among those who had an age-adjusted normal QOL prior to screening and who were found to have the disease, and among those who were found to have normal aortas, no negative effect on QOL was observed. Thus, low QOL before screening is a possible risk factor for negative mental effects of diagnosing an AAA by screening.

▶ One is always concerned that patients knowing about problems will influence their perception of their health and QOL. A positive screening study may negatively affect some patients, but I think it is a minor issue. It was not an issue at all according to the analysis of the US Preventive Services Task Force (Abstract 5–1).

G. L. Moneta, MD

Late Survival After Elective Repair of Aortic Aneurysms Detected by Screening

Taylor JC, Shaw E, Whyman MR, et al (Gloucestershire Royal Hosp, England; Cheltenham Gen Hosp, England)

Eur J Vasc Endovasc Surg 28:270-273, 2004 5–4

Background.—The aim of this study was to examine whether there was any survival advantage in men following elective repair of an abdominal aortic aneurysm (AAA) detected by ultrasound screening compared to those with an AAA detected incidentally.

Methods.—A total of 424 men underwent elective AAA repair between 1990 and 1998; 181 were detected in an aneurysm screening programme and 243 were diagnosed incidentally. Follow-up survival data were collected until 2003 (minimum 5 years) and survival curves were compared using regression analysis.

Results.—The postoperative 30-day mortality rate was significantly lower in men whose aneurysms were detected by screening (4.4%), compared with those detected incidentally (9.0%). Similarly, 5-year survival (78% vs. 65%) and 10-year survival rates (63% vs. 40%) were better after repair of a screen-detected AAA ($p < 0.0003$ at all time intervals, by log rank testing). Multivariate analysis showed that this was largely due to the older age of men who had repair of an incidental AAA (71.2 vs. 67.1 years).

Conclusion.—Men who had elective repair of an AAA detected by screening had a better late survival rate than men whose aneurysm was discovered incidentally because they were younger at the time of surgery.

▶ The greater the patient's potential life span, the greater the possibility of an aneurysm-directed procedure to prolong survival. The article does not necessarily indicate that aneurysm screening programs increase overall survival. It does indicate that participants in aneurysm screening programs get their aneurysms repaired at an earlier age and therefore have greater potential to derive survival benefit from the procedure. The results may also indicate a greater tendency of younger versus older patients to participate in screening programs.

G. L. Moneta, MD

Abdominal Aortic Aneurysm Expansion: Risk Factors and Time Intervals for Surveillance

Brady AR, for the UK Small Aneurysm Trial Participants (MRC Clinical Trials Unit, London; et al)

Circulation 110:16-21, 2004 5–5

Background.—Intervention to reduce abdominal aortic aneurysm (AAA) expansion and optimization of screening intervals would improve current surveillance programs. The aim of this study was to characterize AAA growth in a national cohort of patients with AAA both overall and by cardiovascular risk factors.

Method and Results.—In this study, 1743 patients were monitored for changes in AAA diameter by ultrasonography over a mean follow-up of 1.9 years. Mean initial AAA diameter and growth rate were 43 mm (range 28 to 85 mm) and 2.6 mm/year (95% range, −1.0 to 6.1 mm/year), respectively. Baseline diameter was strongly associated with growth, suggesting that AAA growth accelerates as the aneurysm enlarges. AAA growth rate was lower in those with low ankle/brachial pressure index and diabetes but higher for current smokers (all P<0.001). No other factor (including lipids and blood pressure) was associated with AAA growth. Intervals of 36, 24, 12, and 3 months for aneurysms of 35, 40, 45, and 50 mm, respectively, would restrict the probability of breaching the 55-mm limit at rescreening to below 1%.

Conclusions.—Annual, or less frequent, surveillance intervals are safe for all AAAs ≤45 mm in diameter. Smoking increases AAA growth, but atherosclerosis plays a minor role.

► This article is of immediate practical significance. It provides very reasonable guidelines for surveillance periods for aortic aneurysms. I wonder, however, if these guys really practice medicine. The number of potential intervals for surveillance based on differing aneurysm diameters is too many to be practical. Nevertheless, the proposed screening intervals provide a framework for maximum utilization of screening resources.

G. L. Moneta, MD

Aneurysmal Hypertension and Its Relationship to Sac Thrombus: A Semi-qualitative Analysis by Experimental Fluid Mechanics

Chaudhuri A, Ansdell LE, Grass AJ, et al (Univ College London)

Eur J Vasc Endovasc Surg 27:305-310, 2004 5–6

Objectives.—To ascertain the effect of aneurysm thrombus and luminal diameter on arterial blood pressure within the abdominal aortic aneurysm lumen and at the sac wall.

Methods.—A life-like abdominal aortic aneurysm was incorporated in a pulsatile flow unit (Fig 1), using systemic blood pressure settings of 140/100 mmHg and 130/90 mmHg (denoted the high and low settings, respectively).

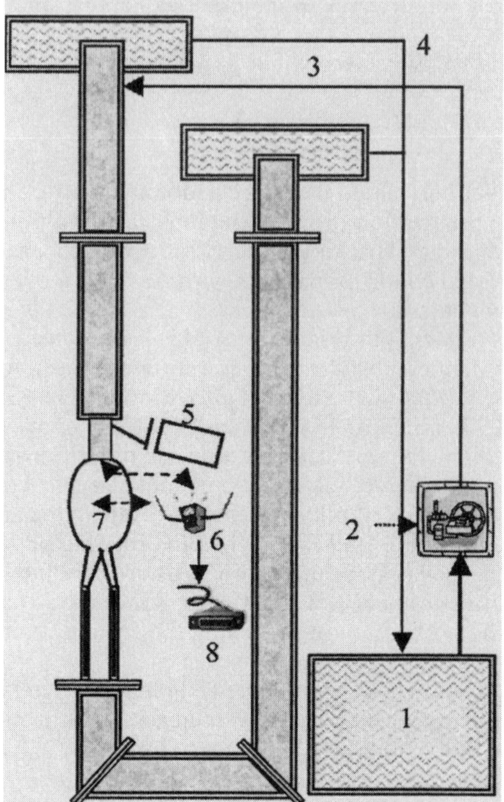

FIGURE 1.—Schematic representation of the pulsatile flow unit (PFU). (*1* = blood analogue in reservoir, *2* = supply pump, *3* = inflow, *4* = outflow, *5* = solenoid angle seat valve coupled to pulse generator, *6* = pressure sensing and display, *7* = abdominal aortic aneurysm [AAA] model test section, *8* = WaveView platform.) (Courtesy of Chaudhuri A, Ansdell LE, Grass AJ, et al: Aneurysmal hypertension and its relationship to sac thrombus: A semi-qualitative analysis by experimental fluid mechanics. *Eur J Vasc Endovasc Surg* 27:305-310, 2004. Copyright 2004, by permission of the publisher.)

Aneurysm sac pressure was measured in the absence of thrombus within the sac. This was repeated after a thrombus analogue (gelatine) was introduced into the aneurysm model in an asymmetric fashion. Luminal and sac wall pressures were compared to the systemic pressure, and to each other, in both blood pressure settings. Statistical analysis was performed using ANOVA in Minitab 13.

Results.—In the empty sac, the luminal and sac wall pressures were identical to the systemic pressures at the high and low settings. After introduction of thrombus, pressure was transmitted in a monophasic pulsatile fashion, measuring 166/142/151 mmHg (SP/DP/MP) at the sac wall, while the corresponding intraluminal pressure was 164/136/145 mmHg ($p < 0.001$, high setting). By contrast, in the low setting, these readings were 157/133/141 (sac wall) and 160/128/138 mmHg (lumen; $p < 0.001$). The sac wall pressures were significantly higher than the luminal pressures for both high and low settings ($p < 0.001$).

Conclusions.—Thrombus has a significant effect on the intraaneurysmal lumen itself and causes localised hypertension with high intraluminal pressures. The differences between the sac wall/luminal pressures may affect regional aneurysm wall biomechanics, but needs further study.

▶ Arterial pressure waves contribute to wall stress within an abdominal aortic aneurysm sac. These pressure waves can be modified by changes in the aneurysm sac and the sac contents. This study, along with studies from the University of Pittsburgh and Dartmouth, suggests areas of increased stress on certain points of the aneurysm wall. At some point, it may be possible to map stress points on the wall of an abdominal aortic aneurysm and to predict the likelihood of rupture with greater certainty than is possible with measurement of aneurysm diameter alone.

G. L. Moneta, MD

Endovascular Aortic Repair or Minimal Incision Aortic Surgery: Which Procedure to Choose for Treatment of High-Risk Aneurysms?

Tefera G, Carr SC, Turnipseed WD, et al (Univ of Wisconsin, Madison)

Surgery 136:748-753, 2004 5–7

Background.—This study evaluates use of endovascular aortic repair (EVAR) and minimal incision aortic surgery (MIAS) for treatment of high-risk patients with infrarenal aneurysms.

Methods.—A retrospective review of patients treated with EVAR or MIAS between 2000 and 2002 was performed. High-risk criteria included age older than 80 years, creatinine level greater than 3.0 mg/dL, recent myocardial infarction, congestive heart failure, severe chronic obstructive pulmonary disease, hostile abdomen, or morbid obesity (body mass index greater than 30). Patient demographics, duration of stay, morbidity, and mortality were compared. Exclusionary criteria for EVAR treatment included neck less than 1.5 cm or greater than 26 mm in diameter, densely calcified iliac arteries less than 6 mm, or creatinine level greater than 3.0 mg/dL. Exclusionary criteria for MIAS included pararenal abdominal aortic aneurysm, aneurysm greater than 10 cm, and morbid obesity.

Results.—Eighty-four patients were treated (61 EVAR, 23 MIAS). Average age for EVAR was 74 years and 72 years for MIAS. Average aneurysm size was 6 cm for both. American Society of Anesthesiologists score was 3.1 for EVAR and 3.0 for MIAS patients. Thirty-two of 61 EVAR patients (52%) had 2 risk factors, and 12 of 61 (20%) had 3 risk factors. Seven of 23 MIAS patients (30%) had 2 risk factors, and 7 had more than 3 risk factors (30%). There were 2 EVAR deaths (3%) from multiorgan failure and 1 MIAS death (4%) from myocardial infarction. Average duration of stay was 5.1 days for both EVAR and MIAS. Thirty-day morbidity was 18% for EVAR and 17% for MIAS patients.

Conclusions.—EVAR and MIAS are comparable for the treatment of high-risk aneurysm patients.

▶ The Wisconsin group has acquired considerable expertise with both EVAR and MIAS. The current study suggests that EVAR and MIAS are comparable in the high-risk aneurysm population. The authors, however, continued to dance around performance of a randomized trial in their institution. They appear to have both the expertise and the patients to perform such a trial, and it is time to do so.

G. L. Moneta, MD

Thoracovisceral Segment Aneurysm Repair After Previous Infrarenal Abdominal Aortic Aneurysm Surgery

Menard MT, Nguyen LL, Chan RK, et al (Brigham & Women's Hosp, Boston)

J Vasc Surg 39:1163-1170, 2004 5–8

Objective.—Repair of thoracovisceral aortic aneurysms (TVAA) after previous open repair of an infrarenal abdominal aortic aneurysm (AAA) poses significant challenges. We sought to better characterize such recurrent aneurysms and to evaluate their operative outcome.

Methods.—We reviewed the records and radiographs of 49 patients who underwent repair of TVAAs between 1988 and 2002 after previous repair of an AAA. Visceral artery reconstructions were completed with combinations of beveled anastomoses, inclusion patches, and side arm grafts (Fig 3). In 14 patients visceral endarterectomy was required to treat associated occlusive

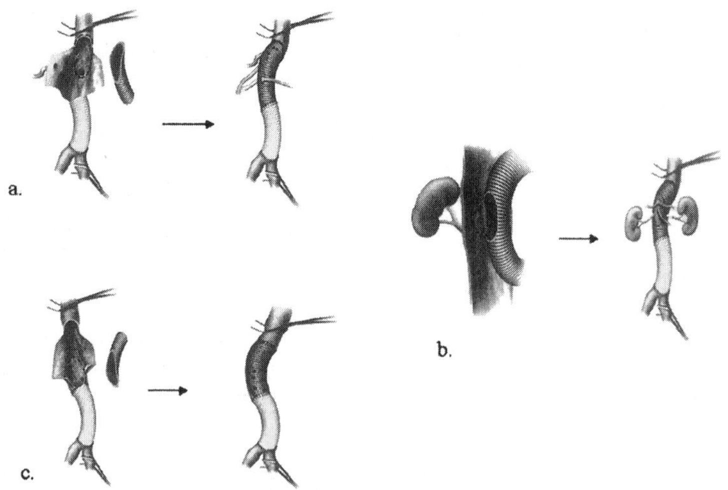

FIGURE 3.—Visceral reconstruction: **a**, Proximal beveled anastomosis, left renal artery Carrel patch. **b**, Visceral inclusion patch, left renal artery side arm. **c**, Distal beveled anastomosis. (Reprinted by permission of the publisher from Menard MT, Nguyen LL, Chan RK, et al: Thoracovisceral segment aneurysm repair after previous infrarenal abdominal aortic aneurysm surgery. *J Vasc Surg* 1163-1170, 2004. Copyright 2004 by Elsevier.)

disease. Sixteen patients had cerebrospinal fluid drainage, and 10 patients had distal perfusion during cross-clamping.

Results.—Patient mean age was 72 years, and 80% were men. Fifty-one percent of patients had symptomatic disease, and average TVAA diameter was 6.2 cm. Mean time between AAA and TVAA repair was 77 months. Twenty-six percent of aneurysms were restricted to the lower visceral aortic segment, 35% extended to the diaphragm, another 35% extended to the distal or middle thoracic aorta, and 4% involved the entire remaining visceral and thoracic aorta. The 30-day operative mortality rate was 4.1% in patients with nonruptured aneurysms and 50% in patients with ruptured aneurysms, for an overall mortality rate of 8.2%. Fifteen patients (30.6%) had major morbidity, including paresis in two patients and dialysis-dependent renal failure in five patients. At late follow-up, three patients required further aortic operations to treat additional aneurysms, and four patients had fatal aortic ruptures. Two-year and 5-year cumulative survival rates were 61% (7.5%) and 37% (7.8%), respectively. At univariate analysis, operative blood loss was the sole significant predictor of major morbidity ($P < .023$), and rupture ($P < .030$, $P < .0001$) and aneurysm extent ($P < .0007$, $P < .0001$) correlated with both operative death and long-term survival. Only aneurysm extent ($P < .010$, relative risk 37.3) remained a significant predictor of long-term survival at multivariate analysis.

Conclusion.—Elective repair of TVAAs after previous AAA repair can be performed with an acceptable level of operative mortality, though with considerable operative morbidity. Limited long-term survival mandates careful patient selection, and the high mortality associated with ruptured TVAA underscores the need for post-AAA surveillance.

► Repair of visceral aortic aneurysms above previous AAA repairs is required with increasing frequency. One wonders how many of these cases could be potentially avoided by repair of dilated visceral aortas at the time of the original AAA operation. The authors' recommendation that visceral aortas dilated to 3.5 cm at the time of AAA repair also be repaired along with the AAA makes sense for surgeons experienced with suprarenal aortic surgery.

G. L. Moneta, MD

Abdominal Aortic Surgery in Patients With Human Immunodeficiency Virus Infection

Lin PH, Bush RL, Yao Q, et al (Methodist Hosp, Houston)

Am J Surg 188:690-697, 2004 5–9

Purpose.—Human immunodeficiency virus (HIV) infection is known to cause acquired immune deficiency syndrome, which has been associated with a wide array of cardiovascular pathologies. This report examined the clinical outcome of patients infected with HIV who underwent abdominal aortic reconstruction for aneurysm or occlusive disease.

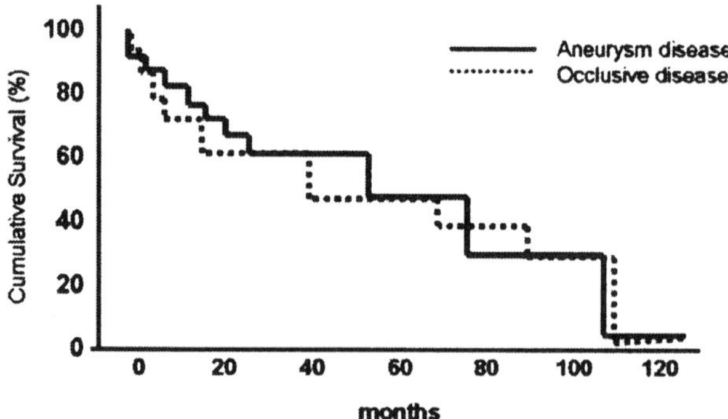

FIGURE 1.—Survival rates of patients with HIV infection who underwent aortic reconstruction for either aneurysmal or aortic occlusive disease. (Reprinted from Lin PH, Bush RL, Yao Q, et al: Abdominal aortic surgery in patients with human immunodeficiency virus infection. *Am J Surg* 188:690-697, 2004. Copyright 2004, with permission from Excerpta Medica Inc.)

Methods.—Hospital and clinic records of all patients with HIV infection who underwent an abdominal aortic operation were reviewed during an 11-year period. Relevant risk factors and clinical variables were assessed for surgical outcome.

Results.—Forty-eight HIV patients (mean age 54 ± 13 years) were identified who underwent abdominal aortic bypass grafting during the study period. Indications for aortic operation included aneurysm (n = 20) and aortoiliac occlusive disease (n = 28). All patients underwent successful aortic reconstructions without intraoperative mortality. Postoperative complications and in-hospital mortality occurred in 16 patients (33%) and 7 patients (15%), respectively. The mean follow-up period was 41 months. Life-table survival rates in aneurysm and occlusive patients at 60 months were 43.2% ± 5.3% and 46.3% ± 7.4% (not significant), respectively (Fig 1). Multivariate analysis showed that low CD4 lymphocyte counts (<200/μL, P <0.05) and hypoalbuminemia (<3.5 g/dL, P <0.05) were risk factors for postoperative complications.

Conclusion.—Perioperative morbidity and mortality rates are high in HIV patients undergoing an abdominal aortic operation. Low CD4 lymphocyte counts and hypoalbuminemia are associated with poor clinical outcomes in HIV patients undergoing abdominal aortic reconstruction.

► Everyone likes to publish good results. It is, however, sometimes the responsible thing to publish horrible results. Clearly, results of aortic surgery in patients with HIV infection are significantly inferior to what one would expect in patients without HIV infection. The message is that aortic reconstruction in patients with HIV infection should be undertaken only for compelling indications.

G. L. Moneta, MD

Abdominal Aortic Surgery and Horseshoe Kidney

Davidović LB, Kostić DM, Jakovljević NS, et al (Clinical Ctr of Serbia, Belgrade)

Ann Vasc Surg 18:725-728, 2004 5–10

Introduction.—Horseshoe kidney presents a special challenge during surgery of the abdominal aorta. The aim of this study was to evaluate the morbidity and define optimal management based on clinical histories of 15 patients with horseshoe kidney who underwent surgical procedures on the abdominal aorta over a 20-year period. There were 2 female and 13 male patients with an average age of 62.66 (50-75) years. The indications for surgery included aortic aneurysms in 10 patients and aortoiliac occlusive disease in 5. The horseshoe kidney was detected before surgery in 12 patients (80%) by ultrasonography, angiography, computed tomography (CT) or excretory urography. Angiography revealed multiple or anomalous renal arteries in 8 of 12 patients studied preoperatively. At surgery, 10 patients (66.6%) were found to have multiple or anomalous renal arteries. Five patients (33.41%) were without multiple or anomalous renal arteries. Ten required renal revascularization (reimplantation with a Carrel patch in 7 patients and aortorenal bypass in 3). Two patients, both with ruptured abdominal aortic aneurysms, died postoperatively. In the other 10 cases the average follow-up period was 5.3 years (6 months to 17 years). During this period there were no signs of graft occlusion, renovascular hypertension, or renal failure. From these results we conclude that aortic surgery can be performed safely in patients with horseshoe kidney without increased mortality. These patients require exact preoperative diagnosis (ultrasonography, CT scan, angiography), reimplantation of anomalous renal arteries, and preservation of the renal isthmus.

► In recent years, the retroperitoneal approach has been advocated for repair of abdominal aortic aneurysms associated with horseshoe kidneys. These guys from Serbia used exclusively a transperitoneal approach. I have repaired several aneurysms associated with horseshoe kidneys using both transperitoneal and retroperitoneal approaches. I have to say that, while not currently popular, the transperitoneal approach seems more versatile. It also has the advantage of less hassle with the ureters and sometimes anomalous renal veins associated with the horseshoe kidney.

G. L. Moneta, MD

Magnetic Resonance Imaging Identifies the Fibrous Cap in Atherosclerotic Abdominal Aortic Aneurysm

Kramer CM, Cerilli LA, Hagspiel K, et al (Univ of Virginia, Charlottesville)

Circulation 109:1016-1021, 2004 5–11

Background.—MRI can distinguish components of atherosclerotic plaque. We hypothesized that contrast enhancement with gadolinium-

DTPA (Gd-DTPA) could aid in the differentiation of plaque components in abdominal aortic aneurysm (AAA).

Method and Results.—Twenty-three patients (19 males, age 70±8 years) with AAA underwent MRI on a 1.5-T clinical scanner 33 days before surgical grafting. T1- and T2-weighted (W) black blood spin echo imaging was performed in 1 axial slice, and the T1-W imaging was repeated after a Gd-DTPA–enhanced 3D magnetic resonance angiogram. A section of the aorta at the site of imaging was resected at surgery for histopathologic examination of tissue components and inflammatory cells. Signal-to-noise and contrast-to-noise ratios (CNR) were measured in visualized plaque components from multispectral MRI, and percent enhancement after contrast on T1-W imaging was calculated. The κ value for agreement between pathology and MRI for the number of tissue components was 0.785. T2-W imaging identified thrombus as regions of high signal and lipid core as low signal, with a CNR of 6.43±3.41. Nine patients had a fibrous cap pathologically, which was visualized as a discrete area of uniform increased signal on T2-W imaging with a CNR of 4.52±1.93 compared with lipid core. Within the cap, the percent enhancement after Gd-DTPA on T1-W imaging was 91±63%.

Conclusions.—Higher signal on T2-W MRI identifies the fibrous cap and thrombus within AAA. Contrast enhancement improves delineation of the fibrous cap. The addition of contrast to MRI plaque imaging may enhance identification of vulnerable plaque.

► I am not sure the authors' efforts are of much use here. The status of the fibrous cap is clearly of importance in carotid artery disease, but aortic aneurysm plaque is usually covered by thrombus. Aortic atheroembolism, while well recognized, is not the major source of morbidity associated with aortic aneurysms. If the fibrous cap of the aortic plaque can somehow be shown to be associated with rupture of the aneurysm, expansion of the aneurysm, or both, this line of investigation may be clinically worthwhile. Otherwise, this appears to be research driven by available technology rather than a clinical question.

G. L. Moneta, MD

6 Abdominal Aortic Endografting

Comparison of Endovascular Aneurysm Repair With Open Repair in Patients With Abdominal Aortic Aneurysm (EVAR Trial 1), 30-Day Operative Mortality Results: Randomised Controlled Trial

Greenhalgh RM, for the EVAR Trial Participants (Imperial College London)

Lancet 364:343-348, 2004 6–1

Background.—Endovascular aneurysm repair (EVAR) is a new technology to treat patients with abdominal aortic aneurysm (AAA) when the anatomy is suitable. Uncertainty exists about how endovascular repair compares with conventional open surgery. EVAR trial 1 was instigated to compare these treatments in patients judged fit for open AAA repair.

Methods.—Between 1999 and 2003, 1082 elective (non-emergency) patients were randomised to receive either EVAR (n=543) or open AAA repair (n=539). Patients aged at least 60 years with aneurysms of diameter 5.5 cm or more, who were fit enough for open surgical repair (anaesthetically and medically well enough for the procedure), were recruited for the study at 41 British hospitals proficient in the EVAR technique. The primary outcome measure is all-cause mortality and these results will be released in 2005. The primary analysis presented here is operative mortality by intention to treat and a secondary analysis was done in per-protocol patients.

Findings.—Patients (983 men, 99 women) had a mean age of 74 years (SD 6) and mean AAA diameter of 6.5 cm (SD 1). 1047 (97%) patients underwent AAA repair and 1008 (93%) received their allocated treatment. 30-day mortality in the EVAR group was 1.7% (9/531) versus 4.7% (24/516) in the open repair group (odds ratio 0.35 [95% CI 0.16-0.77], p=0.009). By per-protocol analysis, 30-day mortality for EVAR was 1.6% (8/512) versus 4.6% (23/496) for open repair (0.33 [0.15-0.74], p=0.007). Secondary interventions were more common in patients allocated EVAR (9.8% vs 5.8%, p=0.02).

Interpretation.—In patients with large AAAs, treatment by EVAR reduced the 30-day operative mortality by two-thirds compared with open repair. Any change in clinical practice should await durability and longer term results.

▶ This trial and the DREAM trial (Abstract 6–2) deliver a clear message. Endovascular AAA repair has a lower risk of 30-day mortality than does open aneurysm repair. However, the durability of EVAR remains unknown. Some reports have suggested that ongoing risk of rupture with EVAR, even though low, may lead to obliteration of the perioperative benefit of lower operative mortality rate. The need for secondary procedures in the EVAR patients and the cost of ongoing treatment and monitoring also remain significant questions. At this point, the results of this trial and the DREAM trial do not mandate change in clinical practice.

G. L. Moneta, MD

A Randomized Trial Comparing Conventional and Endovascular Repair of Abdominal Aortic Aneurysms

Prinssen M, for the Dutch Randomized Endovascular Aneurysm Management (DREAM) Trial Group (Univ Med Ctr, Utrecht, The Netherlands; et al)

N Engl J Med 351:1607-1618, 2004 6–2

Background.—Although the initial results of endovascular repair of abdominal aortic aneurysms were promising, current evidence from controlled studies does not convincingly show a reduction in 30-day mortality relative to that achieved with open repair.

Methods.—We conducted a multicenter, randomized trial comparing open repair with endovascular repair in 345 patients who had received a diagnosis of abdominal aortic aneurysm of at least 5 cm in diameter and who were considered suitable candidates for both techniques. The outcome events analyzed were operative (30-day) mortality and two composite end points of operative mortality and severe complications and operative mortality and moderate or severe complications.

Results.—The operative mortality rate was 4.6 percent in the open-repair group (8 of 174 patients; 95 percent confidence interval, 2.0 to 8.9 percent) and 1.2 percent in the endovascular-repair group (2 of 171 patients; 95 percent confidence interval, 0.1 to 4.2 percent), resulting in a risk ratio of 3.9 (95 percent confidence interval, 0.9 to 32.9). The combined rate of operative mortality and severe complications was 9.8 percent in the open-repair group (17 of 174 patients; 95 percent confidence interval, 5.8 to 15.2 percent) and 4.7 percent in the endovascular-repair group (8 of 171 patients; 95 percent confidence interval, 2.0 to 9.0 percent), resulting in a risk ratio of 2.1 (95 percent confidence interval, 0.9 to 5.4).

Conclusions.—On the basis of the overall results of this trial, endovascular repair is preferable to open repair in patients who have an abdominal aortic aneurysm that is at least 5 cm in diameter. Long-term follow-up is needed to determine whether this advantage is sustained.

▶ This study and the larger EVAR trial (Abstract 6–1) both document lower 30-day mortality rates with endovascular aneurysm repair versus open abdominal aortic aneurysm repair. However, it is not possible to truly compare endovascular repair and open repair without long-term data regarding risk of aneurysm rupture, graft complications, need for follow-up, and costs. There are also indications that larger aneurysms repaired with endovascular techniques may not do as well in the long term as will the smaller aneurysms[1]. All of these concerns, in combination with a recent suppression of a Food and Drug Administration report under pressure from industry,[2] combine to lead one to question the authors' conclusions in the abstract of this article. An insightful editorial on these arguments by Dr Frank Lederle, is included in the same issue of *The New England Journal of Medicine* as this abstract,[3] and is recommended to readers of the YEAR BOOK.

G. L. Moneta, MD

References

1. Ouriel K, Srivasta SD, Sarac TP, et al: Disparate outcome after endovascular treatment of small versus large abdominal aortic aneurysm. *J Vasc Surg* 137:1206-1212, 2003.
2. Cronenwett JL, Seeger JM: Withdrawal of article by the FDA after objection from Medtronic. *J Vasc Surg* 40:209-210, 2004.
3. Lederle FA: Abdominal aortic aneurysm—open versus endovascular repair. *N Engl J Med* 351:1677-1679, 2004.

Perioperative Outcomes After Open and Endovascular Repair of Intact Abdominal Aortic Aneurysms in the United States During 2001

Lee WA, Carter JW, Upchurch G, et al (Univ of Florida, Gainesville; Univ of Michigan, Ann Arbor)

J Vasc Surg 39:491-496, 2004 6–3

Objective.—Small patient numbers, mixed data from clinical trials, and longitudinal series representing institutional learning curves have characterized previous studies of early outcomes after endovascular abdominal aortic aneurysm (AAA) repair. We compared the perioperative outcomes of endovascular and open surgical AAA repair in an unselected sample of patients in a single calendar year using a national administrative database.

Methods.—The 2001 National Inpatient Sample database was retrospectively reviewed. This database represents 20% of all-payer stratified sample of non-federal US hospitals. Patients older than 49 years were identified by primary diagnostic codes (International Classification of Disease, ninth revision [ICD-9], 441.4, intact, nonruptured AAA) and procedure codes (ICD-9 38.44 for open, 39.71 for endovascular repair). Patient demographic data (age, sex), comorbid conditions (ICD-9 coded), inpatient complications (ICD-9 coded), length of stay, final discharge disposition (home vs institution vs death), and hospital charges were examined with univariate and multivariate analyses.

Results.—In calendar year 2001, 7172 patients underwent either open (64%) or endovascular (36%) repair of intact, nonruptured AAAs. Despite comparable rates of preoperative comorbid conditions and a greater proportion of octogenarians (23% vs 16%%; *P* =.0001), morbidity (18% vs 29%; *P* =.0001) and mortality (1.3% vs 3.8%; *P* =.0001) were significantly lower for endovascular repair than for open repair. The median length of stay (2 vs 7 days; *P* =.0001) and the rate of discharge to an institutional facility versus home (6% vs 14%; *P* =.0001) were also much lower in the endovascular group than in the open repair group. At multivariate analysis, open AAA repair and age older than 80 years were strong independent predictors (*P* =.0001 for all) for death (open repair: odds ratio [OR], 3.3; 95% confidence interval [CI], 2.3-4.9; age: OR, 14.2; 95% CI, 3.5-58.1), complications (open repair: OR, 1.9; 95% CI, 1.7-2.1; age: OR, 1.9; 95% CI, 1.5-2.5), and not being discharged to home (open repair: OR, 3.4; 95% CI, 2.9-4.1; age: OR, 12.0; 95% CI, 7.0-20.4). Mean hospital charges were significantly greater (difference, $3337; *P* =.0009) for endovascular repair than for open repair. Extrapolated to the total number of endovascular AAA repairs performed during the single 2001 calendar year, this resulted in a staggering $50.3 million in additional hospital charges.

Conclusions.—Endovascular repair of intact AAAs results in a significantly lower number of complications and deaths, shorter hospital stay, and improved likelihood of discharge to home, even in older patients, when compared with open surgical repair. These impressive gains in clinical outcome, however, are achieved at similarly impressive increases in health care costs.

► This study demonstrates a statistically significant improvement in perioperative mortality after endovascular aneurysm repair (EVAR) versus open surgical repair. The 3-to-1 lower perioperative mortality rate of EVAR over open repair has been duplicated by large retrospective population based studies[1,2] and by prospective randomized trials.[3,4] It is remarkable that only 15 months after FDA approval, endovascular repair of AAA already represents more than a third of all AAA repairs. However, one cannot cheat age. Older patients do worse than younger patients after aneurysm repair, independent of the mode of treatment (see next article, Abstract 6–4).

W. A. Lee, MD

References

1. Anderson PL, Arons RR, Moskowitz AJ, et al: A statewide experience with endovascular abdominal aortic aneurysm repair: Rapid diffusion with excellent early results. *J Vasc Surg* 39:10-19, 2004.
2. Cao P, Verzini F, Parlani G, et al: Clinical effect of abdominal aneurysm endografting: 7-year concurrent comparison with open repair. *J Vasc Surg* 40:841-848, 2004.
3. Prinssen M, Verhoeven EL, Buth J, et al: A randomized trial comparing conventional and endovascular repair of abdominal aortic aneurysms. *N Engl J Med* 351:1607-1618, 2004.

4. Greenhalgh RM, Brown LC, Kwong GP, et al: Comparison of endovascular aneurysm repair with open repair in patients with abdominal aortic aneurysm (EVAR trial I), 30-day operative mortality results: Randomized controlled trial. *Lancet* 364:843-848, 2004.

Endovascular Aortic Aneurysm Repair in the Octogenarian: Is It Worthwhile?

Minor ME, Ellozy S, Carroccio A, et al (Mount Sinai School of Medicine, New York)

Arch Surg 139:308-314, 2004 6–4

Hypothesis.—During the past decade, endovascular stent graft repair (EVSG) of abdominal aortic aneurysms has emerged as a less invasive and less morbid alternative to open surgical repair. We hypothesize that EVSG may become the treatment method of choice among patients older than 80 years.

Design.—Retrospective case series.

Setting.—Major academic medical center with extensive experience in endovascular and open aortic aneurysm surgery

Patients and Methods.—During a 5-year period, EVSG was performed in 595 patients at our institution. One hundred fifty (25.2%) of these patients were older than 80 years. Our prospectively acquired database was reviewed with respect to the demographic, intraoperative, and outcome data of this elderly population.

Main Outcome Measures.—Technical and clinical success, aneurysm-related events (aneurysm-related death, type I or type III endoleaks, aneurysm expansion, or aneurysm rupture), and secondary interventions.

Results.—There were 119 men (79.3%) and 31 women (20.7%) (mean age, 84.6 years). Mean aneurysm diameter was 6.7 cm. Comorbidities including chronic obstructive pulmonary disease, coronary artery disease, chronic renal insufficiency, peripheral vascular disease, hypertension, and hypercholesterolemia were common in these patients, with an average of 2.9 comorbid conditions per patient. Mean follow-up was 16.9 months (range, 1.0-61.4 months). One hundred forty-six patients (97.3%) received only regional anesthesia, and the average intraoperative blood loss was 369 mL. Average hospital and intensive care unit stays were 2.5 days and 0.1 day, respectively. The procedure was performed emergently in 3 patients, and each recovered uneventfully. There were 5 aborted procedures (3.3%) for technical reasons and 4 conversions to open aortic repair (2.6%). In addition to these aborted procedures, there were 2 additional technical failures resulting in a technical success rate of 95.3%. Endoleaks were common and included 9 type I (6.90%), 35 type II (24.10%), and 1 type III (0.69%). The majority either resolved spontaneously (type IIs) or with minimally invasive secondary intervention, which was performed in 13 patients. Perioperative local/vascular and systemic complications occurred in 16 (10.7%) and 8 (5.3%) patients, respectively. There were 5 perioperative deaths (3.3%)(<30 days postoperatively). Forty late deaths (26.7%)(>30 days postoperatively) occurred, which were unrelated to the EVSG procedure.

Conclusions.—Endovascular repair of abdominal aortic aneurysms can be performed safely and successfully in the majority of octogenarians with relatively low complication rates. Improved EVSG devices and operator experience may make this procedure the treatment method of choice for patients in this age group who meet specific anatomical criteria.

▶ The study shows that the presence of an aortic aneurysm represents a sobering marker of systemic cardiovascular disease. Eighty-year-old patients with AAA do not follow the life expectancy curve of an "80-year-old expected to live another 6 to 7 years" but a significantly curtailed one. "Aneurysm-related mortality" may be low, but late all-cause mortality parallels quite closely the natural history of an unrepaired aneurysm. In this segment of the population, the decision to offer therapy should be individualized. "Endo-enthusiasm" should be tempered by a realistic assessment of added quality of life (above and beyond no treatment at all), given all the baggage an endovascular repair carries.

W. A. Lee, MD

Decreased Use of Iliac Extensions and Reduced Graft Junctions With Software-assisted Centerline Measurements in Selection of Endograft Components for Endovascular Aneurysm Repair

Velazquez OC, Woo EY, Carpenter JP, et al (Univ of Pennsylvania, Philadelphia)

J Vasc Surg 40:222-227, 2004 6–5

Objective.—The purpose of this study was to determine the impact of using computerized software-assisted centerline measurements for extensions and graft junctions during the selection of endograft components for modular aortic endografts in endovascular repair of abdominal aortic aneurysms.

Methods.—From April 1998 to December 2002, 289 modular aortic endografts were implanted at our institution. These included 248 grafts (prior to 2002, group 1) with components selected on the basis of manual caliper measurements from combined contrast computed tomography (CT) and marker-catheter arteriography data, and 41 grafts (2002, group 2) with components selected with the use of computerized software that allowed for centerline measurements on 3-dimensional reconstructions based on CT data. These 2 groups were compared for the number and type of extensions required per case. Seventeen other relevant variables were analyzed for their potential influence on selection of endograft components. These variables included age, gender, maximum aneurysm size, level of distal fixation, length and diameter at the fixation points, endograft manufacturer (make), and configuration. The significance of the observed differences was analyzed with a multivariate regression model, adjusting for potentially confounding preoperative measures.

Results.—Multivariate analysis demonstrated that the number of right iliac extensions, left iliac extensions, total extensions, and total graft junctions was significantly reduced by the use of computerized software-assisted centerline measurements (group 2) compared with caliper measurements (group 1), independent of all other 17 preoperative variables. Notably, the mean number of required right iliac extensions was double in group 1 versus group 2.

Conclusions.—Centerline software-assisted measurements can significantly reduce the need for iliac extensions and, concomitantly, the number of required endograft junctions. On average, twice as many extensions were required for right iliac fixation when the manual caliper measurements were used compared with software-assisted measurements. These findings are highly relevant to issues of total endograft cost and long-term endograft integrity and focus attention on the tools that may need to be considered standards of care rather than optional for selection of endograft components.

► Selection of the optimal device length is essential to accurate planning for endovascular aneurysm repair. The problem is complicated by the fact that path length is also dependent on the material properties of the stent graft. Centerline measurements, while an incremental improvement, do not represent the panacea the authors claim. Centerline measurements may be longer than the path length taken by the device. By using a device that is too long, there is a risk of inadvertent hypogastric artery coverage. Centerline measurements have little impact on proximal extension usage. This is primarily a technical issue related to deployment. The 3 things that will ultimately lead to decreased extension use are (1) a trimodular device with 2 separate docking iliac limbs; (2) the ability to "trombone" the limbs within the main body for a variable distance of 1 to 3 cm (vs a fixed overlap zone); and (3) complete iliac limb inventories so intraoperative changes of length can be made as necessary.

W. A. Lee, MD

First Experience in Human Beings With a Permanently Implantable Intrasac Pressure Transducer for Monitoring Endovascular Repair of Abdominal Aortic Aneurysms

Ellozy SH, Carroccio A, Lookstein RA, et al (Mount Sinai School of Medicine, New York)

J Vasc Surg 40:405-412, 2004 6–6

Objectives.—Endovascular stent graft repair of abdominal aortic aneurysms (AAAs) prevents rupture by excluding the aneurysm sac from systemic arterial pressure. Current surveillance protocols after endovascular aneurysm repair (EVAR) follow secondary markers of sac pressurization, namely, endoleak and sac enlargement. We report the first clinical experience with the use of a permanently implantable, ultrasound-activated remote pressure transducer to measure intrasac pressure after EVAR.

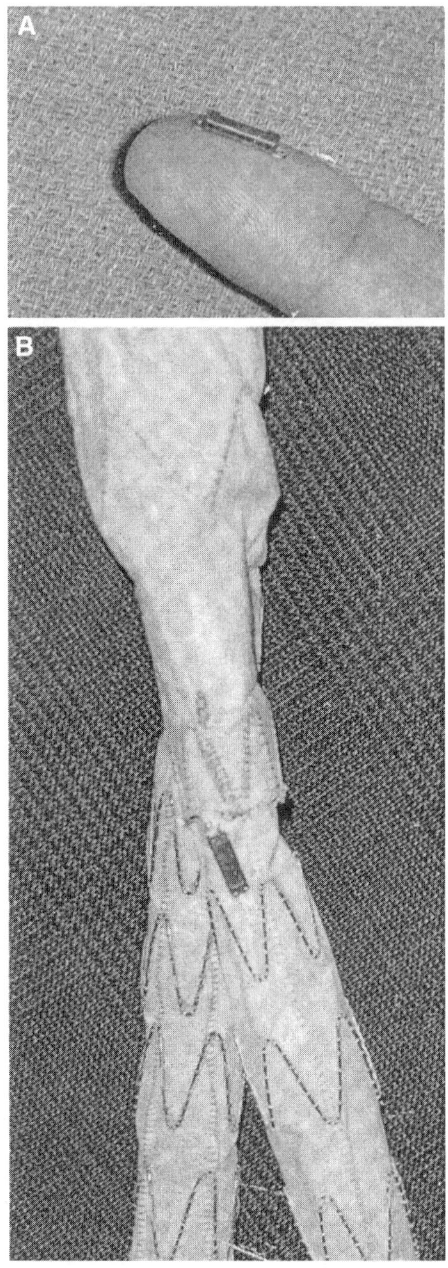

FIGURE 1.—A, Impressure abdominal aortic aneurysm sac pressure transducer (Remon Medical). B, Pressure transducer sewn to contralateral limb of bifurcated Talent device. (Reprinted by permission of the publisher from Ellozy SH, Carroccio A, Lookstein RA, et al: First experience in human beings with a permanently implantable intrasac pressure transducer for monitoring endovascular repair of abdominal aortic aneurysms. *J Vasc Surg* 40:405-412, 2004. Copyright 2004 by Elsevier.)

Methods.—Over 7 months, 14 patients underwent EVAR of an infrarenal abdominal aortic aneurysm with implantation of an ultrasound-activated remote pressure transducer fixed to the outside of the stent graft and exposed to the excluded aortic sac. Twelve patients received modular bifurcated stent grafts, and 2 patients received aortouniiliac devices. Intrasac pressures were measured directly with an intravascular catheter and by the remote sensor at stent-graft deployment. Follow-up sac pressures were measured with a remote sensor and correlated with systemic arterial pressure at every follow-up visit. Mean follow-up was 2.6 ± 1.9 months.

Results.—Excellent concordance was found between catheter-derived and transducer-derived intrasac pressssure intraoperatively. Pulsatile waveforms were seen in all functioning transducers at each evaluation interval. One implant ceased to function at 2 months of follow-up. In 1 patient a type I endoleak was diagnosed on 1-month computed tomography (CT) scans; 3 type II endoleaks were observed. Those patients with complete exclusion of the aneurysm on CT scans had a significant difference in systemic and sac systolic pressures initially (P <.001) and at 1 month (P <.001). Initial sac diastolic pressures were higher than systemic diastolic pressures (P <.001). The ratio of systemic to sac systolic pressure increased over time in those patients with complete aneurysm exclusion (P <.001). Four of 6 patients with no endoleak and greater than 1-month follow-up had diminution of sac systolic pressure to 40 mm Hg or less by 3 months.

Conclusion.—This is the first report of a totally implantable chronic pressure transducer to monitor the results of EVAR in human beings. Aneurysm exclusion leads to gradual diminution of sac pressure over several months. Additional clinical follow-up will be necessary to determine whether aneurysm sac pressure monitoring can replace CT in the long-term surveillance of patients after EVAR (Fig 1).

▶ The hemodynamic environment within the aneurysm sac is complex. There are compartmentalization of pressures and nonuniform distribution of wall strain. Given this, I am uncertain as to how to properly interpret and use the data gathered from this device. An intrasac pressure monitor also only addresses the problem after the fact. Prevention of the endoleak is a far better strategy. Although there may be some role for intrasac pressure detection in surveillance, it is difficult to imagine it substantially supplanting contrast-based cross-sectional imaging and abdominal radiographs.

W. A. Lee, MD

Endoleak Following Endovascular Abdominal Aortic Aneurysm Repair: Implications for Duration of Screening

Corriere MA, Feurer ID, Becker SY, et al (Vanderbilt Univ, Nashville, Tenn)
Ann Surg 239:800-807, 2004 6–7

Objective.—Endovascular abdominal aortic aneurysm repair (EAR) requires long-term surveillance for endoleak or increase in aneurysm diameter.

We analyzed the natural history of and risk factors for endoleak development.

Summary Background Data.—Endoleak is a common complication of EAR that can lead to aneurysm enlargement and even rupture. Following EAR, imaging studies are used to identify leaks since patients with endoleak may require additional endovascular interventions or conversion to open repair. No criteria currently exist for cessation or reduction in frequency of screening imaging studies.

Methods.—Data on 220 patients undergoing EAR were retrospectively reviewed. Kaplan-Meier survival analysis and Cox proportional hazards regression were used with the end point being new endoleak development. Potential risk factors included preoperative aneurysm diameter, number of negative surveillance studies, and postoperative increase in diameter.

Results.—A total of 52 patients (24%) who underwent EAR had endoleak detected during postoperative follow-up, which averaged 19 months (range, 0.4-101 months). One, 6-, 12-, and 24- month endoleak-free survival was 90%, 80%, 77%, and 73%, respectively. Three leaks occurred after year 2, at postoperative months 24, 48, and 85. Increasing number of negative screening studies was negatively associated with risk for endoleak development (B = −3.122, $P < 0.001$), while increase in aneurysm diameter was positively associated with risk for endoleak (B = 0.072, $P = 0.04$).

Conclusion.—Risk for endoleak declines as the number of negative postoperative scans increases, but new endoleaks are identified as late as 7 years following EAR. Reduction in screening frequency cannot be uniformly recommended at this time. Patients with documented aneurysm expansion should be monitored carefully and endoleak should be suspected.

► A major limitation to EAR is the need for long-term follow-up with imaging studies. This study has demonstrated a decreased risk for new endoleak development as the number of negative screening studies increases. However, new endoleaks were discovered as late as 85 months after EAR. At this time, cessation of surveillance for endoleak cannot be recommended.

G. L. Moneta, MD

Two-Year Outcomes After Conventional or Endovascular Repair of Abdominal Aortic Aneurysms

Blankensteijn JD, for the Dutch Randomized Endovascular Aneurysm Management (DREAM) Trial Group (Radboud Univ, Nijmegen, The Netherlands; et al)

N Engl J Med 352:2398-2405, 2005 6–8

Background.—Two randomized trials have shown better outcomes with elective endovascular repair of abdominal aortic aneurysms than with conventional open repair in the first month after the procedure. We investigated whether this advantage is sustained beyond the perioperative period.

Methods.—We conducted a multicenter, randomized trial comparing open repair with endovascular repair in 351 patients who had received a diagnosis of abdominal aortic aneurysm of at least 5 cm in diameter and who were considered suitable candidates for both techniques. Survival after randomization was calculated with the use of Kaplan-Meier analysis and compared with the use of the log-rank test on an intention-to-treat-basis.

Results.—Two years after randomization, the cumulative survival rates were 89.6 percent for open repair and 89.7 percent for endovascular repair (difference, −0.1 percentage point; 95 percent confidence interval, −6.8 to 6.7 percentage points). The cumulative rates of aneurysm-related death were 5.7 percent for open repair and 2.1 percent for endovascular repair (difference, 3.7 percentage points; 95 percent confidence interval, −0.5 to 7.9 percentage points). This advantage of endovascular repair over open repair was entirely accounted for by events occurring in the perioperative period, with no significant difference in subsequent aneurysm-related mortality. The rate of survival free of moderate or severe complications was also similar in the two groups at two years (at 65.9 percent for open repair and 65.6 percent for endovascular repair; difference, 0.3 percentage point; 95 percent confidence interval, −10.0 to 10.6 percentage points).

Conclusions.—The perioperative survival advantage with endovascular repair as compared with open repair is not sustained after the first postoperative year.

▶ The results of this midterm analysis of the DREAM trial are a bit surprising. One would have thought, on the basis of the randomized process, that the initial survival advantage of the endovascular-treated patients would have been maintained. In addition, one might have suspected that the reinterventions for problems with the endovascular repair would have continued to mount over time. Instead, survival advantage was not maintained and reinterventions for endovascular-treated patients after 9 months did not differ from those for patients treated with open repair. Clearly, efforts must be intensified to use medical management to maintain the survival advantage initially conferred by endovascular aneurysm repair. It is unclear whether the stabilization of reinterventions in the endovascular group after 9 months is related to stabilization of the endograft or, perhaps, the changing management practice of endoleaks.

G. L. Moneta, MD

Proximal Type I Endoleak After Endovascular Abdominal Aortic Aneurysm Repair: Predictive Factors

Sampaio SM, Panneton JM, Mozes GI, et al (Mayo Clinic, Rochester, Minn; Vascular and Transplant Specialists, Norfolk, Va)

Ann Vasc Surg 18:621-628, 2004 6–9

Introduction.—Proximal type I endoleaks after endovascular abdominal aortic aneurysm repair (EVAR) are associated with a high risk of rupture.

Risk factors for developing this complication are not fully elucidated. We aimed to define preoperative predictors for proximal type I endoleak and describe its clinical outcome. From a consecutive series of 257 patients who underwent EVAR, we selected 202 who had available pre- and postoperative CT scan studies. Proximal neck diameter, length, angulation, calcification, thrombus load (thickness, percentage of neck circumference coverage, percentage of neck area occupancy), and maximum aneurysm diameter were evaluated on preoperative CT scans. All postoperative CT and duplex ultrasound scans, supplemented with angiograms in selected cases, were reviewed for the presence or absence of endoleak. Device overlap and oversizing (relative to the proximal neck) were also determined. Type I proximal endoleak rates were estimated using the Kaplan-Meier method. The associations between the variables listed above and proximal type I endoleak were evaluated by use of Cox proportional hazards models. Proximal type I endoleak occurred in eight patients, corresponding to a 3-year incidence rate of 4% (SE = 1.5%). The median follow-up was 340 days (range, 22-1954). Univariate analyses found significant associations between proximal type I endoleak and the following variables: percentage of calcified neck circumference (hazards ratio = 2.19 for a 25% increase, p = 0.019), aneurysm maximum diameter (hazards ratio = 1.98 for a 1-cm increase, p = 0.006) and proximal neck and device overlap (hazards ratio =

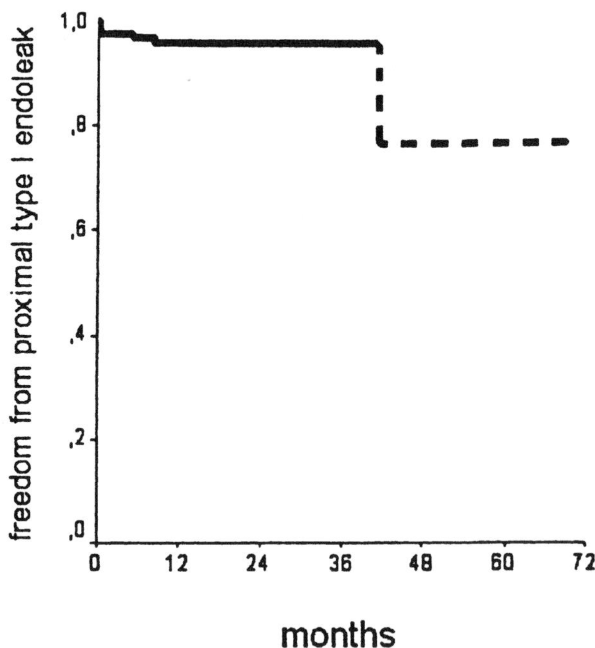

FIGURE 1.—Freedom from proximal type I endoleak: 96% at 3 years, Kaplan-Meier estimate. *Dashed line*, standard error ≥10%. (Courtesy of Sampaio SM, Panneton JM, Mozes GI, et al: Proximal type I endoleak after endovascular abdominal aortic aneurysm repair: Predictive factors. *Ann Vasc Surg* 18:621-628, 2004.)

0.53 for a 5-mm increase, $p = 0.007$). The mean overlap among cases with and without type I proximal endoleak was 15.6 mm and 29.3 mm, respectively. When these variables were included in a multivariate model, all remained statistically significant. No significant association could be documented for neck thrombus-related variables. Thirty-nine (19.3%) patients had a β neck angle inferior to 120°. There was a trend toward a higher incidence of proximal type I endoleaks in these patients ($p = 0.057$). Device oversize relative to proximal neck diameter did not affect the probability of this type of endoleak. One patient survived an emergency open repair of a ruptured aneurysm after significant expansion. Six patients underwent endovascular reinterventions (4 additional proximal cuff placements, 2 proximal angioplasties). The mean interval for reintervention was 389 days. Distal migration (≥5 mm) was identified in four cases (50%). Proximal type I endoleak is a rare complication after EVAR, but it is associated with a high number of reinterventions and potentially serious consequences. Patients with short and heavily calcified aneurysmal necks and large aneurysms are at increased risk of proximal type I endoleaks. (Fig 1)

▶ In the past, it was dogma that one did not leave the operating room with a proximal type I endoleak. Now, if everything short of open conversion has been done, most experienced endovascular surgeons will follow the endoleak expectantly, with the knowledge that more than half will resolve by 1 month and many will resolve by 6 months. The following points should be kept in mind. Fixation and late-failure modes of devices are different. So-called primary type I endoleaks (ie, those present in the perioperative period) cannot be considered along with secondary or late type I endoleaks that have been detected during follow-up when no endoleak was previously present. Primary type I endoleaks represent an error in patient or device selection and/or technical failure of the operation. Secondary type I endoleaks represent device failure as a result of migration or morphologic changes in the aneurysm.

W. A. Lee, MD

Predicting Aneurysm Enlargement in Patients With Persistent Type II Endoleaks

Timaran CH, Ohki T, Rhee SJ, et al (Albert Einstein College of Medicine, New York)

J Vasc Surg 39:1157-1162, 2004 6–10

Objective.—The clinical significance of type II endoleaks is not well understood. Some evidence, however, indicates that some type II endoleaks might result in aneurysm enlargement and rupture. To identify factors that might contribute to aneurysm expansion, we analyzed the influence of several variables on aneurysm growth in patients with persistent type II endoleaks after endovascular aortic aneurysm repair (EVAR).

Methods.—In a series of 348 EVARs performed during a 10-year period, 32 patients (9.2%) developed type II endoleaks that persisted for more than

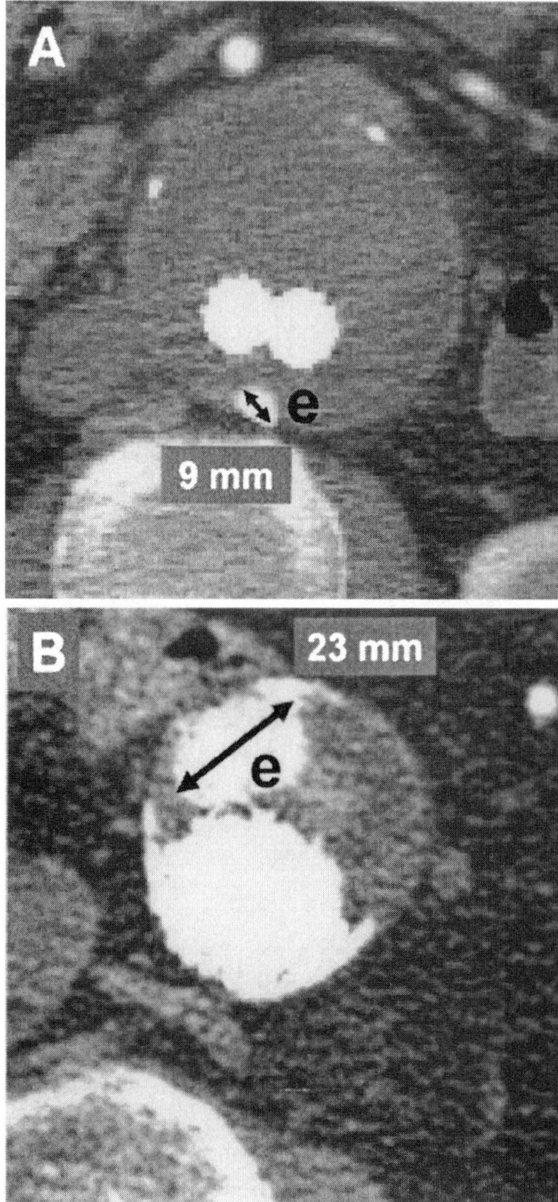

FIGURE 1.—Maximum diameter measurements of the main endoleak cavity or nidus (*e*) was obtained from CT scan images by using calipers or CT imaging analysis software with magnification and precise cursor placement. (**A**, Small endoleak nidus (2) measuring 9 mm. Although the endoleak channel was sometimes irregular and complex, a maximum nidus diameter could be determined in all patients. **B**, Large endoleak nidus measuring 23 mm in maximum diameter. When more than one nidus was seen, the maximum diameter of the largest nidus was selected. (Reprinted by permission of the publisher from Timaran CH, Ohki T, Rhee SJ, et al: Predicting aneurysm enlargement in patients with persistent type II endoleaks. *J Vasc Surg* 39:1157-1162, 2004. Copyright 2004 by Elsevier.)

6 months. Variables analyzed included those defined by the reporting standards for EVAR (SVS/AAVS) as well as other endoleak characteristics. Univariate, receiver operating characteristic curve, and Cox regression analyses were used to determine the association between variables and aneurysm enlargement.

Results.—The median follow-up period was 26.5 months (range, 6-88 months). Thirteen patients (41%) had aneurysm enlargement by 5 mm or more (median increase in diameter, 10 mm), whereas 19 (59%) had stable or shrinking aneurysm diameter. Univariate and Cox regression analyses identified the maximum diameter of the endoleak cavity, ie, the size of the nidus as defined on contrast computed tomography scan, as a significant predictor for aneurysm enlargement (relative risk, 1.12; 95% confidence interval, 1.04-1.19; P =.001). The median size of the nidus was 23 mm (range, 13-40 mm) in patients with aneurysm enlargement and 8 mm (range, 5-25 mm) in those without expansion (Mann-Whitney U test, P <.001). Moreover, receiver operating characteristic curve and Cox regression analyses showed that a maximum nidus diameter greater than 15 mm was particularly associated with an increased risk of aneurysm enlargement (relative risk, 11.1; 95% confidence interval, 1.4-85.8; P =.02). Other risk factors including gender, smoking history, hypertension, need of anticoagulation, aneurysm diameter, type of endograft used, and number or type of collateral vessels were not significant predictors of aneurysm enlargement.

Conclusions.—In patients with persistent type II endoleaks after EVAR, the maximum diameter of the endoleak cavity or nidus is an important predictor of aneurysm growth and might indicate the need for more aggressive surveillance as well as earlier treatment (Fig 1).

▶ "Minimally" controversial statements about type II endoleaks are (1) they comprise the majority of endoleaks; (2) they generally follow a benign course; (3) the only clear indication for intervention is demonstrated aneurysm growth; (4) individually, aneurysms can grow or shrink with or without endoleak; and (5) it remains unpredictable which aneurysms with type II endoleaks will grow or shrink. The authors report the concept of an "endoleak nidus." Their methods for assessing the nidus are suspect given the nidus is a complex 3-dimensional space that cannot be characterized by a 1-dimensional measure. Visualization of this space with CT is dependent on a host of dynamic factors, including timing of the contrast bolus, cardiac output, inflow and outflow state of the aneurysm sac, and specific gravity of the contrast agent relative to the liquefied portions of the sac.

W. A. Lee, MD

Explant Analysis of AneuRx Stent Grafts: Relationship Between Structural Findings and Clinical Outcome

Zarins CK, Arko FR, Crabtree T, et al (Stanford Univ, Calif; Cleveland Clinic Found, Ohio; Cleveland Clinic, Naples, Fla; et al)

J Vasc Surg 40:1-11, 2004 6–11

Objective.—We reviewed the structural findings of explanted AneuRx stent grafts used to treat abdominal aortic aneurysms, and relate the findings to clinical outcome measures.

Methods.—We reviewed data for all bifurcated AneuRx stent grafts explanted at surgery or autopsy and returned to the manufacturer from the US clinical trial and worldwide experience of more than 33,000 implants from 1996 to 2003. Devices implanted for more than 1 month with structural analysis are included in this article. Explant results were analyzed in relation to cause of explantation and pre-explant evidence of endoleak, enlargement, or device migration.

Results.—One hundred twenty explanted stent grafts, including 37 from the US clinical trial, were analyzed. Mean implant duration was 22 ± 13 months (range, 1-61 months). Structural abnormalities included stent fatigue fractures, fabric abrasion holes, and suture breaks. The mean number of nitinol stent strut fractures per explanted device was 3 ± 4, which represents less than 0.2% of the total number of stent struts in each device. The mean number of fabric holes per explanted device was 2 ± 3, with a median hole size of 0.5 mm^2. Suture breaks were seen in most explanted devices, but composed less than 1.5% of the total number of sutures per device. "For cause" explants (n = 104) had a 10-month longer implant duration (P =.007) compared with "incidental" explants (n = 16). "For cause" explants had more fractures (3 ± 5; P =.005) and fabric holes (2 ± 3; P =.008) per device compared with "incidental" explants, but these differences were not significant (P =.3) when adjusted for duration of device implantation. Among clinical trial explants the number of fabric holes in grafts in patients with endoleak (2 ± 3 per device) was no different from those without endoleak (3 ± 4 per device; P = NS). The number of fatigue fractures or fabric holes was no different in grafts in clinical trial patients with pre-explant aneurysm enlargement compared with those without enlargement. Pre-explant stent-graft migration was associated with a greater number of stent strut fractures (5 ± 7 per device; P =.04) and fabric holes (3 ± 3 per bifurcation; P =.03) compared with explants without migration. Serial imaging studies revealed inadequate proximal, distal, or junctional device fixation as the probable cause of rupture or need for conversion to open surgery in 86% of "for cause" explants. Structural device abnormalities were usually remote from fixation sites, and no causal relationship between device findings and clinical outcome could be established.

Conclusions.—Nitinol stent fatigue fractures, fabric holes, and suture breaks found in explanted AneuRx stent grafts do not appear to be related to clinical outcome measures. Longer term studies are needed to confirm these observations (Fig 5).

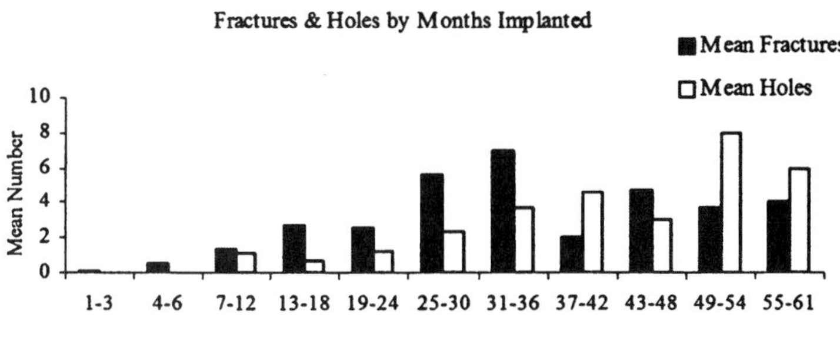

FIGURE 5.—Fractures and holes as a function of number of months the device was implanted. Number of explants at each time point is indicated on the x-axis. (Reprinted by permission of the publisher from Zarins CK, Arko FR, Crabtree T, et al: Explant analysis of AneuRx stent grafts: Relationship between structural findings and clinical outcome. *J Vasc Surg* 40:1-11, 2004. Copyright 2004 by Elsevier.)

▶ This is an observational study of late structural failures of one type of aortic stent graft. There are several important points to consider as follows: (1) stent fractures, fabric holes, and suture breaks are quite common; (2) despite Dr Chuter's (primary Discussant) analogy of "a broken chain is still broken even if 99% of the links remain intact," there is some redundancy intrinsic to any complex mechanical object, and many late structural failures do not lead to an immediate type III endoleak; (3) angulation and tortuosity identify areas of chronic mechanical stress and negatively impact long-term device integrity; and (4) the primary causes of late failure is loss of or inadequate initial fixation and seal, not structural failures of the device itself.

W. A. Lee, MD

Initial Management and Outcome of Aortic Endograft Limb Occlusion

Erzurum VZ, Sampram ESK, Sarac TP, et al (Cleveland Clinic Found, Ohio)

J Vasc Surg 40:419-423, 2004 6–12

Objective.—The purpose of this study was to determine the differences in outcome related to initial management of aortic endograft limb occlusion (ELO).

Methods.—During a 7-year period, 823 endovascular aneurysm repairs (EVARs) resulted in 25 ELOs in 22 patients. The initial management and outcome of these ELOs were reviewed. Median follow-up after ELO was 24.2 ± 16.8 months.

Results.—Initial EVARs included both unsupported unibody (n = 5) and supported modular (n = 17) devices. ELO was significantly more common in the unsupported unibody graft design (P <.024) and with extension of the graft limb to the external iliac artery (P <.001). ELO was managed with an endovascular approach (EVA), including some combination of mechanical thrombectomy (n = 8), angioplasty with or without stenting (n = 8), and thrombolysis (n = 2) in 12 patients and bypass procedures (femoral-femoral bypass, n = 11; axillofemoral bypass, n = 1; and aortofemoral bypass, n =

1) in 13. At 12-month follow-up, freedom from secondary procedures with EVA was 80.2 ± 17.7% versus 53.2 ± 17.1% with extra-anatomic bypass (EB) (P = NS). Secondary patency was 100% with EVA and 80.6 ± 14.4% with EB (P = NS). Of the 12 EVAs, there was 1 (8.3%) perioperative mortality with EVA and none with EB. EB failure was directly attributed to donor limb occlusion in 4 of 6 EVAs (67%), and when this occurred it resulted in bilateral lower extremity ischemia. Amputation was required in 2 of 12 (16.7%) EBs versus none of the 12 EVAs (P = NS). EVA never resulted in graft dislodgement or endoleak but did identify an underlying treatable cause in 8 of 12 (67%).

Conclusion.—Both EVA and EB are acceptable management strategies for ELO. The potential risk of graft dislodgement was not observed with an EVA. If EB is employed, assessment of the donor limb and treatment of any underlying lesions is advisable in an attempt to minimize future donor limb occlusion.

▶ This article supports the observation that limb occlusion is a device-dependent complication with unsupported limbs posing the greatest risk. Indeed, despite comprising only 8% of the endografts in this study, Ancure devices represented 28% of limb occlusions. Now that all approved devices are fully supported, one can anticipate decreased occlusion rates. The groups in the article are too small to make any meaningful recommendations as to the optimal treatment of limb occlusions. The mere detection of an asymptomatic limb occlusion on routine imaging should not prompt treatment. For symptomatic occlusions, 2 small groin incisions with a femoral-femoral bypass is an expedient solution.

W. A. Lee, MD

Effects of Bilateral Hypogastric Artery Interruption During Endovascular and Open Aortoiliac Aneurysm Repair

Mehta M, Veith FJ, Darling C III, et al (Inst for Vascular Health and Disease, Albany, NY; Montefiore Med Ctr, New York)

J Vasc Surg 40:698-702, 2004 6–13

Purpose.—Hypogastric artery interruption is sometimes required during aortoiliac aneurysm repair. We have not experienced some of the life-threatening complications of pelvic ischemia reported by others. Therefore we analyzed our experience to identify factors that help minimize pelvic ischemia with unilateral and bilateral hypogastric artery interruption.

Methods.—From 1995 to 2003, 48 patients with aortoiliac aneurysm required interruption of both hypogastric arteries as part of endovascular (n = 32) or open surgical (n = 16) repair. During endovascular aneurysm repair coils were placed at the origin of the hypogastric arteries, and bilateral hypogastric artery interruptions were staged at 1 to 2 weeks when possible. Open surgery necessitated oversewing or excluding the origins of the hypogastric arteries and extending the prosthetic graft to the external iliac or femoral artery. Collateral branches from the external iliac and femoral arteries were preserved, and patients received systemic heparinization (50 units/kg).

Results.—There was no buttock necrosis, ischemic colitis requiring colon resection, or death with the bilateral hypogastric artery interruption. Initially buttock claudication developed in 20 patients (42%), but persisted in only 7 patients (15%) at 1 year. New onset of impotence occurred in 4 of 28 patients (14%), and there were no neurologic deficits.

Conclusions.—Bilateral hypogastric artery interruptions can be accomplished with limited morbidity. When hypogastric artery interruption is needed during endovascular aneurysm repair, certain principles help minimize pelvic ischemia. These include hypogastric artery interruption at its origin to preserve the pelvic collateral vessels, staging bilateral hypogastric artery interruptions when possible, preserving collateral branches from the femoral and external iliac arteries, and providing adequate heparinization of the patient during these procedures.

► I am dismayed to come across another article proposing the safety of bilateral hypogastric interruption. Although the incidence of life-threatening pelvic ischemia is relatively rare after acute hypogastric interruption, it makes little sense to subject a patient to this risk when alternatives exist. The authors recommend the often practiced but completely unproven method of "staging" bilateral hypogastric interruptions. It does not make sense that 1 to 2 weeks will make any real difference in recruitment of collaterals. It takes at least 6 months for the 40% to 45% of patients who sustain buttock claudication to start noticing any improvement in their symptoms. Truncal versus distal branch embolization has also never been shown to make any difference. This article certainly does not provide additional evidence one way or the other, although, occasionally, bilateral hypogastric interruption may be necessary to facilitate repair of a complex aortoiliac aneurysm. However, these situations are uncommon. Patients with buttock and thigh claudication after endovascular aneurysm repair are some of the most miserable patients. The impact of this complication on quality of life cannot be underestimated.

W. A. Lee, MD

Overt Ischemic Colitis After Endovascular Repair of Aortoiliac Aneurysms

Geraghty PJ, Sanchez LA, Rubin BG, et al (Washington Univ, St Louis)
J Vasc Surg 40:413-418, 2004 6–14

Objective.—Controversy exists as to the cause of ischemic colitis complicating endovascular aneurysm repair. Occlusion of the hypogastric arteries (HAs) during endovascular repair of aortoiliac aneurysms (AIAs) results in a significant incidence of buttock claudication, and has been suggested as a causative factor in the development of postprocedural colonic ischemia, in addition to factors such as systemic hypotension, embolization of atheromatous debris, and interruption of inferior mesenteric artery inflow. To analyze the relationship between perioperative HA occlusion and postoperative ischemic colitis, we reviewed our experience over 2 years with Food and Drug Administration-approved endovascular graft devices for treatment of AIAs.

Methods.—Elective repair of AIAs with bifurcated endovascular grafts was performed in 233 patients over a 2-year period. These included 184 AneuRx grafts, 17 Ancure grafts, and 32 Excluder grafts. During the experience, 44 patients (18.9%) underwent unilateral perioperative HA occlusion (28 right, 16 left) during the course of endovascular AIA repair, and 1 patient (0.4%) underwent bilateral HA occlusion.

Results.—In 4 patients (1.7%) signs and symptoms of ischemic colitis developed 2.0 ± 1.4 days postoperatively. In all patients the diagnosis was confirmed at sigmoidoscopy, and initial treatment included bowel rest, hydration, and intravenous antibiotic agents. Three patients with bilateral patent HAs required colonic resection 14.7 ± 9.7 days after the initial diagnosis, and 2 of these 3 patients died in the postoperative period. Pathologic findings confirmed the presence of atheroemboli in the colonic vasculature in all 3 patients who underwent colonic resection. The fourth patient had undergone multiple manipulations of the left HA in an unsuccessful attempt to preserve patency of this vessel during AIA repair. This patient recovered completely with nonoperative management. Perioperative unilateral HA occlusion was not associated with a significantly higher incidence of postoperative ischemic colitis.

Conclusion.—Perioperative HA occlusion during aortoiliac open or endovascular surgery may contribute to development of the rare but potentially lethal complication of ischemic colitis. However, our extensive experience suggests that embolization of atheromatous debris to the HA tissue beds during endovascular manipulations, rather than proximal HA occlusion, is the primary cause of clinically significant ischemic colitis after endovascular aneurysm repair.

▶ This small case series does not provide enough data to support atheroemboli as the primary reason for colonic ischemia after endovascular aneurysm repair (EVAR). The presence of cholesterol emboli on histologic analysis does not prove cansation. Given the manipulations typically performed in a thrombus-laden aortoiliac system during EVAR, if colonic histologic findings were available for every endograft case, one would likely find a high incidence of asymptomatic atheroemboli. Other factors, such as hypogastric occlusion, may significantly contribute to clinically important colonic ischemia. The author's recommendation for "meticulous interventional technique" is lofty but moot. Rhetorically speaking, who knowingly does not exercise meticulous technique?

W. A. Lee, MD

Late Abdominal Aortic Aneurysm Enlargement After Endovascular Repair With the Excluder Device
Cho J-S, Dillavou ED, Rhee RY, et al (Univ of Pittsburgh, Pa)
J Vasc Surg 39:1236-1242, 2004 6–15

Objectives.—Behavior of the abdominal aortic aneurysm (AAA) sac after endovascular abdominal aortic aneurysm repair (EVAR) is graft-dependent. The Excluder endograft has been associated with less sac regression than some other stent grafts. Long-term follow-up has not been reported.

Methods.—Between May 1999 and July 2002, 50 patients underwent EVAR with the Excluder bifurcated endoprosthesis. These patients were followed up prospectively with computed tomography (CT) at 1, 6, and 12 months and yearly thereafter. One immediate conversion to open surgery and three deaths occurred within 6 months. One additional patient was lost to follow-up. The remaining 45 patients, 35 men and 10 women, were followed up for at least 1 year, and form the basis for this report. Their mean age

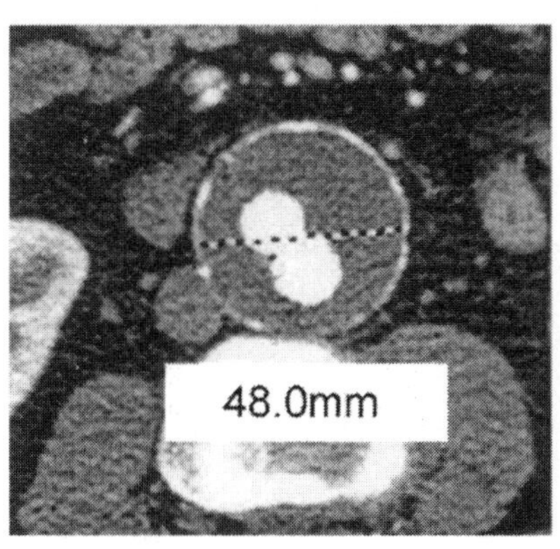

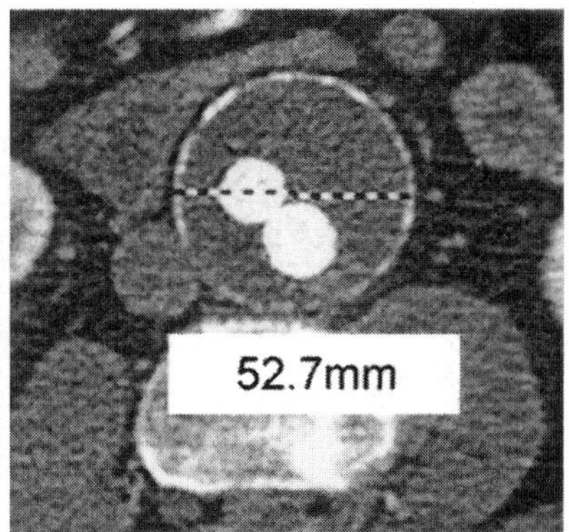

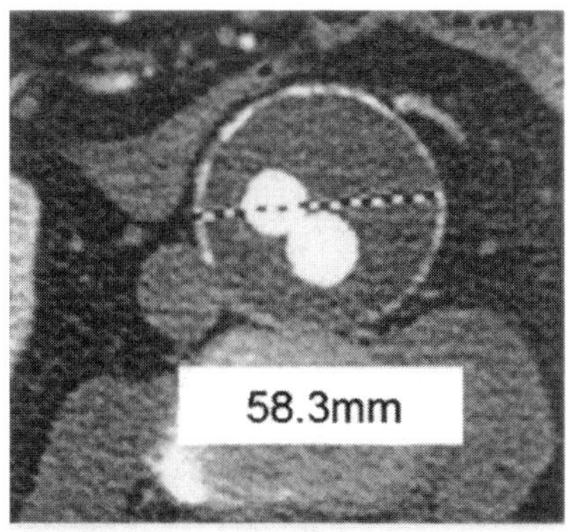

FIGURE 3.—Serial computed tomography scans demonstrate gradual increase in abdominal aortic aneurysm sac size after implantation of the Excluder device. (Reprinted by permission of the publisher from Cho J-S, Dillavou ED, Rhee RY, et al: Late abdominal aortic aneurysm enlargement after endovascular repair with the Excluder device. *J Vasc Surg* 39:1236-1242, 2004. Copyright 2004 by Elsevier.)

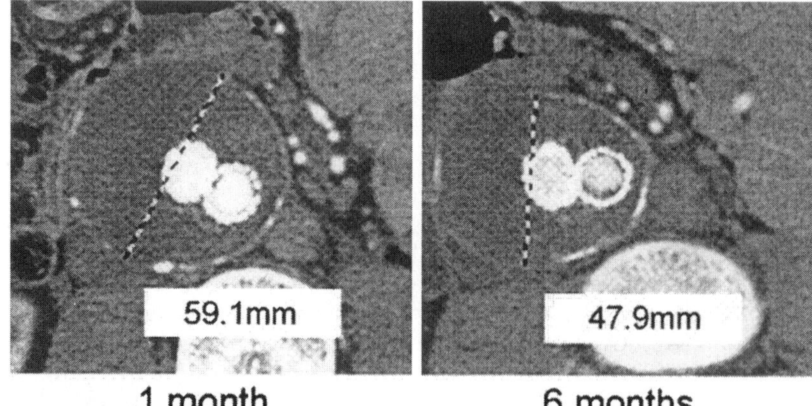

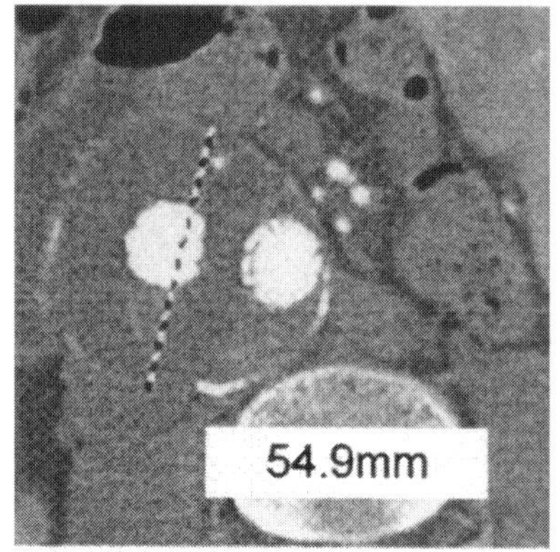

FIGURE 5.—Serial computed tomography scans demonstrate initial decrease in abdominal aortic aneurysm sac size, followed by re-expansion. (Reprinted by permission of the publisher from Cho J-S, Dillavou ED, Rhee RY, et al: Late abdominal aortic aneurysm enlargement after endovascular repair with the Excluder device. *J Vasc Surg* 39:1236-1242, 2004. Copyright 2004 by Elsevier.)

was 73 ± 5.5 years. The minor axis diameter at the largest area of the AAA on CT examination was compared with the baseline measurement at 1 month and to the smallest size previously recorded during follow-up. Change in sac size of 5 mm or greater was considered significant. Mean follow-up was 2.7 ± 1.2 years (range, 1-4 years). Nominal variables were compared with the χ^2 test, and continuous variables with the Student *t* test.

Results.—A significant decrease in average AAA sac diameter was observed at 6-month, 1-year, and 2-year follow-up. These differences were lost by the 3-year evaluation, because of delayed sac growth (n = 9) and re-expansion of once shrunken aneurysms (n = 3). The probability of freedom from sac growth or re-expansion at 4 years was only 43%. At last follow-up, sac expansion occurred in the absence of active endoleak in nine patients. Type II endoleak was associated with sac expansion in three patients (P =.003), resulting in one conversion to open surgery after the 4-year follow-up. No graft migrations, AAA ruptures, or aneurysm-related deaths were noted.

Conclusions.—Late aneurysm sac growth or re-expansion after EVAR with the Excluder device is common, even in the absence of endoleak. Although the incidence of important clinical sequelae is low at this point, the incidence of aneurysm expansion should be taken into consideration during the risk-benefit assessment before EVAR repair with the Excluder device (Fig 3 and Fig 5).

▶ The only thing contributing to sac growth after EVAR that is readily remediable is transgraft transudation. W. L. Gore has subsequently redesigned the Excluder device with a new, extremely low permeable expanded polytetrafluoroethylene. Whether this has "fixed" the problem remains to be seen. I dislike reports like this that focus attention on surrogate markers of EVAR success or failure. The only true end points of any therapy for aortic aneurysms are rupture and aneurysm-related death.

W. A. Lee, MD

Symptomatic Sac Enlargement and Rupture Due to Seroma After Open Abdominal Aortic Aneurysm Repair With Polytetrafluoroethylene Graft: Implications for Endovascular Repair and Endotension

Thoo CHC, Bourke BM, May J (Gosford Hosp, Australia; Univ of Sydney)

J Vasc Surg 40:1089-1094, 2004 6–16

Objective.—We report 5 patients in whom a symptomatic perigraft seroma developed within the aortic sac, without vascular endoleak, after open repair of an abdominal aortic aneurysm (AAA) with a polytetrafluoroethylene (PTFE) graft. We also discuss possible relationships of this phenomenon to endovascular repair of AAAs.

Patients and Methods.—Over 18 years, 1156 patients underwent repair of an AAA by one of the authors (B.M.B.). Of these, 1084 underwent open repair, 256 with PTFE grafts. Five patients in the PTFE group (2.3%) returned at a mean of 4.5 years with acute abdominal or back pain and enlargement of the aortic sac. Mean diameter of the aneurysms was 5.9 cm preoperatively and 8.1 cm at readmission. There was no evidence of vascular endoleak on computed tomography scans, but 1 patient had a retroperitoneal hematoma.

Results.—Laparotomy in 4 patients disclosed a seroma containing firm rubbery gelatinous material under tension, histologically identified as amorphous eosinophilic material containing thrombus and degenerate blood cells in all cases. Rupture of the sac was confirmed in the patient with a retroperitoneal hematoma. The sac contents were evacuated and the integrity of the underlying grafts and anastomoses was confirmed before sac reduction, with imbricating sutures, and closure was performed. One patient died at 8 months of an unrelated cause; the other 3 patients remain well at mean follow-up of 12 months. The fifth patient received conservative treatment and remains asymptomatic 3 years after acute presentation.

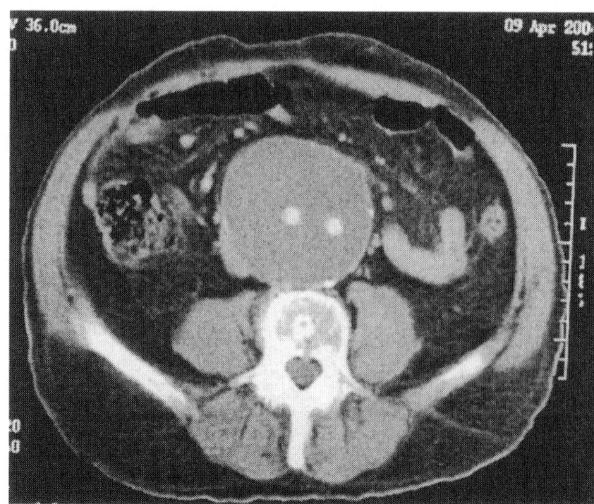

FIGURE 1.—Case 3. Five years after open AAA repair, contrast-enhanced computed tomography scan demonstrates a sac 9 cm in diameter surrounding graft limbs. (Reprinted by permission of the publisher from Thoo CHC, Bourke BM, May J: Symptomatic sac enlargement and rupture due to seroma after open abdominal aortic aneurysm repair with polytetrafluoroethylene graft: Implications for endovascular repair and endotension. *J Vasc Surg* 40:1089-1094, 2004. Copyright 2004 by Elsevier.)

Conclusions.—These findings of sac enlargement without vascular endoleak after open AAA repair are reminiscent of sac enlargement in the absence of endoleak after endovascular AAA repair. This has been referred to as endotension. The comparatively benign outcome in 5 patients with symptomatic sac enlargement, including 2 patients with rupture, after open AAA repair provides data to support a circumspect approach to endotension, especially in patients with asymptomatic disease, which has been reported as occurring in almost half of patients who received a PTFE Excluder endograft (Fig 1).

▶ We do not know the actual incidence of sac enlargement after ePTFE graft replacement. The rate of symptomatic enlargement may be approximately 2% at 4 years. As noted above, we do not know the clinical significance, if any, of sac enlargement, symptomatic or not. A conservative and "circumspect approach" to its management is warranted.

W. A. Lee, MD

Treatment of Short-necked Infrarenal Aortic Aneurysms With Fenestrated Stent-Grafts: Short-term Results

Verhoeven ELG, Prins TR, Tielliu IFJ, et al (Univ Hosp of Groningen, The Netherlands)

Eur J Vasc Endovasc Surg 27:477-483, 2004 6–17

Introduction.—A proximal neck of 15 mm length is usually required to allow endovascular repair of abdominal aortic aneurysms (EVAR). Many

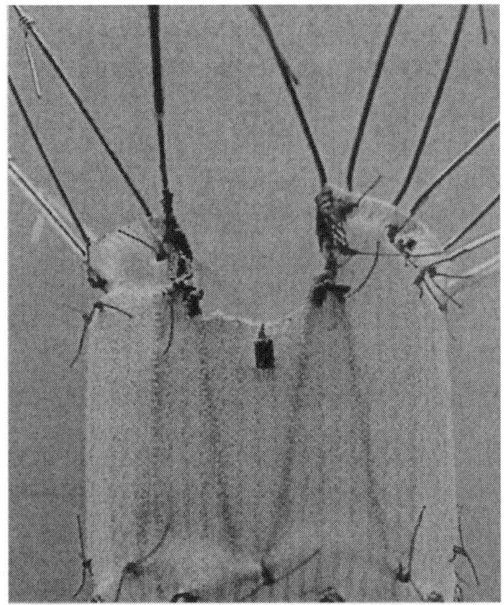

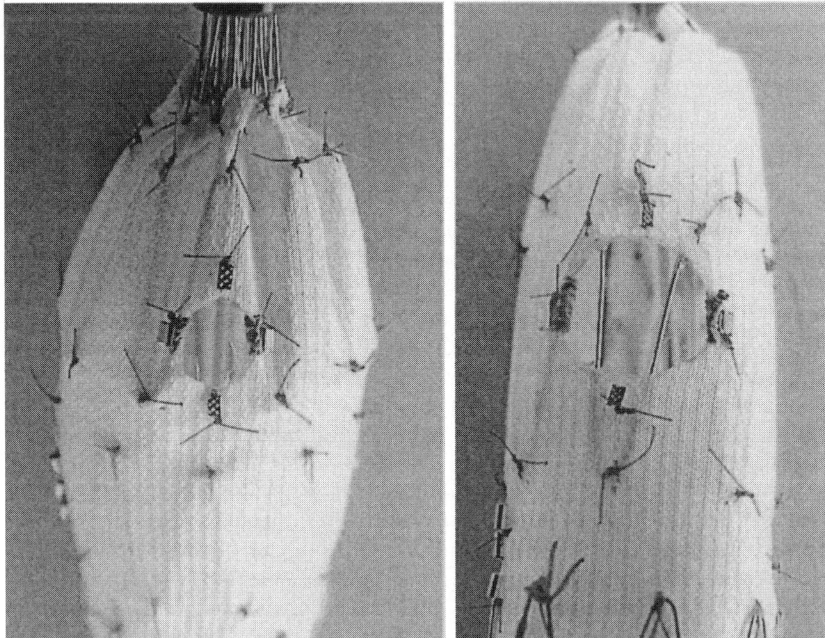

FIGURE 2.—Different types of fenestrations: scallop, large fenestration, and small fenestration. (Reprinted from Verhoeven ELG, Prins TR, Tielliu IFJ, et al: Treatment of short-necked infrarenal aortic aneurysms with fenestrated stent-grafts: Short-term results. *Eur J Vasc Endovasc Surg* 27:477-483, 2004. Copyright 2004 by permission of the publisher.)

patients have been refused EVAR due to a short neck. By customising fenestrated grafts to the patients' anatomy, we can offer an endovascular solution, especially for patients who are unsuitable for open repair.

Methods.—Eighteen patients were selected for fenestrated stent-grafting if they presented with an abdominal aneurysm of at least 55 mm in diameter, a short neck (less than 15 mm), plus contra-indications for open repair (cardiopulmonary impairment or a hostile abdomen). The stent-graft used was a customised fenestrated model based on the Cook Zenith® composite system. We used additional stents to ensure apposition of the fenestrations with the side branches.

Results.—All endovascular procedures were successful. Out of the 46 targeted side branches (10 superior mesenteric arteries, 36 renal arteries), 45 were patent at the end of the procedure. One accessory renal artery became occluded by the stent-graft. There was one possible proximal type I endoleak, which later proved to be a type II endoleak. There was no mortality, but complications occurred in six patients: two cardiac complications, three urinary complications and one occlusion of a renal artery. At follow-up (mean 9.4 months, range 1-18), there were no additional renal complications and all the remaining targeted vessels stayed patent.

Discussion.—By customizing fenestrated stent-grafts, it is possible to position the first covered stent completely inside the proximal neck, thus achieving a more stable position. The additional side-stents may also contribute to a better fixation. This technique may become a valuable alternative for patients who are at high risk from open surgery (Fig 2).

▶ More than 800 fenestrated devices have been implanted worldwide (mainly Europe and Australia). Regulatory constraints have limited their dissemination in the United States. The primary advance has been separation of aortoiliac anatomy into the perivisceral component and the infrarenal component. This simplifies the procedure by using the fenestrated tube device as a "suprarenal aortic adapter" creating an endovascular "neck." A conventional endovascular repair can then be performed without the complexity of simultaneous orientation of the fenestrations and the iliac limbs.

W. A. Lee, MD

Rupture of Abdominal Aortic Aneurysm: Concurrent Comparison of Outcome of Those Occurring After Endovascular Repair Versus Those Occurring Without Previous Treatment in an 11-Year Single-Center Experience

May J, White GH, Stephen MS, et al (Univ of Sydney; Royal Prince Alfred Hosp, Sydney)

J Vasc Surg 40:860-866, 2004 6–18

Objective.—The purpose of this single-center study was to compare findings at presentation and surgical outcome in patients in whom abdominal aortic aneurysms (AAAs) ruptured after endovascular repair and patients in whom AAAs ruptured before any treatment, over a defined period.

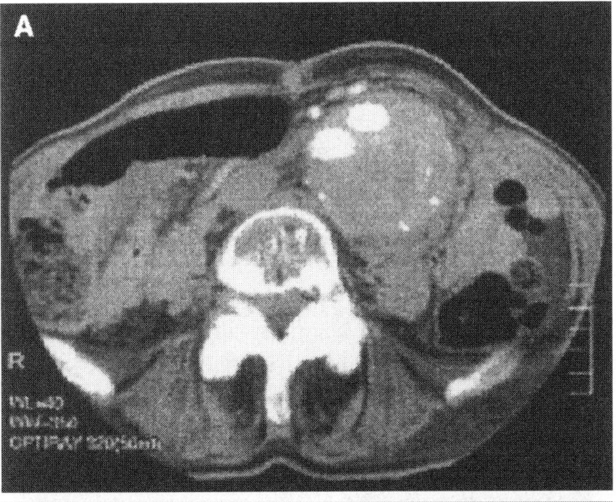

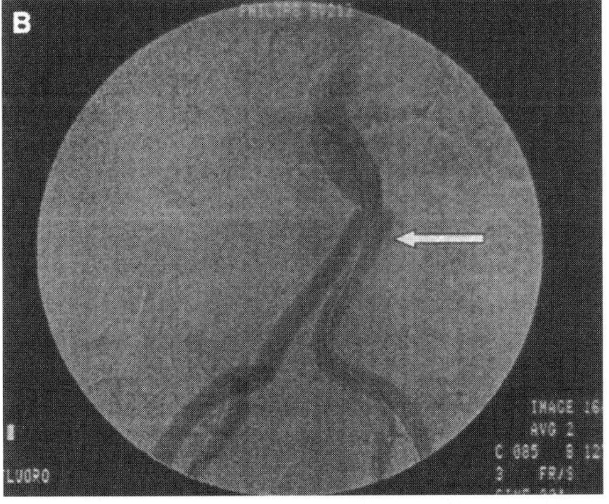

FIGURE 1.—This case illustrates the limitations of surveillance with annual scans and the importance of plain x-ray films in demonstrating separation of radiopaque markers. The patient underwent endovascular abdominal aortic aneurysm (AAA) repair with a Vanguard prosthesis in 1996. Preoperative diameter was 5.4 cm. At follow-up, diameter was 5.00 cm (1998), 5.2 cm (1999), 5.5 cm (2000), 5.5 cm (2002) and 6.1 cm (2003). No endoleak was demonstrated in these studies. **A**, Contrast material-enhanced computed tomography scan of AAA (diameter, 6.5 cm) demonstrates endoleak and rupture, obtained 10 days after annual scan in 2003, which demonstrated no endoleak. **B**, Aortogram demonstrates type III endoleak between contralateral stump and contralateral limb (*arrow*) (Reprinted by permission of the publisher from May J, White GH, Stephen MS, et al: Rupture of abdominal aortic aneurysm: Concurrent comparison of outcome of those occurring after endovascular repair versus those occurring without previous treatment in an 11-year single-center experience. *J Vasc Surg* 40: 860-866, 2004. Copyright 2004 by Elsevier.)

Methods.—From May 1992 to September 2003, 1043 patients underwent elective repair of intact infrarenal AAAs. Endovascular repair was performed in 609 patients, and open repair in 434 patients. Eighteen of 609 patients (3%) who underwent endovascular AAA repair required treatment because of rupture of the aneurysm after a mean of 29 months (group 1). During the same 11-year period, another 91 patients without previous treatment required urgent repair of a ruptured AAA (group 2). Rupture was diagnosed at contrast material-enhanced computed tomography or by presence of extramural extravasation of blood at open repair. Except for a higher incidence of women in group 2, patients in both groups were similar with regard to demographics and clinical characteristics but differed in findings at presentation. Eight patients in group 1 had a known endoleak before AAA rupture, whereas contrast-enhanced computed tomography, performed in 15 patients at presentation, demonstrated an endoleak in all. Hypotension (systolic blood pressure <100 mm Hg) was noted at presentation in 4 of 18 patients (22%) in group 1 and 76 of 91 patients (84%) in group 2. All patients underwent open repair via a transperitoneal approach, except for 4 patients in group 1 and 3 patients in group 2 who underwent endovascular repair of ruptured AAAs.

Results.—The proportion of patients with hypotension at presentation in group 1 (4 of 18) was significantly less than in group 2 (76 of 91; $P < .01$). The difference in perioperative (30 day) mortality rate in group 1 (3 of 18; 16.6%) compared with group 2 (49 of 91; 53.8%) was also significant ($P < .01$). The outcome in group 1 was therefore superior to that in group 2.

Conclusions.—This study confirms that endovascular AAA repair complicated by endoleak does not prevent rupture. The data suggest, however, that rupture, when it occurs in these circumstances, may not be accompanied by such major hemodynamic changes and high mortality as rupture of an untreated AAA. Further long-term follow-up and analysis in a larger group of patients are required to confirm the apparent intermediate level of protection afforded by failed endovascular repair, which does not prevent rupture but enhances survival after operation to treat rupture, possibly by ameliorating the hemodynamic changes associated with the rupture process (Fig 1).

▶ The risk of rupture after EVAR is real, about 1% per year. Aneurysm ruptures after endovascular aneurysm repair (EVAR) are not all equal. Direct large-caliber communication between the aortic circulation and the aneurysm sac is similar to a free rupture in an untreated aneurysm (ie, type I or III endoleak). Rupture that is secondary to a patent branch-vessel or endotension without demonstrable leak is similar to a stable contained rupture (see also Abstract 6–12). The authors correctly point out neither endoleaks nor aneurysm sac changes are reliable markers of impending failure. An examination of stent graft configuration, aneurysm morphology, and stability of fixation, from plain radiographs and other imaging studies, may be most important.

W. A. Lee, MD

Embolization as Cause of Bowel Ischemia After Endovascular Abdominal Aortic Aneurysm Repair

Zhang WW, Kulaylat MN, Anain PM, et al (State Univ of New York at Buffalo; Buffalo Catholic Health System, NY)

J Vasc Surg 40:867-872, 2004 6–19

Objective.—We investigated the incidence, cause, and outcome of large bowel and small bowel ischemia after endovascular abdominal aortic aneurysm (AAA) repair.

Methods.—Medical records for all patients undergoing endovascular AAA repair from December 1999 to December 2003 were reviewed. The incidence, cause, and outcome of clinically detected postoperative bowel ischemia were analyzed.

Results.—Seven hundred two endovascular AAA repairs were performed. In 10 patients (1.4%) acute bowel ischemia developed. Six of these patients

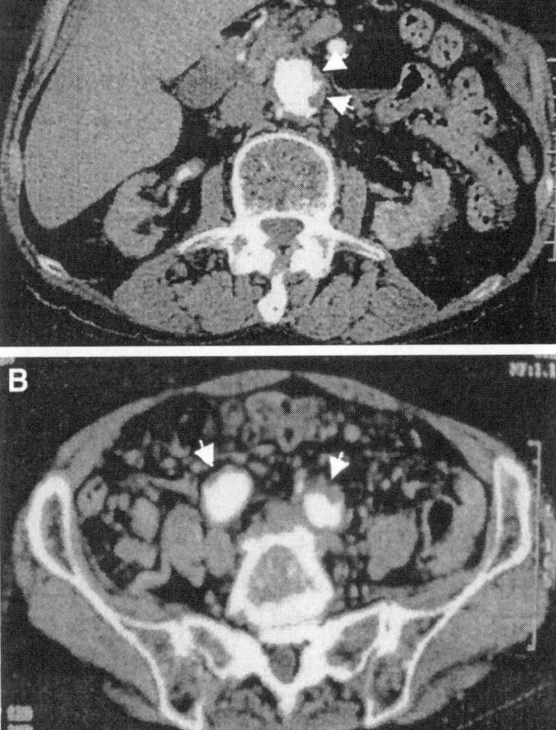

FIGURE 1.—Computed tomography scans show thrombus or atheroma in proximal neck of abdominal aortic aneurysm (*arrows*; **A**), and thrombus or atheroma in bilateral iliac arteries (*arrows*; **B**). These are possible sources of microembolization during endovascular aneurysm repair. (Reprinted by permission of the publisher from Zhang WW, Kulaylat MN, Anain PM, et al: Embolization as cause of bowel ischemia after endovascular abdominal aortic aneurysm repair. *J Vasc Surg* 40:867-872, 2004. Copyright 2004 by Elsevier.)

sustained concurrent small bowel necrosis, and the remaining 4 had isolated colon ischemia. Seven patients underwent exploratory laparotomy. In 6 of these bowel resection was performed, and in 1 patient the ischemic bowel was unsalvageable. Of the 6 patients with small and large bowel ischemia, 4 had segmental or patchy necrosis, which was separated by normal-appearing intestine, and 1 had extensive ischemia that involved most of the small bowel and the entire colon, with pathologic evidence of microembolization. Three patients had preoperative occlusion of the inferior mesenteric artery. One had unilateral and 1 had bilateral hypogastric artery interruption. Five of the 6 patients with small bowel ischemia had thrombus or atheroma in the proximal aneurysmal necks. All patients with isolated colon ischemia survived. All 6 patients with concurrent small bowel ischemia died.

Conclusion.—The total incidence of clinically evident bowel ischemia after endovascular AAA repair is similar to that after open surgery. However, small bowel ischemia occurs more commonly in patients with endovascular repair, and is associated with extremely high mortality. The direct pathologic evidence and the patterns of segmental, skipped, or patchy ischemia in most patients imply that microembolization has an important role (Fig 1).

▶ This article should be read together with Abstract 6–10 in this section. Atheroembolization during endovascular aneurysm repair (EVAR) has always been a concern during the early collective experience of this procedure. I think everyone was surprised to find that the rate of clinically significant atheroembolization was as low as it was. Although the authors present a cogent argument for atheroemboli as the cause of the bowel ischemia, it is likely not the only nor even the major cause. Bowel ischemia is a fatal complication after any vascular procedure, whether endovascular or open. Expeditious diagnosis and definitive treatment provide the best hope of survival.

W. A. Lee, MD

Endovascular Aneurysm Repair Versus Open Repair in Patients With Abdominal Aortic Aneurysm (EVAR Trial 1): Randomised Controlled Trial

Greenhalgh RM, for the EVAR Trial Participants (Imperial College of London; et al)

Lancet 365:2179-2186, 2005 6–20

Background.—Although endovascular aneurysm repair (EVAR) has a lower 30-day operative mortality than open repair, the long-term results of EVAR are uncertain. We instigated EVAR trial 1 to compare these two treatments in terms of mortality, durability, health-related quality of life (HRQL), and costs for patients with large abdominal aortic aneurysm (AAA).

Methods.—We did a randomised controlled trial of 1082 patients aged 60 years or older who had aneurysms of at least 5.5 cm in diameter and who had been referred to one of 34 hospitals proficient in the EVAR technique. We assigned patients who were anatomically suitable for EVAR and fit for an open repair to EVAR (n=543) or open repair (n=539). Our primary endpoint was all-cause mortality, with secondary endpoints of aneurysm related mortality, HRQL, postoperative complications, and hospital costs. Analyses were by intention to treat.

Findings.—94% (1017 of 1082) of patients complied with their allocated treatment and 209 died by the end of follow-up on Dec 31, 2004 (53 of aneurysm-related causes). 4 years after randomisation, all-cause mortality was similar in the two groups (about 28%; hazard ratio 0.90, 95% CI 0.69-1.18, p=0.46), although there was a persistent reduction in aneurysm-related deaths in the EVAR group (4% vs 7%; 0.55, 0.31-0.96, p=0.04). The proportion of patients with postoperative complications within 4 years of randomisation was 41% in the EVAR group and 9% in the open repair group (4.9, 3.5-6.8, p<0.0001). After 12 months there was negligible difference in HRQL between the two groups. The mean hospital costs per patient up to 4 years were UK £13,257 for the EVAR group versus £9946 for the open repair group (mean difference £3311, SE 690).

Interpretation.—Compared with open repair, EVAR offers no advantage with respect to all-cause mortality and HRQL, is more expensive, and leads to a greater number of complications and reinterventions. However, it does result in a 3% better aneurysm-related survival. The continuing need for interventions mandates ongoing surveillance and longer follow-up of EVAR for detailed cost-effectiveness assessment.

► Both the EVAR trial and the DREAM Study indicate short-term perioperative survival benefit for EVARs (Abstracts 6–1 and 6–2). Longer-term results are disappointing. Clearly, EVAR is not a clear winner for many patients and certainly not for the health care system. I suspect, however, that it is a clear winner for those companies that manufacture endovascular grafts. Some will regard this trial (see also Abstract 6–8) and the DREAM Trial as essentially showing overall equivalence of endovascular and open repair of AAAs. Given this interpretation, it is unlikely the results of these 2 trials will have any affect on the frequency of EVAR for AAA.

G. L. Moneta, MD

7 Aortoiliac Disease

Aortofemoral Bypass in Young Patients With Premature Atherosclerosis: Is Superficial Femoral Vein Superior to Dacron?

Jackson MR, Ali AT, Bell C, et al (Univ of Texas, Dallas)

J Vasc Surg 40:17-23, 2004 7–1

Purpose.—Previous studies have documented poor patency rates in "young" patients (age 55 years or younger) with premature atherosclerosis undergoing aortofemoral bypass (AFB) to treat aortoiliac occlusive disease. Given the high reported graft patency rates with superficial femoral vein (SFV) grafts performed because of aortic graft infection, we evaluated the role of SFV grafts for AFB as primary therapy for premature atherosclerosis in a case-control study.

Methods.—Over 10 years 31 patients aged 55 year or younger underwent AFB with use of SFV (V-AFB). Case controls consisted of all patients 55 years of age or younger who underwent AFB with use of Dacron (D-AFB) during the same period (n = 80). In all cases this was the initial therapy (no repeat operations). The two groups were well matched for age, sex, weight, preoperative ankle-brachial index, and the comorbid conditions of smoking, coronary artery disease, chronic obstructive pulmonary disease, hyperlipidemia, hypertension, and renal insufficiency. There were more patients with diabetes in the V-AFB group (34% vs 16%; $P = .05$). Patients in the V-AFB group had more advanced disease, and the surgical indication was more frequently critical ischemia compared with the D-AFB group (90% vs 46%; $P < .001$).

Results.—There was only one perioperative death in each group. There were no differences in cardiac, pulmonary, or gastrointestinal complications. However, fasciotomy occurred more frequently with V-AFB (44% vs 1%; $P < .001$). Surgery time was longer with V-AFB (7.3 vs 4.5 hours; $P < .001$). Despite these short-term drawbacks, V-AFB proved superior at long-term follow-up. The 5-year primary patency rate was significantly higher with V-AFB than with D-AFB (100% vs 56%; $P = .013$). There was also a trend for higher limb salvage at 5 years (90% vs 62%). Four graft infections occurred with D-AFB, and none with V-AFB ($P = .32$).

Conclusions.—AFB performed with SFV grafts is a far more durable operation than standard D-AFB in young patients with aortoiliac occlusive disease. However, V-AFB is far more likely to require lower extremity fasciotomy, and takes almost twice as long to perform (Fig 1 and Fig 2).

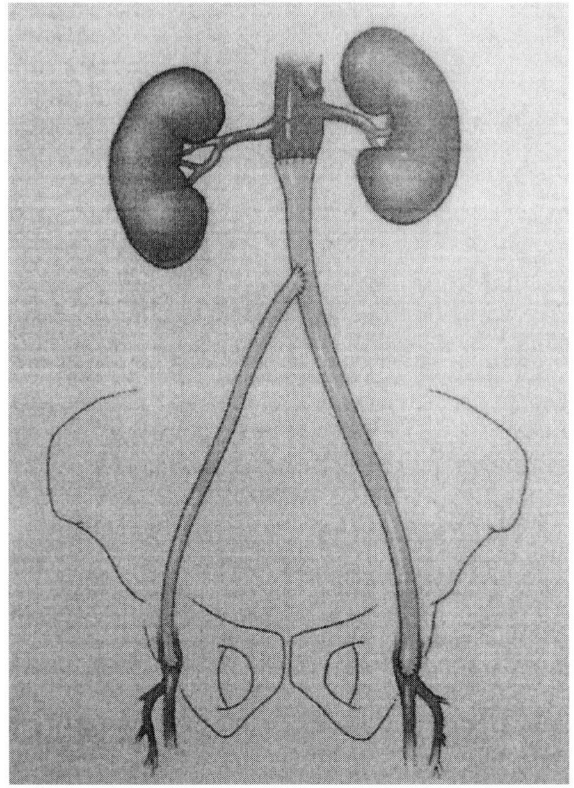

FIGURE 1.—Configuration of V-AFB grafts. Single vein proximal end-to-side, n = 13. Single vein proximal end-to-end, n = 12. (Reprinted by permission of the publisher from Jackson MR, Ali AT, Bell C, et al: Aortofemoral bypass in young patients with premature atherosclerosis: Is superficial femoral vein superior to dacron? *J Vasc Surg* 40:17-23, 2004. Copyright 2004 by Elsevier.)

▶ The immediate thought is to reject this approach for aortoiliac reconstruction because of the need for fasciotomy in almost half the patients. However, the 100% primary patency rate of the neoaortas cannot be ignored. It is reasonable to consider this procedure for certain subgroups of patients with critical ischemia who are not candidates for a prosthetic bypass or endovascular therapy for aortoiliac occlusive disease. Patients with small aortas and hypercoagulable states immediately come to mind.

G. L. Moneta, MD

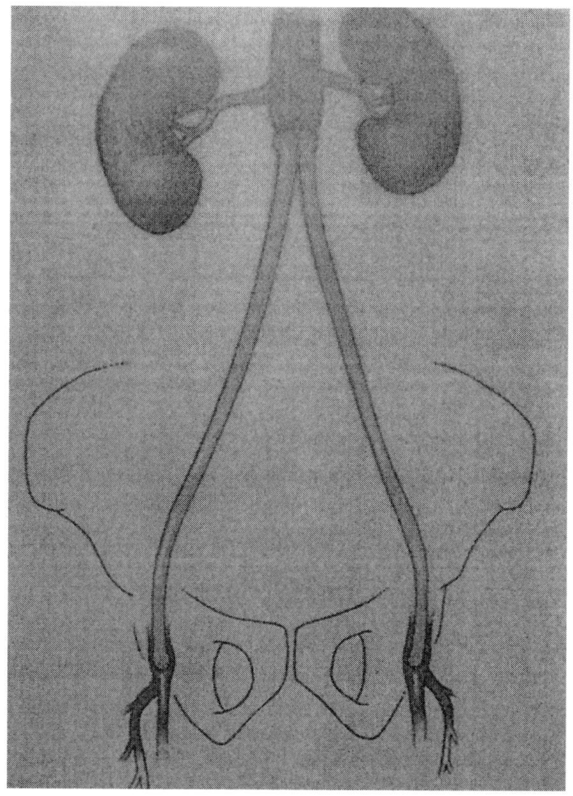

FIGURE 2.—Configuration of V-AFB grafts. Pantaloon veins proximal end-to-end, n = 3. Pantaloon veins proximal end-to-side, n = 1. (Reprinted by permission of the publisher from Jackson MR, Ali AT, Bell C, et al: Aortofemoral bypass in young patients with premature atherosclerosis: Is superficial femoral vein superior to dacron? *J Vasc Surg* 40:17-23, 2004. Copyright 2004 by Elsevier.)

Aortoiliac Insufficiency: Long-term Experience With Stent Placement for Treatment

Murphy TP, Ariaratnam NS, Carney WI Jr, et al (Rhode Island Hosp, Providence; Brown Univ, Providence, RI; Univ of Michigan, Ann Arbor)
Radiology 231:243-249, 2004 7–2

Purpose.—To establish and report the authors' experience with the long-term outcomes of aortoiliac stent placement for treatment of chronic lower-extremity ischemia.

Materials and Methods.—Stents were placed in 505 arterial segment lesions in 365 patients who presented with symptoms of chronic leg ischemia between February 1992 and March 2001. The 505 treated lesions were 88 occlusions and 417 stenoses. Indications for stent placement were claudication in 312 (62%), rest pain in 107 (21%), ulcer in 67 (13%), and gangrene in 19 (4%) arterial segments. Patients were followed up for up to 105 months (mean, 33 months ± 27 [SD]).

Results.—Hemodynamic success was achieved in 484 (98%) of the 496 limbs for which postprocedural translesion pressure gradients were available. Mean ankle-brachial indexes improved from 0.53 ± 0.25 to 0.79 ± 0.23 ($P < .001$). Major complications were seen in 24 (7%) patients. Two patients (0.5%) died within 30 days after stent placement. Twenty (6%) of 355 patients underwent aortic or iliac bypass surgery during the follow-up period. Eight years after stent placement, primary patency was 74%; primary assisted patency, 81%; and secondary patency, 84%. Variables associated with better patency included stenosis (rather than occlusion), shorter lesion length, older age, and limb-threatening ischemia. At the last follow-up examination, 74% of the 466 limbs for which follow-up clinical status data were available were asymptomatic, 22% were associated with claudication, 3% were associated with rest pain, and 1% were associated with ischemic tissue loss. Five patients underwent amputation on the ipsilateral side after stent placement.

Conclusion.—Findings from long-term experience with aortoiliac stent placement for treatment of chronic lower-extremity ischemia confirmed the procedure to be a durable, low-risk revascularization option.

▶ There is nothing new in this article. It is, however, a large series with seemingly good results although the methods of determining clinical success and stent patency were far less than ideal. Bird cage lining.

G. L. Moneta, MD

Total Laparoscopic Bypass for Aortoiliac Occlusive Lesions: 93-Case Experience

Coggia M, Javerliat I, Di Centa I, et al (Ambroise Parè Univ, Boulogne-Billancourt, France; Versailles Saint Quentin en Yvelines Univ, France; Belcolle Hosp, ASL Viterbo, Italy)

J Vasc Surg 40:899-906, 2004 7–3

Objectives.—We describe our experience with a new technique of total laparoscopic bypass surgery to treat aortoiliac occlusive lesions.

Material and Methods.—From November 2000 to December 2003, 93 total laparoscopic bypass procedures were performed to treat TASC (TransAtlantic Inter-Society Consensus document) grade C or D aortoiliac occlusive lesions. We also reimplanted 2 inferior mesenteric arteries, and performed 3 prosthesis-superior mesenteric bypasses and 2 suprarenal aorta endarterectomies. Our technique includes a sloping right lateral decubitus installation, which enables a simple transperitoneal left retrocolic or retrorenal approach to the infrarenal abdominal aorta. In patients with a hostile abdomen a retroperitoneal videoscopic approach was used. Aorta-prosthesis laparoscopic anastomoses are performed simply, which averts any trauma to the suture material.

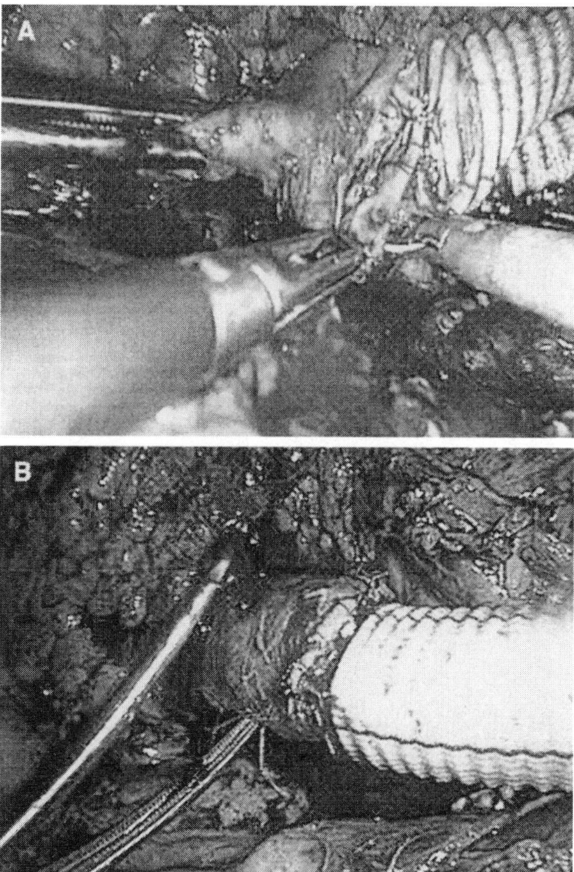

FIGURE 5.—Operative pictures show performance of proximal aorta-prosthesis anastomosis (**A**) and final aspect after aortic unclamping (**B**). (Reprinted by permission of the publisher from Coggia M, Javerliat I, Di Centa I, et al: Total laparoscopic bypass for aortoiliac occlusive lesions: 93-case experience. *J Vasc Surg* 40:899-906, 2004. Copyright 2004 by Elsevier.)

Results.—Patients included 76 men and 17 women, with median patient age 61 years (range, 38-79 years). The approach to the aorta was always possible, in particular, in obese patients. It enabled stable aortic exposure during performance of the laparoscopic aorta-prosthesis anastomosis. Median operative time was 240 minutes (range, 150-450 minutes). Median aortic clamping time measured to unclamping of the first prosthetic limb was 67.5 minutes (range, 30-135 minutes). Median duration of aorta-prosthesis anastomosis was 30 minutes (range, 12-90 minutes). The longest durations were mainly observed during the learning curve. Thirty-day postoperative mortality was 4% (4 of 93 patients). Two patients died of myocardial infarction. One patient with American Society of Anesthesiologists grade 4 disease operated on to treat critical ischemia died of multiple organ system failure, and 1 patient died of colonic ischemia. Major nonlethal postoperative complications were observed in 4 patients, and included lung atelectasia in 2 patients, graft infection in 1 patient operated on emergently to treat aortic occlusion, and secondary spleen rupture at day 5 in 1 patient. Median hospital stay was 7 days (range, 2-57 days). With a mean follow-up of 19 months (range, 1-37 months), complete recovery was observed in 89 patients, and all grafts were patent. One patient had kinking of a prosthetic limb at the groin, and in 1 patient *Staphylococcus epidermidis* graft infection developed, which was treated with in situ replacement with a rifampin-bonded graft.

Conclusion.—Total laparoscopic aortic bypass is feasible. In patients with TASC C and D aortoiliac occlusive lesions, short-term outcomes are comparable to those with conventional aortic bypass. After the initial learning curve, laparoscopic technique may reduce the operative trauma of aortic bypass (Fig 5).

► A few groups have developed amazing technical skill in performing laparoscopic aortic surgery. However, outside these pockets of activity, laparoscopic aortic surgery is not likely to move forward at any significant pace. Virtually everyone is pursuing endovascular aortic techniques. Laparoscopic aortic surgery is currently an interesting novelty. It will remain that way and be washed aside by the endovascular wave. (See Abstract 17–2.)

G. L. Moneta, MD

8 Visceral Renal Disease

Divergent Outcomes After Percutaneous Therapy for Symptomatic Renal Artery Stenosis

Sivamurthy N, Surowiec SM, Culakova E, et al (Univ of Rochester, NY)

J Vasc Surg 39:565-574, 2004 8–1

Objective.—Percutaneous intervention for symptomatic renal artery atherosclerosis is rapidly replacing surgery in many centers. This study evaluated the anatomic and functional outcomes of endovascular therapy for atherosclerotic renal artery stenosis on a combined vascular surgery and interventional radiology service at an academic medical center.

Methods.—This was a retrospective analysis of patients who underwent renal artery angioplasty with or without stenting between January 1990 and June 2002. Indications included hypertension (86%) and rising serum creatinine concentration (55%). One hundred forty-six patients (80 women; average age, 71 years [range, 44-89 years]) underwent 183 attempted interventions (64 to treat bilateral stenosis). Forty-five percent of patients had significant bilateral disease: 27% had greater than 50% bilateral stenosis, and the remainder had nonfunctioning, absent, or occluded vessels.

Results.—Of 183 planned interventions, technical success (<30% residual stenosis) was achieved in 179 vessels (98%) with placement of 137 stents (75%). Thirty-day mortality was 0.7%. The major morbidity rate was 4%, and the procedure-related complication rate was 18%. Five-year cumulative patient mortality was 25%. Primary patency, assisted primary patency, and recurrent stenosis rates were 82% ± 9%, 100% ± 0%, and 30% ± 7%, respectively, at 5 years. Within 3 months of the procedure, 52% of patients who received treatment of hypertension demonstrated clinical benefit (hypertension improved or cured), which was maintained in 68% of patients at 5 years. Serum creatinine concentration was lowered or stabilized in 87% of patients within 3 months of the procedure, but this benefit, including freedom from dialysis, was maintained in only 45% of patients at 5 years (Figure).

Conclusions.—Endovascular intervention for symptomatic atherosclerotic renal artery stenosis is technically successful. There were excellent patency and low recurrent stenosis rates. There is immediate clinical benefit for most patients, but divergent long-term functional outcomes. Endovascular interventions modestly enhance the care of the patient with hypertension,

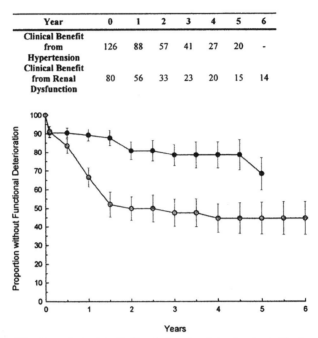

Year	0	1	2	3	4	5	6
Clinical Benefit from Hypertension	126	88	57	41	27	20	-
Clinical Benefit from Renal Dysfunction	80	56	33	23	20	15	14

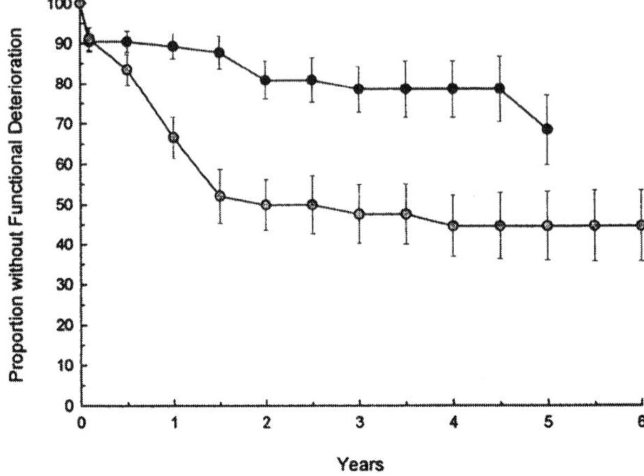

FIGURE.—Life table analysis of the likelihood of continued deterioration in blood pressure (*black circles*) and renal function (*gray circles*) after renal angioplasty with or without stenting. The number of patients or vessels in each interval is given in the table to the left of the corresponding graph. Values represent mean ± SE <10% for all data points. (Reprinted by permission of the publisher from Sivamurthy N, Surowiec SM, Culakova E, et al: Divergent outcomes after percutaneous therapy for symptomatic renal artery stenosis. *J Vasc Surg* 39:565-574, 2004. Copyright 2004 by Elsevier.)

but poorly preserve long-term renal function in the patient with chronic renal impairment.

▶ Treatment of renal artery stenosis does not always achieve the goal of improved hypertension or improved renal function. However, some patients do benefit. Because renal angioplasty can be done with high technical success rates and low morbidity, and the fact that renal artery stenoses "can't be a good thing," it is tempting to treat all renal artery lesions with angioplasty. This article and others indicate this is clearly a waste of resources. We must try to identify patients most likely to benefit.

G. L. Moneta, MD

Delay of Dialysis in End-Stage Renal Failure: Prospective Study on Percutaneous Renal Artery Interventions

Korsakas S, Mohaupt MG, Dinkel HP, et al (Swiss Cardiovascular Ctr, Bern, Switzerland)

Kidney Int 65:251-258, 2004 8–2

Background.—Renal artery stenosis (RAS) is a cause of end-stage renal failure. We studied the effect of percutaneous renal artery intervention (PRI) in patients with advanced, progressive disease at risk for renal failure, hypothesizing a beneficial effect.

Methods.—Thirty-nine primary and 14 secondary PRIs were performed on 28 patients with atherosclerotic RAS, serum creatinine >300 µmol/L, and progressive loss of renal function ≥1 year before PRI. Renal function and RA patency were prospectively followed for 12 months after primary and secondary PRI. The intervention's effect on the progressive loss of renal function was calculated by comparing reciprocal slopes of serum creatinine against time before and after PRI.

Results.—Progression of renal failure slowed significantly following PRI. Mean (±SE) slopes of reciprocal serum creatinine values were: 6.69 ± 0.97 L μmol^{-1} day^{-1} ($\times 10^{-6}$) before and 6.76 ± 3.03 L μmol^{-1} day^{-1} ($\times 10^{-6}$) after PRI ($P = 0.0007$). Fifteen patients (53.5%) showed improvement or stabilization of progressive renal dysfunction. Out of 11 patients expected to become dialysis dependent within one year, 8 (72.7%) experienced an improvement in renal function sufficient to remain dialysis-free. Favorable outcome correlated with a lower creatinine level ($P = 0.0137$) and a more negative slope of progression ($r = 0.49$, $P = 0.020$) at entry. Mortality was 10.7%, and rate of local complications was 7.1%. Deterioration of renal function following PRI was suspected in 17.9% of patients.

Conclusion.—PRI may improve renal function and ultimately delay dialysis in patients with advanced renal failure. Possible advantages must be weighed against the risk of renal failure advancement and high procedure-related complication rate.

► One would expect more favorable outcomes for renal artery angioplasty in patients with milder impairment of renal function. That is a feature of percutaneous series for RAS and surgical series. Plotting reciprocal slopes of creatinine levels to select patients for percutaneous intervention is interesting. Longer follow-up than is presented in this article will be required to fully assess this approach (see also Abstract 8–1).

G. L. Moneta, MD

Surgical Management of Renal Artery Aneurysms
English WP, Pearce JD, Craven TE, et al (Wake Forest Univ, Winston-Salem, NC)
J Vasc Surg 40:53-60, 2004 8–3

Purpose.—This retrospective review describes the surgical management and clinical outcome for renal artery aneurysms (RAAs) in 62 consecutive patients.

Methods.—From January 1987 through July 2003, 804 patients had operative renal artery (RA) repair involving 1206 kidneys at our center. A subgroup of 62 patients (42 women, 20 men; mean age 46 ± 18 years) received repair of 72 RAAs. Demographic data, comorbidity, and surgical technique were examined. Blood pressure and renal function response were determined. Patency of repair was evaluated by renal duplex sonography. Primary patency and patient survival were estimated by life-table methods. Tests of association were performed using χ^2 and the Student t tests.

Results.—Seventy-two RAs were repaired for RAA with a mean diameter of 2.6 cm (range, 1.3 to 5.5 cm). Bilateral RAAs were present in 21 patients. Associated conditions included fibromuscular dysplasia, atherosclerosis, and arteritis in 54%, 35%, and 7%, respectively. Hypertension was present in 89% (mean blood pressure, 171 ± 35/95 ± 19 mm Hg; mean medications, 2.2 ± 1.2 drugs) and renal insufficiency was present in 8% (mean serum creatinine, 1.9 ± 0.6 mg/dL). RAA repair included bypass (67%), aneurysmorrhaphy (15%), or a combination (17%). One planned nephrectomy (1%) was performed for un-reconstructable disease. Branch RA reconstruction in 78% used ex vivo cold perfusion in 50%, in situ cold perfusion in 29%, and warm in situ repair in 21%. Of 9 bilateral RAA repairs, 7 (78%) were staged and 2 (22%) were simultaneous. Combined aortic reconstruction was required in 6 (10%) patients. Perioperative death occurred in 1 patient (1.6%), and significant morbidity was observed in 8 patients (12%). Hypertension was considered improved in 54%, cured in 21%, and unchanged in 25% at mean follow-up of 48 months (range, 1-156 months). Among patients with renal insufficiency, renal function was improved in 3 (60%), unchanged in 1 (20%), and declined in 1 (20%). Follow-up patency (mean, 33 months; range, 1-118 months) was determined for 64 (91%) RA reconstructions. Product-limit estimate of primary patency at 48 months was 96%. Product-limit estimate of survival was 91% at 120 months.

Conclusion.—RAAs were repaired with low morbidity and mortality. Complex branch RAA repair using cold perfusion preservation and ex vivo techniques resulted in no unplanned nephrectomy, with an estimated primary patency of 96% at 48 months. Beneficial blood pressure response was observed in the majority of hypertensive patients. These results support selective surgical management of RAA.

▶ I don't know why an RAA should have an effect on blood pressure anymore than an aneurysm of the suprarenal aorta or the thoracic aorta should affect blood pressure. The authors' article is important primarily because it demonstrates the technical results that can be achieved with repair of RAAs. Readers should note the description of in vivo renal preservation with cold perfusion. This permits complex repairs without having to divide the vein and ureter and autotransplant the kidney.

G. L. Moneta, MD

A Simple But Useful Method of Screening for Mesenteric Ischemia Secondary to Acute Aortic Dissection

Kurimoto Y, Morishita K, Fukada J, et al (Sapporo Med Univ, Japan)
Surgery 136:42-46, 2004 8–4

Background.—In spite of recent improvements in treatment for acute aortic dissection, mesenteric ischemia secondary to aortic dissection is still challenging. We propose a simple screening method to detect mesenteric ischemia secondary to acute aortic dissection.

Methods.—From 1991 to 2002, 245 patients with acute aortic dissection were admitted to our hospital. Nine (3.7%) of those were complicated with mesenteric ischemia. The clinical records of those 9 patients were retrospectively analyzed. The ratios of the diameter of the superior mesenteric vein (SMV) to that of the superior mesenteric artery (SMA) were calculated in patients with mesenteric ischemia (group M) and in patients without mesenteric ischemia (group C) (Fig 1). Blood test data, including results of arterial blood gas analysis, in the 2 groups were also compared.

Results.—The SMV/SMA ratios in groups M and C were 1.16 ± 0.33 and 1.78 ± 0.29, respectively (P = .003) (Fig 2). A cutoff value of the SMV/SMA ratio was 1.5 (sensitivity, 88.9%; specificity, 88.9%) with an odds ratio of 64.0. Although there were differences between the 2 groups in glutamate oxaloacetate transaminase, lactate dehydrogenase, creatine phosphate kinase, pH, and lactate values, the measurement of lactate was especially useful (P = .002).

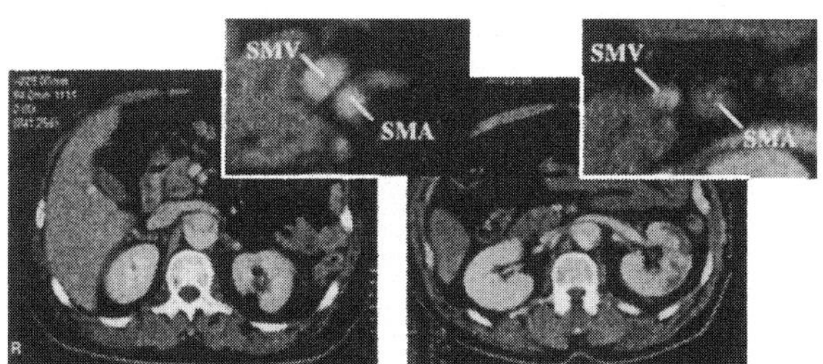

FIGURE 1.—Contrast CT images at the level of the left renal vein in patients with acute aortic dissection. The images show a large difference in the diameter of the SMV between group C (**left side**) and group M (**right side**). *Abbreviations: SMV,* Superior mesenteric vein; *SMA,* superior mesenteric artery. (Reprinted by permission of the publisher from Kurimoto Y, Morishita K, Fukada J, et al: A simple but useful method of screening for mesenteric ischemia secondary to acute aortic dissection. *Surgery* 136:42-46, 2004. Copyright 2004 by Elsevier.)

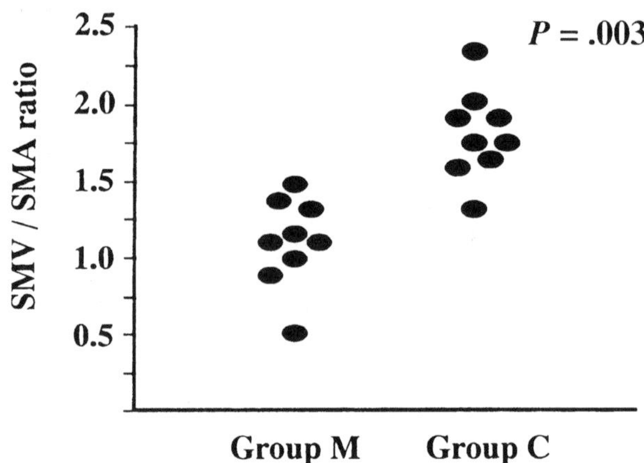

FIGURE 2.—The SMV/SMA ratio in group M is significantly smaller than that in group C ($P = .003$). *Abbreviations: SMV,* Superior mesenteric vein; *SMA,* superior mesenteric artery. (Reprinted by permission of the publisher from Kurimoto Y, Morishita K, Fukada J, et al: A simple but useful method of screening for mesenteric ischemia secondary to acute aortic dissection. *Surgery* 136:42-46, 2004. Copyright 2004 by Elsevier.)

Conclusions.—The combination of the SMV/SMA ratio and lactate concentration is a useful screening method to detect mesenteric ischemia secondary to acute aortic dissection.

► In essence, the authors are suggesting mesenteric venous volume, as measured by CT-derived measurements of SMV diameter, is an indicator of adequate intestinal perfusion. It makes sense that if less blood is being returned from the mesenteric circulation, that less blood must have been delivered to the mesenteric circulation. The study is obviously too small to influence clinical practice. It is, however, intriguing, basically makes sense, and the information required is routinely available in patients with aortic dissection.

G. L. Moneta, MD

Mesenteric Artery Disease in the Elderly

Hansen KJ, Wilson DB, Craven TE, et al (Wake Forest Univ, Winston-Salem, NC)

J Vasc Surg 40:45-52, 2004 8–5

Purpose.—The purpose of this study was to estimate the population-based prevalence of mesenteric artery stenosis (MAS) and occlusion among independent elderly Americans.

Method.—As part of an ancillary investigation to the Cardiovascular Health Study (CHS), participants in the Forsyth County, NC cohort had visceral duplex sonography of the celiac arteries and superior mesenteric arteries (SMAs). Critical MAS was defined by celiac peak systolic velocity ≥2.0 m/s and/or SMA peak systolic velocity ≥2.7 m/s. Occlusion of either vessel was defined by lack of a Doppler-shifted signal within the imaged artery. Demographic data, blood pressures, and blood lipid levels were collected as part of the baseline CHS examination. Participants' weights were measured at baseline and before the duplex exam. Univariate tests of association were performed with two-way contingency tables, Student *t* tests, and Fisher exact tests. Multivariate associations were examined with logistic regression analysis.

Results.—A total of 553 CHS participants had visceral duplex sonography technically adequate to define the presence or absence of MAS. The study group had a mean age of 77.2 ± 4.9 years and comprised 63% women and 37% men. Participant race was 76% white and 23% African-American. Ninety-seven participants (17.5%) had MAS. There was no significant difference in age, race, gender, body mass index, blood pressure, cholesterol, or low-density lipoproteins for participants with or without MAS. Forward stepwise variable selection found renal artery stenosis (*P* =.008; odds ratio [OR], 2.85; 95% confidence interval [CI], 1.31, 6.21) and high-density lipoprotein >40 (*P* =.02; OR, 3.03; 95% CI, 1.17, 7.81) significantly associated with MAS in a multivariate logistic regression model. Eighty-three of the 97 participants with MAS (15.0% of the cohort) had isolated celiac stenosis. Seven participants (1.3% of the cohort) had combined celiac and SMA stenosis. Five participants (0.9% of the cohort) had isolated SMA stenosis. Two participants (0.4% of the cohort) had celiac occlusion. Considering all participants with MAS, there was no association with weight change. However, SMA stenosis and celiac occlusion demonstrated an independent association with annualized weight loss (*P* =.028; OR, 1.54; 95% CI, 1.05, 2.26) and with renal artery stenosis (*P* =.001; OR, 9.48; 95% CI, 2.62, 34.47).

Conclusion.—This investigation provides the first population-based estimate of the prevalence of MAS among independent elderly Americans. MAS existed in 17.5% of the study cohort. The majority had isolated celiac disease. SMA stenosis and celiac artery occlusion demonstrated a significant and independent association with weight loss and concurrent renal artery disease.

► This study formalizes what we already know—that is, celiac stenosis is far more common than SMA stenosis, and visceral artery stenosis is far more common than the clinical entity of chronic mesenteric ischemia. The association of mesenteric artery disease with renal artery stenosis makes sense given that SMA, celiac artery, and renal artery stenoses are usually "spillover" lesions from atherosclerosis of the visceral aorta. We have recognized this association for some time. Renal duplex studies in our vascular laboratory include assessment of the celiac artery and SMA.

G. L. Moneta, MD

Chronic Visceral Ischemia: Symptom-Free Survival After Open Surgical Repair

English WP, Pearce JD, Craven TE, et al (Wake Forest Univ, Winston-Salem, NC)

Vasc Endovasc Surg 38:493-503, 2004 8–6

Introduction.—A retrospective review of patients treated with a history of chronic visceral ischemia (CVI) was made to determine primary patency of open surgical repair and estimated symptom-free survival. Patients with CVI between 1990 and 2003 were reviewed. Included were those with chronic symptoms alone (C-CVI) and acute-on-chronic symptoms (A-CVI). Data were obtained from a vascular database. Symptom-free survival and graft patency were estimated by using product limit estimates. Fifty-eight patients (13 men, 45 women; mean age: 63 years) were treated surgically for C-CVI (34 patients) and A-CVI (24 patients). All patients had postprandial abdominal pain and weight loss (mean: 17 kg). One fourth reported food fear. Preoperative imaging demonstrated disease of the superior mesenteric artery (SMA) (100%; 64% occluded), celiac axis (89%; 37% occluded), and inferior mesenteric artery (IMA) (54%; 60% occluded). Multiple vessels were involved in 95% of patients (mean: 2.3 vessels/patient). Operative management included antegrade revascularization of 80 vessels. Combined aortic

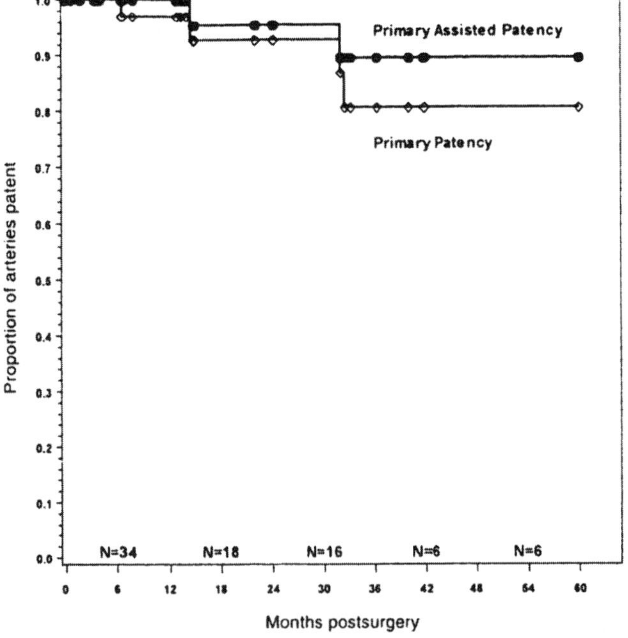

FIGURE 3.—Product-limit estimates of primary and assisted patencies of visceral artery reconstruction (SE < 10% for all distinct failure times). (Courtesy of English WP, Pearce JD, Craven TE, et al: Chronic visceral ischemia: symptom-free survival after open surgical repair. *Vasc Endovasc Surg* 38:493-503, 2004.)

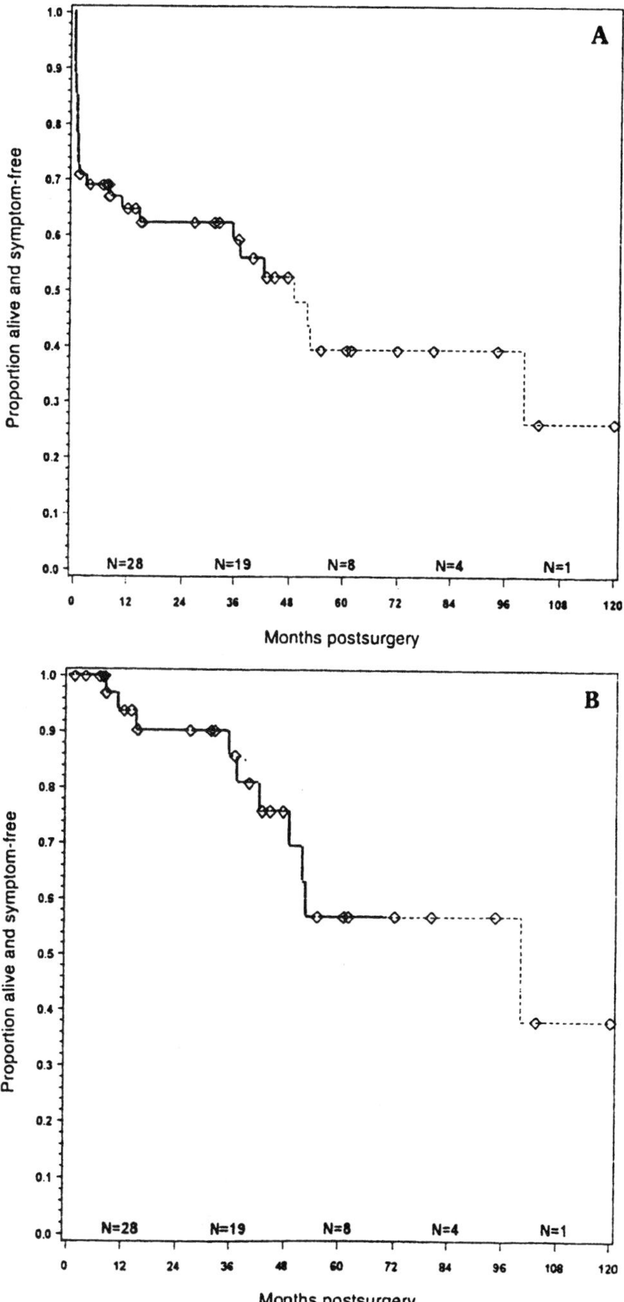

FIGURE 1.—A, Product-limit estimates of symptom-free survival (includes perioperative deaths); SE > 10% at 48.1 months. B, Product-limit estimates of ssymptom-free survival (perioperative deaths excluded); SE > 10% at 69.7 months. (Courtesy of English WP, Pearce JD, Craven TE, et al: Chronic visceral ischemia: symptom-free survival after open surgical repair. *Vasc Endovasc Surg* 38:493-503, 2004.)

and/or renal procedures were performed in 7 patients. Patient demographics and visceral disease did not differ for C-CVI and A-CVI; however, perioperative mortality differed significantly (10% for C-CVI vs 54% for A-CVI [$p < 0.001$]). Intestinal gangrene at presentation was associated with perioperative (hazard ratio [HR]: 7.6; 95% CI: 2.7-21.6; $p = 0.0002$) and follow-up death (HR: 7.8; CI 2.8-21.9; $p < 0.0001$). Follow-up (mean: 34 months) was complete for 54/68 vessels (79%). Estimated primary and primary assisted patency at 5 years were 81% and 89% respectively (Fig 3). Estimated symptom-free survival for hospital survivors was 57% at 70 months (Fig 1). Open antegrade methods of visceral artery repair for CVI were durable and associated with 57% symptom-free survival at 70 months. Patient demographics and distribution of visceral artery anatomy were similar; however, perioperative mortality for C-CVI and A-CVI differed dramatically. Improved outcomes for A-CVI require recognition and treatment of CVI before onset of intestinal gangrene.

▶ This is a single institutional review of the experience at Wake Forest University with surgical treatment of CVI. Patency rates for mesenteric bypass are what should be achieved by experienced surgeons.

G. L. Moneta, MD

Outcomes After Redo Procedures for Failed Mesenteric Revascularization

Giswold ME, Landry GJ, Taylor LM Jr, et al (Oregon Health and Sciences Univ, Portland)

Vasc Endovasc Surg 38:315-319, 2004 8–7

Introduction.—This report examines results of mesenteric revascularization following a failed splanchnic revascularization. Patients undergoing repeat mesenteric revascularization from January 1985 to July 2002 were identified from a prospectively maintained registry. Data recorded included procedures performed, perioperative mortality, complications, and operative indications. Patients who had embolic events were excluded. Eighty-six patients underwent 105 mesenteric interventions in this time period; 22 patients underwent 33 repeat mesenteric revascularization procedures. There were 25 single-vessel bypasses, 3 multivessel reconstructions, 3 angioplasty procedures (1 open, 2 percutaneous), and 2 graft thrombectomies. Complications occurred in 33.3%. Perioperative mortality was 6.1%, all in patients with acute mesenteric ischemia. One- and 4-year primary patency for repeat mesenteric revascularization was 73.5% and 62.2%, respectively, and survival for repeat mesenteric revascularization was 85.9% and 75.5%, respectively. Patients surgically treated for mesenteric ischemia can require additional interventions. Repeat revascularization effectively prolongs survival when an earlier intervention fails (Fig 2).

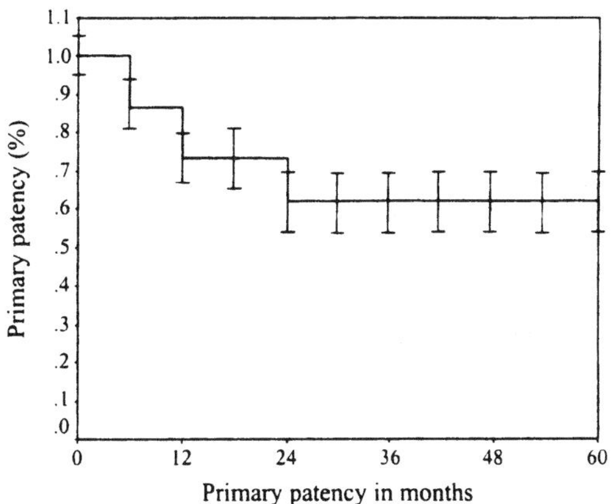

FIGURE 2.—Life-table-determined primary patency of 33 mesenteric revascularization procedures for treatment of a failed mesenteric intervention. (Courtesy of Giswold ME, Landry GJ, Taylor LM Jr, et al: Outcomes after redo procedures for failed mesenteric revascularization. *Vasc Endovasc Surg* 38:315-319, 2004.)

▶ It is important to know what to expect when patients with failed mesenteric reconstructions require reoperation for mesenteric graft failure. Important points are symptomatic recurrence involves failure of the superior mesenteric artery graft, and repeat procedures, sometimes involving unusual target arteries, can be lifesaving. Reasonable patency can be achieved with these repeat operations.

G. L. Moneta, MD

9 Thoracic Aorta

Endovascular Treatment of Thoracic Aortic Aneurysms: Results of the Phase II Multicenter Trial of the GORE TAG Thoracic Endoprosthesis

Makaroun MS, for the GORE TAG Investigators (Univ of Pittsburgh, Pa; et al)

J Vasc Surg 41:1-9, 2005 9–1

Objective.—A decade after the first report of descending thoracic aortic aneurysm (DTA) repair with endografts, a commercial device is yet to be approved in the United States. The GORE TAG endoprosthesis, an investigational nitinol-supported expanded polytetrafluoroethylene tube graft with

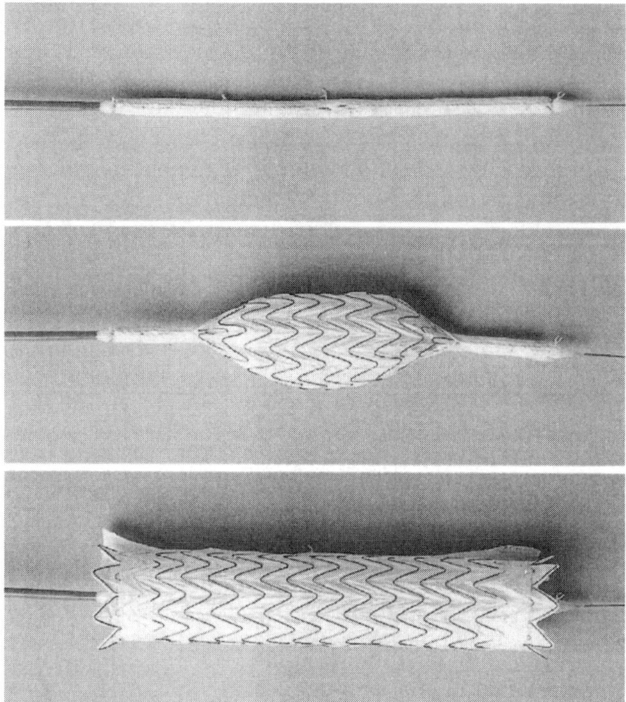

FIGURE 1.—Deployment sequence of the GORE TAG device. (Reprinted by permission of the publisher from Makaroun MS, for the GORE TAG Investigators: Endovascular treatment of thoracic aortic aneurysms: Results of the phase II multicenter trial of the GORE TAG thoracic endoprosthesis. *J Vasc Surg* 41:1-9, 2005. Copyright 2005 by Elsevier.)

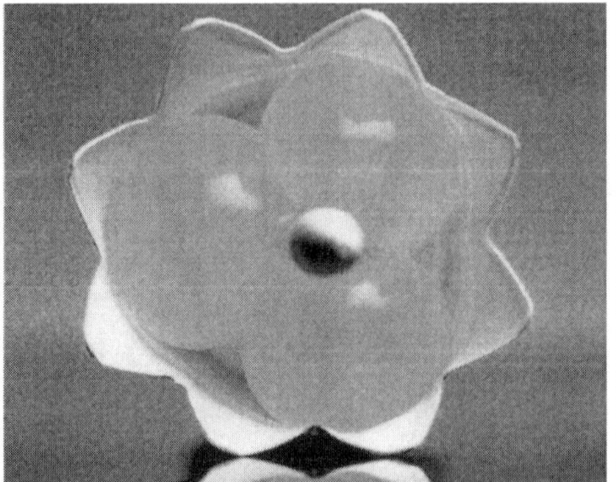

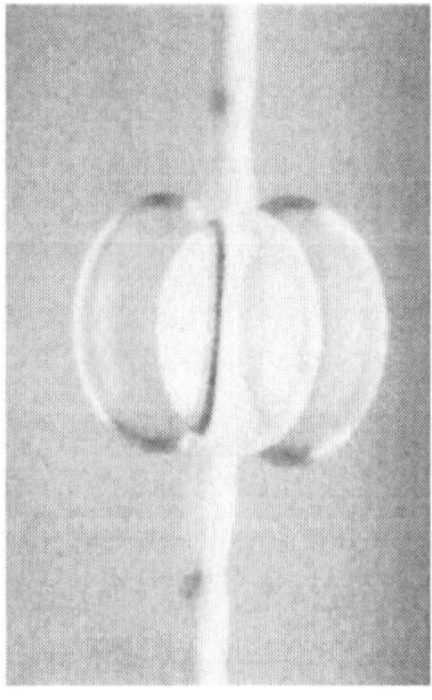

FIGURE 2.—Trilobed ballon with *arrows* illustrating flow-through channels. (Reprinted by permission of the publisher from Makaroun MS, for the GORE TAG Investigators: Endovascular treatment of thoracic aortic aneurysms: Results of the phase II multicenter trial of the GORE TAG thoracic endoprosthesis. *J Vasc Surg* 41:1-9, 2005. Copyright 2005 by Elsevier.)

diameters of 26 to 40 mm, is the first DTA device to enter phase II trials in the United States and has been used worldwide for a host of thoracic pathologies (Figs 1 and 2).

Methods.—A multicenter prospective nonrandomized phase II study of the GORE TAG endoprosthesis was conducted at 17 sites. Enrollment was from September 1999 to May 2001. Preoperative workup included arteriography and spiral computed tomography scans of the chest, abdomen, and pelvis. Follow-up radiographs and computed tomography scans were obtained at 1, 6, and 12 months and yearly thereafter.

Results.—A total of 139 (98%) of 142 patients had a successful implantation of the device. Inadequate arterial access was responsible for the 3 failures. The mean DTA size was 64.1 ± 15.4 mm. Men slightly outnumbered women (57.7%), with an average age of 71 years, and 88% of the patients were white. Ninety percent were American Society of Anesthesiologists category III or IV. One device was used in 44% of patients, and 56% required two or more devices to bridge the thoracic aorta. The left subclavian artery was covered in 28 patients, with planned carotid-subclavian transposition. The procedure time averaged 150 minutes, estimated blood loss averaged 506 mL, intensive care unit stay averaged 2.6 days, and hospital stay averaged 7.6 days. Within 30 days, 45 (32%) patients had at least 1 major adverse event: 5 (4%) experienced a stroke, 4 (3%) demonstrated temporary or permanent paraplegia, 20 (14%) experienced vascular trauma or thrombosis, and 2 (1.5%) died. Mean follow-up was 24.0 months. Four patients had aneurysm-related deaths. Three patients underwent endovascular revisions for endoleak. No ruptures have been reported. Twenty wire fractures have been identified in 19 patients; 18 (90%) of these occurred in the longitudinal spine, and only 1 patient required treatment. At 2 years, aneurysm-related and overall survival rates are 97% and 75%, respectively.

Conclusions.—The GORE TAG thoracic endoprosthesis provides a safe alternative for the treatment of DTAs, with low mortality, relatively low morbidity, and excellent 2-year freedom from aneurysm-related death. Longitudinal spine fractures have so far been associated with rare clinical events.

▶ The device studied here is different than the device now approved by the Food and Drug Administration (FDA). This trial was halted because of wire fractures in the longitudinal spine of the device. Nevertheless, the deployment device and the basics of the design minus the longitudinal spine, are similar to that approved by the FDA. Crucial points to be noted from this study are the incidence of paraplegia, strokes associated with carotid subclavian bypass, and the advisability of using delivery conduits to avoid arterial injury. Thoracic endografting has more difficulties and complexities than endografting of the abdominal aorta. Still, overall complications with this device will be lower than that with open surgery for diseases of the thoracic aorta.

G. L. Moneta, MD

Endovascular Treatment of Thoracic Aortic Diseases: Combined Experience From the EUROSTAR and United Kingdom Thoracic Endograft Registries

Leurs LJ, for the EUROSTAR and the UK Thoracic Endograft Registry Collaborators (Catharina Hosp, Eindhoven, The Netherlands; et al)

J Vasc Surg 40:670-680, 2004 9–2

Purpose.—The objective of this study was to assess the initial and 1-year outcome of endovascular treatment of thoracic aortic aneurysms and dissections collated in the European Collaborators on Stent Graft Techniques for Thoracic Aortic Aneurysm and Dissection Repair (EUROSTAR) and the United Kingdom Thoracic Endograft registries.

Methods.—Four hundred forty-three patients underwent endovascular repair of thoracic aortic disease between September 1997 and August 2003 (EUROSTAR, 340 patients; UK, 103 patients). Patients represented 4 major disease groups: degenerative aneurysm (n = 249), aortic dissection (n = 131), false anastomotic aneurysm (n = 13), and traumatic aortic injury (n = 50).

Results.—Mean age in the entire study group was 63 years. Fifty-two percent of patients were deemed at high risk for open surgery because of major comorbidity. Sixty percent of patients underwent an elective procedure, and 35% required emergency treatment. Conventional indications for treatment of aortic dissection, including aortic expansion, continuous pain, rupture, or symptoms of branch occlusion constituted the basis for endograft placement in 57% of patients, whereas in 43% of patients aortic dissections were asymptomatic. Primary technical success was obtained in 87% of patients with degenerative aneurysm and in 89% with aortic dissection. Paraplegia was a postoperative complication in 4.0% of patients with degenerative aneurysm and 0.8% of patients with aortic dissection (not significant). Thirty-day mortality in the entire study group was 9.3%, with mortality rates after elective procedures of 5.3% for degenerative aneurysms and 6.5% for aortic dissection. Mortality for degenerative aneurysm after emergency repair was higher (28%; $P < .0001$) then after elective procedures. For aortic dissection the emergency repair rate was 12% (not significant compared with elective repair of aortic dissection, and $P = .025$ compared with emergency repair of degenerative aneurysm). One-year follow-up was complete in 195 patients. The outcome at 1 year was more favorable for aortic dissection than for degenerative aneurysm with regard to aortic expansion (0% vs 15%; $P = .001$) and late survival (90% vs 80%; $P = .048$). In the groups with false anastomotic aneurysm and traumatic aortic injury, 30-day mortality rates were 8% and 6%, respectively.

Conclusion.—This multicenter experience demonstrates acceptable rates for operative mortality and paraplegia after endovascular repair of thoracic aortic disease. Outcome after 30 days and 1 year was more favorable for aortic dissection than for degenerative aneurysm. However, the durability of this technique is currently unknown, and continued use of registries should provide data from long-term follow-up.

► Clearly there was more action in Europe than in the United States with regard to evaluating the efficacy and feasibility of stent graft repair of the thoracic aorta. Thoracic aortic pathology is more varied than that of the abdominal aorta (aneurysm, dissection, traumatic rupture, intramural hematoma, penetrating ulcer). There will need to be specific trials to evaluate thoracic stent grafts with regard to the individual types of thoracic aortic pathology.

G. L. Moneta, MD

Endoluminal Stent–Graft Placement for Acute Rupture of the Descending Throacic Aorta

Scheinert D, Krankenberg H, Schmidt A, et al (Univ of Leipzig, Germany; Centre for Cardiology and Vascular Intervention, Hamburg, Germany)

Eur Heart J 25:694-700, 2004 9–3

Aims.—To investigate the results of endovascular stent-graft placement for the treatment of acute perforating lesions of the descending thoracic aorta.

Method and Results.—A total of 31 consecutive patients underwent interventional treatment for perforating lesions of the descending aorta (Fig 2). In 21 cases (group A), the aortic perforation was due to rupture of a descending thoracic aneurysm or dissection, whereas 10 patients (group B) were treated for traumatic transection of the descending aorta. A total of 42 endoprostheses were implanted. The implantation procedure was successful in all cases without peri-interventional complications. In one case, implantation of a second endoprosthesis became necessary due to type I endoleak. Overall, the 30-day mortality was 9.7%. As all three deaths occurred in group A, the mortality rate in this group was 14.3% versus 0% in group B. Similarly,

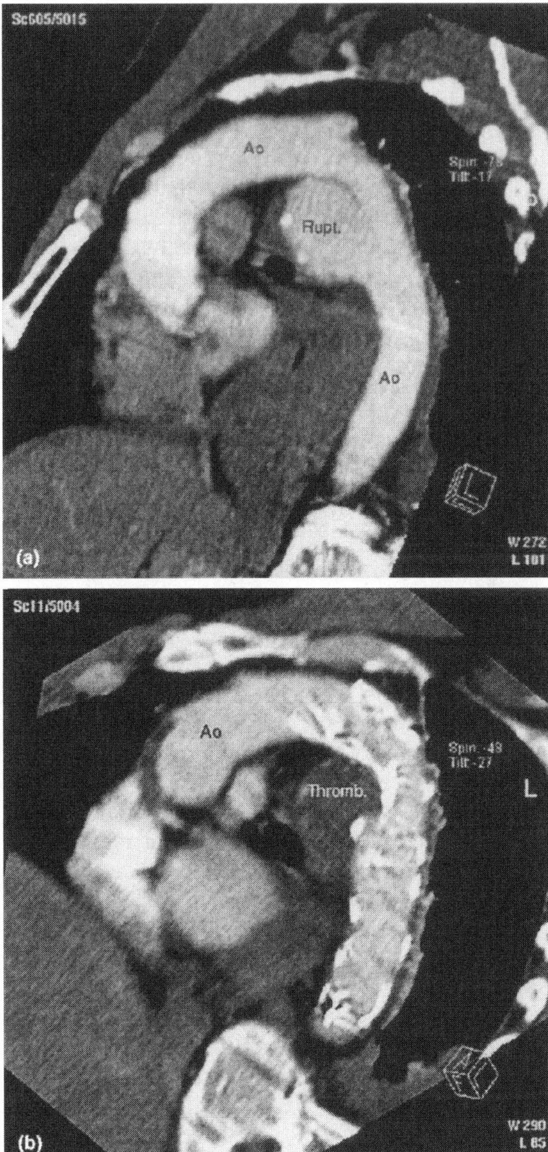

FIGURE 2.—Two-dimensional CT reconstruction (multiplanar reconstruction) before (**a**) and after successful stent-graft repair (**b**) of an aortic rupture (LAO-like view, reconstruction axis varies slightly because of variations in the patient's position). *Abbreviations: LAO,* Left anterior oblique; *Ao,* aorta; *Rupt,* rupture; *Thromb,* thrombosis. (Courtesy of Scheinert D, Krankenberg H, Schmidt A, et al: Endoluminal stent–graft placement for acute rupture of the descending throacic aorta. *Eur Heart J* 25:694-700, 2004. Copyright 2004, by permission of Oxford University Press.)

postinterventional complications were more prevalent, with 28.6% in group A (renal failure $n = 4$; stroke $n = 2$) versus 10.0% in group B (renal failure $n = 1$). No paraplegia and no further deaths or ruptures occurred during follow-up (mean 17 months).

Conclusion.—Interventional stent-graft placement is an effective treatment option for the emergency repair of descending aortic perforations.

► Clearly, endograft repair of thoracic aortic disruption is feasible with excellent short-term results in selected patients. It is still unclear what percentage of patients with acute thoracic disruption will be eligible for endograft therapy. Nevertheless, as these devices become available, endograft therapy for acute thoracic aortic disruption will be the preferred treatment for selected patients.

G. L. Moneta, MD

Complications of Endovascular Repair of High-Risk and Emergent Descending Thoracic Aortic Aneurysms and Dissections

Hansen CJ, Bui H, Donayre CE, et al (Harbor-UCLA Med Ctr, Torrance)

J Vasc Surg 40:228-234, 2004 9–4

Purpose.—The advent of endovascular prostheses to treat descending thoracic aortic lesions offers an alternative approach in patients who are poor candidates for surgery. The development of this approach includes complications that are common to the endovascular treatment of abdominal aortic aneurysms and some that are unique to thoracic endografting.

Methods.—We conducted a retrospective review of 60 emergent and high-risk patients with thoracic aortic aneurysms (TAAs) and dissections treated with endovascular prostheses over 4 years under existing investigational protocols or on an emergent compassionate use basis.

Results.—Fifty-nine of the 60 patients received treatment, with one access failure. Thirty-five patients received treatment of TAAs. Four of these procedures were performed emergently because of active hemorrhage. Twenty-four patients with aortic dissections (16 acute, 8 chronic) also received treatment. Eight of the patients with acute dissection had active hemorrhage at the time of treatment. Three devices were used: AneuRx (Medtronic; n = 31), Talent (Medtronic; n = 27), and Excluder (Gore; n = 1). Nineteen secondary endovascular procedures were performed in 14 patients. Most were secondary to endoleak (14 of 19), most commonly caused by modular separation of overlapping devices (n = 8) (Figure). Other endoleaks included 4 proximal or distal type I leaks and 2 undefined endoleaks. The remaining secondary procedures were performed to treat recurrent dissection (n = 1), pseudoaneurysm enlargement (n = 3), and endovascular abdominal aortic aneurysm repair (n = 1). One patient underwent surgical repair of a retrograde ascending aortic dissection after endograft placement. Procedure-related mortality was 17% in the TAA group and 13% in the dissection group, including 2 acute retrograde dissections that resulted in death from cardiac tamponade. Overall mortality was 28% at 2-year follow-up.

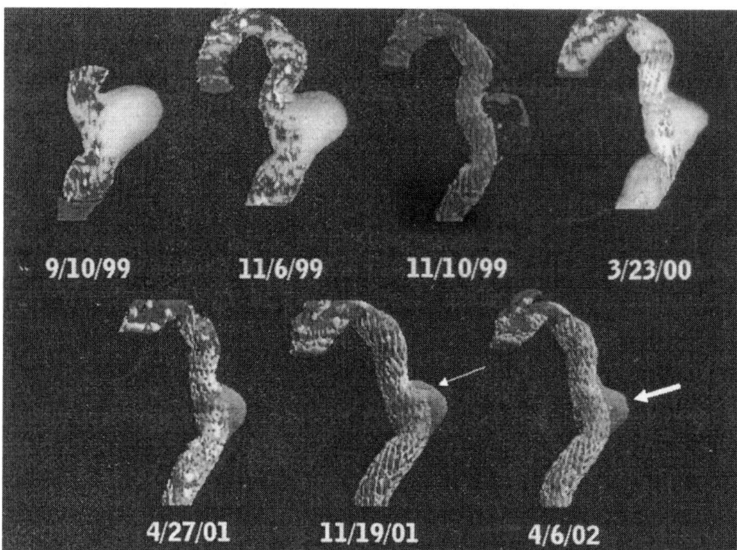

FIGURE.—Composite sequential computed tomography angiogram reconstructions demonstrate follow-up of patient treated for descending thoracic aneurysm. Regression occurred until 11/01, when a new endoleak was identified (*small arrow*) originating from device separation. Additional thoracic endografts were deployed. Six-month follow-up (4/02) demonstrated continued regression with absence of endoleak. (Reprinted by permission of the publisher from Hansen CJ, Bui H, Donayre CE, et al: Complications of endovascular repair of high-risk and emergent descending thoracic aortic aneurysms and dissections. *J Vasc Surg* 40:228-234, 2004. Copyright 2004 by Elsevier.)

Conclusion.—Although significant morbidity and mortality remain, endovascular repair of descending TAAs and dissections in high-risk patients can be accomplished with acceptable outcomes compared with traditional open repair. The major cause for repeat intervention in these patients was endoleak, most commonly caused by device separation. Improved understanding of these complications may result in a decrease in secondary procedures, morbidity, and mortality in these patients. The need for secondary interventions in a significant number of patients underscores the necessity for continued surveillance.

► High risk is high risk. Thoracic stent grafts are a definite improvement over open surgery for thoracic aortic disease, but there will be some vicious bumps in the road. The complication rates reported here by very experienced endovascular aneurysm surgeons are significant. Those newly embarking upon this procedure will do well to closely study this article so that they can provide appropriate informed consent to their patients and themselves.

G. L. Moneta, MD

Number Needed to Treat: Analyzing of the Effectiveness of Thoracoabdominal Aortic Repair

Miller CC III, Porat EE, Estrera AL, et al (Univ of Texas, Houston)
Eur J Vasc Endovasc Surg 28:154-157, 2004 9–5

Background.—Number needed to treat (NNT) is a method used to calculate the number of patients who need to be treated to prevent one adverse outcome. To analyze the effectiveness of thoracoabdominal and descending thoracic aortic aneurysm repair, we computed the NNT required to prevent one death.

Methods.—Between Jan 1991 and Feb 2003, we repaired 1004 aneurysms of the descending thoracic and thoracoabdominal aorta. We followed the patients from surgery until death. Five-year actuarial survival in our population was computed by the Kaplan-Meier method. Natural history data for comparison were taken from the population-based work of Bickerstaff et al., 1982. NNT was calculated as the reciprocal of the risk difference at 5 years. 95% confidence intervals were computed by the method of Daly.

Results.—Five-year mortality in the population-based cohort was 87 vs. 39% in our treated population, for a risk difference of 48% (Fig 1). 1/0.48 = 2, indicating that two patients need to be treated to prevent one death at 5 years (95% CI 1.8-2.5, $p < 0.0001$).

Conclusion.—An NNT of two demonstrates the effectiveness of surgical repair of descending thoracic and thoracoabdominal aortic aneurysms when compared to the natural history. By comparison, carotid endarterectomy for symptomatic lesions >70% has an NNT of 15 to prevent a single stroke or death. NNT can also be applied to aneurysm size criteria to estimate the effort required to prevent death or rupture for a given aneurysm size.

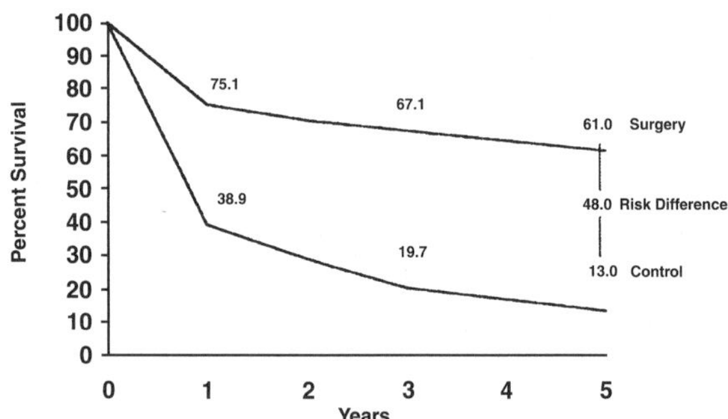

FIGURE 1.—Actuarial survival in our thoracoabdominal aortic aneurysm (TAAA) repair population compared to the population-based control described by Bickerstaff et al, 1982. The risk difference is shown. (Reprinted from Miller CC III, Porat EE, Estrera AL, et al: Number needed to treat: Analyzing of the effectiveness of thoracoabdominal aortic repair. *Eur J Vasc Endovasc Surg* 28:154-157, 2004. Copyright 2004 by permission of the publisher.)

▶ As much as we all like and admire Dr Safi and his work, this analysis is too simplistic. The number needed to treat to prevent death from thoracoabdominal and descending thoracic aneurysms is only part of the story. One must balance the morbidity incurred by the treatment with prevention of death in elderly patients, many of whom have accepted death as inevitable. An interesting question would be to ask how many patients would have had thoracoabdominal aneurysm repair if they truly knew preoperatively what they experienced postoperatively?

G. L. Moneta, MD

Biochemical Markers of Cerebrospinal Ischemia After Repair of Aneurysms of the Descending and Thoracoabdominal Aorta

Anderson RE, Winnerkvist A, Hansson L-O, et al (Karolinska Hosp, Stockholm; CanAg Diagnostics AB, Gothenburg, Sweden; Sahlgrenska Hosp, Gothenburg, Sweden)

J Cardiothorac Vasc Anesth 17:598-603, 2003 9–6

Objective.—To investigate the clinical potential of several markers of spinal cord ischemia in cerebrospinal fluid (CSF) and serum during aneurysm repair of the descending thoracic or thoracoabdominal aorta.

Design.—Observational study of consecutive patients. Nonblinded, nonrandomized.

Setting.—University hospital thoracic surgical unit.

Participants.—Eleven consecutive elective patients.

Interventions.—Distal extracorporeal circulation and maintenance of CSF pressure <10 mmHg until intrathecal catheter removal.

Measurements and Main Results.—CSF and serum levels of S100B (and its isoforms S100A1B and S100BB), neuronal-specific enolase (NSE), and the CSF levels of glial fibrillary acidic protein (GFAp) and lactate were determined. Two patients had postoperative neurologic deficit. One with a stroke showed a 540-fold increased GFAp, a 6-fold NSE, and S100B increase in CSF. One with paraplegia had a 270-fold increase in GFAp, a 2-fold increase in NSE, and 5-fold increased S100B in CSF. One patient without deficit increased GFAp 10-fold, NSE 4-fold, and S100B 23-fold in CSF. CSF lactate increased >50% in 6 of 9 patients without neurologic deficit. Serum S100B increased within 1 hour of surgery in all patients without any concomitant increase in CSF. S100A1B was about 70% of total S100B in both serum and CSF in patients with or without neurologic defects. S100B in CSF increased 3-fold in 3 of 9 asymptomatic patients.

Conclusions.—In patients with neurologic deficit, GFAp in CSF showed the most pronounced increase. Biochemical markers in CSF may increase without neurologic symptoms. There is a significant increase in serum S100B from surgical trauma alone without any increase in CSF.

▶ There appear to be chemical markers of neurologic injury in patients after thoracoabdominal aneurysm repair. For biochemical markers of neurologic injury to be clinically useful, they must provide prognostic information beyond that available from clinical assessment. The data presented in this article, however, suggest that increases in biochemical markers of neurologic injury after thoracoabdominal aortic aneurysm repair occur in a wide spectrum of patients, from those with no neurologic symptoms to those with neurologic impairment. The information is interesting but does not have much clinical relevance at this time.

G. L. Moneta, MD

Descending Thoracic and Thoracoabdominal Aortic Aneurysm in Patients With Takayasu's Disease

Kieffer E, Chiche L, Bertal A, et al (Pitié-Salpêtrière Univ, Paris; Docteur Maouche EMS, Algiers, Algeria)

Ann Vasc Surg 18:505-513, 2004 9–7

Introduction.—From June 1974 to December 2001 we performed operative treatment on 33 patients with descending thoracic or thoracoabdominal aortic aneurysm in association with Takayasu disease (Fig 3). There were 25

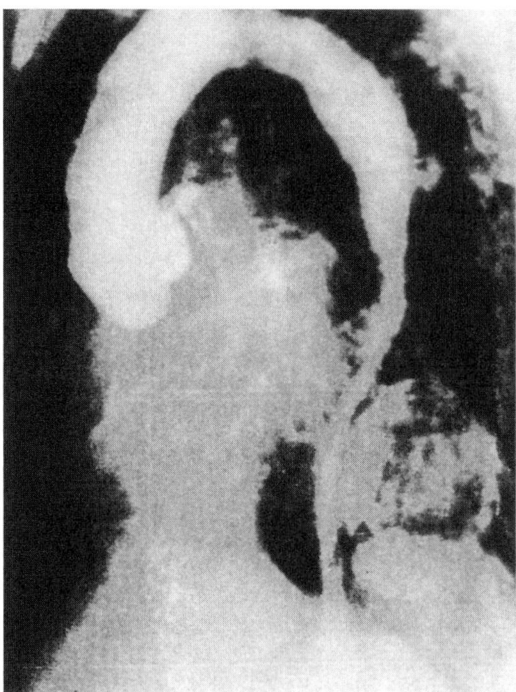

FIGURE 3.—Aortogram showing a saccular descending thoracic aortic aneurysm in a patient with Takayasu disease (TD). Note long associated stenosis involving the whole descending thoracic aorta. (Courtesy of Kieffer E, Chiche L, Bertal A, et al: Descending thoracic and thoracoabdominal aortic aneurysm in patients with Takayasu's disease. *Ann Vasc Surg* 18[5]:505-513, 2004.)

men and 8 women with a mean age of 40.2A years (range 16-64A years). Nineteen patients came from North Africa, 6 were from France, and 8 were from various locations in the world. The revealing symptom was hypertension in 12 cases, thoracic or abdominal pain in 7, isolated inflammatory syndrome in 5, neurologic or ocular manifestations in 3, rupture in 3, and embolization to the lower extremity in 1. In the remaining two cases discovery was coincidental. The aneurysm was confined to the thoracic aorta in 10 cases and involved both the thoracic and abdominal aorta in 23 cases. There were 8 type I, 6 type II, 4 type III, and 5 type IV aneurysms according to Crawford's classification. Two patients had undergone previous repair of the thoracoabdominal aorta. Four patients required first-stage treatment of a renal artery lesion to control hypertension. Six patients had associated aneurysms of the proximal aorta, including five treated via the distal elephant trunk technique in first-stage procedures. Aneurysm repair consisted of prosthetic replacement of the thoracoabdominal aorta in 31 cases, exclusion bypass in 1 case, and stent graft placement in 1 case. The procedure was performed with cross-clamping alone in 13 cases, distal perfusion in 17 cases, and deep hypothermic circulatory arrest in 3 cases. Twenty patients (61%) had associated renal and/or intestinal artery lesions that were treated during the same procedure as that for the thoracoabdominal aorta in 19 patients (58%). A total of 24 procedures were performed on renal arteries (17 revascularizations, 7 nephrectomies). Associated supraaortic trunks lesions were present in 15 patients (45%) and were treated in 12 patients, including 8 in first-stage procedures prior to thoracoabdominal aortic aneurysm repair. Three patients died of multiple organ failure, after reoperation in two cases and infection in one case involving prior long-term corticosteroid therapy. Three patients developed paraplegia, including one who had undergone emergency treatment following rupture. Two patients required reoperation, for hematoma in one case and bowel necrosis in one. Four patients developed respiratory complications requiring artificial ventilation for more than 48 hr. During follow-up, two patients died from complications after repair of the proximal aorta and one patient required nephrectomy. Despite the extent of aneurysmal lesions and high frequency of association with visceral and supraaortic vessel lesions, the outcome of surgery in patients presenting with descending thoracic or thoracoabdominal aortic aneurysm in association with Takayasu disease was satisfactory.

▶ These sorts of articles indicate what can be done. They don't help much with individual patients other than to emphasize that individual patients need individual solutions.

G. L. Moneta, MD

10 Leg Ischemia

Inflammatory and Thrombotic Blood Markers and Walking-Related Disability in Men and Women With and Without Peripheral Arterial Disease

McDermott MM, Guralnik JM, Greenland P, et al (Northwestern Univ, Chicago; Natl Inst on Aging, Bethesda, Md; Harvard Med School, Boston; et al)

J Am Geriatr Soc 52:1888-1894, 2004 10–1

Objectives.—To determine whether higher circulating levels of thrombotic and inflammatory markers are associated with greater disability.

Design.—Cross-sectional.

Setting.—Academic medical center.

Participants.—A total of 346 men and women with peripheral arterial disease (PAD) and 203 without PAD.

Measurements.—Disability measures were the Walking Impairment Questionnaire (WIQ) distance, speed, and stair-climbing scores and the 36-item Short-Form (SF-36) physical functioning score. The SF-36 and WIQ are scored on a 0 to 100 scale (100=best).

Results.—In persons with PAD, higher D-dimer levels were associated with lower WIQ speed scores ($P<.001$), lower stair-climbing scores ($P<.04$), and poorer SF-36 physical functioning scores ($P<.01$), adjusting for known and potential confounders. In participants without PAD, higher D-dimer levels were associated with lower WIQ distance scores ($P<.03$), lower speed scores ($P<.05$), and poorer SF-36 physical functioning scores ($P<.02$) (Fig 2). Higher high-sensitivity C-reactive protein (hsCRP) levels were associated with lower WIQ distance ($P<.02$) and speed scores ($P<.001$) in persons without PAD. Most of these associations were attenuated after additional adjustment for objectively measured functional limitations.

Conclusion.—Higher circulating D-dimer and hsCRP levels are associated with greater disability in walking and physical functioning in individuals with and without PAD. Physiological changes that result in walking disability may mediate these associations.

▶ It is unlikely the inflammatory markers studied here are causing the disabilities measured or the perceived lower measures of health. More likely, the inflammatory markers are so intricately associated with factors impairing health that they cannot be statistically separated.

G. L. Moneta, MD

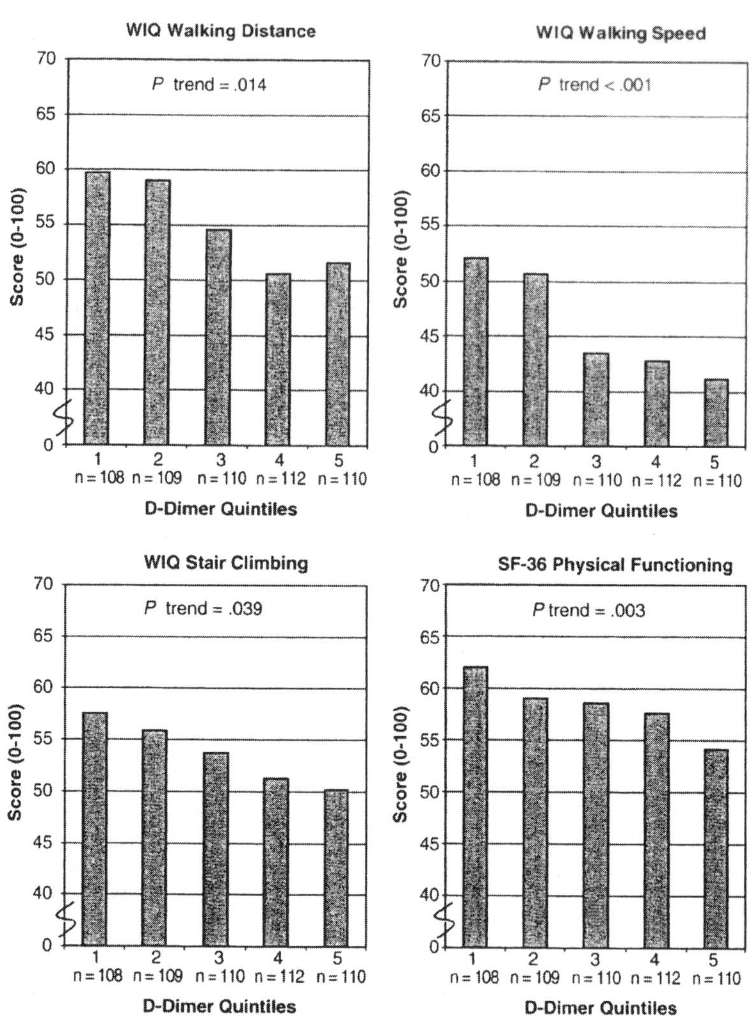

FIGURE 2.—Adjusted associations between D-dimer and Walking Impairment Questionnaire (WIQ) and 36-item Medical Outcome Study Short Form (SF-36) Physical Functioning Scores in men and women with and without peripheral arterial disease (n = 549). Quintiles (μg/mL): 1 = 0.06<0.36, 2 = 0.36<0.50, 3 = 0.50<0.67, 4 = 0.67<0.95, 5 = 0.95<9.64. (Courtesy of McDermott MM, Guralnik JM, Greenland P, et al: Inflammatory and thrombotic blood markers and walking-related disability in men and women with and without peripheral arterial disease. *J Am Geriatr Soc* 52:1888-1894, 2004. Reprinted by permission of Blackwell Publishing.)

Changes in Blood Coagulability as It Traverses the Ischemic Limb

Shankar VK, Chaudhury SR, Uthappa MC, et al (John Radcliffe Hosp, Oxford, England)

J Vasc Surg 39:1033-1042, 2004 10–2

Objective.—We undertook this study to determine whether changes in blood coagulability associated with peripheral arterial occlusive disease are due to contact with the atherosclerotic arterial wall or passage through distal ischemic tissue.

Methods.—Thirty patients with peripheral arterial occlusive disease undergoing angiography participated in the study. Ankle-brachial pressure index was recorded before intervention. Blood samples taken from the aorta, common femoral artery, and common femoral vein were analyzed at thromboelastography. Angiograms were scored for stenotic disease by a radiologist blinded to the other results.

Results.—When femoral artery samples were compared with aortic samples there was a decrease in reaction time (R; $P < .05$), an increase in maximum amplitude (MA; $P < .05$), and an increase in coagulation index (CI; $P < .002$), indicating an increase in coagulability as blood flowed down the iliac segment. These changes also correlated (ΔR, $r = 0.442$, $P < .05$; ΔMA, $r = 0.379$, $P < .05$; ΔCI, $r = 0.429$, $P < .05$) with the severity of disease in the ipsilateral iliac segment. Significant differences in R ($P < .05$), angle ($P < .05$), MA ($P < .005$), and CI ($P < 001$) between common femoral arterial and venous samples confirmed that venous samples were more coagulable in this group of patients. This difference in thromboelastography parameters

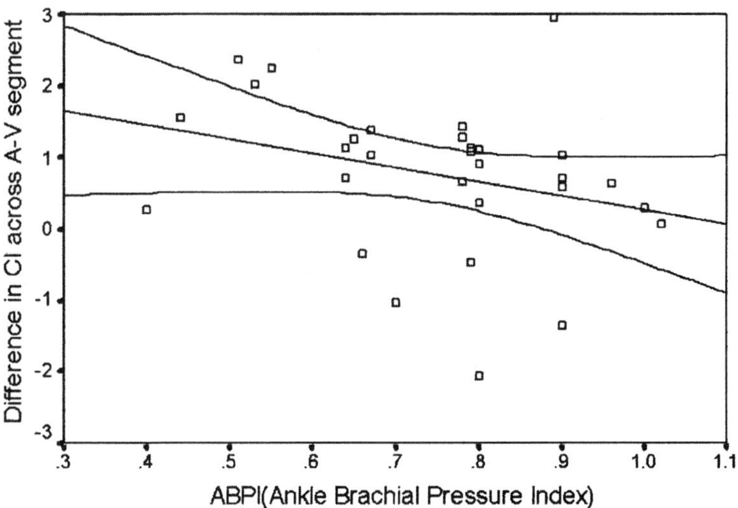

FIGURE 6.—Correlation between change in coagulation index (*CI*) and ankle-brachial pressure index (*ABPI*). (Reprinted by permission of the publisher from Shankar VK, Chaudhury SR, Uthappa MC, et al: Changes in blood coagulability as it traverses the ischemic limb. *J Vasc Surg* 39:1033-1042, 2004. Copyright 2004 by Elsevier.)

across the arteriovenous segment correlated inversely with the degree of ischemia (represented by ankle-brachial pressure index; δCI, $r = -0.427$, $P < .05$; ΔMA, $r = -0.370$, $P < .05$) in the puncture side limb (Fig 6).

Conclusion.—Passage of blood down an atherosclerotic artery leads to an increase in coagulability proportional to the degree of stenosis in that vessel. Passage of blood through ischemic tissue may also contribute to increased coagulability in peripheral arterial occlusive disease.

▶ The authors have performed elegant measurements of hypercoagulability as blood returns from a diseased limb. Obviously, these changes in coagulability are diluted by the general circulation. It is interesting to speculate if this localized hypercoagulability is required or merely associated with thrombosis of an atherosclerotic artery. Given the decreased flow rates and severe stenosis associated with thrombosis of lower extremity arteries, the observations presented here, while interesting, are probably of little true pathologic significance.

G. L. Moneta, MD

Effects of Warm-up on Exercise Capacity, Platelet Activation and Platelet–Leucocyte Aggregation in Patients With Claudication

Pasupathy S, Naseem KM, Homer-Vaniasinkam S (Leeds Gen Infirmary, England; Univ of Bradford, England)

Br J Surg 92:50-55, 2005 10–3

Background.—The effects of exercise and warm-up were investigated in patients with claudication.

Methods.—This case–control crossover study involved two treadmill exercise tests, one preceded by a warm-up. Exercise continued until maximal leg pain (patients with claudication) or exhaustion (controls). Blood was taken before, and 5 and 60 min after exercise for flow cytometric analysis of platelet activation and platelet–leucocyte aggregation.

Results.—Both cohorts (eight patients with claudication of median age 63 years and eight healthy controls of median age 63.5 years) demonstrated improvement in exercise capacity after warm-up (13.1 per cent, $P = 0.012$ and 15.6 per cent, $P = 0.008$ respectively). Platelet activation increased after exercise in patients with claudication (fibrinogen binding: 1.11 per cent before exercise *versus* 2.63 per cent after exercise, $P = 0.008$; P-selectin: 0.68 *versus* 1.11 per cent, $P = 0.028$) (Fig 1). Neither agonist stimulation nor warm-up altered this trend. Platelet–leucocyte (PLA) and platelet–neutrophil (PNA) aggregation were similarly increased immediately after exercise in patients with claudication (PLA: 7.6 *versus* 13.0 per cent, $P = 0.004$; PNA: 6.8 *versus* 10.2 per cent, $P = 0.012$) (Fig 2). These remained high 60 min after exercise only in patients with claudication, but recovered to baseline levels when preceded by warm-up. Warm-up significantly desensitized PNA after stimulation with 10 μmol/l adenosine 5'-diphosphate at all time points.

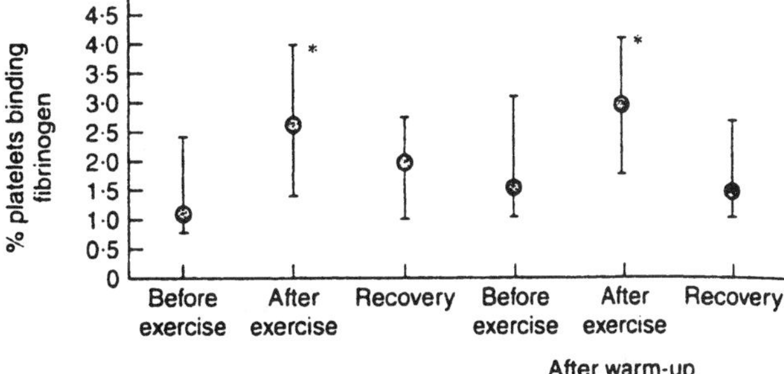

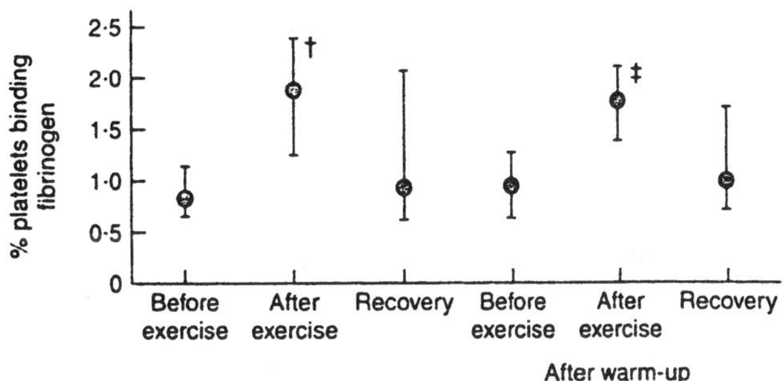

FIGURE 1.—Median (interquartile range platelet fibrinogen binding with and without warm-up in patients with claudication and age-matched controls. **P* = 0.008, †*P* = 0.004, ‡*P* = 0.025 *versus* before exercise (Wilcoxon signed rank test). (Courtesy of Pasupathy S, Naseem KM, Homer-Vaniasinkam S: Effects of warm-up on exercise capacity, platelet activation and platelet–leucocyte aggregation in patients with claudication. *Br J Surg* 92:50-55, 2005. Reprinted by permission of Blackwell Publishing.)

Conclusion.—Warm-up increased the exercise capacity of patients with claudication. Exercise induced a thromboinflammatory response, with PLA and PNA persistently increased after 60 min in patients with claudication, an effect diminished after warm-up.

▶ This small case-controlled study compared 8 patients with claudication on aspirin and a statin against healthy volunteers with a treadmill to evaluate what effects warming up before exercise might have on platelet aggregation and exercise capacity. Subjects did three 5-minute warm-ups on the treadmill, followed by a 20-minute rest before performing exhaustive exercise. Warm-up provided significant increases in exercise capacity in both claudicants and controls (13.1% and 15.6%, respectively). Platelet aggregation and inflammatory response abrogated with warm-up as opposed to without warm-up.

Perhaps the personal trainers are right after all: warm-up helps. Now if we can just get those claudicants to the gym.

A. B. Reed, MD

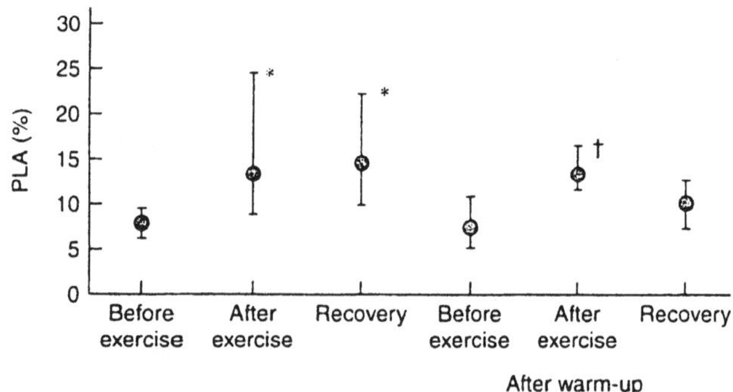

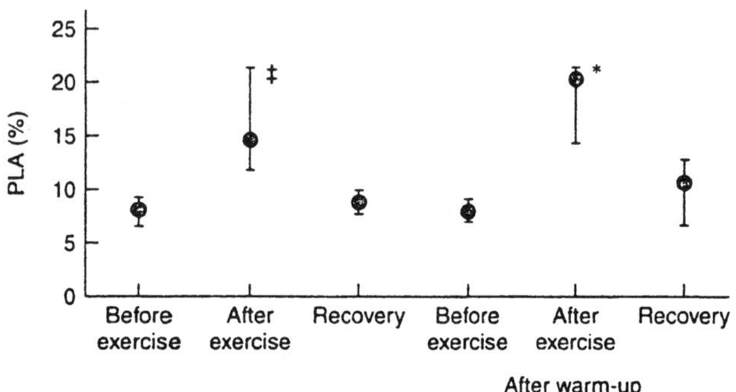

FIGURE 2.—Median (interquartile range) platelet–leukocyte aggregation (PLA) with and without warm-up in patients with claudication and age-matched controls. $^{*}P = 0.004$, $^{\dagger}P = 0.036$, $^{\ddagger}P = 0.017$ *versus* before exercise (Wilcoxon signed rank test). (Courtesy of Pasupathy S, Naseem KM, Homer-Vaniasinkam S: Effects of warm-up on exercise capacity, platelet activation and platelet–leucocyte aggregation in patients with claudication. *Br J Surg* 92:50-55, 2005. Reprinted by permission of Blackwell Publishing.)

Picotamide, a Combined Inhibitor of Thromboxane A_2 Synthase and Receptor, Reduces 2-Year Mortality in Diabetics With Peripheral Arterial Disease: The DAVID Study

Serneri GGN, for the Committees and the Investigators of the Drug Evaluation in Atherosclerotic Vascular Disease in Diabetics (DAVID) Study Group (Univ of Florence, Italy; et al)

Eur Heart J 25:1845-1852, 2004 10–4

Aims.—Patients with diabetes are at excessive risk of mortality and cardiovascular morbidity. Previous studies suggest that aspirin may be less effective in diabetic patients. In this multi-centre, randomized, double blind trial picotamide, a dual inhibitor of thromboxane A_2 synthase and receptor, was compared with aspirin for the prevention of mortality and major cardiovascular events in diabetics with peripheral arterial disease (PAD).

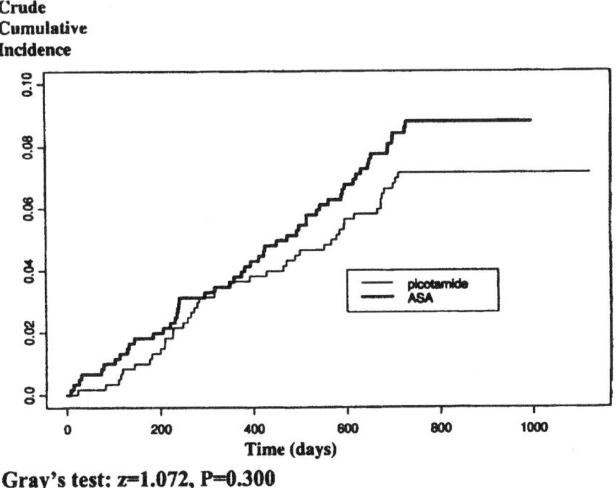

Gray's test: z=1.072, P=0.300

FIGURE 3.—Crude cumulative incidence curves of first event for combined endpoint, considering lost to follow-up a competing risk. (Courtesy of Serneri GGN, for the Committees and the Investigators of the Drug Evaluation in Atherosclerotic Vascular Disease in Diabetics (DAVID) Study: Picotamide, a combined inhibitor of thromboxane A_2 synthase and receptor, reduces 2-year mortality in diabetics with peripheral arterial disease: The DAVID study. *Eur Heart J* 25:1845-1852, 2004. Reprinted by permission of Oxford University Press.)

Method and Results.—A total of 1209 adults aged 40–75 years with type 2 diabetes and PAD were randomized to receive picotamide (600 mg bid) or aspirin (320 mg od) for 24 months. The cumulative incidence of the 2 years overall mortality was significantly lower amongst patients who received picotamide (3.0%) than in those who received aspirin (5.5%) with a relative risk ratio for picotamide versus aspirin of 0.55 (95% CI: 0.31–0.98%) (Fig 3). Events were reported in 43 patients (7.1%) on picotamide and 53 (8.7%) on aspirin. The combined endpoint of mortality and morbidity had a slightly lower incidence in the picotamide group but this difference did not reach statistical significance.

Conclusion.—Picotamide is significantly more effective than aspirin in reducing overall mortality in type 2 diabetic patients with associated PAD.

▶ The Caprie study showed an advantage of clopidogrel over aspirin in preventing vascular death. The results were largely driven by patients with PAD. The FDA has also found insufficient evidence to allow PAD as an approved labeling for aspirin. Caprie and the FDA findings, combined with the results of this study, suggest that while aspirin may have some effect in PAD patients, it is likely relatively weak compared with what may be achieved with other types of antiplatelet drugs.

G. L. Moneta, MD

Comparison of Generic and Disease-Specific Questionnaires for the Assessment of Quality of Life in Patients With Peripheral Arterial Disease

de Vries M, Ouwendijk R, Kessels AG, et al (Maastricht Univ, The Netherlands; Erasmus MC Rotterdam, The Netherlands)

J Vasc Surg 41:261-268, 2005 10–5

Objective.—This study compared the ability of generic and disease-specific questionnaires to assess quality of life (QOL) at baseline and to detect change in QOL after treatment in patients with peripheral arterial disease (PAD).

Methods.—This prospective multicenter trial recruited 514 patients with PAD who needed an imaging workup and had an ankle brachial pressure index of less than 0.90. Patients with severe comorbidity were excluded, leaving a study population of 450 patients. Patients completed two generic questionnaires, the Short Form 36 (SF-36) and the European Quality of Life 5D (EuroQol-5D), and one disease-specific questionnaire, the Vascular Quality of Life (VascuQol) at baseline and after 6 months of follow-up. Rutherford classification and treadmill walking distance were determined at baseline and after 6 months of follow-up and were considered indicators of disease severity. Receiver operating characteristic (ROC) curves and areas under the curves (AUCs) were used to evaluate each of the three questionnaires for its ability to discriminate between severe and mild disease at baseline and to discriminate between a large and small change in disease severity after follow-up (Fig 3). The underlying assumption was that disease severity is a major determinant of QOL. This implies that the validity of a QOL questionnaire is reflected by its ability to discriminate between mildly and severely diseased patients.

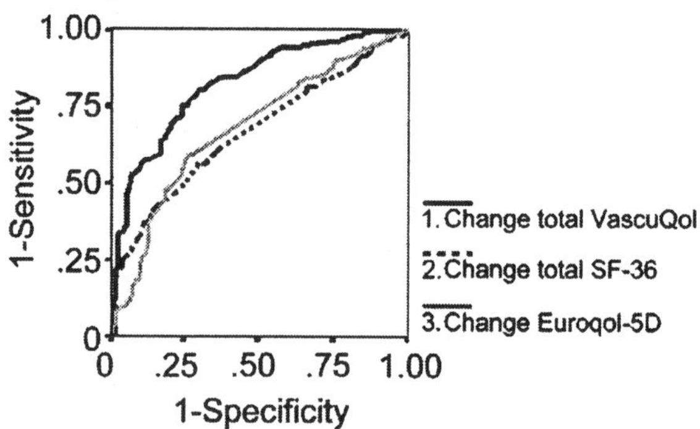

FIGURE 3.—Receiver operating characteristic (ROC) curve after follow-up for patients with claudication. *P* 1-2 < .001; (*P* value comparing AUCs VascuQol with SF-36). *P* 1-3 < 001; (*P* value comparing AUCs VascuQol with EuroQol-5D). *P* 2-3 = .7; (*P* value comparing AUCs SF-36 with EuroQol-5D). (Reprinted by permission of the publisher from de Vries M, Ouwendijk R, Kessels AG, et al: Comparison of generic and disease-specific questionnaires for the assessment of quality of life in patients with peripheral arterial disease. *J Vasc Surg* 41:261-268, 2005. Copyright 2005 by Elsevier.)

Results.—At baseline, 443 patients and after follow-up, 386 patients completed questionnaires. At baseline, no significant ($P > .05$) differences were observed among AUCs for the total scores of the three questionnaires, indicating that all three questionnaires assessed the disease severity equally well. After follow-up, the AUCs for the VascuQol were significantly higher than the AUCs for the SF-36 and EuroQol-5D with respect to detection of improvement in Rutherford classification ($P < .05$), indicating that change in disease severity after follow-up was best detected by the VascuQol.

Conclusion.—The VascuQol is the preferred questionnaire as outcome measure for QOL in future trials and clinical follow-up of patients with PAD.

► Questionnaires are boring subjects for research, but they are assuming more and more importance as we move from lesion- and graft-oriented measures of success of intervention to patient-oriented measures of success. It is a bit of a difficult concept that the patient does not really care if the graft is open. What patients want is freedom from pain, freedom from repeat procedures, and improved well-being. These are difficult to measure with a life table, and you also need the appropriate questionnaire!

G. L. Moneta, MD

Functional Decline in Peripheral Arterial Disease: Associations With the Ankle Brachial Index and Leg Symptoms

McDermott MM, Liu K, Greenland P, et al (Northwestern Univ, Chicago; Natl Inst on Aging, Bethesda, Md; Univ of California, San Diego; et al)

JAMA 292:453-461, 2004 10–6

Context.—Among individuals with lower-extremity peripheral arterial disease (PAD), specific leg symptoms and the ankle brachial index (ABI) are cross-sectionally related to the degree of functional impairment. However, relations between these clinical characteristics and objectively measured functional decline are unknown.

Objective.—To define whether PAD, ABI, and specific leg symptoms predict functional decline at 2-year follow-up.

Design, Setting, and Participants.—Prospective cohort study among 676 consecutively identified individuals (aged ≤55 years) with and without PAD (n=417 and n=259, respectively), with baseline functional assessments occurring between October 1, 1998, and January 31, 2000, and follow-up assessments scheduled 1 and 2 years thereafter. PAD was defined as ABI less than 0.90, and participants with PAD were categorized at baseline into 1 of 5 mutually exclusive symptom groups.

Main Outcome Measures.—Mean annual changes in 6-minute walk performance and in usual-paced and fast-paced 4-m walking velocity, adjusted for age, sex, race, prior-year functioning, comorbid diseases, body mass index, pack-years of cigarette smoking, and patterns of missing data.

Results.—Lower baseline ABI values were associated with greater mean (95% confidence interval) annual decline in 6-minute walk performance (−73.0 [−142 to −4.2] ft for ABI <0.50 vs −58.8 [−83.5 to −34.0] ft for ABI 0.50 to <0.90 vs −12.6 [−40.3 to 15.1] ft for ABI 0.90-1.50, P=.02). Compared with participants without PAD, PAD participants with leg pain on exertion and rest at baseline had greater mean annual decline in 6-minute walk performance (−111 [−173 to −50.0] ft vs −8.67 [−36.9 to 19.5] ft, P=.004), usual-pace 4-meter walking velocity (−0.06 [−0.09 to −0.02] m/sec vs −0.01 (−0.03 to 0.003] m/sec, P=.02), and fastest-pace 4-meter walking velocity (−0.07 [−0.11 to −0.03] m/sec vs −0.02 [−0.04 to −0.006] m/sec, P=.046). Compared with participants without PAD, asymptomatic PAD was associated with greater mean annual decline in 6-minute walk performance (−76.8 (−135 to −18.6] ft vs −8.67 (−36.9 to 19.5] ft, P=.04) and an increased odds ratio for becoming unable to walk for 6 minutes continuously (3.63; 95% confidence interval, 1.58-8.36; P=.002).

Conclusions.—Baseline ABI and the nature of leg symptoms predict the degree of functional decline at 2-year follow-up. Previously reported lack of worsening in claudication symptoms over time in patients with PAD may be more related to declining functional performance than to lack of disease progression.

► It is very difficult to adjust for the effects of comorbidities on functional decline in patients with PAD. This study did not stratify for worsening or improvement of comorbidities. The consistent message, however, is that PAD patients with lower ABIs have greater functional decline than PAD patients with higher ABIs (see also Abstracts 10–5 and 10–7). The source of this functional decline does not appear to be decreasing ABI. We need to determine if functional decline in PAD patients is attributable to worsening comorbidities or deconditioning secondary to PAD-induced restrictions on activity and walking.

G. L. Moneta, MD

Natural History of Physical Function in Older Men With Intermittent Claudication

Gardner AW, Montgomery PS, Lillewich LA (Univ of Oklahoma, Norman; Univ of Texas, Galveston; Univ of Maryland, Baltimore)

J Vasc Surg 40:73-78, 2004 10–7

Purpose.—This study was undertaken to determine the natural history of physical function in older men limited by intermittent claudication.

Methods.—Forty-three men limited by intermittent claudication (mean age, 69 ± 7 years) were recruited and followed up for 18 months. At baseline the patients reported a history of intermittent claudication for 6.1 ± 6.1 years, and were able to walk for 1.9 ± 1.6 blocks before experiencing claudication pain. Measurements during the 18-month study included ankle-brachial index (ABI), calf blood flow, 6-minute walk performance, monitored and self-reported physical activity, self-reported stability while walking, and summary performance score of physical function determined from a 4-m walk test, a chair stand test, and a tandem stand test.

Results.—Pain-free walking distance during the 6-minute walk test decreased by 22% ($P < .05$) from baseline (185 ± 96 m) to follow-up (144 ± 93 m), and the total 6-minute walk distance decreased by 9% ($P < .05$), from 368 ± 106 m to 334 ± 90 m. Furthermore, monitored physical activity decreased by 31% ($P < .05$), from 159 ± 151 kcal/d to 110 ± 137 kcal/d; self-reported physical activity declined by 27% ($P <$ 05), from 1.5 ± 1.0 units to 1.1 ± 0.8 units; tandem stance time declined by 14% ($P < .05$), from 9.46 ± 1.83 seconds to 8.12 ± 2.10 seconds; summary performance score of physical function decreased by 12% ($P <$ 05), from 6.8 ± 2.4 units to 6.0 ± 2.4 units; and the percentage of patients reporting ambulatory unsteadiness and stumbling increased from 28% to 43% ($P < .05$). Calf blood flow measured at rest declined by 18% ($P < .05$), from 3.72 ± 1.81 (mL/100 mL^{-1}/min^{-1}) to 3.04 ± 1.43 mL/100 mL^{-1}/min^{-1}, whereas ABI did not change ($P > .05$).

Conclusion.—Older men limited by intermittent claudication experienced decline in ambulatory function, physical activity, physical function, stability, and calf blood flow over 18 months of follow-up, despite no change in ABI.

▶ Older men experience decline in physical activity and ambulatory function as they age even if their ABIs don't change. I am not sure I needed this article to tell me something my 85-year-old neighbor could have expounded upon. Nonetheless, the authors carefully monitored a group of 43 male claudicants for 18 months to determine what happened to their exercise capabilities, physical function, and gait stability. I suspect many of the usual vascular-associated comorbidities—coronary artery disease, congestive heart failure, chronic obstructive pulmonary disease—got in the way of physical activity as well, making it hard to discern whether functional decline is caused by progression of peripheral arterial disease or overall deconditioning. Despite these limitations, this study is an excellent reminder for those who are considering intervention on aging claudicants.

A. B. Reed, MD

Walking Exercise in Patients With Intermittent Claudication. Experience in Routine Clinical Practice

Bartelink M-L, Stoffers HEJH, Biesheuvel CJ, et al (Univ Med Centre Utrecht, The Netherlands; Julius Centre for Health Sciences and Primary Care, Utrecht, The Netherlands; Univ of Maastricht, The Netherlands)

Br J Gen Pract 54:196-200, 2004 10–8

Background.—In patients with intermittent claudication, exercise in the form of walking is effective in reducing pain and maximising achievable walking distance. However, data are lacking on the implementation of walking exercise in these patients.

Aims.—To explore the current behaviour and views of patients with intermittent claudication towards taking walking exercise. DESIGN OF STUDY: Postal questionnaire and focus group meetings.

Setting.—Two academic general practice networks (Utrecht and Maastricht Universities) in The Netherlands.

Method.—Three hundred and seventy-five patients with intermittent claudication, selected from the files of general practitioners participating in two academic general practice networks, were sent a postal questionnaire; 216 (58%) were returned. Nine of these responders also attended a focus group meeting.

Results.—Seventy per cent (151/216) of the patients reported having received advice about walking exercise. If specified, the advice given most often recommended walking in the local neighbourhood (56%, 84/151). Fifty-two per cent (113/216) of all patients actually performed walking exercise and only 32%of them received any kind of supervision. Among the barriers for taking walking exercise, 'comorbidity', 'lack of (specific) advice' and 'lack of supervision' were often mentioned. Among the stimuli to start and continue walking, 'following the doctor's advice', 'relief of complaints' and 'a better general condition' were often mentioned by patients.

Conclusions.—Walking exercise was not carried out by almost half of patients with intermittent claudication in this study. Lack of specific advice and supervision were found to be important barriers to taking walking exercise.

► Walking works, but unfortunately many patients cannot or do not participate in walking programs. On an intention to treat basis, therefore, walking is poor therapy for claudication. This study points out some of the barriers to walking therapy. Knowledge of a problem is the first stage of solving the problem. Giving the patient specific instructions seems like an easy way to improve results of walking therapy for claudication.

G. L. Moneta, MD

Response to Exercise Rehabilitation in Smoking and Nonsmoking Patients With Intermittent Claudication

Gardner AW, Killewich LA, Montgomery PS, et al (Univ of Oklahoma, Norman; Univ of Texas, Galveston; Univ of Maryland, Baltimore; et al)

J Vasc Surg 39:531-538, 2004 10–9

Background.—The purpose was to compare the changes in claudication pain, ambulatory function, daily physical activity, peripheral circulation, and health-related quality of life following a program of exercise rehabilitation in smoking and nonsmoking patients with peripheral arterial disease (PAD) limited by intermittent claudication.

Methods and Results.—Thirty-nine smokers (63 ± 4 pack-year smoking history; mean ± SE) and 46 nonsmokers (former smokers who had a 51 ± 7 pack-year smoking history who quit 14 ± 2 years prior to investigation) completed the study. The 6-month exercise rehabilitation program consisted of intermittent treadmill walking to near maximal claudication pain 3 days per week, with progressive increases in walking duration and intensity during the program. Measurements were obtained on each patient before and after rehabilitation. Following exercise rehabilitation the smokers and nonsmokers had similar improvements in these measures, as initial claudication distance increased by 119% in the smokers (P < .001) and by 97% in the nonsmokers (P < 001), and absolute claudication distance increased by 82% (P < .001) and 59% (P < .001) in the smokers and nonsmokers, respectively. Furthermore, exercise rehabilitation improved (P < .05) ambulatory function, daily physical activity, peripheral circulation, and health-related quality of life in the smokers and nonsmokers.

Conclusion.—Exercise rehabilitation is an effective therapy to improve functional independence in both smoking and nonsmoking patients with PAD limited by intermittent claudication. Therefore, smokers with intermittent claudication are prime candidates for exercise rehabilitation because their relatively low baseline physical function does not impair their ability to regain lost functional independence to levels similar to nonsmoking patients with PAD.

► I suspect many vascular surgeons doubt significant improvement in physical function with walking programs will occur in patients with intermittent claudication if they continue to smoke. This study, however, finds similar improvements in ambulatory function, physical activity, and health-related quality of life in smokers and nonsmokers after a 6-month exercise program. In fact, since smokers start out with lower functional status and greater impairments, they appear to gain even more. However, I think we still need to try to get our patients to stop smoking.

A. B. Reed, MD

Outcome of Conservative Therapy of Patients With Severe Intermittent Claudication

Amighi J, Sabeti S, Schlager O, et al (Vienna Gen Hosp, Austria)
Eur J Vasc Endovasc Surg 27:254-258, 2004 10–10

Background.—Intermittent claudication due to peripheral artery disease (PAD) can be treated conservatively, or by revascularization.

Objectives.—To assess the short-term outcome of conservatively-treated claudicants, and determine predictors for clinical improvement. Design. A retrospective cohort study.

Methods.—We evaluated Fontaine stage, walking distance and ankle brachial index (ABI) at baseline and after median 9 months (interquartile range (IQR) 6–24) in 181 patients with severe claudication.

Results.—We found clinical improvement by at least one Fontaine stage in 38 patients (21%) with an increased walking distance from baseline median 100 m (IQR 50–150) to follow-up median 650 m (IQR 300 to unlimited; $p < 0.001$), but without changes in ABI (median 0.57, IQR 0.48–0.73 vs. median 0.54, IQR 0.45–0.81; $p = 0.10$). One hundred and thirty-eight patients (76%) remained clinically and hemodynamically stable. A worsening of the clinical stage but without amputation was recorded in five patients (3%). Female gender (hazard ratio (HR) 0.51, $p = 0.052$), diabetes (HR 0.35, $p = 0.020$), and baseline ABI below 0.44 (HR 0.31, $p = 0.019$) were associated with a reduced probability of clinical improvement.

Conclusion.—Certain patients with intermittent claudication show substantial clinical improvement with conservative medical therapy, despite any lack of hemodynamic improvement. Given the low number of patients with clinical deterioration in the short term, primarily conservative therapy should be the preferred initial option for most claudicants.

▶ This article reinforces the wisdom of conservative management of even those patients with severe symptoms of intermittent claudication. Based on the authors' analysis, patients who are female, have diabetes, and have a baseline ABI less than 0.4 can be advised that they are less likely to improve than other patients with similar symptoms. They are also very unlikely to deteriorate in short-term follow-up.

G. L. Moneta, MD

Bypass to Plantar and Tarsal Arteries: An Acceptable Approach to Limb Salvage

Hughes K, Domenig CM, Hamdan AD, et al (Harvard Med School, Boston)

J Vasc Surg 40:1149-1157, 2004 10–11

Objective.—This study was undertaken to evaluate our experience with distal arterial bypass to the plantar artery branches and the lateral tarsal artery for ischemic limb salvage.

Methods.—This was a retrospective analysis of data prospectively entered into our vascular surgery database from January 1990 to January 2003 for all consecutive patients undergoing bypass grafting to the plantar artery branches or the lateral tarsal artery. Median follow-up was 9 months (range, 1-112 months). Demographic data, indications for surgery, outcomes, and patency were recorded, and statistical analysis was performed to assess significance.

Results.—Ninety-eight bypass procedures to either the medial plantar artery, lateral plantar artery, or lateral tarsal artery were performed in 90 patients. Eighty-one patients (83%) were men. Mean age was 67.5 ± 11.6 years. Indications for operation were tissue loss in 93 patients (95%), rest pain in 3 patients (3%), and failing graft in 2 patients (2%). Eighteen patients (18%) had previously undergone vascular reconstruction, and 5 patients (5%) had undergone previous bypass to the dorsalis pedis artery. Seventy-one grafts (72%) had inflow from the popliteal artery, 25 grafts had inflow from a femoral artery or graft (26%), and 2 grafts had inflow from a tibial artery (2%). Conduits used were greater saphenous vein in 67 patients (69%), arm vein in 20 patients (20%), composite vein in 10 patients (10%),

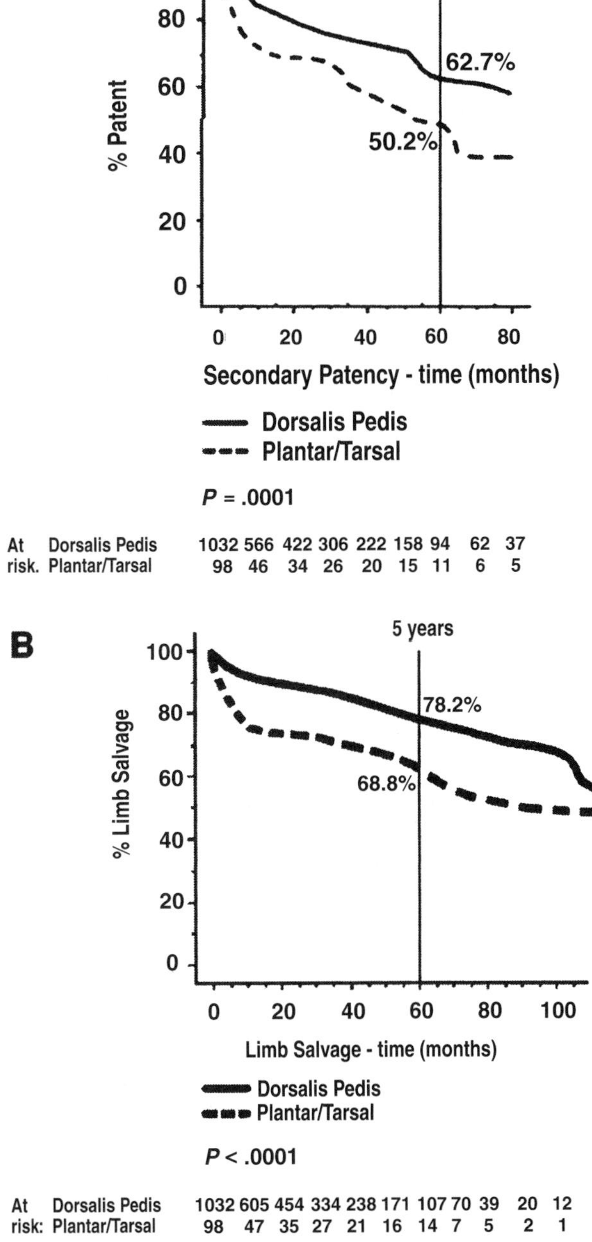

FIGURE 5.—Comparison of secondary patency (**A**) and limb salvage (**B**) between dorsalis pedis bypass and plantar or tarsal bypass patient populations. (SE <10% at all time intervals.) (Reprinted by permission of the publisher from Hughes K, Domenig CM, Hamdan AD, et al: Bypass to plantar and tarsal arteries: An acceptable approach to limb salvage. *J Vasc Surg* 40:1149-1157, 2004. Copyright 2004 by Elsevier.)

and polytetrafluoroethylene conduit in 1 patient (1%). There were 77 bypasses (79%) to plantar artery branches, and 21 bypasses (21%) to the lateral tarsal artery. Thirty-day mortality was 1% (1 of 98 procedures). Early graft failure within 30 days occurred in 11 patients (11%). In the subset of patients with a previous arterial reconstruction, there were 2 early graft failures within 30 days (11%). Both occurred in patients who had undergone previous bypass to the dorsalis pedis artery. Primary patency, secondary patency, limb salvage, and patient survival were 67%, 70%, 75%, and 91%, respectively, at 12 months, and 41%, 50%, 69%, and 63%, respectively, at 5 years, as determined from Kaplan-Meier survival curves (Fig 5). Greater saphenous vein grafts performed better than all other conduits, with a secondary patency rate of 82% versus 47% at 1 year ($P = .009$).

Conclusion.—Inframalleolar bypass to plantar artery branches and the lateral tarsal artery, even in patients with a previously failed revascularization, can be undertaken with acceptable patency and limb salvage rates. Early graft failure, however, is higher, whereas patency and limb salvage rates are lower, compared with bypass to the dorsalis pedis artery. The use of saphenous vein as a conduit results in the best patency for plantar or lateral tarsal bypass procedures.

► This group continues to persevere and provide excellent results with distal autogenous bypass, this time evaluating their experience to the plantar and tarsal arteries. While these grafts are likely subcutaneous and easily palpable, it worries me when groups report graft patency based on physical examination by an attending physician rather than objective examination by duplex. In these days of outcomes assessment and analysis, routine trips to the vascular lab are a necessity.

A. B. Reed, MD

Infrainguinal Vein Bypass Graft Revision: Factors Affecting Long-term Outcome

Nguyen LL, Conte MS, Menard MT, et al (Harvard Med School, Boston)
J Vasc Surg 40:916-923, 2004 10–12

Objectives.—We sought to determine the long-term results of revision procedures performed for repair of stenotic lesions in infrainguinal vein bypass grafts.

Methods.—A retrospective review of 188 vein grafts, from a total series of 1260 bypasses, undergoing revision of stenotic lesions between January 1, 1987, and December 31, 2002, at Brigham & Women's Hospital was undertaken. Lesions were identified by recurrence of symptoms, change in examination findings, or with routine duplex ultrasound graft surveillance. Demographic and medical risk factors, and surgical variables were analyzed with respect to patency outcomes after the initial graft revision, with descriptive statistics, logistic regression, and life table analysis. Primary and secondary patency rates were determined from the time of graft revision.

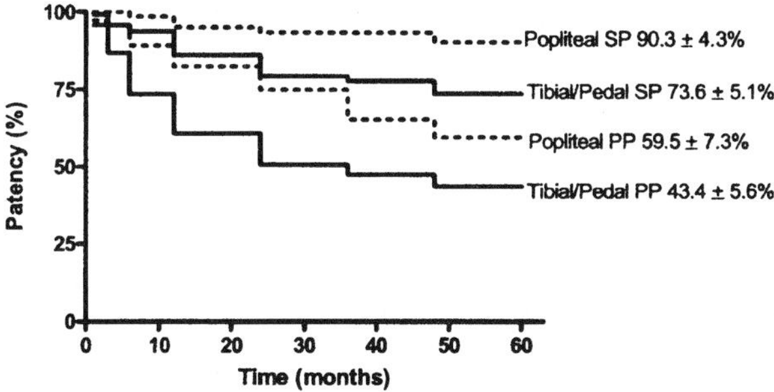

FIGURE 2.—Primary and secondary revision graft patency for popliteal versus tibial or pedal distal anastomosis sites. (Reprinted by permission of the publisher from Nguyen LL, Conte MS, Menard MT, et al: Infrainguinal vein bypass graft revision: Factors affecting long-term outcome. *J Vasc Surg* 40:916-926, 2004. Copyright 2004 by Elsevier.)

Results.—Patients included 108 men (57%) and 80 women (42%) who underwent revision at a mean age of 67.8 years. One hundred thirty grafts required only a single revision, whereas 58 required subsequent additional revisions. Revision procedures included 99 vein patches (52.7%), 23 jump grafts (12.2%), 23 interposition grafts (12.2%), 8 transpositions to new outflow vessels (4.3%), and 35 balloon angioplasty procedures (18.6%). During a mean follow-up of 1535 days, 5-year primary patency rate was 49.3% ± 4.5% (SE) and 5-year secondary patency rate was 80.3% ± 3.6% (Fig 2). There was no difference in patency rate for different revision procedures, type of vein graft, indication for the original procedure, or for patients with diabetes mellitus or renal disease (Fig 3). The overall limb salvage rate was 83.2% ± 3.5% 5 years after graft revision. With COX proportional hazard analysis of time to failure of the revision procedure, the outflow level of the original bypass and the time of revision proved to be an important predictor of durability of the graft revision. Revision of popliteal bypass grafts resulted in a 60% 5-year primary patency rate, whereas revision of tibial grafts resulted in a 42% 5-year primary patency rate (P = 004; hazard ratio [HR], 2.06). Five-year secondary patency rates were 90% and 76%, respec-

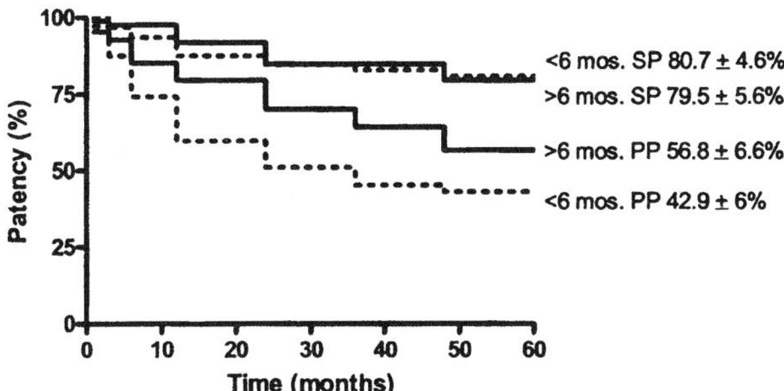

FIGURE 3.—Primary graft patency for grafts revised less than 6 months versus greater than 6 months after index operation. (Reprinted by permission of the publisher from Nguyen LL, Conte MS, Menard MT, et al: Infrainguinal vein bypass graft revision: Factors affecting long-term outcome. *J Vasc Surg* 40:916-926, 2004. Copyright 2004 by Elsevier.)

tively (P = .009; HR = 3.43). The timing of the graft revision proved an additional predictor. Grafts revised within 6 months of the index operation had lower primary patency than those with later revisions (42.9% vs 80.7%, respectively; HR = 1.754; P = .0152).

Conclusions.—Vein graft revisions offer durable patency and limb salvage rates after repair of stenotic infrainguinal bypass grafts. Vigilant ongoing surveillance is essential, because 30.9% of revised grafts will develop additional lesions that will require repair. Tibial level bypass grafts that require early repeat intervention to treat graft stenosis are at particular risk for development of subsequent lesions.

▶ Of the 1629 autogenous infrainguinal bypasses performed over a 15-year period, only an impressive 188 grafts (11.5 %) had to undergo revision—the majority being a one-time event. The majority of grafts undergoing revision required an open patch—56.9% of single revision grafts and 43.1% of multiple revisions—versus 16.9% and 22.4%, respectively, for percutaneous angioplasty. As cutter balloons come onto the market and technology advances, I suspect more revisions will become percutaneous. One thing that will not change, however, is the ongoing need for objective graft surveillance with duplex or other imaging modalities.

A. B. Reed, MD

Optimizing Infrainguinal Arm Vein Bypass Patency With Duplex Ultrasound Surveillance and Endovascular Therapy

Armstrong PA, Bandyk DF, Wilson JS, et al (Univ of South Florida, Tampa)

J Vasc Surg 40:724-731, 2004 10–13

Objective.—Infrainguinal bypass grafting with arm vein is associated with lower patency rates compared with saphenous vein conduits. In this study the effect of a duplex ultrasound surveillance program to enable identification and treat graft lesions with open or endovascular repair on patency was analyzed.

Methods.—Over 9 years 89 infrainguinal arm vein (26% spliced vein) bypasses were performed to treat critical lower limb ischemia in 89 patients without adequate saphenous vein conduits. Seventy-six (85%) of the bypasses were repeat procedures. Grafts were assessed at operation with duplex ultrasound scanning, then enrolled in a surveillance program. Graft stenoses with peak systolic velocity greater than 300 cm/s and velocity ratio greater than 3.5, detected at duplex ultrasound scanning, were repaired with percutaneous transluminal balloon angioplasty (PTA) if specific criteria were met, including greater than 3 months since primary procedure, lesion length less than 2 cm, and graft diameter greater than 3.5 mm, or with open surgical repair for early appearing or extensive graft lesions.

Results.—During a mean 26-month follow-up, duplex surveillance resulted in a 48% (43 bypasses) intervention rate. Primary patency rate was 43% at 3 years (Fig 1). Twenty-six (43%) of 61 lesions identified and re-

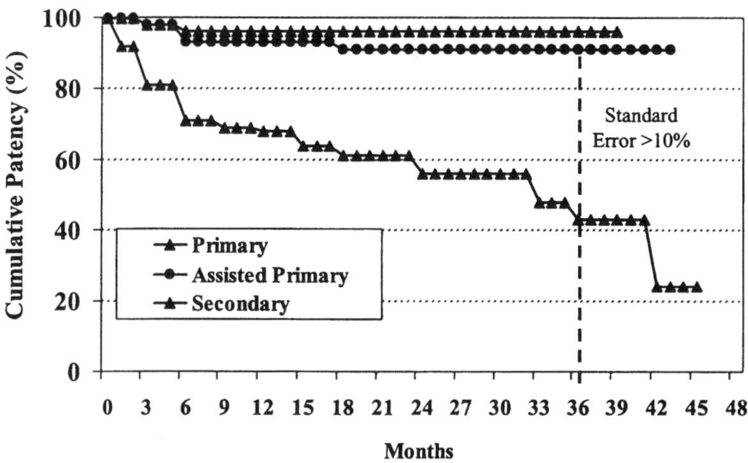

FIGURE 1.—Life table analysis of primary, assisted primary, and secondary patency rates for 88 infrainguinal arm vein bypasses. (Reprinted by permission of the publisher from Armstrong PA, Bandyk DF, Wilson JS, et al: Optimizing infrainguinal arm vein bypass patency with duplex ultrasound surveillance and endovascular therapy. *J Vasc Surg* 40:724-731, 2004. Copyright 2004 by Elsevier.)

paired met criteria for PTA; the remaining 35 graft lesions (stenosis, n = 30; vein graft aneurysm, n = 5) were surgically corrected with vein patch angioplasty (n = 15), interposition grafting (n = 13), jump graft bypass (n = 6), or open repair (n = 1). At 3 years the assisted primary patency rate was 91% (7 graft failures). Multiple interventions were performed in 18 (42%) revised grafts because of metachronous (n = 6) or repair site stenosis (n = 12). In 18 graft interventions (PTA, n = 9; surgery, n = 9) recurrent stenosis developed, and endovascular therapy was used in one third (n = 6). At 3 years the

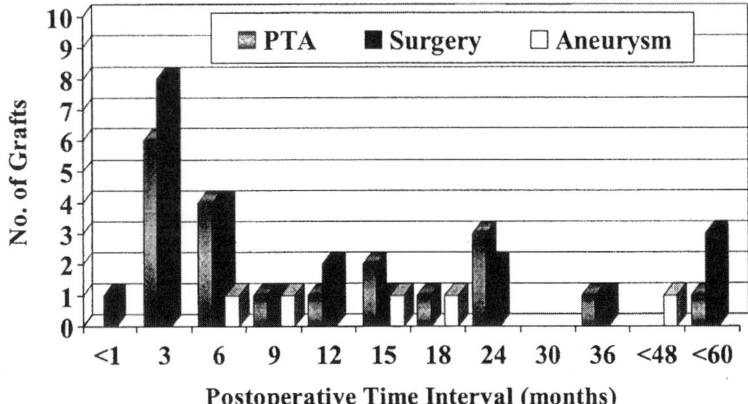

FIGURE 2.—Time to repair of 32 primary and 6 metachronous graft stenosis with percutaneous transluminal angioplasty (*PTA*) or surgery, and of 5 identified vein graft aneurysms with interpositional grafting. (Reprinted by permission of the publisher from Armstrong PA, Bandyk DF, Wilson JS, et al: Optimizing infrainguinal arm vein bypass patency with duplex ultrasound surveillance and endovascular therapy. *J Vasc Surg* 40:724-731, 2004. Copyright 2004 by Elsevier.)

stenosis-free patency rate for PTA (48%) and surgically repaired (53%) graft lesions was similar (Fig 2).

Conclusions.—Arm veins used in lower limb bypass procedures are prone to development of stenosis and aneurysm, lesions easily detected with a lifelong duplex ultrasound surveillance program. Excellent long-term patency (91%) was achieved despite graft intervention being performed in nearly half of all bypasses and one third of revised grafts. Endovascular treatment was possible in half of all graft stenosis, with outcomes similar to those with surgical repair.

▶ This is an excellent report on not only the use of arm vein, but what to expect in terms of duplex surveillance and treatment of graft stenoses. Duplex scanning, as opposed to just physical examination (see Abstract 10–11), is clearly the preferred approach to follow grafts long term. The relatively equivalent results of percutaneous versus open revision are encouraging.

A. B. Reed, MD

Statin Therapy Is Associated With Improved Patency of Autogenous Infrainguinal Bypass Grafts

Abbruzzese TA, Havens J, Belkin M, et al (Harvard Med School, Boston)
J Vasc Surg 39:1178-1185, 2004 10–14

Objective.—HMG-CoA reductase inhibitors (statins) broadly reduce cardiovascular events, effects that are only partly related to cholesterol lowering. Recent studies suggest important anti-inflammatory and antiproliferative properties of these drugs. The purpose of this study was to determine the influence of statin therapy on graft patency after autogenous infrainguinal arterial reconstructions.

Methods.—A retrospective analysis of consecutive patients (1999-2001) who underwent primary autogenous infrainguinal reconstructions with a single segment of greater saphenous vein was performed. Patients were categorized according to concurrent use of a statin. Graft lesions (identified by duplex surveillance) and interventions were tabulated. Comparisons between groups were made by using the Fisher exact test for categorical variables and the Student t test for continuous variables. Patency, limb salvage, and survival were compared by log rank test. A stepwise Cox proportional hazards analysis was then employed to ascertain the relative importance of factors influencing graft patency.

Results.—A total of 172 patients underwent 189 primary autogenous infrainguinal arterial reconstructions (94 statin, 95 control) during the study period. The groups were well matched for age, indication, and atherosclerotic risk factors. Procedures were performed primarily for limb salvage (92%), with 65% to an infrapopliteal target. Perioperative mortality (2.6%) and major morbidity (3.2%) were not different between groups. There was no difference in primary patency (74% ± 5% vs 69% ± 6%; $P = .25$), limb salvage (92% ± 3% vs 90% ± 4%; $P = .37$), or survival (69% ± 5% vs 63%

± 5%; $P = .20$) at 2 years. However, patients on statins had higher primary-revised (94% ± 2% vs 83% ± 5%; $P < .02$) and secondary (97% ± 2% vs 87% ± 4%; $P < .02$) graft patency rates at 2 years. Of all factors studied by univariate analysis, only statin use was associated with improved secondary patency ($P = .03$) at 2 years. This was confirmed by multivariate analysis. The risk of graft failure was 3.2-fold higher (95% confidence interval, 1.04-10.04) for the control group. Perioperative cholesterol levels (available in 47% of patients) were not statistically different between groups.

Conclusions.—Statin therapy is associated with improved graft patency after infrainguinal bypass grafting with saphenous vein.

▶ The conclusions of this study are a bit of a stretch given its retrospective design, the wide confidence intervals of the data, and the unknown and previously unpostulated mechanism of how statins may influence intimal hyperplasia. However, the data are the data, and this group is widely respected for its contributions to the literature regarding infrainguinal bypass. Results of similar analyses from other groups are eagerly awaited.

G. L. Moneta, MD

Patency and Limb Salvage Rates After Distal Revascularization to Unclampable Calcified Outflow Arteries

Ballotta E, Renon L, Toffano M, et al (Univ of Padua, Italy)

J Vasc Surg 39:539-546, 2004 10–15

Purpose.—Severe circumferential calcification of the outflow artery during lower-extremity distal revascularization is considered a poor prognostic factor for bypass graft patency. The aim of this study was to assess the influence of circumferential infrapopliteal arterial calcification on bypass graft patency and limb salvage rates, comparing patency and limb salvage rates in unclampable calcified distal outflow arteries with those observed in uncalcified distal outflow arteries.

Methods.—From July 1990 to July 1997, of 441 distal bypass graft procedures performed by the same surgeon, 69 (16%, group I) involved unclampable calcified outflow vessels, whereas 83 (19%, group II) outflow vessels were uncalcified; the other 289 (65%) had varying intermediate degrees of calcification and were not included in this analysis. All procedures were performed for limb-threatening ischemia and involved standard vein patch angioplasty of the distal anastomotic site, irrespective of the conduit used (Fig 1). Primary and secondary patency, limb salvage, and survival rates were assessed by using Kaplan-Meier analysis.

Results.—Groups were similar with regard to age, sex, and atherosclerotic risk factors except for a higher incidence of diabetes mellitus (88% vs 65%, $P = .001$) and renal failure (17% vs 5%, $P = .01$), including dialysis dependency ($P = .01$) in group I. Gangrene as an indication for surgery was statistically more frequent in group I (49% vs 29%, $P = .01$). The distal anastomotic locations and types of conduit involved were similar in the two

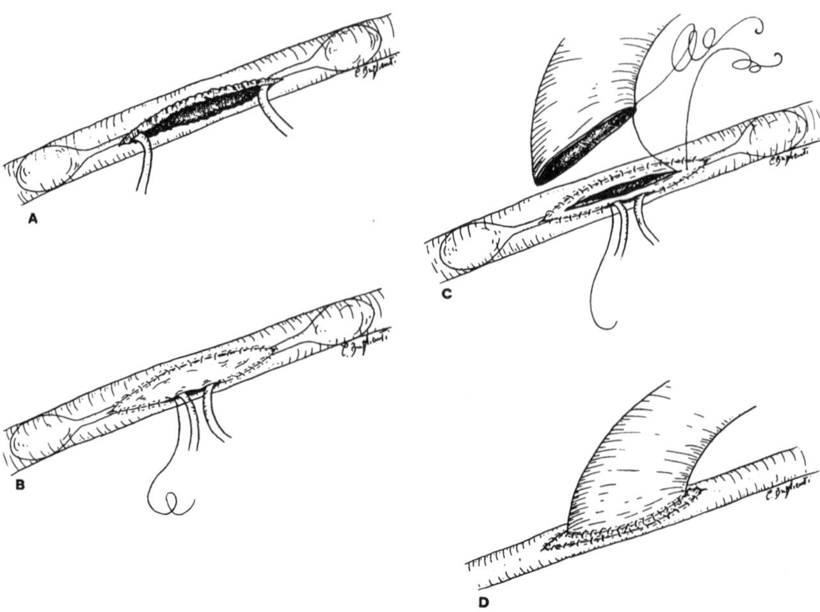

FIGURE 1.—A, After performing a longitudinal arteriotomy in the unclampable calcified vessel, olive-type metal intraluminal occluders are placed to control proximal and distal backflow. B, A vein patch is routinely sutured to the calcified artery with simple running stitches on cardiovascular needles. C, Before the patch anastomosis is completed, the chosen conduit is implanted in the vein patch. D, Intraluminal occluders are removed from the primitive anastomosis and then the suture is tied. (Reprinted by permission of the publisher from Ballotta E, Renon L, Toffano M, et al: Patency and limb salvage rates after distal revascularization to unclampable calcified outflow arteries. *J Vasc Surg* 39:539-546, 2004. Copyright 2004 by Elsevier.)

groups. The femoral inflow level was used more often in group II (63% vs 38%, $P = .003$), the popliteal in group I (32% vs 17%, $P = .03$). Follow-up ranged from 30 days to 144 months, with a mean of 69 months. None of the patients were lost during the follow-up period. None of the patients died during the perioperative (30-day) period. Primary patency rates at 1, 3, and 5 years were 84%, 65%, and 52% for group I and 89%, 76%, and 69% for group II ($P = .07$). Secondary patency rates at 1, 3, and 5 years were 96%, 82%, and 78% for group I and 96%, 85%, and 82% for group II ($P = .58$). Limb salvage rates at 1, 3, and 5 years were 93%, 83%, and 81% for group I and 97%, 90%, and 86% for group II ($P = .39$).

Conclusions.—Distal revascularization to unclampable, severely calcified outflow arteries can achieve much the same results to those obtained in uncalcified outflow arteries. A circumferentially calcified distal recipient artery should not be considered a major obstacle to an attempt at limb salvage bypass graft surgery.

▶ The technique of sewing a vein cuff to a calcified tibial or pedal vessel before performing the distal anastomosis makes sense. However, if the vein cuff can be sewn to the vessel, why not just go straight to constructing the distal anastomosis, particularly when there is no patency advantage?

A. B. Reed, MD

Randomized Clinical Trial of Distal Anastomotic Interposition Vein Cuff in Infrainguinal Polytetrafluoroethylene Bypass Grafting

Griffiths GD, for the Joint Vascular Research Group (Ninewells Hosp, Dundee, Scotland)

Br J Surg 91:560-562, 2004 10–16

Background.—The aim was to examine the effect of a Miller vein cuff at the distal anastomosis on the medium- to long-term patency and limb salvage rates of femoral to above-knee and femoral to below-knee popliteal artery polytetrafluoroethylene (PTFE) bypasses.

Methods.—This study involved extended follow-up of the original cohort of patients included in a previously reported multicentre randomized clinical study. Outcome measures were bypass graft patency and limb salvage.

Results.—Two hundred and sixty-one bypass operations were originally randomized. For this study, full data were available on 235 (120 with a Miller cuff, 115 without). The cumulative 5-year patency rate for above-knee bypasses with a Miller cuff was 40 per cent, compared with 42 per cent for non-cuffed bypasses ($P = 0.702$) (Fig 1). The cumulative 3-year patency rate for below-knee bypasses with a Miller cuff was 45 per cent, compared with 19 per cent for non-cuffed bypasses ($P = 0.018$) (Fig 2). A Miller cuff had no significant effect on limb salvage for above-knee or below-knee bypasses.

Conclusion.—Three-year patency rates of femoral to below-knee popliteal PTFE bypasses were improved by a Miller cuff. Miller cuffs had no effect

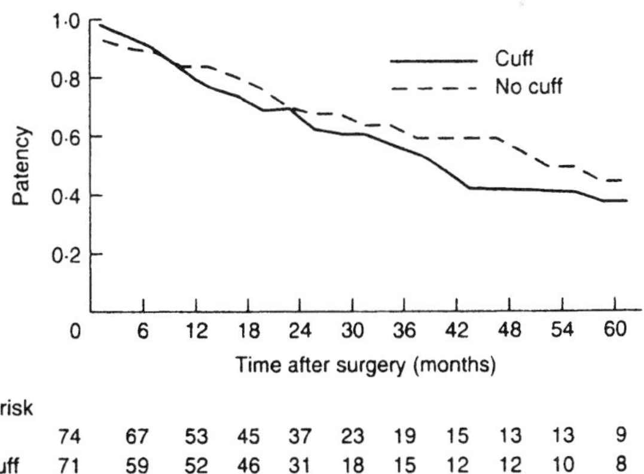

No. at risk											
Cuff	74	67	53	45	37	23	19	15	13	13	9
No cuff	71	59	52	46	31	18	15	12	12	10	8

FIGURE 1.—Cumulative 5-year patency for above-knee bypasses with and without a Miller cuff. $P = 0.702$ (generalized Wilcoxon test). (Courtesy of Griffiths GD, for the Joint Vascular Research Group: Randomized clinical trial of distal anastomotic interposition vein cuff in infrainguinal polytetrafluoroethylene bypass grafting. *Br J Surg* 91:560-562, 2004. Reprinted by permission of Blackwell Publishing.)

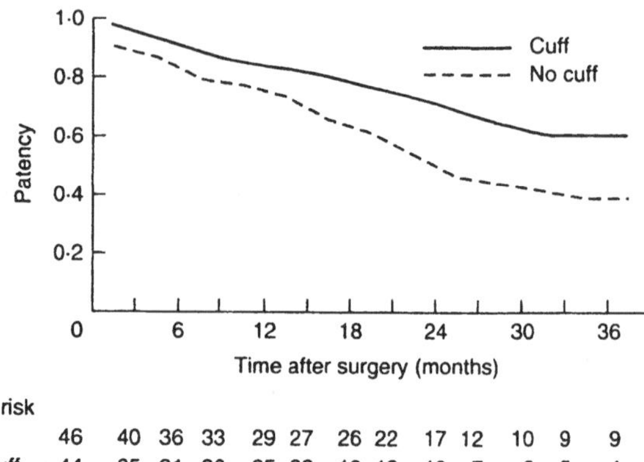

No. at risk													
Cuff	46	40	36	33	29	27	26	22	17	12	10	9	9
No cuff	44	35	31	26	25	23	18	13	10	7	6	5	4

FIGURE 2.—Cumulative 3-year patency for below-knee bypasses with and without a Miller cuff. $P = 0.018$ (generalized Wilcoxon test). (Courtesy of Griffiths GD, for the Joint Vascular Research Group: Randomized clinical trial of distal anastomotic interposition vein cuff in infrainguinal polytetrafluoroethylene bypass grafting. *Br J Surg* 91:560-562, 2004. Reprinted by permission of Blackwell Publishing.)

on patency rates for femoral to above-knee popliteal bypasses at 5 years and did not improve limb salvage in either group.

► The results indicate that when PTFE bypasses are performed to the below-knee popliteal artery in a primarily limb salvage population, a Miller cuff should be utilized. The results also confirm PTFE bypass to the popliteal artery for limb salvage, whether it be above or below the knee, has poor long-term patency.

G. L. Moneta, MD

Heparin-Bonded Dacron or Polytetrafluorethylene for Femoropopliteal Bypass: Five-Year Results of a Prospective Randomized Multicenter Clinical Trial

Devine C, for the North West Femoro-Popliteal Trial Participants (Wythenshawe Hosp, Manchester, England)
J Vasc Surg 40:924-931, 2004 10–17

Objective.—Dacron was largely abandoned for femoropopliteal bypass 30 years ago, because better patency rates were achieved with saphenous vein. Despite the range of potential prosthetics, polytetrafluoroethylene (PTFE) clearly predominates in current femoropopliteal practice. We compared heparin-bonded Dacron (HBD) with PTFE in a randomized multicenter clinical trial.

Method.—Over 28 months, 209 patients (179 above-knee disease, 30 below-knee disease) were randomized to receive HBD (n = 106) or PTFE (n = 103) grafts. Aspirin, 300 mg/d, was started before surgery, and was continued if tolerated.

Results.—At follow-up for a minimum of 5 years (mean, 76 months; range, 60-89 months), 37 patients (17.7%) had died with patent grafts and

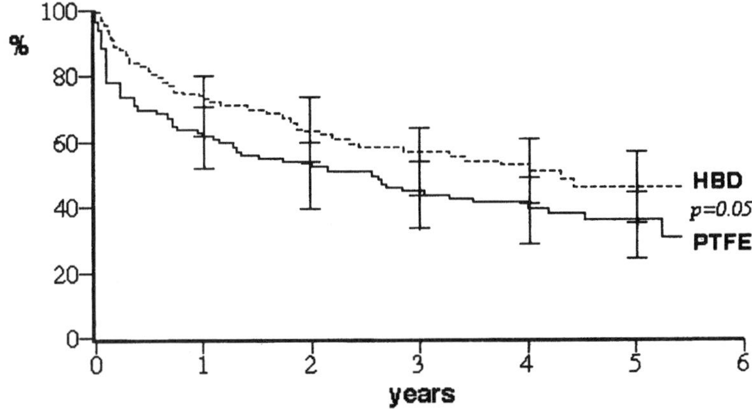

FIGURE 1.—Primary patency at life table analysis for heparin-bonded Dacron (*HBD*) was 71%, 54%, and 46%, respectively, for years 1, 3, and 5, compared with 62%, 44%, and 35% for polytetrafluoroethylene (*PTFE*). (Reprinted by permission of the publisher from Devine C, for the North West Femoro-Popliteal Trial: Heparin-bonded Dacron or polytetrafluorethylene for femoropopliteal bypass: Five-year results of a prospective randomized multicenter clinical trial. *J Vasc Surg* 40:924-931, 2004. Copyright 2004 by Elsevier.)

121 (58%) grafts were occluded. Primary patency rate, measured with Kaplan-Meier survival analysis, was 46% (95% confidence interval [CI], 35%-57%) at year 5 for HBD, compared with 35% for PTFE (CI, 25%-45%; $P < .055$). Long-term patency was achieved in only 4 of 78 interventions performed in 55 thrombosed grafts. Secondary patency rate for HBD was 47% (CI, 36%-58%), and for PTFE was 36% (CI, 26%-46%). Risk factors for arterial disease did not significantly influence prosthetic patency. Major limb amputation was necessary in 9 patients with HBD grafts and 20 patients with PTFE grafts ($P < .025$). Two amputations in the HBD group and 8 amputations in the PTFE group were in patients undergoing bypass surgery to treat claudication only. Limb salvage rate was 86% (CI, 77%-95%) and 74% (CI, 64%-84%), respectively.

Conclusions.—Significantly better patency rates were achieved with HBD than with PTFE at 3 years ($P < .044$), but the difference was no longer statistically significant at 5 years ($P < .055$). The incidence of major limb amputation, however, was significantly greater ($P < .025$) in the PTFE group compared with the HBD group at both 3 and 5 years of follow-up (Fig 1).

▶ This important clinically relevant study answers the question of differences in graft patencies with respect to femoral to above-knee popliteal artery bypass grafts. HBD had a significantly better patency at 3 years compared with PTFE ($P < .044$), with no difference by 5 years. This is good news to those of us who become impatient with the inevitable needle-hole bleeding that seems prominent with PTFE. The number of femoral to above-knee popliteal artery bypass grafts will decrease as minimally invasive technology improves. However, when percutaneous superficial femoral artery interventions fail, it seems reasonable to reach for HBD if no autogenous vein is available.

A. B. Reed, MD

Haemodynamic Effect of Intermittent Pneumatic Compression of the Leg After Infrainguinal Arterial Bypass Grafting

Delis KT, Husmann MJ, Szendro G, et al (Imperial College, London)

Br J Surg 91:429-434, 2004 10–18

Background.—Intermittent pneumatic compression (IPC) may increase blood flow through infrainguinal arterial grafts, and has potential clinical application as blood flow velocity attenuation often precedes graft failure. The present study examined the immediate effects of IPC applied to the foot (IPC_{foot}), the calf (IPC_{calf}) and to both simultaneously ($IPC_{foot+calf}$) on the haemodynamics of infrainguinal bypass grafts.

Methods.—Eighteen femoropopliteal and 18 femorodistal autologous vein grafts were studied; all had a resting ankle : brachial pressure index of 0.9 or more. Clinical examination, graft surveillance and measurement of graft haemodynamics were conducted at rest and within 5 s of IPC in each

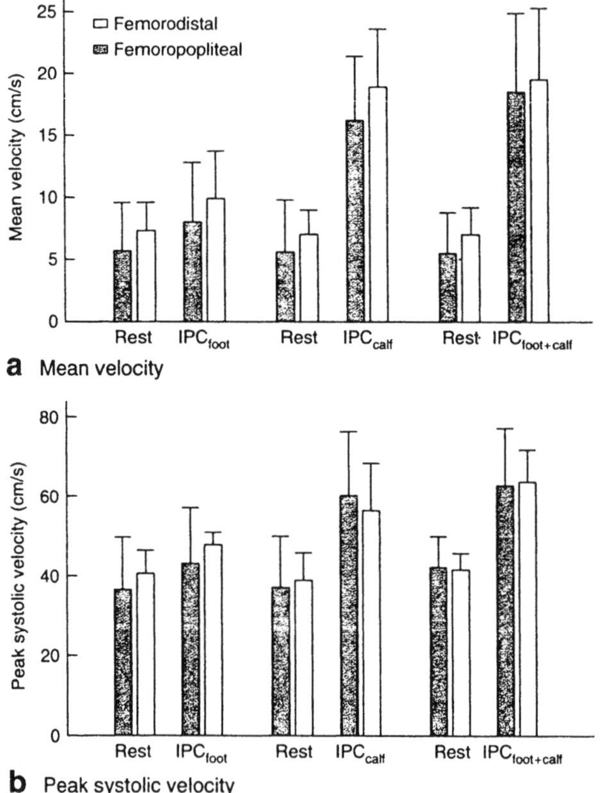

FIGURE 1.—Effects of intermittent pneumatic compression of the foot and calf ($IPC_{foot+calf}$) calf (IPC_{calf}), and foot (IPC_{foot}) on a mean velocity and b peak systolic velocity in 18 femoropopliteal and 18 femorodistal grafts. Values are expressed as median and interquartile range. (Courtesy of Delis KT, Husmann MJ, Szendro G, et al: Haemodynamic Effect of Intermittent Pneumatic Compression of the Leg After Infrainguinal Arterial Bypass Grafting. *Br J Surg* 91:429-434, 2004. Reprinted by permission of Blackwell Publishing.)

mode using duplex imaging. Outcome measures included peak systolic (PSV), mean (MV) and end diastolic (EDV) velocities, pulsatility index (PI) and volume flow in the graft.

Results.—All IPC modes significantly enhanced MV, PSV, EDV and volume flow in both graft types; $IPC_{foot+calf}$ was the most effective (Fig 1). $IPC_{foot+calf}$ enhanced median volume flow, MV and PSV in femoropopliteal grafts by 182, 236 and 49 per cent, respectively, and attenuated PI by 61 per cent. Enhancement in femorodistal grafts was 273, 179 and 53 per cent respectively, and PI attenuation was 63 per cent.

Conclusion.—IPC was effective in improving infrainguinal graft flow velocity, probably by reducing peripheral resistance. IPC has the potential to reduce the risk of bypass graft thrombosis.

► The article is interesting but of little practical significance. Despite what the authors believe, no one will do this! To achieve significant enhancement of graft flow with intermittent pneumatic compression, the limb must be dependent and therefore is more subject to postoperative swelling. I would not want to apply the device directly to the anastomotic area or to surgical wounds. It is unclear to me whether these devices would increase postoperative discomfort in the operated extremity. Pedal devices might be contraindicated in patients with pedal gangrene and calf devices contraindicated in patients with calf wounds. Finally, it is unclear whether the short-term increase in flow velocities provided by these devices will result in long-term graft patency.

G. L. Moneta, MD

Expansion Rates of Asymptomatic Popliteal Artery Aneurysms

Pittathankal AA, Dattani R, Magee TR, et al (Royal Berkshire Hosp, Reading, England)

Eur J Vasc Endovasc Surg 27:382-384, 2004 10–19

Objectives.—In the absence of symptoms the decision to operate on popliteal artery aneurysms (PA) is often made on PA diameter. Little information exists on growth rate and therefore optimum scanning intervals. The aim of this paper is to define growth rate of PA managed conservatively.

Methods.—A prospective study of patients with asymptomatic PA was carried out. Patients were invited for ultrasound scanning at 6–12 months intervals. Diameter changes between consecutive pairs of scans were measured. A decision to operate was made in fit patients if PA became symptomatic and/or had a diameter above 3 cm.

Results.—Twenty-one men (24 aneurysms) with a median age of 69 years (46–86) underwent 78 scans. Sixteen PA were on the right and eight on the left. Eighteen patients had bilateral aneurysms, 15 of which were complicated on one side at presentation and were dealt with surgically on that side. The median size at first scan was 19 mm (14–36). The median time interval to the first follow-up scan was 9 months and subsequent scans were 12 months. The mean rate of expansion at aneurysm sizes below 20 mm diam-

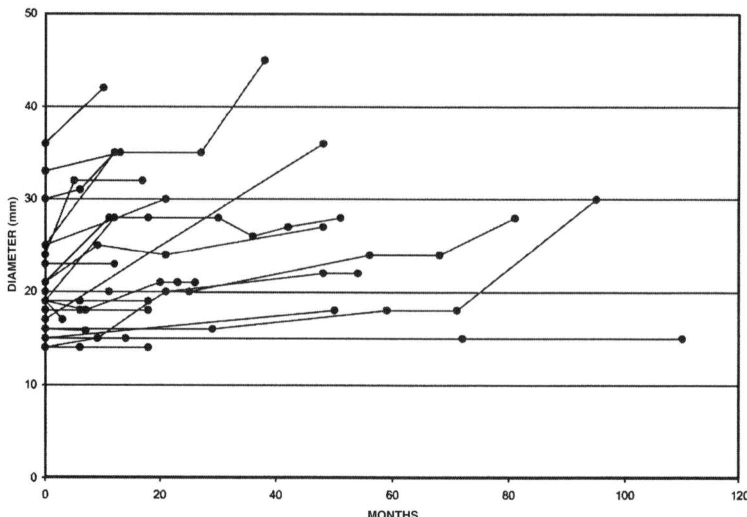

FIGURE 1.—Serial ultrasound scans of 24 aneurysms. *X*-axis represents time since diagnosis. *Y*-axis the diameter in mm. Each USS episode is represented by a circle. (Reprinted from Pittathankal AA, Dattani R, Magee TR, et al: Expansion rates of asymptomatic popliteal artery aneurysms. *Eur J Vasc Endovasc Surg* 27:382-384, 2004. Copyright 2004 by permission of the publisher.)

eter was 1.5 mm/year (Fig 1). PA grew by 3.0 mm/year at sizes 20–30 mm and by 3.7 mm/year at sizes >30 mm. Among the risk factors analysed, hypertension appeared to increase the risk of aneurysm growth.

Conclusion.—The expansion rate of PA increases with increasing size of the PA. This rate of growth in relation to size at previous scan and threshold diameter for intervention should be borne in mind when planning surveillance intervals.

▶ I suppose it is nice to know expansion rates of popliteal aneurysms. But popliteal aneurysms cause trouble by thrombosis and embolization and not rupture. There are some, but not much, data suggesting popliteal aneurysms greater than 3 cm are at greatest risk for thrombosis.[1] Of perhaps more interest would have been information on the accumulation of thrombus within the aneurysm.

G. L. Moneta, MD

Reference

1. Ramesh S, Michaels JA, Galland RB: Popliteal aneurysm: Morphology and management. *Br J Surg* 80:1531-1533, 1993.

Popliteal Artery Aneurysms: A Comparison of Outcomes in Elective Versus Emergent Repair

Aulivola B, Hamdan AD, Hile CN, et al (Beth Israel Deaconess Med Ctr, Boston)
J Vasc Surg 39:1171-1177, 2004 10–20

Objective.—The purpose of this study was to assess and compare outcomes of elective versus emergent operative repair of popliteal artery aneurysms.

Design.—A retrospective analysis of a prospectively recorded vascular surgery database from June 1992 to December 2002 was performed with chart review.

Main Outcome Measures.—Patient survival, limb salvage, and graft patency were evaluated.

Results.—Fifty-one popliteal artery aneurysms were repaired in 39 patients, all male and ranging in age from 18 to 87 years (mean 67.1). Mean follow-up was 47.8 months. Repair was elective in 37 (72.5%) and emergent in 14 (27.5%) limbs, 13 with acute ischemia and one with aneurysm rupture. Thrombolytic therapy was utilized in four ischemic limbs with no suitable bypass target vessel identified on initial arteriogram. Outflow vessels included the popliteal artery in 22 (43.1%) and infrapopliteal vessels in 29 (56.9%) limbs. Cardiac morbidity and 30-day mortality rates were 0%. Overall primary patency, secondary patency, limb salvage, and actuarial survival were 95.6%, 100%, 98.0%, and 98.0% at 1 year and 85.1%, 96.9%, 98.0%, and 83.8% at 5 years, respectively (Fig 3). Bypass graft redo or revi-

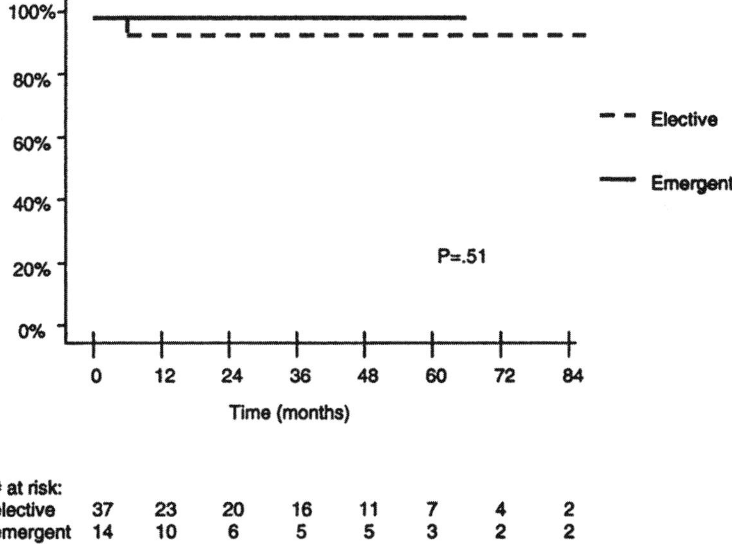

FIGURE 3.—Kaplan-Meier life table analysis of secondary graft patency. Graphs are truncated where SE exceeds 10%. (Reprinted by permission of the publisher from Aulivola B, Hamdan AD, Hile CN, et al: Popliteal artery aneurysms: A comparison of outcomes in elective versus emergent repair. *J Vasc Surg* 39:1171-1177, 2004. Copyright 2004 by Elsevier.)

sion was performed for stenosis in one and occlusion in four limbs. Two amputations were performed at 6 days and 63.6 months after initial aneurysm repair. No difference was noted between elective and emergent groups with regard to patency, limb salvage, or survival ($P > 26$), and no association between the number of identified target vessels and limb salvage or patency was demonstrated ($P = .12$).

Conclusion.—In our experience, the outcome of the popliteal artery aneurysm repair was comparable in the emergent and elective settings. Aggressive tibial reconstruction plays a crucial role in the treatment of popliteal artery aneurysms, especially in those presenting with acute limb ischemia. Thrombolytic therapy is infrequently required in the acute setting, although it may be useful in patients with no identifiable outflow target vessel on initial arteriogram.

▶ As long as there is a target vessel, a good vein, and a leg that is not dead, one should get good results with even emergent repair of popliteal artery aneurysms. Only 1 patient in this series had any motor dysfunction at all. The "emergent" cases in this series do not appear all that emergent. The statement "elective and emergent repairs give equal results" applies only to the not very emergent, emergent repairs.

G. L. Moneta, MD

Operative Repair of Popliteal Aneurysms: Effect of Factors Related to the Bypass Procedure on Outcome

Blanco E, Serrano-Hernando FJ, Moñux G, et al (Universidad Complutense, Madrid)

Ann Vasc Surg 18:86-92, 2004 10–21

Introduction.—The objective of this study was to compare patency rates following the repair of popliteal aneurysms according to the site of inflow, material of bypass graft and quality of distal runoff. Seventy bypasses were performed over an 11-year period. Autogenous saphenous vein was used in 53 procedures (75.7%) and prosthetic material was used in 17 (24.3%). Early mortality was 2.8%. Early primary and secondary patency rates were 95.7% and 97.1%, respectively (Fig 3). Autogenous vein showed better 10-year patency than prosthetic material (86% vs. 57%; $p = 0.02$). No significant differences in patency were observed according to the inflow site (87.8% groin vs. 74.7% supragenicular). Bypasses that originated in the groin showed improved patency when a saphenous vein was used (84.8% vs. 43.7%; $p = 0.01$). However, no influence of the graft material was noted in supragenicular bypasses (90.4% vs. 84.8%; $p = 0.6$). Bypasses in extremities with good runoff showed better patency than those in limbs showing poor runoff (86% vs. 55%; $p = 0.003$). The use of saphenous vein for the repair of popliteal aneurysms showed better results than those with prosthetic material, although in bypasses originating from the distal superficial femoral or above-knee popliteal artery, no significant differences in patency

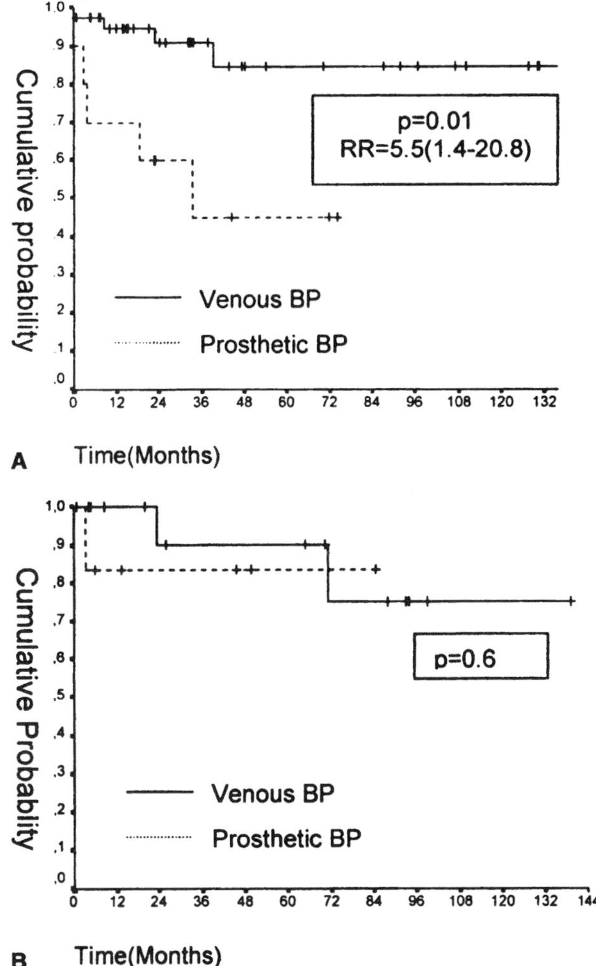

FIGURE 3.—**A** Secondary patency of long BPs according to graft material. **B** Secondary patency of short BPs according to graft material. (Courtesy of Blanco E, Serrano-Hernando FJ, Moñux G, et al: Operative repair of popliteal aneurysms: Effect of factors related to the bypass procedure on outcome. *Ann Vasc Surg* 18:86-92, 2004.)

were observed. Good distal runoff was associated with improved overall outcome.

▶ It is no surprise to learn that when a graft must originate from the groin for treatment of a popliteal aneurysm that autogenous is better than prosthetic. What is striking is the lack of a significant difference when comparing the 2 for short bypasses beginning in the distal superficial femoral or proximal popliteal artery. With an endovascular option available, many may go the way of our vice president.

A. B. Reed, MD

Surgical Management of Popliteal Artery Embolism at the Turn of the Millennium

Raut CP, Cambria RP, LaMuraglia GM, et al (Massachusetts Gen Hosp, Boston)
Ann Vasc Surg 18:79-85, 2004 10–22

Introduction.—Popliteal artery embolism has been a focus of study at the Massachusetts General Hospital for over 60 years. It is a formidable vascular problem with significant limb loss and mortality. To assess the impact of advances in cardiac and vascular therapies, we reviewed our outcomes over 12 years. A retrospective review from our databases identified 66 patients with 72 popliteal artery emboli between January 1989 and October 2000. Patients undergoing nonsurgical therapy or with in situ atherosclerotic thrombosis were excluded. Demographics, comorbidities, presentation, duration, etiology, treatment, and outcomes were analyzed. Patients were classified into those with acute (AP; symptoms <7 days; 59 of 72, 82%) or delayed (DP; symptoms >7 days; 13 of 72, 18%) presentation. The presentation was typically acute ischemia (85%) in the AP group and claudication (69%), rest pain (15.5%), or gangrene (15.5%) in the DP group. The most common etiology was embolism secondary to atrial fibrillation (17 of 72, 24%). Femoral artery access (15 of 72, 21%) was more prevalent than in our prior experience. In the AP group, 9 of 59 (15%) were treated with a femoral artery approach, 44 of 59 (75%) with a popliteal artery approach, and 6 of 59 (10%) with bypass. In the DP group, 11 of 13 (85%) were treated with a popliteal approach and 2 of 13 (15%) with bypass. Completion angiography was done in 17 cases (24%). Limb salvage rate was 88% (88% AP, 85% DP); the rate was 94% with angiography and 85% without it ($p > 0.1$). There were seven deaths (10%). The mortality rate was 33% after amputation and 7% after limb salvage ($p < 0.05$). Except for a greater prevalence of femoral artery access as an etiology, the demographics of patients with popliteal embolism were similar to those of prior reports. Although a femoral approach may be appropriate in select AP cases, a popliteal approach is preferred in most patients and is necessary in DP cases. Completion angiography should be performed to ensure adequacy of the embolectomy. Outcomes are unchanged. Future therapies should aim to improve limb salvage and mortality rates.

► Limb salvage rates are high with surgical treatment of popliteal embolism, but the surgeon is best to use a popliteal approach rather than a femoral approach. This makes perfect sense. Almost everyone hits the target more frequently the closer they stand to the target.

G. L. Moneta, MD

Subintimal Angioplasty in the Treatment of Patients With Intermittent Claudication: Long Term Results

Flørenes T, Bay D, Sandbaek G, et al (Aker Univ, Oslo, Norway)

Eur J Vasc Endovasc Surg 28:645-650, 2004 10–23

Objectives.—Reporting the long-term results of subintimal angioplasty (SA) in patients with intermittent claudication (IC).

Design.—A prospective study.

Patients.—One hundred and sixteen SA procedures were performed in 104 patients, from February 1997 to January 2000 (Fig 3).

Methods.—This is a prospective study of patients treated for IC with infrainguinal SA. Primary assisted patency rates were calculated, also on intention to treat basis. Univariate and multivariate Cox regression tests were used to assess whether patency was correlated with co-morbidities, run-off or occlusion length.

Results.—There was no early mortality. Technical success was achieved in 101 cases (87%). Primary assisted patency rates on intention to treat basis (116 cases) at 6, 12, 36 and 60 months were 69, 62, 57 and 54%, respectively. For successfully recanalized patients (101 cases) these respective numbers are 79, 70, 66 and 64%. Length of occlusion, age and male gender were independent risk factors for reocclusion.

Conclusions.—The satisfactory results obtained in the present study are probably due to two main factors. First, the three participating radiologist are highly skilled and experienced. Secondly, a conscientious surveillance was adhered to, so that restenoses could be diagnosed and treated early. SA is

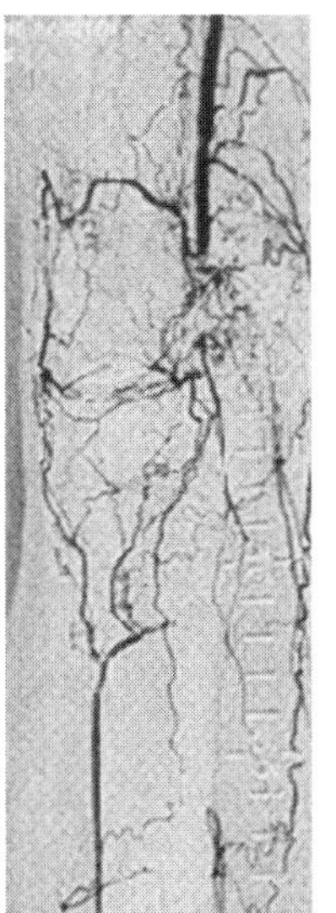

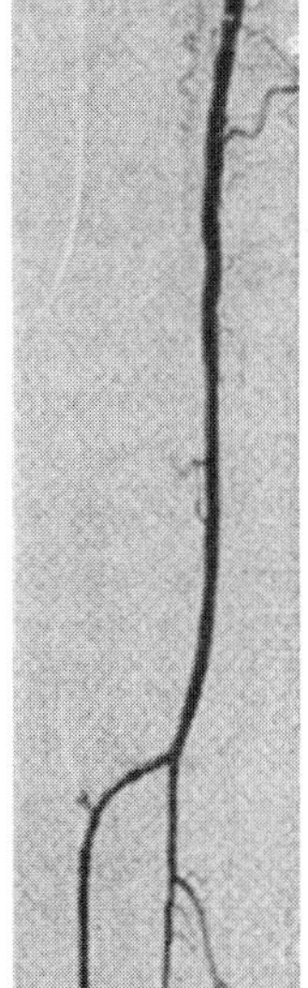

FIGURE 3.—SA of right popliteal artery and crural arteries. (Reprinted from Flørenes T, Bay D, Sandbaek G, et al: Subintimal angioplasty in the treatment of patients with intermittent claudication: Long term results. *Eur J Vasc Endovasc Surg* 28:645-650, 2004. Copyright 2004 by permission of the publisher.)

a relevant alternative to bypass surgery in patients with disabling IC due to long femoro-popliteal occlusions. It is far less traumatic than conventional vascular reconstructions, complications are few and not serious. Very importantly, SA never interfered with later successful vascular surgery. Therefore, we have adopted SA as the primary treatment for patients with IC when medical treatment alone has not been satisfactory.

► The patency results in this study are reasonable, but overall the study is not all that helpful. We already know subintimal angioplasty can be successful. The goal of treatment in patients with intermittent claudication, however, is improvement in walking and quality of life. The authors don't even present hemodynamic data, much less data regarding walking and quality of life. In a prospective study of treatment for intermittent claudication, more functional data, not just simple patency analysis, should be included.

G. L. Moneta, MD

Percutaneous Intentional Extraluminal Recanalization in Patients With Chronic Critical Limb Ischemia

Spinosa DJ, Leung DA, Matsumoto AH, et al (Univ of Virginia, Charlottesville)
Radiology 232:499-507, 2004 10–24

Purpose.—To review percutaneous intentional extraluminal recanalization (PIER) for treatment of patients who are poor candidates for infrainguinal arterial bypass surgery (IABS) and have arterial occlusions and chronic critical limb ischemia (CCLI).

Materials and Methods.—Patients with CCLI who were poor candidates for IABS were candidates for PIER. PIER was performed to create continuous arterial flow to the foot for limb salvage. PIER was attempted in 40 patients (22 men, 18 women; median age, 69 years; age range, 44–87 years) (Fig 1). Of these patients, 24 (60%) had diabetes, 17 (42%) had renal disease, and 26 (66%) had coronary artery disease. Wound healing was evaluated at follow-up. Kaplan-Meier curves were constructed to evaluate limb salvage, survival, and amputation-free survival.

Results.—Fifty procedures were attempted in 44 limbs. Tissue loss was present in 40 (91%) limbs, and rest pain was present in four (9%); technical success occurred in 38 (86%). Thirty-seven (84%) of 44 limbs treated with PIER involved tibial vessels (tibial vessels only, $n = 15$; tibial and superior femoral artery [SFA] and/or popliteal vessels, $n = 22$). Sixty-six infrainguinal arterial vessel segments (SFA, $n = 29$; tibial, $n = 37$) in 38 limbs (1.7 segments per limb) were successfully treated with PIER. Thirty-five (95%) of 37 tibial occlusions and 24 (83%) of 29 SFA and/or popliteal occlusions were longer than 10 cm. Median run-off scores were 5.3 (range, 3–8) and 6.6 (range, 3–9) for patients with tibial occlusions and SFA and/or popliteal occlusions, respectively, as scored with modified Rutherford weighting of run-off arteries. Median follow-up was 7.8 months (range, 1–24 months). Twelve months after PIER, Kaplan-Meier analysis showed limb salvage rate

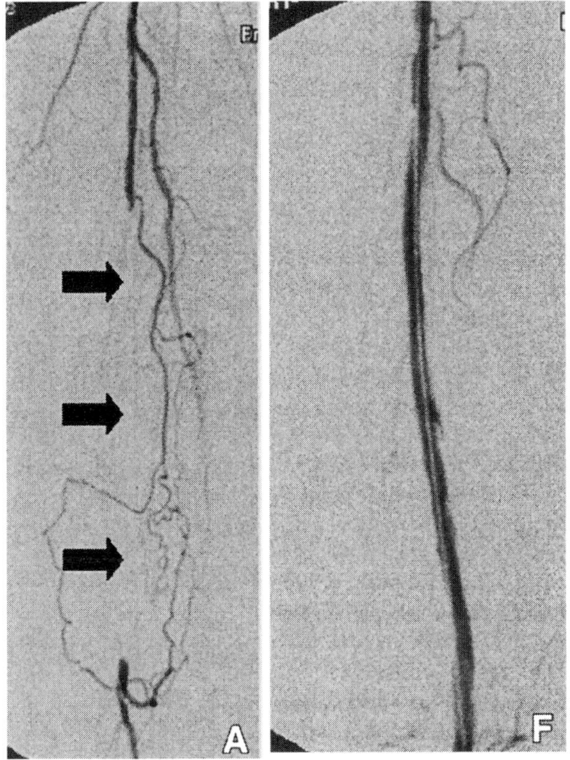

FIGURE 1.—Arteriogram obtained in a 74-year-old woman with a nonhealing ulcer of the left first toe and rest pain. *A*, Posteroanterior projection shows long left SFA occlusion (arrows). *F*, Posteroanterior projection shows successful antegrade SFA PIER. (Courtesy of Spinosa DJ, Leung DA, Matsumoto AH, et al: Percutaneous intentional extraluminal recanalization in patients with chronic critical limb ischemia. *Radiology* 232:499-507, 2004. Radiological Society of North America.)

was 66%, survival rate was 71%, and amputation-free survival rate was 48% in these patients. The 30-day mortality rate was 2.5%. Major complications occurred in four (10%) patients, and minor complications occurred in an additional four (10%).

Conclusion.—PIER is a useful percutaneous technique for limb salvage in patients with CCLI.

► Is it just me, or do most vascular surgeons find it difficult to imagine percutaneously cannulating a reconstituted distal tibial vessel in a retrograde fashion, let alone placing a 3F sheath in it? The SAFARI (subintimal arterial flossing with antegrade-retrograde approach) technique proposed by the authors would surely get the camel dung award if Dr John Porter were still alive. Nonetheless, despite the fact these techniques seem outlandish, I remember when our specialty thought percutaneous superficial femoral and tibial artery interventions were heresy. Stay tuned?

A. B. Reed, MD

Primary Patency of Femoropopliteal Arteries Treated With Nitinol Versus Stainless Steel Self-expanding Stents: Propensity Score-Adjusted Analysis

Sabeti S, Schillinger M, Amighi J, et al (Univ of Vienna)

Radiology 232:516-521, 2004 10–25

Purpose.—To evaluate, in a propensity score–adjusted analysis, the intermediate-term primary patency rates associated with nitinol versus stainless steel self-expanding stent placement for treatment of atherosclerotic lesions in femoropopliteal arteries.

Materials and Methods.—The authors analyzed the clinical and imaging data of 175 consecutive patients with peripheral artery disease and either intermittent claudication ($n = 150$) or critical limb ischemia ($n = 25$) who underwent femoropopliteal artery implantation of nitinol ($n = 104$) or stainless steel ($n = 123$) stents in a nonrandomized setting. The stents were placed owing to either significant residual stenosis (ie, >30% lumen diameter reduction) or flow-limiting dissection after initial balloon angioplasty of the femoropopliteal artery. Patients were followed up for a median period of 9 months (mean, 13 months; range, 6–66 months) for the detection of a first in-stent restenosis, defined as a greater than 50% lumen diameter reduction that was seen at color-coded duplex ultrasonography and confirmed at angiography.

Results.—Cumulative patency rates at 6, 12, and 24 months were 85%, 75%, and 69%, respectively, after nitinol stent placement versus 78%, 54%, and 34%, respectively, after stainless steel stent placement ($P = .008$, log-rank test). There were no statistically significant differences in associated patency among the three different nitinol stents used ($P = .72$, log-rank test). Multivariate Cox proportional hazard analysis, in which the effect of propensity to receive a nitinol stent was considered, revealed a significantly reduced risk of restenosis with the nitinol stents compared with the risk of restenosis with the stainless steel stents (adjusted hazard ratio, 0.44; 95% confidence interval: 0.22, 0.85; $P = .014$).

Conclusion.—Nitinol stents are associated with significantly improved primary patency rates in femoropopliteal arteries compared with stainless steel stents. Randomized controlled trials are needed to confirm these results.

► Perhaps I missed it, but there was no information as to whether the patients could walk better or if improvement in ankle-brachial index was maintained. Shame on them.

G. L. Moneta, MD

De Novo Femoropopliteal Stenoses: Endovascular Gamma Irradiation Following Angioplasty—Angiographic and Clinical Follow-up in a Prospective Randomized Controlled Trial

Krueger K, Zaehringer M, Bendel M, et al (Univ of Cologne, Germany)

Radiology 231:546-554, 2004 10–26

Purpose.—To assess and report the follow-up results of a randomized controlled trial on centered endovascular gamma irradiation performed after percutaneous transluminal angioplasty (PTA) for de novo femoropopliteal stenoses.

Materials and Methods.—Thirty patients who underwent PTA for de novo femoropopliteal stenoses were randomly assigned to undergo 14-Gy centered endovascular irradiation (irradiation group, $n = 15$) or no irradiation (control group, $n = 15$). Intraarterial angiography was performed 6, 12, and 24 months after treatment; duplex ultrasonography (US), the day before and after PTA and 1, 3, 6, 9, 12, 18, and 24 months later. Treadmill tests and interviews were performed the day before PTA and 1, 3, 6, 9, 12, 18, and 24 months later. Results of angiography, duplex US, treadmill tests, and interviews were evaluated with the nonpaired *t* or the Fisher exact test.

Results.—Baseline characteristics did not differ significantly between the two groups. Mean absolute individual changes in degree of stenosis, compared with the degrees of stenosis shortly after PTA, in the irradiation group versus in the control group were −10.6% ± 22.3 versus 39.6% ± 24.6 ($P < .001$) at 6 months, −2.0% ± 34.2 versus 40.6% ± 32.6 ($P = .002$) at 12 months, and 7.4% ± 43.2 versus 37.7% ± 34.5 ($P = .043$) at 24 months. The rates of target lesion restenosis at 6 ($P = .006$) and 12 ($P = .042$) months were significantly lower in the irradiation group. The numbers of target lesion re-treatments were similar between the groups, but target vessel retreatments were more frequent in the irradiation group. There were no significant differences in interview or treadmill test results between the two groups at *t* test analysis.

Conclusion.—The degree of stenosis was significantly reduced 6, 12, and 24 months after angioplasty of de novo femoropopliteal stenoses in the patients who underwent endovascular irradiation.

▶ The irradiated arteries stayed open longer than the nonirradiated arteries, but functional parameters in follow-up in the 2 patient groups were not different. This suggests that "lesion"-only evaluation in studies assessing the efficacy of catheter-based treatment of the superior femoral artery may not be of much value.

G. L. Moneta, MD

Effect of Smoking on Restenosis During the 1st Year After Lower-Limb Endovascular Interventions

Schillinger M, Exner M, Mlekusch W, et al (Univ of Vienna)
Radiology 231:831-838, 2004 10–27

Purpose.—To investigate whether smoking has an effect on recurrent lumen narrowing after percutaneous transluminal angioplasty (PTA) or stent placement in lower-limb arteries.

Materials and Methods.—A total of 650 patients (median age, 70 years; 389 men) with peripheral artery disease who underwent iliac artery PTA (n = 95), iliac artery stent placement (n = 83), femoropopliteal PTA (n = 406), or femoropopliteal stent placement (n = 66) were selected from a prospective database. Patients were categorized according to their preintervention smoking habits as nonsmokers (n = 352), light smokers (one to nine cigarettes daily) (n = 54), habitual smokers (10–20 cigarettes daily) (n = 82), or heavy smokers (>20 cigarettes daily) (n = 162). Multivariate Cox proportional hazards analysis was used to determine whether there was an association between smoking habits and restenosis (≥50%) in the treated vessel segment within 1 year after treatment.

Results.—Cumulative restenosis rates at 6 and 12 months according to patients' smoking habits were 99 and 190 nonsmokers, 18 and 22 light smokers, 16 and 29 habitual smokers, and 26 and 47 heavy smokers, respectively (P < .001) (Fig 2). Adjusted hazard ratios for restenosis in smokers compared with nonsmokers were 1.51 (95% CI: 0.92, 2.50) for light smokers, 0.49 (95% CI: 0.28, 0.87) for habitual smokers, and 0.46 (95% CI: 0.30, 0.71) for heavy smokers, indicating a reduced restenosis risk in patients who smoked 10 or more cigarettes daily. These patients had reduced

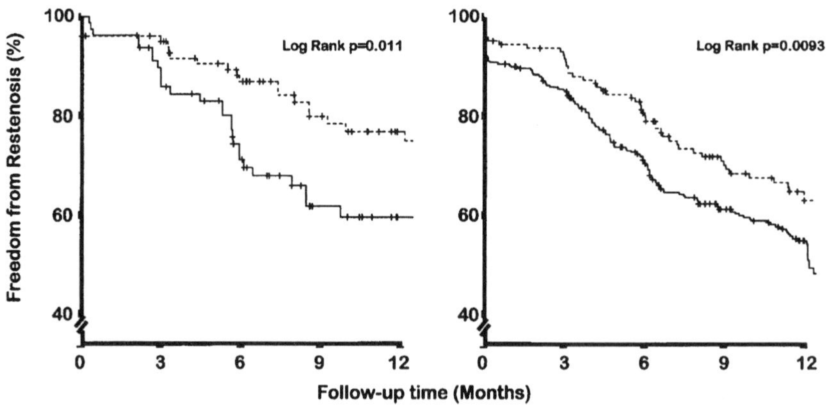

FIGURE 2.—Graphs show cumulative freedom from restenosis at 24 hours and at 3, 6, 9, and 12 months after endovascular treatment of iliac artery (left) (n = 178) or femoropopliteal artery (right) (n = 472) stenosis in habitual smokers and heavy smokers (≥10 cigarettes daily; continuous line) versus nonsmokers and light smokers (<10 cigarettes daily; dashed line). Reduced postintervention restenosis rates were observed for habitual smokers and heavy smokers, compared with those for nonsmokers and light smokers. (Courtesy of Schillinger M, Exner M, Mlekusch W, et al: Effect of smoking on restenosis during the 1st year after lower-limb endovascular interventions. *Radiology* 231:831-838, 2004. Radiological Society of North America.)

restenosis rates after either iliac (P = .011) or femoropopliteal intervention (P = .009). However, endovascular treatment at a younger age, coronary artery disease, and history of myocardial or cerebrovascular infarction were more frequently found in smokers.

Conclusion.—Smoking 10 or more cigarettes daily is associated with a reduced rate of intermediate-term restenosis after lower-limb endovascular interventions.

▶ This retrospective study claims that smoking 10 or more cigarettes per day is associated with a reduced restenosis rate after lower-limb endovascular interventions. What? Closer evaluation of the data reveals that smokers had nearly twice as many iliac interventions as opposed to nonsmokers. Further inspection of the statistical analysis reveals that the light smokers (10 or less cigarettes per day) were grouped with the nonsmokers because of low numbers when trying to perform a stratified analysis based on vessel treated. This mixing of apples and oranges makes it difficult to justify the authors' conclusion. I believe it is safe to say that recommending "smoking in moderation" to vascular surgery patients is probably not a good idea.

A. B. Reed, MD

Homocysteine Levels, Haemostatic Risk Factors and Patency Rates After Endovascular Treatment of the Above-Knee Femoro-Popliteal Artery

Laxdal E, Eide GE, Wirsching J, et al (Haukeland Univ, Bergen, Norway; Univ of Bergen, Norway)

Eur J Vasc Endovasc Surg 28:410-417, 2004 10–28

Objectives.—To investigate the relationship between plasma homocysteine and other haemostatic variables and restenoses or reocclusions after endovascular treatment of symptomatic atherosclerosis of the above-knee femoro-popliteal artery.

Design.—Prospective observational study.

Setting.—University hospital.

Patients and Methods.—The study included 103 patients (116 limbs), treated with subintimal angioplasty in 58 cases (50%) and with intraluminal PTA in 58 (50%): 39 (34%) patients were treated for critical limb ischaemia. Blood samples for analyses of fasting plasma values of homocysteine, fibrinogen, D-dimer, activated protein C resistance were drawn upon admission. Median follow-up for all procedures was 11 months (range 0–42 months). Outcome events (arterial patency) were defined as ≥50% restenosis or reocclusion in the treated arterial segment. Patency rates were estimated with the product limit method and Kaplan-Meier curves. Variables found to be related significantly to patency were included in multivariate analysis performed with the Cox proportional hazard model.

Results.—The 1-year cumulative primary patency rate for all procedures was 48% (Fig 1). One-year limb salvage rate in cases of critical ischaemia was 74%. Multivariate analysis demonstrated significant independent asso-

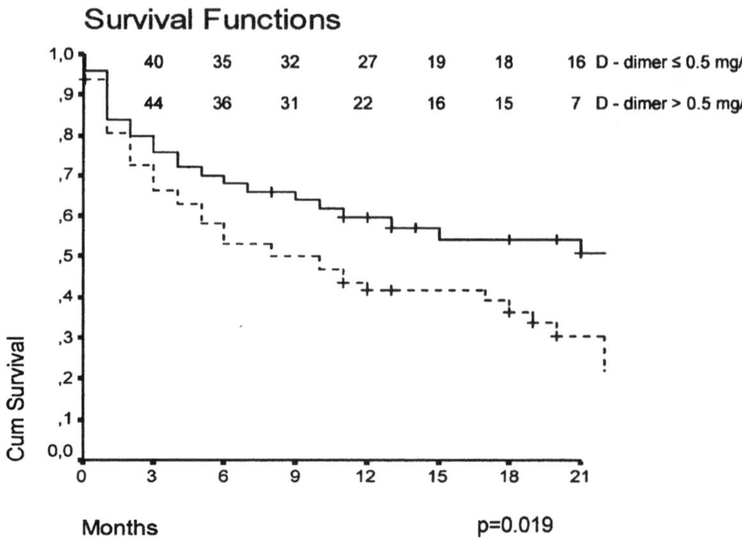

FIGURE 1.—Comparison of patency rates after 116 above-knee femoro-popliteal endovascular procedures in patients with D-dimer >0.5 mg/l (broken line) and patients with D-dimer ≤0.5 mg/l (unbroken line). (Reprinted from Laxdal E, Eide GE, Wirsching J, et al: Homocysteine levels, haemostatic risk factors and patency rates after endovascular treatment of the above-knee femoro-popliteal artery. *Eur J Vasc Endovasc Surg* 28:410-417, 2004. Copyright 2004 by permission of the publisher.)

ciations between patency rates and plasma D-dimer, diabetes mellitus, the nature of the lesion treated (stenosis vs. occlusion) and antithrombotic therapy with aspirin after the procedure. Plasma levels of homocysteine, fibrinogen or activated protein C resistance were not associated with patency rates. Homocysteine levels were higher in patients with critical limb ischaemia than those with intermittent claudication.

Conclusions.—Early restenosis or reocclusion after endovascular intervention of lesions in the above-knee femoro-popliteal artery was more frequent following treatment of occlusion (versus stenosis), for patients with diabetes, patients with elevated D-dimer and those without antithrombotic therapy after the procedure. Plasma homocysteine did not appear to influence the outcome of endovascular intervention.

► Inconsistent follow-up and no consistent protocol incorporating imaging studies of the treated artery are major and obvious weaknesses of this study. In addition, the mixing of 2 types of angioplasty techniques and the mixing of clinical indications are also serious methodologic weaknesses that preclude any definitive conclusions. However, the idea that different hematologic factors may have variable effects on the outcome of angioplasty is interesting and deserves further study.

G. L. Moneta, MD

Remote Superficial Femoral Artery and Endarterectomy and Distal aSpire Stenting: Multicenter Medium-term Results

Rosenthal D, Martin JD, Schubart PJ, et al (Atlanta Med Ctr, Ga; Anne Arundel Med Ctr, Annapolis, Md; O'Conner Hosp, San Jose, Calif)

J Vasc Surg 40:67-72, 2004 10–29

Objective.—The purpose of this study was to examine the results of remote superficial femoral artery endarterectomy (RSFAE) in conjunction with distal aSpire stenting (Fig 1).

Methods.—RSFAE is a minimally invasive procedure performed through a limited groin incision. Forty patients were included in the study. The indications for the procedure were claudication in 36 patients and limb salvage in 4 patients. RSFAE was performed with the MollRing Cutter device through a femoral arteriotomy. The distal atheromatous plaque was "tacked" with the aSpire stent, which is an expandable polytetrafluoroethylene-covered nitinol stent with high radial strength, yet is flexible and able to withstand compressive forces proximal to the knee joint. Before stent deployment, if the stent position is not optimal it can be wrapped down, repositioned, and re-expanded. Therefore, not only is the plaque end point tacked, but the collateral vessels may be preserved. All patients underwent follow-up examination with serial color-flow ultrasound scanning.

Results.—The mean length of endarterectomized superficial femoral artery was 26.2 cm ± 6.2 cm (range, 13-41 cm). The primary cumulative patency rate by means of life table analysis was 68.6% ± 13.5% (SE) at 18 months (mean, 13.2 months; range, 1-31 months). During follow-up percutaneous transluminal balloon or stent angioplasty was necessary in 6 patients, for a primary assisted patency rate of 88.5% ± 8.5% at 18 months. The locations of recurrent stenoses after RSFAE were evenly distributed

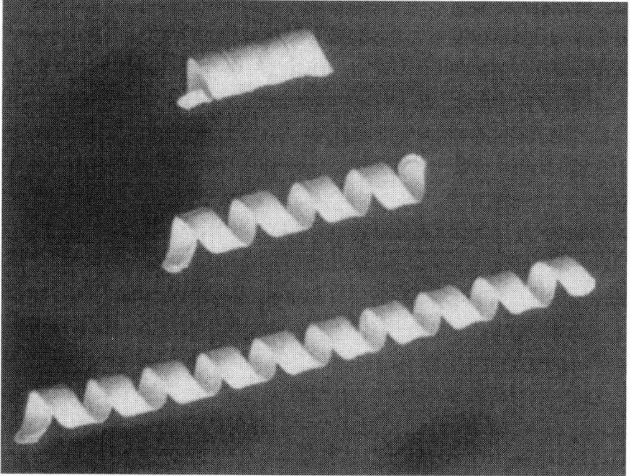

FIGURE 1.—aSpire stent. (Reprinted by permission of the publisher from Rosenthal D, Martin JD, Schubart PJ, et al: Remote superficial femoral artery and endarterectomy and distal aSpire stenting: Multicenter medium-term results. *J Vasc Surg* 40:67-72, 2004. Copyright 2004 by Elsevier.)

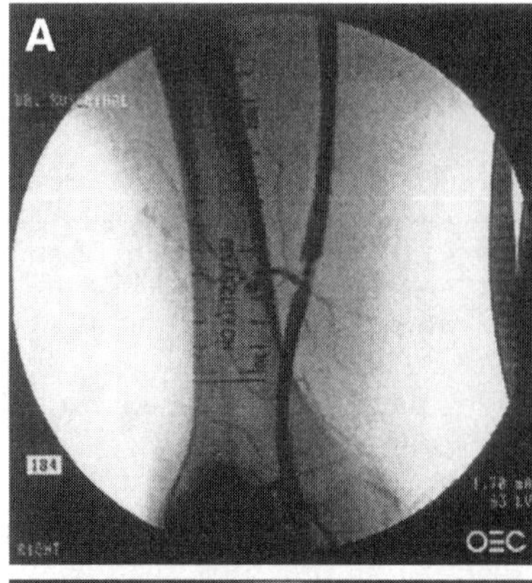

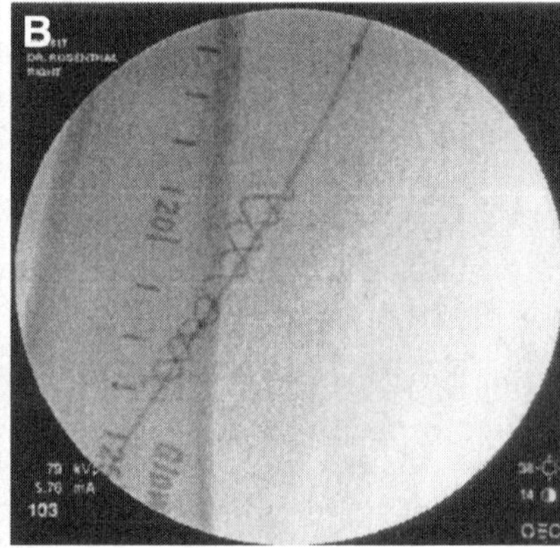

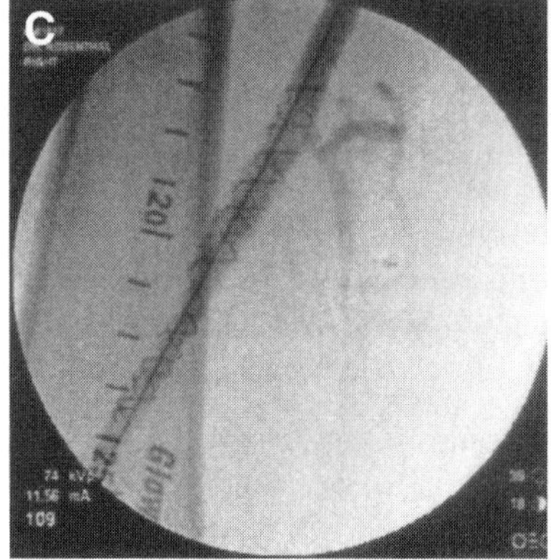

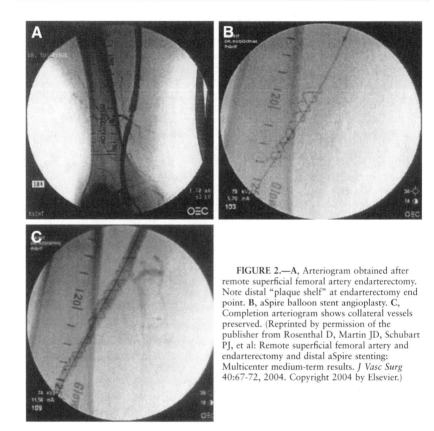

FIGURE 2.—A, Arteriogram obtained after remote superficial femoral artery endarterectomy. Note distal "plaque shelf" at endarterectomy end point. B, aSpire balloon stent angioplasty. C, Completion arteriogram shows collateral vessels preserved. (Reprinted by permission of the publisher from Rosenthal D, Martin JD, Schubart PJ, et al: Remote superficial femoral artery and endarterectomy and distal aSpire stenting: Multicenter medium-term results. *J Vasc Surg* 40:67-72, 2004. Copyright 2004 by Elsevier.)

along the endarterectomized artery. There were no deaths and one wound complication, and mean hospital length of stay was only 2.1 ± 0.5 days.

Conclusions.—RSFAE with distal aSpire stenting is a safe and moderately durable procedure. If long-term patency rates are similar to those of above-knee femoropopliteal bypass graft, this procedure may prove to be a minimally invasive adjunct for the treatment of superficial femoral artery occlusive disease (Fig 2).

► Minimally invasive therapies for treatment of superficial femoral artery disease are abundant. The idea of debulking the vessel of its atherosclerotic burden, then offering a supportive structure with nitinol and expandable polytetrafluoroethylene–covered stents, as in this trial, seems to make sense. However, superficial femoral artery reconstruction with remote endarterectomy and aSpire stenting, as with all our other vascular interventions, is still plagued by restenosis and neointimal hyperplasia. Everything looks good at 18 months. Longer-term data are required to recommend this as a reasonable treatment for claudication.

A. B. Reed, MD

National Audit of Thrombolysis for Acute Leg Ischemia (NATALI): Clinical Factors Associated With Early Outcome

Earnshaw JJ, for the Thrombolysis Study Group (Gloucestershire Royal Hosp, Gloucester, England)

J Vasc Surg 39:1018-1025, 2004 10–30

Objective.—The National Audit of Thrombolysis for Acute Leg Ischemia (NATALI) database is a consecutive series of patients who underwent intra-arterial thrombolysis to treat acute leg ischemia in one of 11 centers in the United Kingdom. The purpose of the study was to analyze the factors associated with outcome after 30 days.

Methods.—The data were collected over 10 years on standard pro formas, and registration was completed at the end of 1999. Since then, data from each unit have been verified and missing data included when available. Univariate and multivariate analyses were performed, with the outcomes of amputation-free survival (AFS), amputation with survival, and death.

Results.—A total of 1133 thrombolytic events were included. Outcome results at 30 days for the entire group were AFS, 852 (75.2%); amputation, 141 (12.4%); and death, 140 (12.4%). Results for the entire group improved from the first half of the database, when AFS ranged from 65% to 75%, to almost 80% for the last few years of the study, although this was not statistically significant. Preintervention factors associated with lower AFS at multivariate analysis included diabetes (P = .002), increasing age (P < .001), short-duration ischemia (P = .027), Fontaine grade (P = .001), and ischemia with neurosensory deficit (P = .004). AFS was improved in patients receiving warfarin sodium at the time of the arterial occlusion (P = .04). Mortality was higher in women (P = .006) and in older patients (P < .001), and in patients with native vessel occlusion (P < .001), emboli (P = 02), or a history of ischemic heart disease (P < .001). Amputation risk was greatest in younger men (P < .001) and in patients with more severe ischemia (P = .02), graft occlusion (PP < .001), or native vessel thrombotic occlusion (P = .02).

Conclusion.—Experienced surgeons and radiologists can achieve an AFS of about 80% in selected patients with acute leg ischemia. Information from the NATALI database can be used in selection of an appropriate intervention in the individual patient.

▶ This interesting study makes use of national United Kingdom database outcomes after arterial thrombolysis. Enthusiasm for the use of thrombolysis in acute limb ischemia has waxed and waned over the years, given the availability of particular agents. Nonetheless, this is a tool all vascular surgeons should have in their armamentarium. Death and hemorrhagic stroke with thrombolytic use were found to be low and typically correlated with underlying patient comorbidities.

A. B. Reed, MD

Comparative Roles of Microvascular and Nerve Function in Foot Ulceration in Type 2 Diabetes

Krishnan STM, Carrington AL, Baker NR, et al (Ipswich Hosp Natl Health Service Trust, England)

Diabetes Care 27:1343-1348, 2004 10–31

Objective.—To determine the relative roles of different modalities of sensory nerve function (large and small fiber) and the role of microvascular dysfunction in foot ulceration in type 2 diabetic subjects.

Research Design and Methods.—A total of 20 control subjects and 18 type 2 diabetic subjects with foot ulceration and 20 without were studied. None of the subjects had clinical features of peripheral vascular disease. The Computer-Aided Sensory Evaluator IV (CASE IV) was used to determine vibration detection threshold (VDT), cold detection threshold (CDT), warm detection threshold (WDT), and heat pain onset threshold (HPO). Vibration perception threshold (VPT) was also assessed by a neurothesiometer. Microvascular function (maximum hyperemia to skin heating to 44°C) was assessed using laser Doppler flowmetry (mean maximum hyperemia using laser Doppler flowmeter [LDF_{max}]), laser Doppler imaging (mean maximum hyperemia using laser Doppler imager [LDI_{max}]), and skin oxygenation with transcutaneous oxygen tension ($TcpO_2$).

Results.—VPT, VDT, CDT, and HPO were all significantly higher in individuals with ulceration than in those without (VPT and VDT: $P < 0.0001$) (CDT and HPO: $P = 0.01$). LDF_{max}, LDI_{max}, and $TcpO_2$ were significantly lower in the two diabetic groups than in the control subjects, but there was no difference between individuals with and without ulceration. Univariate logistic regression analysis revealed similar odds ratios for foot ulceration for VDT, CDT, HPO, and VPT (OR 1.97 [95% CI 1.30–2.98], 1.58 [1.20–2.08], 2.30 [1.21–4.37], and 1.24 [1.08–1.42], respectively). None of the microvascular parameters yielded significant odds ratios for ulceration.

Conclusions.—This study found that there was no additional value in measuring small-fiber function with the CASE IV over measuring vibration by either CASE IV or the inexpensive neurothesiometer in discriminating between individuals with and without ulceration. Furthermore, none of the tests of microvascular function including the $TcpO_2$ were able to discriminate between individuals with and without ulceration, suggesting that such tests may not be of benefit in identifying subjects at greater risk of foot ulceration.

► I do not believe in the concept of "microvascular" disease leading to foot ulcers in patients with diabetes. I think the problem is ischemia or neuropathy, or both. For all practical purposes, one or the other or both are seen in virtually all patients with diabetes and foot ulcers. It is not necessary to invoke a mysterious microangiopathy as the primary etiology of diabetic foot ulceration.

G. L. Moneta, MD

Systematic Review and Meta-analysis of Controlled Trials Assessing Spinal Cord Stimulation for Inoperable Critical Leg Ischaemia

Ubbink DT, Vermeulen H, Spincemaille GHJJ, et al (Academic Med Ctr, Amsterdam; Academic Hosp Maastricht, The Netherlands; Univ Hosp, Lausanne, Switzerland; et al)

Br J Surg 91:948-955, 2004 10–32

Background.—Spinal cord stimulation (SCS) may have a place in the treatment of patients with inoperable chronic critical leg ischaemia.

Methods.—A systematic review and meta-analysis was performed of all controlled studies comparing SCS in addition to any form of conservative treatment for inoperable chronic critical leg ischaemia. Main endpoints were limb salvage, pain relief and clinical situation. Systematic methodological appraisal and data extraction were performed by independent reviewers.

Results.—Of the 18 reports found, nine trials, comprising 444 patients, matched the selection criteria. After pooling, limb salvage at 12 months appeared significantly greater in the SCS group (risk difference (RD) −0.13 (95 per cent confidence interval (c.i.) −0.04 to −0.22)). Significant pain relief occurred in both treatment groups, but patients who received SCS required significantly less analgesia and reached Fontaine stage 2 more often than those who did not have SCS (RD 0.33 (95 per cent c.i. 0.19 to 0.47)). Complications of SCS were problems of implantation (8.2 per cent), changes in stimulation requiring reintervention (14.8 per cent) and infection (2.9 per cent).

Conclusion.—The addition of SCS to standard conservative treatment improves limb salvage, ischaemic pain and the general clinical situation in patients with inoperable chronic critical leg ischaemia. These benefits should be weighed against the cost and the (minor) complications associated with the technique.

► The bulk of the data would suggest that this works in some patients with critical limb ischemia. We probably should be trying it a bit more often.

G. L. Moneta, MD

Survival After Lower-Extremity Amputation

Sandnes DK, Sobel M, Flum DR (Univ of Washington, Seattle; VA Med Ctr, Seattle)

J Am Coll Surg 199:394-402, 2004 10–33

Background.—Lower extremity amputation has long been considered an end-of-life event and it is unclear if survival after amputation has improved over time.

Study Design.—A retrospective cohort comprised from a statewide, hospital discharge database was used to determine if survival after amputation improved with time. The cohort included all patients (older than 18 years)

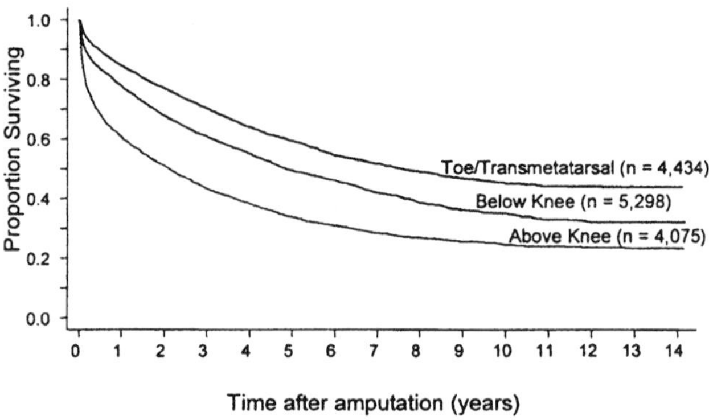

FIGURE 2.—Kaplan-Meier survival estimates, by level of amputation, using log-rank test for equality of survival curves. p < 0.001. (Reprinted from Sandnes DK, Sobel M, Flum DR: Survival after lower-extremity amputation. *J Am Coll Surg* 199:394-402, 2004. Copyright 2004, with permission from the American College of Surgeons.)

with nontraumatic, lower extremity amputations (1987 to 2000). Survival analysis was used to determine the adjusted hazard ratio of survival as it related to the era of amputation.

Results.—A total of 13,807 patients (mean age ± SD, 67 ± 15, 58.5% men) underwent amputation. The gender and age standardized frequency of amputation remained essentially stable, with a 0.01% increase per year (95% CI, 0.006–0.01%). During followup, 49.2% (6,795/13,807) of patients died, with significantly (p < 0.001) worse outcomes for more proximal levels of amputation. After controlling for potential confounders, including age, gender, level of amputation, comorbid illness, emergency status of procedure, hospital type, and payer of the procedure, patients undergoing amputation in more recent years (1995 to 2000) had a 28% lower hazard of dying (hazard ratio 0.72 [95% CI, 0.67–0.77%) during the study period than

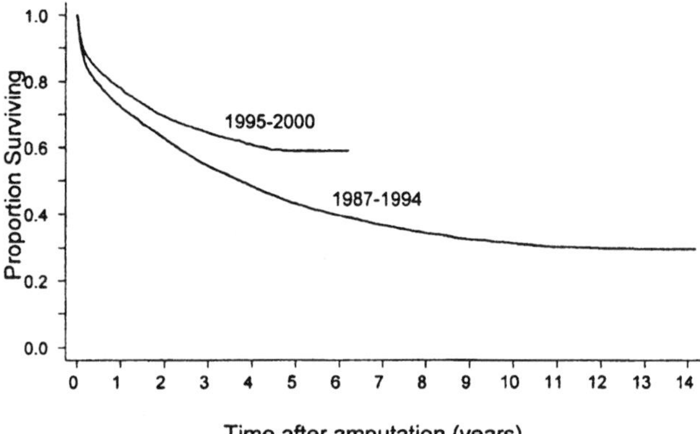

FIGURE 3.—Kaplan-Meier survival estimates, by calendar-year groups, using log-rank test for equality of survival curves. p < 0.001. (Reprinted from Sandnes DK, Sobel M, Flum DR: Survival after lower-extremity amputation. *J Am Coll Surg* 199:394-402, 2004. Copyright 2004, with permission from the American College of Surgeons.)

those undergoing operation before 1995 (Figs 2 and 3). Thirty-day survival did not improve by era ($p = 0.2$), although 1- and 5-year survival after amputation was significantly greater for all levels of amputation ($p < 0.001$).

Conclusions.—Although 30-day survival associated with amputation has remained stable in the state of Washington over the past 14 years, longterm survival after amputation has improved considerably with time. The reasons underlying this improvement should be explored so that further gains may be achieved.

► Statewide hospital discharge data registries—and even national ones, for that matter—are often suspect for research purposes as many data points documenting comorbidities can be missed by the nonclinical personnel who glean the charts. Nonetheless, this study attempts a look at the survival of amputees by era. It is encouraging to see improved long-term survival in the latter half of the 1990s. In this time of complex infrainguinal revascularizations and percutaneous interventions, it will be interesting to see whether the amputee survival advantage can continue to be improved by medical management and risk factor modification.

A. B. Reed, MD

11 Upper Extremity Ischemia/Dialysis Access

Relationship Among Catheter Insertions, Vascular Access Infections, and Anemia Management in Hemodialysis Patients

Roberts TL, Obrador GT, St Peter WL, et al (Minneapolis Med Research Found; Tufts-New England Med Ctr, Boston; Universidad Panamericana, Mexico City; et al)

Kidney Int 66:2429-2436, 2004 11–1

Background.—Arteriovenous fistulas are the recommended permanent vascular access (VA) for chronic hemodialysis. However, in the United States most patients begin chronic hemodialysis with a catheter. Recent data suggest that VA type contributes to recombinant human erythropoietin (rHuEPO) resistance. We examined catheter insertions, VA infections, and anemia management in Medicare, rHuEPO-treated, chronic hemodialysis patients.

Methods.—We compared hemoglobin values and rHuEPO and intravenous iron dosing with concurrent catheter insertions and VA infections in 186,348 period-prevalent patients in 2000. We studied anemia management after catheter insertions and VA infections in 67,410 incident patients from 1997 to 1999. Multiple linear regression models examined follow-up hemoglobin and rHuEPO dose per week (rHuEPO/wk) by numbers of catheter insertions and hospitalizations for VA infection.

Results.—In the prevalent cohort, increasing temporary and permanent catheter insertions and VA infections were associated with slightly lower hemoglobin (Fig 1), higher rHuEPO doses, and higher intravenous iron doses. In the incident cohort, compared to patients with no VA infections or no catheter insertions (temporary or permanent), respectively, patients with 2+ VA infections or 2+ catheter insertions had 0.12 g/dL and 0.06 g/dL lower mean hemoglobin ($P = 0.0028$ and $P < 0.0001$), and 25.7% and 12.2% higher mean rHuEPO/wk ($P < 0.0001$).

Conclusion.—Higher rHuEPO doses may be required to maintain similar or slightly lower mean hemoglobin values among chronic hemodialysis pa-

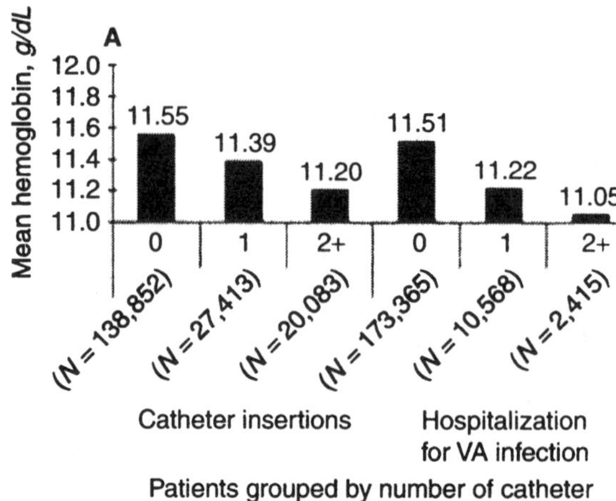

FIGURE 1.—Mean hemoglobin by number of catheter insertions (temporary or permanent) and hospitalizations for vascular access (*VA*) infection during 2000. Includes prevalent recombinant human erythropoietin (rHuEPO)-treated hemodialysis patients in 2000. (Courtesy of Roberts TL, Obrador GT, St Peter WL, et al: Relationship among catheter insertions, vascular access infections, and anemia management in hemodialysis patients. *Kidney Int* 66:2429-2436, 2004. Reprinted by permission of Blackwell Publishing.)

tients with higher numbers of catheter insertions and VA infections, compared to patients without any.

▶ rHuEPO is less effective in the presence of inflammation. Associated inflammation with VA infections may therefore result in lower hemoglobin values in dialysis patients treated with rHuEPO, which is almost all such patients at my institution. The bottom line is there are many obvious and some subtle reasons to avoid catheters and prosthetic grafts for dialysis access. Unresponsiveness to rHuEPO is another addition to a very long list.

G. L. Moneta, MD

Basilic Vein Transposition Fistula: A Good Option for Maintaining Hemodialysis Access Site Options?

Rao RK, Azin GD, Hood DB, et al (Univ of Southern California, Los Angeles)

J Vasc Surg 39:1043-1047, 2004 11–2

Purpose.—The primary use of autogenous arteriovenous access for chronic hemodialysis is recommended by the National Kidney Foundation–Dialysis Outcomes Quality Initiative practice guidelines. We review the outcomes of basilic vein transposition (BVT) to assess its value as a primary upper arm arteriovenous access option.

Methods.—A retrospective review of 56 patients undergoing BVT was performed. Thirty patients were men; average age was 56 years. Etiology of end-stage renal disease, complications, and time to maturation were tabu-

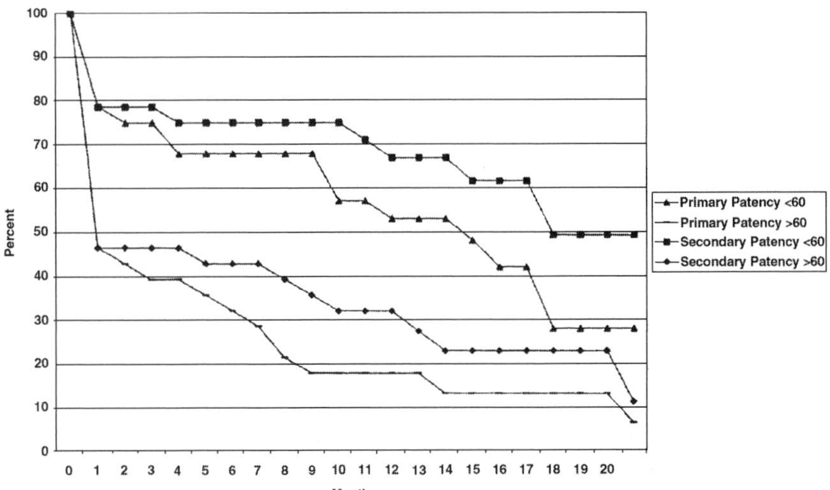

FIGURE 2.—Patency by age. (Reprinted by permission of the publisher from Rao RK, Azin GD, Hood DB, et al: Basilic vein transposition fistula: A good option for maintaining hemodialysis access site options? *J Vasc Surg* 39:1043-1047, 2004. Copyright 2004 by Elsevier.)

lated. Primary and secondary patency rates were determined by using life table methods. Multivariate regression analysis was performed to assess risk factors for fistula failure.

Results.—Renal failure was associated with diabetes in 32 (57%) patients, and BVT was the primary access procedure in 22 (39%) patients. Perioperative complications occurred in 5 (9%) patients and included hematoma (n = 3), myocardial infarction (n = 1), and death (n = 1). The average time to maturation was 74 days (range, 12-265 days), and maturation failure occurred in 21 (38%) patients. Logistic regression analysis showed that age older than 60 years was associated with poorer maturation and patency rates (Fig 2). On an intent-to-treat basis, 1-year primary and secondary patencies were 35% and 47%, respectively, but only 18% and 28%, respectively, for age >60 years. Forty-two percent of failed BVT were subsequently replaced with a prosthetic graft by using the same upper arm vessels.

Conclusion.—BVT frequently do not mature in patients older than 60 years, which compromises its utility as a primary access. However, fistulas that mature provide acceptable patency rates, and subsequent conversion to a prosthetic access is frequently possible. Selective use of BVT might improve the utilization of available access sites.

► A bit of shine is off BVTs. These are significant procedures, and they do not appear to work as well as original reports suggested. Like most operations, some patients are more suitable than others for the procedure. Older patients are not ideal candidates for BVTs. There may still be a role for primary prosthetic grafts in some patients, but don't tell anyone I said that!

G. L. Moneta, MD

Outcome After Autogenous Brachial-Axillary Translocated Superficial Femoropopliteal Vein Hemodialysis Access

Huber TS, Hirneise CM, Lee A, et al (Univ of Florida, Gainesville)
J Vasc Surg 40:311-318, 2004 11–3

Objective.—The optimal configuration for patients with "complex" or "tertiary" hemodialysis access needs remains undefined. This study was designed to examine the utility of the autogenous brachial-axillary translocated superficial femoropopliteal vein access (SFV ACCESS) in this subset of patients.

Methods.—Patients presenting for permanent hemodialysis access without a suitable upper extremity vein for autogenous access identified by duplex ultrasound mapping and those with repeated prosthetic access failures were considered candidates for SFV ACCESS (Fig 1). Ankle-brachial indices were obtained, and duplex scanning of the superficial femoropopliteal and saphenous veins was performed. Patients deemed candidates for SFV ACCESS also underwent preoperative upper extremity arteriography and venography. A retrospective review of the complete medical record was performed, and a follow-up telephone or personal interview was conducted.

Results.—Thirty patients (mean age ± SD, 54 ± 15 years; male, 33%; white, 37%; with diabetes, 50%; obese, 21%) underwent SFV ACCESS among approximately 650 access-related open surgical procedures during

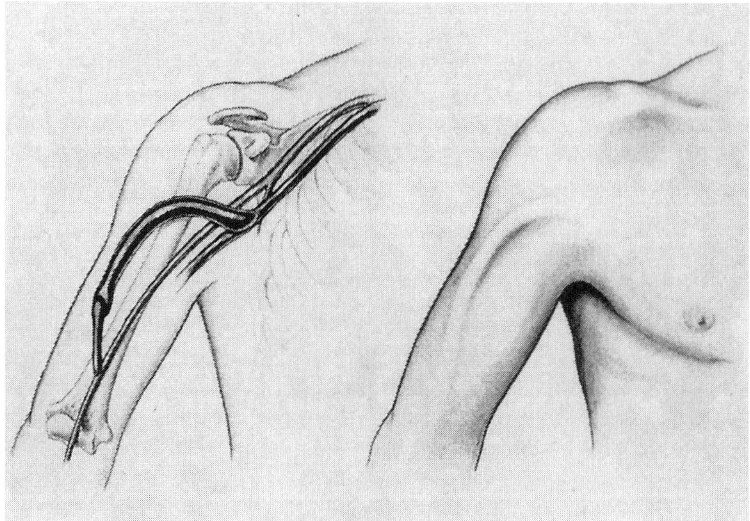

FIGURE 1.—Original artist rendition of the autogenous brachial-axillary translocated superficial femoropopliteal vein access (SFV ACCESS) depicts a composite configuration with saphenous and superficial femoropopliteal vein, although this has rarely been necessary in our more recent experience. As noted in the text, the SFV ACCESS has the appearance of a mature brachiocephalic autogenous access. (From Huber TS, Hirneise CM, Lee A, et al: Outcome after autogenous brachial-axillary translocated superficial femoropopliteal vein hemodialysis access. *J Vasc Surg* 40:311-318, 2004. Reprinted by permission of the publisher from Huber TS, Ozaki CK, Flynn TC, et al: Use of superficial femoral vein for hemodialysis arteriovenous access. *J Vasc Surg* 31:1038-1041, 2000. Copyright 2000 by Elsevier.)

the study period. The patients had been receiving dialysis for 4 ± 5 years (range, 0-24 years), and had 3 ± 3 (range, 0-17) prior permanent accesses, whereas 90% were actively dialyzed through tunneled catheters. In-hospital 30-day mortality was 3%, and the hospital length of stay was 7 ± 7 days. Fifty-seven percent of the patients experienced some type of perioperative complication, and 38+ACU- required a remedial surgical procedure. Hand ischemia developed in 43% of the patients (severity grade: 1, 10%; 2, 7%; 3, 27%), and a distal revascularization, interval ligation was performed in all those with grade 3 ischemia. Thigh wound complications or hematomas developed in 23% of the patients, and arm wound complications or hematomas developed in 17%. The incidence of thigh wound complications was significantly greater (57% vs 9%; *P* = .03) in obese patients, but the other perioperative complications analyzed could not be predicted on the basis of age, gender, or comorbid conditions. The SFV ACCESS was cannulated 7 ± 1 weeks postoperatively. The primary, primary assisted, and secondary patency rates were 96% ± 4%, 100% ± 0%, and 100% ± 0%, respectively, at 6 months; 79% ± 8%, 91% ± 6%, and 100% ± 0%, respectively, at 12 months; and 67% ± 13%, 86% ± 9%, and 100% ± 0%, respectively, at 18 months (life table analysis; % ± SE).

Conclusions.—The intermediate term functional patency rate after SFV ACCESS is excellent, although the magnitude of the procedure and the complication rate are significant. SFV ACCESS should only be considered in patients with limited access options.

► This access provides excellent patency but at the considerable cost of a very high incidence of "steal." Gradman et al[1] reported use of the femoral vein as a dialysis access, leaving the femoral vein in the leg. They subsequently modified the technique of the proximal anastomosis to narrow the vein and decrease steal.[2] Perhaps this technique should also be considered when the femoral vein is translocated to the upper extremity.

G. L. Moneta, MD

References

1. Gradman WS, Cohen W, Haji-Aghaii M: Arteriovenous fistula construction in the thigh with transposed superficial femoral vein: Our initial experience. *J Vasc Surg* 33:968-975, 2001.
2. Gradman WS, Laub J, Cohen W: Femoral vein transposition for arteriovenous hemodialysis access: Improved patient selection and intraoperative measures reduce postoperative ischemia. *J Vasc Surg* 41:279-284, 2005.

Experience With Cryopreserved Cadaveric Femoral Vein Allografts Used for Hemodialysis Access

Madden RL, Lipkowitz GS, Browne BJ, et al (Baystate Med Ctr, Springfield, Mass; Tufts Univ, Boston)

Ann Vasc Surg 18:453-458, 2004 11–4

Introduction.—The purpose of this study was to review the patency and complications of cryopreserved vein allografts used for hemodialysis access, and to compare them to a group with polytetrafluoroethylene (PTFE) grafts. Patients without adequate vasculature for native fistula were implanted with vein allografts or PTFE grafts at the surgeon's discretion. Only cryopreserved (CRY) veins were used until January 2001, when decellularized, cryopreserved Synergraft (SYN) veins became available. The CRY group had 48 patients; the SYN group, 42 patients; the PTFE group, 100 patients, who were selected from billing records listing PTFE graft insertion. Patient demographics were similar. Primary and secondary patencies were not significantly different at 1 or 2 years between groups. Complications in PTFE versus CRY and SYN groups were as follows: infection, 10% vs. 0% ($p < 0.01$); aneurysm, 2% vs. 18% ($p < 0.001$); and steal syndrome, 12% vs. 12% ($p =$ NS). Significantly more vein allograft patients lost their accesses to aneurysm ($p < 0.01$) and multiple stenoses ($p < 0.05$), whereas PTFE patients lost significantly more accesses to infection ($p < 0.01$) and recurrent thrombosis ($p < 0.05$). We conclude that cadaver vein allografts have similar patency to PTFE grafts. These allografts are more resistant to infection but significantly more susceptible to aneurysms. When used, vein allografts should be monitored aggressively for the development of aneurysms.

▶ There is no free lunch when it comes to dialysis access. This is especially so with dialysis access with prosthetic material. (Cryopreserved grafts are basically prosthetic material.) Overall, cryopreserved grafts do not have any advantage over standard PTFE dialysis prosthetic grafts. The rates of thrombosis are the same, and the decreased infection rate of the cryopreserved grafts is offset by more aneurysmal degeneration. The primary role for cryopreserved dialysis access grafts appears to be in patients with recurrent graft infections of other types of prosthetic dialysis access.

G. L. Moneta, MD

Outcomes of Upper Arm Arteriovenous Fistulas for Maintenance Hemodialysis Access

Fitzgerald JT, Schanzer A, Chin AI, et al (Univ of California, Sacramento)

Arch Surg 139:201-208, 2004 11–5

Hypothesis.—Radiocephalic fistulas for maintenance hemodialysis access are not feasible in all patients with end-stage renal disease. Our aim was to review our experience with 3 types of upper arm arteriovenous fistula

(AVF) to ascertain whether they are reasonable alternatives to radiocephalic fistulas and which, if any, have superior performance.

Patients and Methods.—Patient medical records were retrospectively reviewed. The main outcomes were maturation rate, time to maturation, assisted maturation rate, complication rates, reintervention rates, primary and assisted primary patency rates, and effects of comorbidities.

Results.—Eighty-six patients with end-stage renal disease underwent creation of a brachiocephalic, brachiobasilic, or brachial artery–to–median antecubital vein AVF. Overall, 80% matured, with 23% requiring an intervention to achieve maturity. The mean time to maturation was 3.8 months; 47% had a complication (inability to access, thrombosis, and so on), and 43% required additional interventions. The overall primary patency and assisted primary patency rates at 12 months were 50% and 74%, respectively. Brachiobasilic AVFs not superficialized immediately often needed a second operation. There were no significant differences in patency rates among the 3 AVF types. The AVFs in patients with diabetes took 2 months longer to mature than did those in patients without diabetes.

Conclusions.—An upper arm AVF is a reasonable alternative for maintenance hemodialysis access when a radiocephalic AVF is not possible. There are 3 valid options from which to choose to best accommodate each patient's antecubital anatomy. Diabetes may adversely affect outcomes. Our data suggest that brachiobasilic AVFs should be superficialized at the initial procedure, if feasible.

► Most of the secondary procedures required to achieve maturation of upper arm AVFs in this article were superficialization of brachial-basilic fistulas. All these superficialization procedures can obviously be avoided by superficialization of the basilic vein at the time of construction of the original brachiobasilic anastomosis. The need for secondary procedures to achieve upper arm fistula maturity should be uncommon.

G. L. Moneta, MD

Intra-access Blood Flow in Patients With Newly Created Upper-Arm Arteriovenous Native Fistulae for Hemodialysis Access

Chin AI, Chang W, Fitzgerald JT, et al (Univ of California, Sacramento)

Am J Kidney Dis 44:850-858, 2004 11–6

Background.—The upper-arm native arteriovenous fistula for hemodialysis (HD) vascular access is an important option in the long-term HD population. This single-center cohort study evaluated intra-access blood flow (Q_{AC}) in 3 variants of newly created upper-arm fistulae.

Methods.—Fifty-three patients with mature, working, upper-arm fistulae composed of brachial artery to cephalic vein (n = 27), brachial artery to basilic vein (n = 13), and brachial artery to median antecubital vein (n = 13) fistulae were included. Nine of 13 brachio-median antecubital fistulae were of the Gracz type and used the deep perforating vein. Q_{AC} was measured by means of ultrasound velocity dilution during HD. In brachio-median antecubital fistulae, additional flow in the alternate draining vein was measured by means of duplex ultrasound, with 9 of 11 studied patients showing a patent alternate outflow, of whom 7 patients showed substantial flow (median, 0.7 L/min).

Results.—Q_{AC} in the HD-used primary vein in brachio-median antecubital fistulae (0.85 L/min) was significantly less than those of brachiocephalic and brachiobasilic fistulae (1.4 and 1.7 L/min, respectively). However, when the additional flow provided by the patent alternate vein in brachio-median antecubital fistulae was considered, flow rates provided by all 3 variants of fistulae appeared similar. The inverse correlation between alternate-vein and primary-vein flows ($r = -0.70$; $P = 0.017$) suggested there was competitive flow between the 2 venous outlets. There was no instance of access recirculation.

Conclusion.—Upper-arm fistulae, regardless of type, provide excellent blood flows and should be considered routinely if a wrist fistula is not feasible. The patent alternate vein in the brachio-median antecubital or Gracz fistula may continue to drain a substantial amount of blood.

► In this and the previous article (Abstract 11–5), the authors report their results with upper arm arteriovenous fistulas. It appears all types of upper arm arteriovenous fistulas behave about the same in terms of maturation (see Abstract 11–5) and ultimate flow rates and volume flow.

G. L. Moneta, MD

Impaired Hyperemic Response Is Predictive of Early Access Failure

Wall LP, Gasparis A, Callahan S, et al (State Univ of New York at Stony Brook)

Ann Vasc Surg 18:167-171, 2004 11–7

Introduction.—The aim of this study was to demonstrate that hyperemic response is a predictor of access failure. We conducted a review of a prospective database of dialysis access patients with preoperative hyperemia studies from June 1998 to August 2002. These consisted of bilateral brachial artery pressures followed by flow velocity measurements of the brachial artery and radial artery at rest and after 3 min of arm ischemia. Measurements were taken by using a cuff placed above the antecubital fossa and inflated to 20 mmHg above systolic pressure. There were no differences recorded in brachial artery pressures for the bilateral studies. Hyperemic response was entered into a stepwise Cox regression to determine its effect on access failure. Access failure was defined as failure to mature or thrombosis. Accesses were placed according to Dialysis Outcome Quality Intiatives (DOQI) guidelines. Kaplan-Meier survival analysis was performed. Log-rank testing was used to compare patency results. Censored end points were death, renal transplant, and access survival to the end of the study period. Fistulas that failed to mature were considered failures at 3 months. Arteries with a <5 cm/sec increase in peak systolic velocity were defined as nonresponders. The 59 ar-

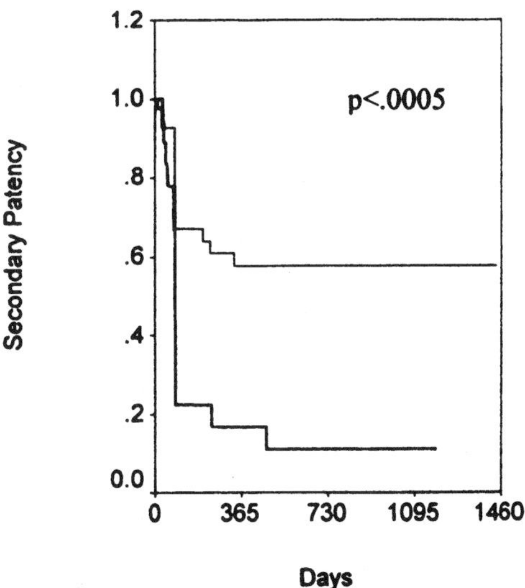

FIGURE 1.—Access survival by hyperemic response. *Top line*, >5 cm/sec; *bottom line*, <5 cm/sec. (Courtesy of Wall LP, Gasparis A, Callahan S, et al: Impaired hyperemic response is predictive of early access failure. *Ann Vasc Surg* 18[2]167-171, 2004.)

teries used for dialysis access were divided into two groups on the basis of their hyperemic response in cm/sec. The nonresponders were compared with the remainder of accesses performed. Accesses based on arteries with absent or minimal hyperemic response had significantly lower ($p < 0.0005$) secondary patencies by Kaplan-Meier analysis (Fig 1). Upon further stratification into radial and brachial arteries, the significant difference in secondary patency remained for radial artery–based accesses ($p = 0.024$) and approached statistical significance for brachial artery–based accesses ($p = 0.057$). A significant difference was not seen in primary patencies, indicating that accesses based on arteries with an acceptable hyperemic response are more likely to be salvaged by revisions. A nonresponsive radial artery was not a significant predictor of a nonresponsive brachial artery in the same extremity by binary logistic regression ($p = 0.111$), and a nonresponsive artery was not a significant predictor of nonresponsiveness in the corresponding artery in the contralateral extremity ($p = 0.137$). Cox regression analysis revealed that the hyperemic response is a significant predictor of failure to mature or thrombosis. Hyperemic testing is a useful means of evaluating adequate arterial inflow for dialysis access. Reduced or absent hyperemic response is an independent predictor of access failure.

▶ Most surgeons prefer radial artery–based arteriovenous fistulas as the initial form of arteriovenous fistula in a patient requiring dialysis access. Failure of a radiocephalic arteriovenous fistula has been associated with decreased size of the cephalic vein. The current study suggests failure of radial artery–based arteriovenous fistulas may be predicted by an impaired hyperemic response of the radial artery. When the radial artery has poor hyperemic response, the patient may be best off initially using a brachial rather than radial artery–based arteriovenous fistula.

G. L. Moneta, MD

Timing of First Cannulation and Vascular Access Failure in Haemodialysis: An Analysis of Practice Patterns at Dialysis Facilities in the DOPPS

Saran R, Dykstra DM, Pisoni RL, et al (Univ of Michigan, Ann Arbor; Veterans Affairs Med Ctr, Ann Arbor, Mich; Lapeyronie Univ, Montpellier, France; et al)

Nephrol Dial Transplant 19:2334-2340, 2004 11–8

Background.—Optimal waiting time before first use of vascular access is not known.

Methods.—Two practices—first cannulation time for fistulae and grafts, and blood flow rate—were examined as potential predictors of vascular access failure in the Dialysis Outcomes and Practice Patterns Study (DOPPS). Access failure (defined as time to first failure or first salvage intervention) was modelled using Cox regression.

Results.—Among 309 haemodialysis facilities, 2730 grafts and 2154 fistulae were studied. For grafts, first cannulation typically occurred within 2-4 weeks at 62% of US, 61% of European and 42% of Japanese facilities (Fig 2). For fistulae, first cannulation occurred <2 months after placement in 36% of US, 79% of European and 98% of Japanese facilities (Fig 3). Overall, the relative risk (RR) of graft failure in Europe was lower compared with the USA (RR = 0.69, P = 0.04) (Fig 1). The RR of graft failure (reference group = first cannulation at 2-3 weeks) was 0.84 with first cannulation at <2

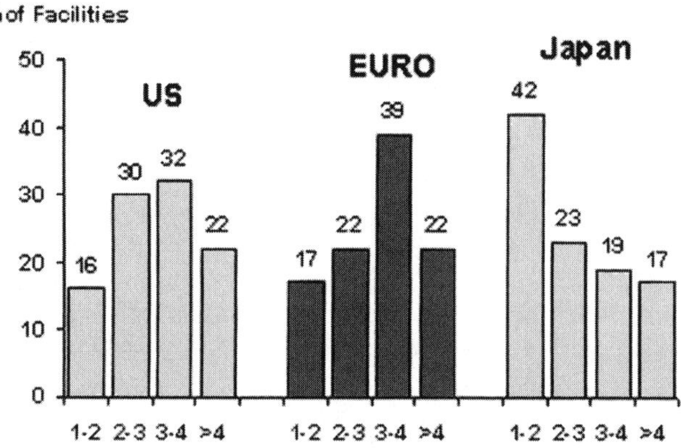

FIGURE 2.—Number of weeks from placement to first cannulation of grafts as a facility-level practice pattern. Bar graph displaying facility typical time to first cannulation of arteriovenous grafts in US, European and Japanese hemodialysis facilities enrolled in the Dialysis Outcomes and Practice Patterns Study (DOPPS). (Courtesy of Saran R, Dykstra DM, Pisoni RL, et al: Timing of first cannulation and vascular access failure in haemodialysis: An analysis of practice patterns at dialysis facilities in the DOPPS. *Nephrol Dial Transplant* 19:2334-2340, 2004. By permission of Oxford University Press.)

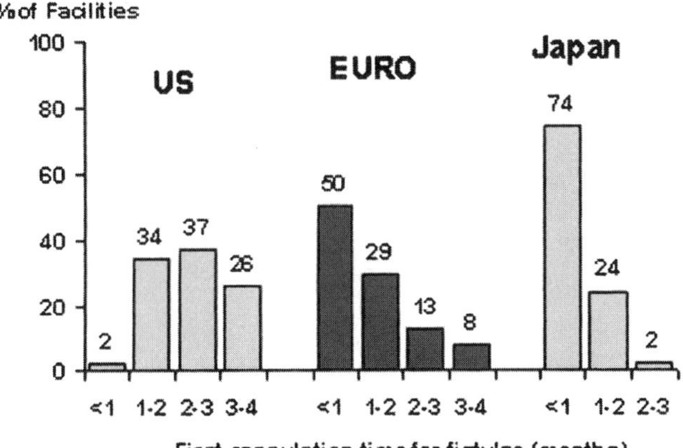

FIGURE 3.—Number of months from placement to first cannulation of fistulae as a facility-level practice pattern. Bar graph displaying facility typical time to first cannulation of arteriovenous fistulae in US, European and Japanese hemodialysis facilities enrolled in the Dialysis Outcomes and Practice Patterns Study (DOPPS). (Courtesy of Saran R, Dykstra DM, Pisoni RL, et al: Timing of first cannulation and vascular access failure in haemodialysis: An analysis of practice patterns at dialysis facilities in the DOPPS. *Nephrol Dial Transplant* 19:2334-2340, 2004. By permission of Oxford University Press.)

weeks ($P = 0.11$), 0.94 with first cannulation at 3-4 weeks ($P = 0.48$) and 0.93 with first cannulation at >4 weeks ($P = 0.48$). The RR of fistula failure was 0.72 with first cannulation at <4 weeks ($P = 0.08$), 0.91 at 2-3 months ($P = 0.43$) and 0.87 at >3 months ($P = 0.31$) (reference group = first cannulation at 1-2 months). Facility median blood flow rate was not a significant predictor of access failure.

Conclusions.—Earlier cannulation of a newly placed vascular access at the haemodialysis facility level was not associated with increased risk of vascular access failure. Potential for confounding due to selection bias cannot

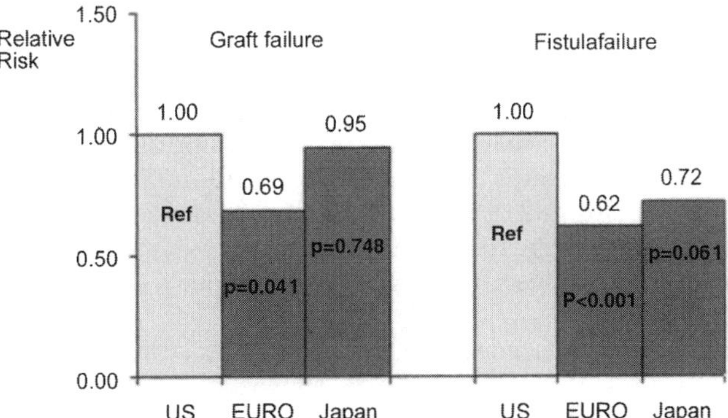

FIGURE 1.—Relative risk of fistula and graft failure by continent. Models were adjusted for patient age, race, sex, body mass index, diabetes mellitus, congestive heart failure, coronary artery disease, peripheral vascular disease and hypertension at study entry, as well as for the number of prior accesses and incidence to end-stage renal disease. (Courtesy of Saran R, Dykstra DM, Pisoni RL, et al: Timing of first cannulation and vascular access failure in haemodialysis: An analysis of practice patterns at dialysis facilities in the DOPPS. *Nephrol Dial Transplant* 19:2334-2340, 2004. By permission of Oxford University Press.)

be excluded, implying the importance of clinical judgement in determining time to first use of vascular access.

▶ These are not randomized data. I suspect the failure of first cannulation time to correlate with fistula failure has more to do with the fact that early maturing fistulas were cannulated early. The implied message is that a fistula can be cannulated when it is "ready," and there is no fixed waiting period required. I am not sure I agree. If you are wrong and cannulate too early, there is a risk of loss of the fistula.

G. L. Moneta, MD

Randomized Controlled Trial of Prophylactic Repair of Hemodialysis Arteriovenous Graft Stenosis

Dember LM, Holmberg EF, Kaufman JS (Boston Univ; VA Boston Healthcare System)

Kidney Int 66:390-398, 2004 11–9

Background.—Previous nonrandomized studies suggest that prophylactic repair of hemodialyisis arteriovenous (AV) graft stenosis reduces thrombosis rates and increases cumulative graft survival. The present study is a randomized trial comparing prophylactic repair of AV graft stenosis with repair at the time of thrombosis.

Methods.—Sixty-four patients with elevated static venous pressure measured in an upper extremity AV graft were randomized to Intervention or Observation. Monthly static venous pressure/systolic blood pressure ratios (SVPR) were determined for all patients throughout the duration of study participation. Patients in the Intervention group underwent angiography and repair of identified stenoses if the monthly SVPR was elevated ($\geq$0.4). Patients in the Observation group underwent stenosis repair only in the event of access thrombosis or clinical evidence of access dysfunction. The primary end point was access abandonment.

Results.—Access abandonment occurred in 14 patients in the Intervention group and 14 patients in the Observation group during the 3.5-year study period. Time to access abandonment did not differ significantly between the treatment groups (hazard ratio for randomization to Intervention 1.75, 95% CI 0.80-3.82, $P = 0.16$). The proportion of patients with a thrombotic event was greater in the Observation group (72%) than in the Intervention group (44%) ($P = 0.04$), but overall thrombosis rates were similar in the groups.

Conclusion.—Compared with a strategy of observation and repair of accesses only in the event of thrombosis, prospective static venous pressure monitoring with prophylactic stenosis repair did not prolong graft survival.

▶ This article fails to confirm a relationship between access survival and access monitoring with prophylactic intervention for identified stenoses. The findings are in direct conflict with results of previously nonrandomized studies. This study was small and occurred at a single institution. In addition, the authors' method for monitoring for access graft stenosis is not universally utilized. The article does suggest the need for a larger multicentered trial evaluating the merits of prophylactic dialysis access intervention. Recommendations for prophylactic repair of stenoses identified in dialysis access grafts may need to be reconsidered.

G. L. Moneta, MD

Can Blood Flow Surveillance and Pre-emptive Repair of Subclinical Stenosis Prolong the Useful Life of Arteriovenous Fistulae? A Randomized Controlled Study

Tessitore N, Lipari G, Poli A, et al (Istituto di Radiologia, Verona, Italy)

Nephrol Dial Transplant 19:2325-2333, 2004 11–10

Background.—Stenosis is the main cause of arteriovenous fistula (AVF) failure. It is unclear, however, if surveillance for stenosis enhances AVF function and longevity and if there is an ideal time for intervention.

Methods.—In a 5-year randomized, controlled, open trial we compared blood flow surveillance and pre-emptive repair of subclinical stenoses (one or both of angioplasty and open surgery) with standard monitoring and intervention based upon clinical criteria alone to determine if the former prolonged the longevity of mature forearm AVFs. Surveillance with blood pump flow (Qb) monitoring during dialysis sessions and quarterly shunt blood flow (Qa) or recirculation measurements identified 79 AVFs with angiographically proven, significant (>50%) stenosis. The AVFs were randomized to either a control group (intervention done in response to a decline in the delivered dialysis dose or thrombosis; n = 36) or to a pre-emptive treatment group (n = 43). To evaluate a possible relationship between outcome and haemodynamic status of the access, AVFs were divided into functional and failing subgroups, according to Qa values higher or lower than 350 ml/min or the absence or presence of recirculation.

Results.—A Kaplan-Meier analysis showed that pre-emptive treatment reduced failure rate ($P = 0.003$) and the Cox hazards model identified treatment ($P = 0.009$) and higher baseline Qa ($P = 0.001$) as the only variables associated with favourable outcome (Fig 3). Primary patency rates were higher in treatment than in control AVFs in both functional ($P = 0.021$) and failing subgroups ($P = 0.005$). They were also higher in functional than in failing AVFs in both control ($P < 0.001$) and treatment groups ($P = 0.023$). Access survival was significantly higher in pre-emptively treated than in control AVFs ($P = 0.050$), a higher post-intervention Qa being the only variable associated with improved access longevity ($P = 0.044$). Secondary patency rates were similar in pre-emptively treated and control AVFs in both functional ($P = 0.059$) and failing subgroups ($P = 0.394$). They were also similar in functional and failing AVFs in controls ($P = 0.082$), but were higher in pre-emptively treated functional AVFs than in pre-emptively treated failing AVFs ($P = 0.033$) or in the entire control group ($P = 0.019$).

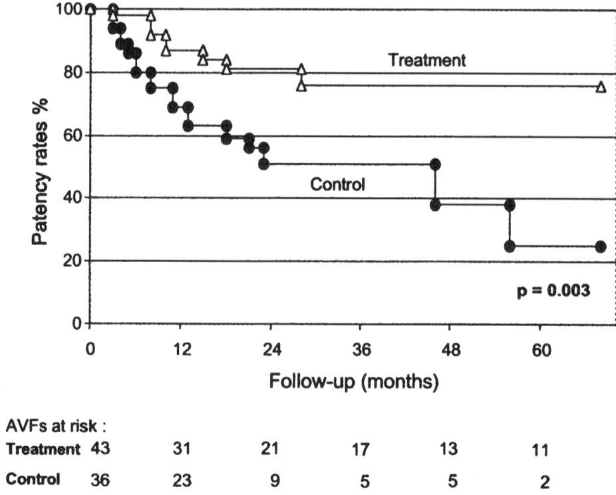

FIGURE 3.—Unadjusted primary patency rates of controls (*closed circles*) compared with unadjusted assisted primary patency rates in the treatment group (*open triangles*). *Abbreviation: AVF,* Arteriovenous fistula. (Courtesy of Tessitore N, Lipari G, Poli A, et al: Can blood flow surveillance and pre-emptive repair of subclinical stenosis prolong the useful life of arteriovenous fistulae? A randomized controlled study. *Nephrol Dial Transplant* 19:2325-2333, 2004. By permission of Oxford University Press.)

Conclusions.—We provide evidence that active blood flow surveillance and pre-emptive repair of subclinical stenosis reduce the thrombosis rate and prolong the functional life of mature forearm AVFs. We also show that Qa is a crucial indicator of access patency and a Qa >350 ml/min portends a superior outcome with pre-emptive action in AVFs.

► The "don't poke a skunk" philosophy is prevalent in most dialysis centers. AVFs that are functioning well are not routinely monitored for signs of stenosis. Data, however, are accumulating that monitoring of flow rates should be routine in AVFs. This is the first study to suggest preemptive repair of subclinical stenoses in well-functioning AVFs identified to be at risk for thrombosis by a Qa of less than 350 mL/min. Note that the previous abstract (Abstract 11–9) indicating no benefit for prophylactic repair of dialysis access focused on grafts, not fistulas, as in this abstract.

G. L. Moneta, MD

Use of Short PTFE Segments (<6 cm) Compares Favorably With Pure Autologous Repair in Failing or Thrombosed Native Arteriovenous Fistulas

Georgiadis GS, Lazarides MK, Lambidis CD, et al (Demokritos Univ, Alexandroupolis, Greece; Athens Univ, Greece)

J Vasc Surg 41:76-81, 2005 11–11

Objective.—The re-establishment of patency in a stenosed or thrombosed native arteriovenous fistula (AVF) is fundamental to regaining adequate hemodialysis through the same cannulable vein. Many surgeons have been reluctant to use even small segments of synthetic grafts in AVF revisions because of a perception that these would lead to poor results; however, studies comparing various treatment options are scarce. This study compared the use of short (<6 cm) polytetrafluoroethylene (PTFE) segments with pure autologous repair in stenosed or thrombosed native fistulas.

Methods.—The cumulative postintervention primary patency rates of two groups of hemodialysis patients receiving different surgical revision operations of their vascular accesses were prospectively compared. Group I (n = 30) comprised patients who presented with stenosed or thrombosed native fistulas and received short (2 to 6 cm) interposition PTFE grafts placed after the stenosed or thrombosed outflow vein segment was resected. These short PTFE grafts were not used for cannulation. Group II (n = 29) comprised patients who presented with dysfunctional or failed AVFs and underwent various types of pure autogenous corrections. AVF dysfunction or thrombosis was detected with clinical examination and color duplex ultrasound scanning. In all cases, on-table arteriography-fistulography was performed before surgical repair. Access adequacy was assessed in all patients postoperatively after the first puncture and every month thereafter (mean follow up 16.7 months).

Results.—No statistically significant difference in patency was observed between the two groups. Postintervention cumulative patencies were 100%, 88%, and 82% for group I and 90%, 82%, and 71% for group II at 6, 12, and 18 months, respectively ($P = .8$).

Conclusions.—Short (<6 cm) interposition PTFE segments used for the revision of failing or failed AVFs compare favorably to purely native repair and do not alter the autologous behavior of the initial access. These short PTFE revisions resulted in satisfactory midterm primary patency without further consumption of the venous capital by harvesting segments of vein from other locations and without compromising more proximal access sites. This practice is recommended and is justified as part of an aggressive access salvage policy addressed by many authors so far.

▶ With increased monitoring of native AVFs, more stenoses are going to be discovered. Use of short segments of PTFE to bridge stenoses not suitable to angioplasty makes revision of stenosed AVFs a relatively simple procedure with minimal morbidity and excellent outcome. This was the method of surgical revision utilized in the previous article (Abstract 11–10).

G. L. Moneta, MD

Hemodialysis-Related Venous Stenosis: Treatment With Ultrahigh-Pressure Angioplasty Balloons

Trerotola SO, Stavropoulos SW, Shlansky-Goldberg R, et al (Univ of Pennsylvania, Philadelphia)

Radiology 231:259-262, 2004 11–12

Background.—Hemodialysis-related stenosis can be resistant to balloon angioplasty and can necessitate the use of high-pressure angioplasty balloons for successful treatment. A retrospective review was presented of experience with ultra–high-pressure angioplasty balloons at pressures equal to or exceeding manufacturer recommendations in the treatment of hemodialysis-related venous stenosis.

Methods.—A total of 87 hemodialysis access revascularization procedures were performed in 75 patients with ultra–high-pressure angioplasty balloons at atmospheric pressures at or above the manufacturer-recommended burst pressure of 30 atm for the treatment of hemodialysis-related venous stenosis. All the procedures were performed in a 4-month period from August through November 2002.

Results.—High-pressure angioplasty was unsuccessful in 7 of 87 procedures. However, the combination of new balloon technology with aggressive inflation procedures provided a 100% technical success rate in the treatment of stenoses that were resistant to high-pressure angioplasty in the 7 failed high-pressure angioplasty procedures.

Conclusions.—The use of ultra–high-pressure angioplasty balloons in the treatment of hemodialysis-related venous stenosis could provide cost savings compared with the costs of other previously described approaches for resistant lesions.

▶ This is a very small series (N = 7). The authors got away with extraordinary inflation pressures in this limited series. We have not been so lucky at our institution and have observed fistula rupture with overaggressive angioplasty pressures.

G. L. Moneta, MD

Percutaneous Treatment of Symptomatic Central Venous Stenosis Angioplasty

Sprouse LR II, Lesar CJ, Meier GH III, et al (Easter Virginia Med School, Norfolk)

J Vasc Surg 39:578-582, 2004 11–13

Objectives.—The increased use of central venous access primarily for hemodialysis has led to a significant increase in clinically relevant central venous occlusive disease (CVOD). The magnitude of and the optimal therapy for CVOD are not clearly established. The purpose of this study is to define the problem of CVOD and determine the success of percutaneous therapy for relieving symptoms and maintaining central venous patency.

Methods.—Patients presenting with disabling upper-extremity edema suggestive of central venous stenosis or occlusion during a 3-year period were evaluated by venography of the upper extremity and central veins. Percutaneous venous angioplasty (PTA) and/or stent placement was performed as clinically indicated. The success of therapy was assessed, and the patients were observed to determine the incidence of recurrence and additional procedures. Recurrent lesions underwent similar evaluation and treatment.

Results.—A total of 32 sides were treated in 29 patients with a mean of 1.9 interventions per side treated. Hemodialysis-related lesions were the underlying cause in 87% with the remaining 13% related to previous central venous catheterization. The lesions involved the axillary, subclavian, and innominate veins with complete venous occlusion in six (19%) cases. Percutaneous angioplasty was followed by stent placement in six (19%) cases. The procedure was a technical success and was performed without complications in all cases (100%). Mean follow-up was 16.5 months (range, 4-36 months). On average, patient symptoms were controlled for 6.5 months after the initial intervention. Recurrent edema led to additional PTA in 20 (63%) cases. Fifty percent (n = 14) of patients with an arteriovenous fistula (AVF) experienced recurrent symptoms after initial and/or repeat PTA and required AVF ligation. Complete resolution after the initial PTA was predictive of long-term success.

Conclusions.—Central venous occlusive disease has emerged as a significant clinical problem. Percutaneous venous angioplasty can provide temporary symptomatic relief; however, multiple procedures are often required and long-term relief is rarely achieved.

► Percutaneous treatment of central stenoses in patients with dialysis access grafts is not a durable procedure. This is an example of doing something because there is not much else to do.

G. L. Moneta, MD

Effectiveness and Safety of Dialysis Vascular Access Procedures Performed by Interventional Nephrologists

Beathard GA, for the Physician Operators Forum of RMS Lifeline, Inc (RMS Lifeline, Austin, Tex; et al)

Kidney Int 66:1622-1632, 2004 11–14

Background.—The purpose of this report was to analyze the results obtained from a group of interventional nephrologists working in multiple centers performing basic procedures that are used routinely in the management of vascular access problems, with an effort toward establishing standards for evaluating success, complication rates, and acceptable times for procedure duration and fluoroscopy.

Methods.—Data on six basic procedures were analyzed—angioplasty of arteriovenous fistulas (AVF-PTA), angioplasty of synthetic grafts (graft-PTA), thrombectomy of arteriovenous fistulas (AVF declot), thrombectomy

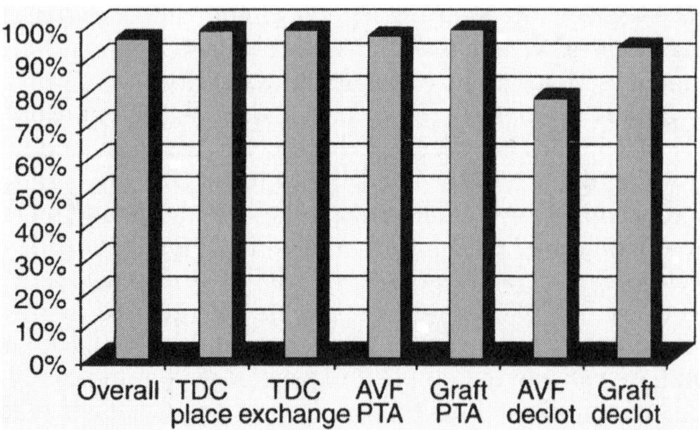

FIGURE 2.—Success rate for each category. *Abbreviations: TDC place,* Tunneled dialysis catheter placement; *TDC exchange,* tunneled dialysis catheter exchange; *AVF-PTA,* arteriovenous fistula angioplasty; *Graft-PTA,* graft angioplasty; *AVF declot,* arteriovenous fistula thrombectomy; *Graft declot,* graft thrombectomy; *overall,* combined group. (Courtesy of Beathard GA, for the Physician Operators Forum of RMS Lifeline, Inc: Effectiveness and safety of dialysis vascular access procedures performed by interventional nephrologists. *Kidney Int* 66:1622-1632, 2004. Reprinted by permission of Blackwell Publishing.)

of synthetic grafts (graft declot), placement of tunneled dialysis catheters (TDC placement), and tunneled dialysis catheter exchange (TDC exchange). These data were examined both as a group and by individual physician operator.

Results.—A total of 14,067 cases were performed under the six categories of procedure that were the subject of this report; 13,503 cases (96.18%) were successful. The overall complication rate for the combined group of procedures was 3.54%, with 3.26% falling within the minor category and 0.28% within the major. The number of cases performed in each individual category with success rates for each were as follows: TDC placement—1765 cases, 98.24% successful; TDC exchange—2262 cases, 98.36% successful; AVF-PTA—1561 cases, 96.58% successful; graft-PTA—3560 cases, 98.06% successful; AVF declot—228 cases, 78.10% successful; graft declot—4671 cases, 93.08% successful (Fig 2).

Conclusion.—This study demonstrates that appropriately trained interventional nephrologists can perform these basic procedures in both a safe and effective manner.

► These cases were performed in an angiography suite. There were no open surgical procedures. These guys wrote like yesteryear's radiologists. The report is very simplistic in that long-term results were not considered. No life-table analysis is presented. However, it does appear nonsurgically trained and nonradiologically trained physicians can learn catheter-based procedures pertinent to maintenance of dialysis access. Interventional radiology appears to be under attack from yet another front. The era of techniques as a specialty may be drawing to a close.

G. L. Moneta, MD

Heparin-Associated Antiplatelet Antibodies Increase Morbidity and Mortality in Hemodialysis Patients

Mureebe L, Coats RD, Silliman WR, et al (Univ of Missouri, Columbia)

Surgery 136:848-853, 2004 11–15

Background.—Patients are frequently exposed to heparin during hemodialysis (HD) to prevent thrombosis of the extracorporeal circuit. Other groups with frequent heparin exposures have a high rate of development of heparin-associated antiplatelet antibodies (HAAb). We sought to define the prevalence of HAAb in HD patients and evaluate their effects.

Methods.—A chart listing of all patients undergoing HD at our tertiary care institution during a six-year period was obtained. Charts of patients who tested positive for HAAb were reviewed. A cohort of randomly selected HD patients who tested negative for HAAb was analyzed as a control group.

Results.—In our sample, 3.7% of HD patients were positive for HAAb. Morbidity, as defined by thromboembolic (TEC) or hemorrhagic complications, was higher in the HAAb-positive group compared with the control patients (60% vs 8.7%, $P < .05$), and the mortality rate (mortality directly related to TECs) was also higher in the HAAb-positive patients (28.6% vs 4.35%, $P < .05$).

Conclusions.—Contrary to reports of HAAb in patients undergoing HD without increased morbidity and mortality, we found significant increases in both morbidity and mortality. The elevated morbidity and mortality may represent ongoing endothelial and platelet activation from repeated heparin exposures. Reduced morbidity and mortality will likely require early recognition of HAAb and alteration of anticoagulation in HD patients.

▶ The primary thrombotic morbidity in dialysis patients with HAAb was thrombosis of permanent dialysis access—both fistulas and grafts. Patients with repeated dialysis access thrombosis probably should be investigated for HAAb, and if positive, alternative forms of anticoagulation be employed during hemodialysis.

G. L. Moneta, MD

Transhepatic Catheter Access for Hemodialysis

Smith TP, Ryan JM, Reddan DN (Duke Univ, Durham, NC)

Radiology 232:246-251, 2004 11–16

Purpose.—To retrospectively review the authors' experience regarding the safety and functionality of transhepatic hemodialysis catheters.

Materials and Methods.—Sixteen patients (seven men and nine women aged 21-77 years; mean age, 51.6 years) underwent placement of 21 transhepatic hemodialysis catheters. Transhepatic catheters were placed in the absence of an available peripheral venous site (11 patients) or for preservation of a single remaining venous site to achieve permanent vascular access. Safety was assessed by means of complications encountered, and catheter functionality was assessed by means of total access site service interval. Catheter patency was described by using a Kaplan-Meier survival curve, and number of catheter days were compared according to patient sex by using a two-sample *t* test.

Results.—Technical success was achieved in all patients. The mean total access site service interval was 138 catheter days (range, 0-599 days), and there was no significant difference according to patient sex ($P = .869$). Of the 16 catheters placed initially, five became dislodged and required an additional access procedure to be performed. These 21 catheters required 30 exchanges in 10 patients (48%) (range, 1-6 exchanges per patient). The most common reason for catheter exchange was device failure. There were six complications among 21 catheters placed (29%), including one death from massive intraperitoneal hemorrhage on the day after catheter placement.

Conclusion.—Transhepatic hemodialysis catheters offer a viable option to patients with limited options; however, there are maintenance issues and complications.

▶ The potential to kill the patient with this procedure has to make this an approach of desperation. Can it really be justified in a very end-stage dialysis patient? These sorts of things are close to being more about doctor ego than patient benefit.

G. L. Moneta, MD

Long-term Outcome Following Thrombembolectomy in the Upper Extremity

Licht PB, Balezantis T, Wolff B, et al (Southern Danish Univ, Odense, Denmark; Odense Univ Hosp, Denmark)

Eur J Vasc Endovasc Surg 28:508-512, 2004 11–17

Objectives.—To evaluate short- and long-term mortality and morbidity in patients that were treated for acute upper extremity ischemia.

Design.—Single center retrospective study.

Patients.—A consecutive series of 148 patients who were admitted with a diagnosis of acute ischemia of the upper extremity during an 11-year period.

Methods.—All charts were reviewed retrospectively and 96% of all survivors participated in clinical follow-up.

Results.—The median age was 78 years and 64% of patients were females. The 30-day mortality was 8% and the overall 5-year survival 37% (Fig 1). The observed mortality during the follow-up period was significantly higher than expected. Survival was not significantly different in patients who received anticoagulant drugs following discharge from the hospital. The duration of ischemia did not significantly influence long-term arm-function (Table 1).

Conclusions.—Acute embolic episodes in the upper extremity primarily occur in elderly and the peri-operative mortality is high. Mortality following

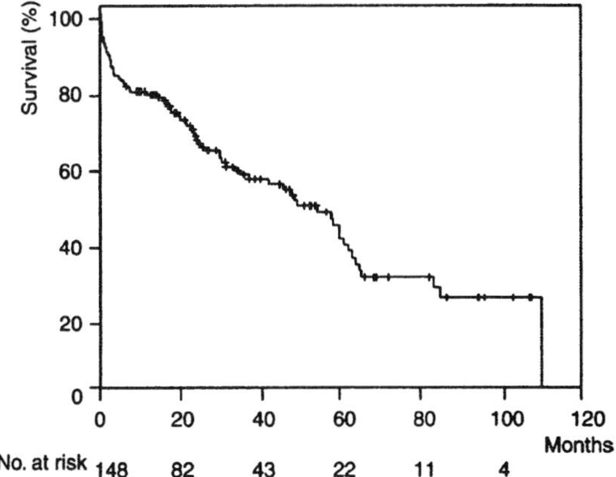

FIGURE 1.—Kaplan-Meier survival curve of all patients who were admitted with acute ischemia of the upper extremity. (Reprinted from Licht PB, Balezantis T, Wolff B, et al: Long-term outcome following thrombembolectomy in the upper extremity. *Eur J Vasc Endovasc Surg* 28:508-512, 2004. Copyright 2004 by permission of the publisher.)

discharge from the hospital remains significantly higher than that of the background population.

▶ This article indicates that embolism to the upper extremity can be treated with good surgical outcome with respect to the limb but poor short- and long-term outcome with respect to patient survival. Despite the fact the authors confirmed an embolic cardiac source in only 61% of their patients, it is very likely emboli large enough to occlude the brachial artery virtually always originate from a cardiac chamber. Unless there is a specific contraindication, long-term anticoagulation would seem reasonable in any patient with a major upper extremity embolus. Perhaps survival is not improved, but repeat embolism may be avoided.

G. L. Moneta, MD

TABLE 1.—The Relationship Between Arm-Function and Duration of Ischemia (147 Available Patient Charts)

	Armfunction			Total
	Normal Armfunction	Slightly Decreased Armfunction	Severely Decreased Armfunction	
Less than 12 h	33 (87%)	4 (11%)	1 (2%)	38
12-24 h	13 (93%)	1 (7%)		14
More than 24 h	11 (69%)	4 (25%)	1 (6%)	16
Total	57 (84%)	9 (13%)	2 (3%)	68

(Reprinted from Licht PB, Balezantis T, Wolff B, et al: Long-term outcome following thrombembolectomy in the upper extremity. *Eur J Vasc Endovasc Surg* 28:508-512, 2004. Copyright 2004 by permission of the publisher.)

12 Carotid and Cerebrovascular Disease

Short Telomeres Are Associated With Increased Carotid Atherosclerosis in Hypertensive Subjects

Benetos A, Gardner JP, Zureik M, et al (Centre d'Investigations Préventives et Cliniques, Paris; Med School of Nancy, France; INSERM U258, Villejuif, France; et al)

Hypertension 43:182-185, 2004 12–1

Introduction.—Recent studies have shown that individuals with shorter telomeres present a higher prevalence of arterial lesions and higher risk of cardiovascular disease mortality. As a group, patients with high blood pressure are at an increased risk for cardiovascular diseases. However, some hypertensive patients are more prone than others to atherosclerotic lesions. The main objective of this study was to examine the relationship between telomere length, as expressed in white blood cells, and carotid artery atherosclerotic plaques in hypertensive males. Data from 163 treated hypertensive men who were volunteers for a free medical examination were analyzed. Extracranial carotid plaques were assessed with B-mode ultrasound. Telomere length was measured from DNA samples extracted from white blood cells. The results of this study show that telomere length was shorter in hypertensive men with carotid artery plaques versus hypertensive men without plaques (8.17±0.07 kb versus 8.46±0.07 kb; $P<0.01$). Multivariate analysis showed that in addition to age, telomere length was a significant predictor of the presence of carotid artery plaques. The findings from this study suggest that in the presence of chronic hypertension, which is a major risk factor for atherosclerotic lesions, shorter telomere length in white blood cells is associated with an increased predilection to carotid artery atherosclerosis.

► The authors have attempted to answer, at least partially, the question as to why some hypertensive patients are more prone to developing atherosclerotic lesions than others. There is a complex relationship between telomere length, oxidative stress, and antioxidant capacity. Overall, the data indicate telomere length may be an indicator of cardiovascular risk in aging of blood vessels.

G. L. Moneta, MD

Elastin and Calcium Rather than Collagen or Lipid Content Are Associated With Echogenicity of Human Carotid Plaques

Gonçalves I, Lindholm MW, Pedro LM, et al (Lund Univ, Malmö, Sweden; Gothenburg Univ, Sweden; Instituto Cardiovascular de Lisboa, Lisbon, Portugal)

Stroke 35:2795-2800, 2004 12–2

Background and Purpose.—Echolucent carotid plaques have been associated with increased risk for stroke. Histological studies suggested that echolucent plaques are hemorrhage- and lipid-rich, whereas echogenic plaques are characterized by fibrosis and calcification. This is the first study to relate echogenicity to plaque composition analyzed biochemically.

Methods.—Echogenicity of human carotid plaques was analyzed by standardized high-definition ultrasound and classified into echolucent, with gray-scale median (GSM) <32 and echogenic with GSM ≥ 32. The biochemical composition of the plaques was assessed by fast-performance liquid chromotography and high-performance thin-layer chromotography.

Results.—As assessed biochemically (milligrams per gram [mg/g]), echolucent plaques contained less hydroxyapatite (43.8 [SD 41.2] mg/g versus 121.6 [SD 106.2] mg/g; $P=0.018$), more total elastin (1.7 [SD 0.4] mg/g versus 1.2 [SD 0.4] mg/g; $P=0.008$), and more intermediate-size elastin forms (1.2 [SD 0.3] mg/g versus 0.8 [SD 0.4] mg/g; $P=0.018$). There was no difference in collagen amount between echogenic and echolucent plaques, neither biochemically (15.3 [SD 3.7] mg/g versus 14.4 [SD 3.4] mg/g) nor histologically (13.4 [SD 4.9] % versus 13.0 [SD 5.6] %). Cholesterol esters, unesterified cholesterol, and triglycerides were increased in plaques associated with symptoms (22.5 [SD 23.3] mg/g versus 13.3 [SD 3.2]; $P=0.04$), but no differences were detected between echolucent and echogenic plaques (13.5 [SD 4.0] versus 20.2 [SD 21.5] mg/g). Similar results were obtained by Oil Red O staining (symptomatic 7.6 [SD 4.7] % versus asymptomatic 4.2 [SD 3.6] %; $P=0.03$; echolucent 5.9 [SD 4.1] % versus echogenic 5.0 [SD 4.0] % of area).

Conclusions.—Echogenicity of carotid plaques is mainly determined by their elastin and calcium but not collagen or lipid content. In addition, echolucency is associated to higher elastin content.

► This is the first study to relate carotid plaque echogenicity to a biochemical analysis of plaque composition. The results suggest that calcification rather than collagen content is the prime determinant of plaque echogenicity. This report is in contradiction to previous reports of histologic analysis relating echogenicity to fibrous tissue content. This is another in a long series of studies hoping to ultimately identify plaque characteristics associated with future neurologic symptoms.

G. L. Moneta, MD

Sex Differences in Carotid Plaque and Stenosis

Iemolo F, Martiniuk A, Steinman DA, et al (Catania Univ, Italy; Univ of Western Ontario, London, Canada; Robarts Research Inst, London, Ont, Canada)

Stroke 35:477-481, 2004 12–3

Background and Purpose.—Women are relatively protected from cardiovascular events; they are 3 times as likely as men to survive to age 90 years. Although clinical trials show an excess of thrombotic events with estrogen/progestin hormone replacement therapy, much experimental and epidemiological evidence suggests that estrogen may have beneficial effects on endothelial function and atherosclerosis, raising the possibility of sex differences in arterial remodeling. We studied sex differences in carotid plaque and stenosis in relation to survival free of stroke, death, and myocardial infarction.

Methods.—A total of 1686 patients from an atherosclerosis prevention clinic were followed annually for up to 5 years (mean, 2.5±1.3 years) with baseline and follow-up measurements; there were 45 strokes, 94 myocardial infarctions, and 41 deaths.

Results.—Carotid stenosis and plaque increased with age. Women had greater stenosis compared with men (P=0.001), whereas men had greater plaque area than did women at all ages (P<0.0001). Stroke, myocardial infarction, and death combined were predicted significantly by plaque area (P=0.004) but not by stenosis (P=0.042).

Conclusions.—Women have more stenosis but less plaque than men, suggesting that differences in sex hormones may affect remodeling of atherosclerosis. Plaque area was a stronger predictor of outcomes than was stenosis.

► It is perplexing why stroke, myocardial infarction, and death were not predicted by carotid stenosis. Perhaps carotid plaque area is a better measure of overall burden of atherosclerosis than carotid artery stenosis. In that regard, it would have been interesting if the authors would have included other measures of atherosclerosis, such as the ankle brachial index, in their study. The study raises the question of whether the vascular laboratory should consider measurement of total plaque burden as part of the assessment of the carotid bifurcation.

G. L. Moneta, MD

Serum Values of Metalloproteinase-2 and Metalloproteinase-9 as Related to Unstable Plaque and Inflammatory Cells in Patients With Greater Than 70% Carotid Artery Stenosis

Alvarez B, Ruiz C, Chacón P, et al (Hosp Universitario Vall d'Hebron, Barcelona)
J Vasc Surg 40:469-475, 2004 12–4

Objective.—Unstable carotid plaques, characterized by increased levels of macrophages and T lymphocytes, have high emboligenic potential and carry a risk for producing cerebral ischemic events. It has been suggested that plaque instability may be mediated by the family of metalloproteinases (MMPs). The purpose of this study was to analyze the relationship between concentrations of MMP-2 and MMP-9 and unstable carotid plaques, presence of macrophages and T-lymphocytes in the plaques, and neurologic symptoms, to establish additional risk markers in patients with greater than 70% carotid artery stenosis. This was a cross-sectional study carried out in a referral center and institutional practice in hospitalized patients.

Methods.—The study included 40 patients with carotid artery stenosis treated with carotid endarterectomy. Of these patients, 67.5% had experienced a previous neurologic event and 32.5% exhibited no symptoms. MMP-2 and MMP-9 levels were determined with enzyme-linked immunosorbent assay 48 hours before surgery. Histopathologic analysis (stable or unstable) and immunohistochemistry (macrophage count, T lymphocytes, activated T lymphocytes) were carried out on the plaques.

Results.—Mean MMP-2 and MMP-9 serum concentrations in the population studied were 1138.27 ± 326.08 ng/mL and 1026.10 ± 412.90 ng/mL, respectively. MMP-2 levels were significantly higher in patients with symptoms compared with patients without symptoms (1247.30 ± 276.80 ng/mL vs 911.80 ± 311.84 ng/mL; $P = .001$). MMP-9 was also significantly higher in the symptomatic group (1026.10 ± 412.90 ng/mL vs 377.84 ± 164.08 ng/mL; $P = .001$) and in patients with unstable plaques compared with those with stable plaques (1006.98 ± 447.09 ng/mL vs 496.16 ± 292.78 ng/mL; $P = .001$). In addition, we found a strong association between elevated MMP-9 concentration and presence of macrophages in plaque (Spearman rho, 0.45; $P = .004$). At logistic regression analysis, variables that best predicted the presence of unstable plaque were a previous neurologic event and MMP-9 level greater than 607 ng/mL (sensitivity, 96%; specificity, 92%; negative predictive value, 94.7%; positive predictive value, 93%).

Conclusion.—Elevated MMP-9 concentration is associated with carotid plaque instability and the presence of macrophages, factors that indicate increased risk for a neurological event. Determination of this gelatinase may enable identification of high-risk subgroups of patients with carotid artery stenosis.

► Two holy grails of carotid research are plaque regression agents and prediction of symptomatic plaques. This article addresses the second. The authors found a high correlation between serum MMP-9, symptoms, and unstable plaques.

Although this is a very intriguing study, in my book it goes down in the "not ready for prime time category." It is a small study that needs to be replicated in a much larger number of patients. Someone needs to show that a person with no symptoms and an elevated MMP-9 level either has or is at risk of having an unstable plaque and that removing the plaque reduces the risk of stroke. We are a long way off from routinely measuring MMP-9 levels in patients.

J. M. Edwards, MD

Progression of Early Carotid Atherosclerosis Is Only Temporarily Reduced After Antibiotic Treatment of *Chlamydia pneumoniae* Seropositivity

Sander D, Winbeck K, Klingelhöfer J, et al (Technical Univ of Munich; Klinikum Chemnitz, Munich)

Circulation 109:1010-1015, 2004 12–5

Background.—*Chlamydia pneumoniae* (Cp) infection has been associated with atherosclerosis and cardiovascular events. There are controversial results regarding the beneficial effects of antibiotic therapy on future cardiovascular end points.

Method and Results.—We determined the long-term effect of a 30-day roxithromycin therapy on intima-to-media thickness (IMT) progression of the common carotid artery in 272 consecutive Cp-positive and Cp-negative patients with ischemic stroke in a prospective, double-blind, randomized trial with a follow-up of 4 years. Cp IgG (≥1:64) or IgA (≥1:16) antibodies were initially found in 125 (46%) patients. During the 3 years before antibiotic therapy, Cp-positive patients showed an enhanced IMT progression even after adjustment for other cardiovascular risk factors (0.12 [0.11 to 0.14] versus 0.07 [0.05 to 0.09] mm/year; $P<0.005$). The 62 Cp-positive patients given roxithromycin showed a reduced IMT progression during the first 2 years compared with the Cp-positive patients without therapy (0.07 [0.045 to 0.095] versus 0.11 [0.088 to 0.132] mm/year; $P<0.01$). However, IMT progression increased again during the third and fourth year to similar values as before treatment. No significant difference in the occurrence of future cardiovascular events was found between both groups during follow-up.

Conclusions.—The only limited positive impact of antibiotic therapy on early atherosclerosis progression in Cp-positive patients observed in our study may explain the negative results of most antibiotic trials on clinical end points.

► Epidemiologic, histopathologic, and in-vitro animal models suggest Cp is an agent that causes or facilitates the development of atherosclerosis. However, several large antibiotic studies have failed to detect a clinical benefit of antibiotic therapy in the prevention of clinical events secondary to atherosclerosis.[1,2] The authors' data suggest long treatments may be required to demonstrate the benefit of antibiotic therapy in reduction of clinical events associated with atherosclerosis. Trials assessing therapy for 2 years are currently in progress.[3]

G. L. Moneta, MD

References

1. Zahn R, Schneider S, Frilling B, et al: Antibiotic therapy after an acute myocardial infarction: A prospective randomized study. *Circulation* 107:1253-1259, 2003.
2. Stone AF, Mendall MA, Kaski JC, et al: Effect of treatment for *Chlamydia pneumoniae* and *Helicobacter pylori* on markers of inflammation and cardiac events in patients with acute coronary syndromes: South Thames Trial of Antibiotics in Myocardial Infarction and Unstable Angina (STAMINA). *Circulation* 106:1219-1223, 2002.
3. Grayston JT: Antibiotic treatment of atherosclerotic cardiovascular disease. *Circulation* 107:1228-1230, 2003.

Focused High-Risk Population Screening for Carotid Arterial Stenosis After Radiation Therapy for Head and Neck Cancer

Steele SR, Martin MJ, Mullenix PS, et al (Madigan Army Med Ctr, Fort Lewis, Wash)

Am J Surg 187:594-598, 2004 12–6

Background.—Cervical radiation for head and neck cancer has been associated with an increased incidence of carotid arterial stenosis. Modern radiation therapy delivers higher doses with increasing long-term survival. Accordingly, the prevalence of radiation-associated carotid stenosis may be higher than previously reported. Phase I of this prospective study was to establish the prevalence of carotid artery stenosis after high-dose cervical radiation.

Methods.—From a prospectively maintained database, we identified patients who had received cervical high-dose radiotherapy (minimum 5,500 cGy). All patients were screened with bilateral carotid arterial duplex ultrasonography. We defined disease as "normal or mild" if the carotid stenosis was <50%, and "significant" if >50%. The relationship between standard demographic risk factors and screening outcomes was then analyzed.

Results.—Screening was performed in 40 patients (mean age 68.2 years, range 26 to 87). Patients received a mean cumulative radiation dose of 6,420 cGy (range 5,500 to 7,680), with a mean duration of 10.2 years since their last radiation treatment. Sixteen patients (40%) had significant carotid artery stenosis. Patients with and without significant stenosis were comparable in terms of age, radiation dose, tobacco use, comorbidities, and postradiation interval (P = not significant). Six patients (15%) had unilateral complete carotid occlusion and 6 patients (15%) had significant bilateral carotid stenosis. Three patients (7.5%) had sustained a previous stroke after radiation therapy.

Conclusions.—The prevalence of carotid arterial disease in patients with prior cervical radiation therapy is clinically significant and warrants aggressive screening as part of routine preradiation and postradiation care. Focused screening of this high-risk population may be cost effective and medically beneficial in terms of risk factor modification and stroke prevention, and will be examined in phase II of this study.

► The authors argue the prevalence of carotid artery disease after radiation therapy warrants aggressive screening as part of postradiation care. However, only 3 (7.5%) patients suffered a stroke after radiation therapy. There is increased risk of carotid intervention in patients with previous radiation therapy and, perhaps, decreased durability of carotid interventions in patients with radiation therapy. It may be the authors' data actually suggest screening for asymptomatic carotid artery stenosis is not indicated after radiation therapy.

G. L. Moneta, MD

Effects of Cholesterol-Lowering With Simvastatin on Stroke and Other Major Vascular Events in 20 536 People With Cerebrovascular Disease or Other High-Risk Conditions

Collins R, for the Heart Protection Study Collaborative Group (Radcliffe Infirmary, Oxford, England)

Lancet 363:757-767, 2004 12–7

Background.—Lower blood cholesterol concentrations have consistently been found to be strongly associated with lower risks of coronary disease but not with lower risks of stroke. Despite this observation, previous randomised trials had indicated that cholesterol-lowering statin therapy reduces the risk of stroke, but large-scale prospective confirmation has been needed.

Methods.—3280 adults with cerebrovascular disease, and an additional 17 256 with other occlusive arterial disease or diabetes, were randomly allocated 40 mg simvastatin daily or matching placebo. Subgroup analyses were prespecified of first "major vascular event" (ie, non-fatal myocardial infarction or coronary death, stroke of any type, or any revascularisation procedure) in prior disease subcategories. Subsidiary outcomes included any stroke, and stroke sub-type. Comparisons are of all simvastatin-allocated versus all placebo-allocated participants (ie, "intention-to-treat"), which yielded an average difference in LDL cholesterol of 1.0 mmol/L (39 mg/dL) during the 5-year treatment period.

Findings.—Overall, there was a highly significant 25% (95% CI 15-34) proportional reduction in the first event rate for stroke (444 [4.3%] simvastatin vs 585 [5.7%] placebo; $p<0.0001$), reflecting a definite 28% (19-37) reduction in presumed ischaemic strokes ($p<0.0001$) and no apparent difference in strokes attributed to haemorrhage (51 [0.5%] vs 53 [0.5%]; rate ratio 0.95 [0.65-1.40]; $p=0.8$). In addition, simvastatin reduced the numbers having transient cerebral ischaemic attacks alone (2.0% vs 2.4%; $p=0.02$) or requiring carotid endarterectomy or angioplasty (0.4% vs 0.8%; $p=0.0003$). The reduction in stroke was not significant during the first year, but was already significant ($p=0.0004$) by the end of the second year. Among patients with pre-existing cerebrovascular disease there was no ap-

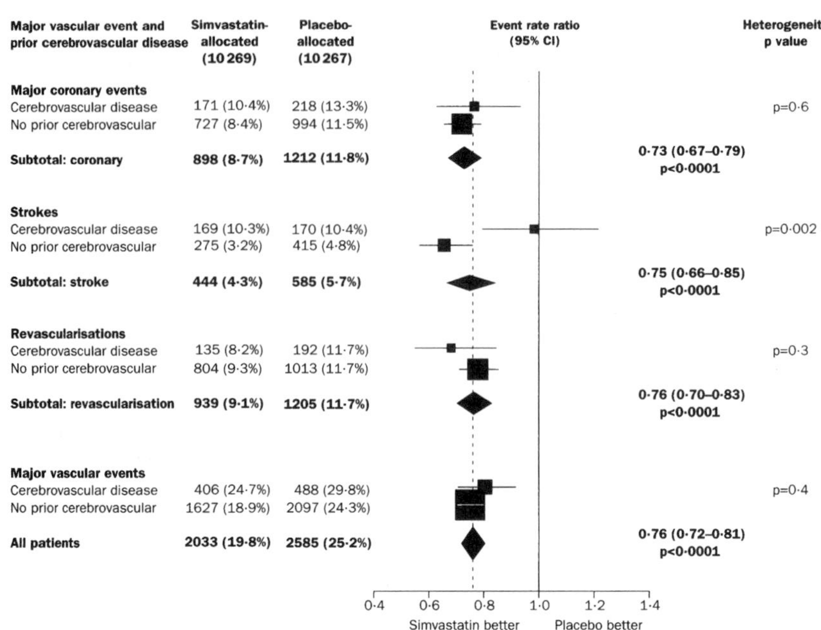

FIGURE 1.—Effects of simvastatin allocation on first major coronary event, stroke, or revascularization in participants subdivided by prior cerebrovascular disease. Analyses are of numbers of participants having a first event of each type during follow-up, so there is some overlap between different types of event. Rate ratios (RRs) are plotted (black squares with area approximately proportional to number of people having events in each subdivision) comparing outcome among participants allocated simvastatin versus placebo, along with 95% CIs (horizontal lines; ending with arrow head when CI extends beyond scale). For particular subtotals and totals, RR and 95% CI are represented by a diamond with values given alongside. P values for χ^2 tests of heterogeneity between RRs in different subcategories are given. Squares or diamonds to the left of the solid vertical line indicate benefit with simvastatin, which is conventionally significant ($p<0.05$) within a particular subcategory considered on its own if the horizontal line or diamond does not overlap the solid vertical line. Broken vertical line indicates the overall RR. (Courtesy of Collins R, for the Heart Protection Study Collaborative Group: Effects of cholesterol-lowering with simvastatin on stroke and other major vascular events in 20 536 people with cerebrovascular disease or other high-risk conditions. *Lancet* 363:757-767, 2004. Reprinted with permission from Elsevier.)

parent reduction in the stroke rate, but there was a highly significant 20% (8-29) reduction in the rate of any major vascular event (406 [24.7%] vs 488 [29.8%]; p=0.001). The proportional reductions in stroke were about one-quarter in each of the other subcategories of participant studied, including: those with coronary disease or diabetes; those aged under or over 70 years at entry; and those presenting with different levels of blood pressure or lipids (even when the pretreatment LDL cholesterol was below 3.0 mmol/L [116 mg/dL]).

Interpretation.—Much larger numbers of people in the present study suffered a stroke than in any previous cholesterol-lowering trial. The results demonstrate that statin therapy rapidly reduces the incidence not only of coronary events but also of ischaemic strokes, with no apparent effect on cerebral haemorrhage, even among individuals who do not have high cholesterol concentrations. Allocation to 40 mg simvastatin daily reduced the rate of ischaemic strokes by about one-quarter and so, after making allowance for non-compliance in the trial, actual use of this regimen would probably reduce the stroke rate by about a third. HPS also provides definitive evidence that statin therapy is beneficial for people with pre-existing cerebrovascular disease, even if they do not already have manifest coronary disease (Fig 1).

► There has been debate regarding the ability of cholesterol-lowering medications to favorably influence stroke rates. This study provides definitive evidence that statin therapy is beneficial for people with cerebrovascular disease and results in reduction of stroke in all categories of patients with extracranial arterial disease.

G. L. Moneta, MD

Different Effects of Antihypertensive Regimens Based on Fosinopril or Hydrochlorothiazide With or Without Lipid Lowering by Pravastatin on Progression of Asymptomatic Carotid Atherosclerosis: Principal Results of PHYLLIS—A Randomized Double-blind Trial

Zanchetti A, for the PHYLLIS Investigators (Univ of Milan, Italy; et al)
Stroke 35:2807-2812, 2004 12–8

Background and Purpose.—The Plaque Hypertension Lipid-Lowering Italian Study (PHYLLIS) tested whether (1) the angiotensin-converting enzyme (ACE) inhibitor fosinopril (20 mg per day) was more effective on carotid atherosclerosis progression than the diuretic hydrochlorothiazide (25 mg per day), (2) pravastatin (40 mg per day) was more effective than placebo when added to either hydrochlorothiazide or fosinopril, and (3) there were additive effects of ACE inhibitor and lipid-lowering therapies.

Methods.—A total of 508 hypertensive, hypercholesterolemic patients with asymptomatic carotid atherosclerosis were randomized to: (A) hydrochlorothiazide; (B) fosinopril; (C) hydrochlorothiazide plus pravastatin; and (D) fosinopril plus pravastatin, and followed up blindly for 2.6 years. B-Mode carotid scans were performed yearly by certified sonographers in 13 hospitals and read centrally. Corrections for drift were calculated from readings repeated at study end. Primary outcome was change in mean maximum intima-media thickness of far and near walls of common carotids and bifurcations bilaterally (CBM_{max}).

Results.—CBM_{max} significantly progressed (0.010±0.004 mm per year; $P=0.01$) in group A (hydrochlorothiazide alone) but not in groups B, C, and D. CBM_{max} changes in groups B, C, and D were significantly different from changes in group A. Changes in group A were concentrated at the bifurcations. "Clinic" and "ambulatory" blood pressure reductions were not significantly different between groups, but total and low-density lipoprotein cholesterol decreased by approximately 1 mmol/L in groups C and D.

Conclusions.—Progression of carotid atherosclerosis occurred with hydrochlorothiazide but not with fosinopril. Progression could also be avoided by associating pravastatin with hydrochlorothiazide.

► We are rapidly moving toward a "cocktail" of drugs for patients with atherosclerosis or at risk of atherosclerosis. This study demonstrates that an ACE inhibitor and a statin can inhibit progression of atherosclerosis at the carotid bifurcation. The effects of ACE inhibitors and statins on cerebrovascular clinical events cannot be determined. Nevertheless, this is another bit of support for essentially routine use of a statin, β-blocker, and now an ACE inhibitor in patients who are at significant risk of progression of atherosclerosis.

G. L. Moneta, MD

Association of Lacunar Infarcts With Small Artery and Large Artery Disease: A Comparative Study

Roquer J, Rodríguez CA, Gomis M (Hosp del Mar, Barcelona)
Acta Neurol Scand 110:350-354, 2004 12–9

Objectives.—Patients with lacunar infarcts (LI) and ipsilateral large artery disease (LAD) greater than 50% must be classified according to the Trial of ORG 10172 in Acute Stroke Treatment (TOAST) criteria as strokes of undetermined etiology. The purpose of this study was to compare the vascular risk factors, clinical symptoms, and outcome characteristics of LI associated with LAD with those patients with LI who fulfilled the TOAST criteria of small artery disease (SAD).

Methods.—Among 1754 consecutive first ever stroke patients admitted to our department, we analyzed age, gender, vascular risk factors (hypertension, diabetes, ischemic heart disease, arterial peripheral disease, hypercholesterolemia, smoking, alcohol, or illicit drug use), clinical data (motor or sensitive deficit and presence of dysarthria), and outcome (hospitalization length, in-hospital medical complications rate, need of rehabilitation, treatment at discharge, in-hospital mortality, and modified Rankin Scale at discharge) of those patients classified as LI associated with LAD as compared with those with SAD.

Results.—After a strict application of the TOAST criteria, we found 144 patients with LI associated with SAD and 73 patients with LI associated with LAD. Univariate analysis showed statistical differences in gender (OR: 0.46; 95% CI: 0.23-0.89; $P = 0.014$), past history of ischemic heart disease (OR: 0.32; 95% CI: 0.13-0.78; $P = 0.004$), and smoking (OR: 0.56; 95% CI: 0.31-1.04; $P = 0.048$). After logistic regression analysis only ischemic heart disease (OR: 0.31; 95% CI: 0.11-0.78; $P = 0.013$), and gender (OR: 0.51; 95% CI: 0.28-0.98; $P = 0.05$) showed statistical differences. During the follow-up, six patients (all with LI associated with LAD) experienced stroke recurrences (OR: 0.32; 95% CI: 0.26-0.39; $P < 0.001$).

Conclusions.—1) There are no differences in clinical presentation and in-hospital outcome between patients with LI associated with SAD and patients with LI associated with LAD. 2) Risk factors are very similar in both groups, and the only differences observed (gender and ischemic heart disease) are related to the atherosclerotic factor. 3) Stroke recurrence seems to be more frequent in LI associated with LAD than in LI associated with SAD, but large follow-up studies are needed to be able to decide whether clinical recurrence of stroke allows to differentiate both clinical entities.

▶ I was taught LIs are due to SAD. The authors of this article point out they may also be due to larger artery and cardioembolic disease. In a series of 1754 first-time stroke patients, 336 were found to have LIs, of which 73 were believed to be due to LAD and 144 due to SAD. Between the groups, very few differences were noted, the most noticeable of which was a higher likelihood of recurrence in the large artery group.

Do not dismiss the lacunar stroke patient as a candidate for carotid evaluation or intervention. The yield may be low—I calculate about 4%—but this is likely a cost-effective range for the use of carotid duplex as a screening tool.

J. M. Edwards, MD

Aspirin and Clopidogrel Compared With Clopidogrel Alone After Recent Ischaemic Stroke or Transient Ischaemic Attack in High-Risk Patients (MATCH): Randomised, Double-Blind, Placebo-Controlled Trial

Diener H-C, for the MATCH Investigators (Univ of Essen, Germany; et al)

Lancet 364:331-337, 2004 12–10

Background.—Clopidogrel was superior to aspirin in patients with previous manifestations of atherothrombotic disease in the CAPRIE study and its benefit was amplified in some high-risk subgroups of patients. We aimed to assess whether addition of aspirin to clopidogrel could have a greater benefit than clopidogrel alone in prevention of vascular events with potentially higher bleeding risk.

Methods.—We did a randomised, double-blind, placebo-controlled trial to compare aspirin (75 mg/day) with placebo in 7599 high-risk patients with recent ischaemic stroke or transient ischaemic attack and at least one additional vascular risk factor who were already receiving clopidogrel 75 mg/day. Duration of treatment and follow-up was 18 months. The primary endpoint was a composite of ischaemic stroke, myocardial infarction, vascular death, or rehospitalisation for acute ischaemia (including rehospitalisation for transient ischaemic attack, angina pectoris, or worsening of peripheral arterial disease). Analysis was by intention to treat, using logrank test and a Cox's proportional-hazards model.

Findings.—596 (15.7%) patients reached the primary endpoint in the group receiving aspirin and clopidogrel compared with 636 (16.7%) in the clopidogrel alone group (relative risk reduction 6.4%, [95% CI −4.6 to 16.3]; absolute risk reduction 1% [−0.6 to 2.7]). Life-threatening bleedings were higher in the group receiving aspirin and clopidogrel versus clopidogrel alone (96 [2.6%] vs 49 [1.3%]; absolute risk increase 1.3% [95% CI 0.6 to

1.9]). Major bleedings were also increased in the group receiving aspirin and clopidogrel but no difference was recorded in mortality.

Interpretation.—Adding aspirin to clopidogrel in high-risk patients with recent ischaemic stroke or transient ischaemic attack is associated with a non-significant difference in reducing major vascular events. However, the risk of life-threatening or major bleeding is increased by the addition of aspirin.

▶ The CAPRIE study established that clopidogrel was more effective than aspirin in reducing cardiovascular end points in patients with vascular disease. This study highlights the old axiom that the enemy of good may be better. The results do not support the use of clopidogrel and aspirin in patients with recent transient ischemic attacks or stroke. At this time, clopidogrel alone appears to be the optimal antiplatelet therapy in such patients.

G. L. Moneta, MD

Stroke Risk After Transient Ischemic Attack in a Population-based Setting

Lisabeth LD, Ireland JK, Risser JMH, et al (Univ of Michigan, Ann Arbor; Univ of Texas, Houston)

Stroke 35:1842-1846, 2004 12–11

Background and Purpose.—Stroke risk after transient ischemic attack (TIA) has not been examined in an ethnically diverse population-based community setting. The purpose of this study was to identify stroke risk among TIA patients in a population-based cerebrovascular disease surveillance project.

Methods.—The Brain Attack Surveillance in Corpus Christi (BASIC) Project prospectively ascertains stroke and TIA cases in a geographically isolated Southeast Texas County. The community is approximately half Mexican American and half nonHispanic white. Cases are validated by board-certified neurologists using source documentation. Cumulative risk for stroke after TIA was determined using Kaplan-Meier estimates. Cox proportional hazards regression was used to test for associations between stroke risk after TIA and demographics, symptoms, risk factors, and history of stroke/TIA.

Results.—BASIC identified 612 TIA cases between January 1, 2000, and December 31, 2002; 60.9% were female and 48.0% were Mexican American. Median age was 73.8 years. Stroke risk within 2 days, 7 days, 30 days, 90 days, and 12 months was 1.64%, 1.97%, 3.15%, 4.03%, and 7.27%, respectively. Stroke risk was not influenced by ethnicity, symptoms, or risk factors.

Conclusions.—Using a population-based design, we found that early stroke risk after TIA was less than previously reported in this bi-ethnic population of Mexican Americans and nonHispanic whites. Approximately half of the 90-day stroke risk after TIA occurred within 2 days.

► Previous reports have indicated the risk of stroke after TIA may be as high as 10% in the first week. This has not been my experience. Although I take TIAs seriously, it is not my practice to rush patients with TIAs off to surgery. I am willing to allow a week or more to pass to evaluate their medical comorbidities when needed. I do not cancel other cases to perform carotid revascularization. This article serves to reinforce this practice pattern. It indicates the risk of stroke is quite low. On the other hand, patients with multiple TIAs, who do not respond to antiplatelet agents and/or anticoagulation, should be treated more urgently.

J. M. Edwards, MD

Transient Ischemic Attacks Are More Than "Ministrokes"

Daffertshofer M, Mielke O, Pullwitt A, et al (Univ Heidelberg, Mannheim, Germany; Landesärztekammer Baden-Wr̈ttemberg, Stuttgart, Germany)

Stroke 35:2453-2458, 2004 12–12

Background and Purpose.—Transient ischemic attacks (TIAs) are warning signs of stroke. Recently, the hypothesis was raised that TIA bears a significant risk for death and dependence and requires the same complex diagnostic workup as a complete stroke.

Methods.—We prospectively collected pre- and in-hospital procedures, symptoms, outcome, complications, and therapies from a representative sample of all stroke-treating hospitals ($n=82$) in southwest Germany. Follow-up was attempted 6 months after discharge. End points were death or dependence in activities of daily living (Barthel Index <95, modified Rankin Scale (mRS) of 3 to 6, or institutionalization in a nursing home).

Results.—1380 TIA patients and 3855 stroke patients entered the database. During hospital stay, stroke incidence was 8% for TIA patients and another 5% within the first half-year. Similarly, for ischemic stroke (IS) patients these figures were 7% and 6% ($P>0.05$), respectively. Two percent of TIA patients died in hospital (5% afterward) compared with 9% of stroke patients (10% afterward, $P<0.001$). Seventeen percent TIA compared with 38% IS patients ($P<0.05$) were dependent at follow-up. Whereas an estimated preexisting deficit (mRS >2) was the strongest predictor for death or disability (baseline mRS odds ratio, 4.1; 95% CI, 2.3 to 7.2), admission to a stroke unit was a valid predictor for survival and independence (odds ratio, 0.4; 95% CI, 0.2 to 0.9).

Conclusions.—These data from a large, multicenter, nonselected, observational study underscore the "not so benign" prognosis for TIA patients. There is a relevant individual risk of early stroke, death, or disability in TIA patients. Management and treatment strategies are similar for both TIA and acute stroke.

► The data indicate hospitalized patients with TIA have a better outcome than hospitalized patients with stroke. This is not surprising. Nevertheless, the risk for death or disability was quite remarkable in the TIA patients. TIA patients perhaps should be treated in a manner similar to acute stroke patients with respect to urgency of evaluation and appropriate therapy. This study is a bit difficult to reconcile with the previous abstract (Abstract 12–11).

G. L. Moneta, MD

Reduced Neuropsychological Test Performance in Asymptomatic Carotid Stenosis: The Tromsø Study

Mathiesen EB, Waterloo K, Joakimsen O, et al (Univ of Tromsø, Norway; Natl Hosp, Oslo, Norway; St Olav's Hosp, Trondheim, Norway)

Neurology 62:695-701, 2004 12–13

Objective.—To assess the relationship between asymptomatic carotid stenosis, neuropsychological test performance, and silent MRI lesions.

Methods.—Performance on several neuropsychological tests was compared in 189 subjects with ultrasound-assessed carotid stenosis and 201 control subjects without carotid stenosis, recruited from a population health study. Subjects with a previous history of stroke were excluded. The test battery included tests of attention, psychomotor speed, memory, language, speed of information processing, motor functioning, intelligence, and depression. Sagittal T1-weighted and axial and coronal T2-weighted spin echo MRI was performed, and presence of MRI lesions (white matter hyperintensities, lacunar and cortical infarcts) was recorded.

Results.—Subjects with carotid stenosis had significantly lower levels of performance in tests of attention, psychomotor speed, memory, and motor functioning, independent of MRI lesions. There were no significant differences in tests of speed of information processing, word association, or depression. Cortical infarcts and white matter hyperintensities were equally distributed among persons with and without carotid stenosis. Lacunar infarcts were more frequent in the stenosis group ($p = 0.03$).

Conclusions.—Carotid stenosis was associated with poorer neuropsychological performance. This could not be explained by a higher proportion of silent MRI lesions in persons with asymptomatic carotid stenosis, making it less likely that the cognitive impairment was caused by silent emboli.

► The impact of carotid stenosis on cognitive function continues to be debated. This article indicates carotid stenosis is associated with adverse performance of some aspects of neuropsyschologic testing. We do not know if it is the carotid stenosis itself or the conditions that lead to carotid stenosis that actually affect neuropsychologic performance. The study does not address whether correction of carotid stenosis results in improvement of neuropsychologic testing or slowed degeneration of neuropsychologic function.

G. L. Moneta, MD

Cognitive Impairment and Decline Are Associated With Carotid Artery Disease in Patients Without Clinically Evident Cerebrovascular Disease

Johnston SC, O'Meara ES, Manolio TA, et al (Univ of California, San Francisco: Univ of Washington, Seattle; Natl Heart, Lung, and Blood Inst, Bethesda, Md; et al)

Ann Intern Med 140:237-247, 2004 12–14

Background.—Whether carotid artery disease is a cause of cognitive impairment in persons who have not had stroke is unknown. If this is the case, diminished performance on the Modified Mini-Mental State Examination should be more common in persons with left carotid artery disease than in those with right carotid artery disease.

Objective.—To determine whether left carotid artery disease is associated with cognitive impairment.

Design.—Cross-sectional and cohort study.

Setting.—Four U.S. communities participating in the Cardiovascular Health Study.

Patients.—4006 right-handed men and women 65 years of age or older without history of stroke, transient ischemic attack, or carotid endarterectomy.

Measurements.—Internal carotid artery stenosis and intima-media thickness of the common carotid artery were assessed by using duplex ultrasonography. Cognitive impairment was defined as a score less than 80 on the Modified Mini-Mental State Examination, and cognitive decline was defined as an average decrease of more than 1 point annually in Modified Mini-Mental State Examination score during up to 5 years of follow-up. Multivariate logistic regression models were used to estimate the risk for cognitive impairment and decline associated with left internal carotid artery stenosis and intima-media thickness, after adjustment for measures of right-sided disease and risk factors for vascular disease.

Results.—After adjustment for right-sided stenosis, high-grade (≥75% narrowing of diameter) stenosis of the left internal carotid artery (32 patients) was associated with cognitive impairment (odds ratio, 6.7 [95% CI, 2.4 to 18.1] compared with no stenosis) and cognitive decline (odds ratio, 2.6 [CI, 1.1 to 6.3]). Intima-media thickness of the left common carotid artery was associated with cognitive impairment and decline in univariate analysis, but this effect did not persist after adjustment.

Conclusions.—Cognitive impairment and decline are associated with asymptomatic high-grade stenosis of the left internal carotid artery. The persistence of the association after adjustment for right-sided stenosis indicates that the association is not due to underlying vascular risk factors or atherosclerosis in general.

▶ I am not quite sure what to make of this study. Thirty-two of the patients had a high-grade left internal carotid artery stenosis and were found to have a significant decrease in cognitive ability during the 5-year follow-up. Clearly, there are multiple reasons for cognitive decline, including alcoholism and Alzheimer's disease, which may not be detectable until later in life or at autopsy.

The authors clearly caution, and I agree, that this study is not evidence for performance of asymptomatic carotid surgery to improve cognition. The topic warrants further study before and after carotid intervention, perhaps as an add-on to another trial of carotid surgery.

J. M. Edwards, MD

Cognition and Quality of Life in Patients With Carotid Artery Occlusion: A Follow-up Study

Bakker FC, Klijn CJM, van der Grond J, et al (Univ Med Ctr Utrecht, The Netherlands; Rudolf Magnus Inst of Neuroscience, Utrecht, The Netherlands)

Neurology 62:2230-2235, 2004 12–15

Background.—Little is known about long-term cognitive functioning and quality of life (QoL) in patients with symptomatic carotid artery occlusion who do not undergo revascularization surgery.

Objective.—To assess the course of cognitive impairment and changes in QoL in these patients and whether impaired cerebral metabolism predicts the course of cognitive functioning.

Methods.—In 73 consecutive patients with TIA or a minor stroke associated with an occlusion of the internal carotid artery (ICA), cognition and health-related QoL in a 1-year follow-up study were examined. The presence of cerebral ischemic lesions was examined by MRI; the metabolic *N*-acetyl aspartate/creatine ratio and the presence of lactate were measured by ^{1}H-MR spectroscopy in the centrum semiovale ipsilateral to the symptomatic ICA occlusion.

Results.—Seventy percent of patients with a stroke and 40% of patients with a TIA were cognitively impaired. In patients with recurrent TIAs during follow-up, cognitive functioning remained at the same (impaired) level (mean impairment score: at baseline 0.7, at 1-year follow-up 0.6; $p = 0.646$). In patients without lactate at baseline and without recurrent symptoms during follow-up, cognitive functioning improved (mean impairment score: at baseline 1.1, at 1-year follow-up 0.7; $p < 0.001$). Self-perceived QoL remained affected at 12 months' follow-up, although not to a large extent (mean SD from norm scores <1).

Conclusions.—In patients with a symptomatic ICA occlusion, cognitive functioning improved within 1.5 years after the ischemic event, if no further symptoms occurred and patients had no lactate at baseline. Self-perceived QoL remained slightly affected.

▶ This was a study of acute cognitive impairment associated with a primary motor event. The results suggest cerebral hypoperfusion associated with an acute event can contribute to cognitive dysfunction. The effects of ICA occlusion appear to extend beyond the temporary motor deficits of TIAs and the permanent motor deficits of stroke.

G. L. Moneta, MD

Vascular Analysis of Individuals With Drop Attacks

Welsh LW, Welsh JJ, Lewin B, et al (Meadowbrook, Pa)

Ann Otol Rhinol Laryngol 113:245-251, 2004 12–16

Background.—There are many and disparate causes of drop attacks, which are described as an abrupt fall to the ground due to a loss of motor tone while maintaining consciousness. The potential mechanisms of drop attacks have been categorized into 5 major divisions for the purpose of clinical analysis. These divisions are cardiac diseases, regional ischemic or perfusion deficits, neurocardiogenic factors, seizure disorders, and miscellaneous factors. The structural arterial abnormalities and perfusion factors that contribute to the drop attack were analyzed, and additional mechanisms relating to other cerebral or cardiogenic disorders that result in abrupt falling were considered.

Methods.—Magnetic resonance angiography (MRA) was chosen for use in this investigation because it can provide a low-risk depiction of the cere-

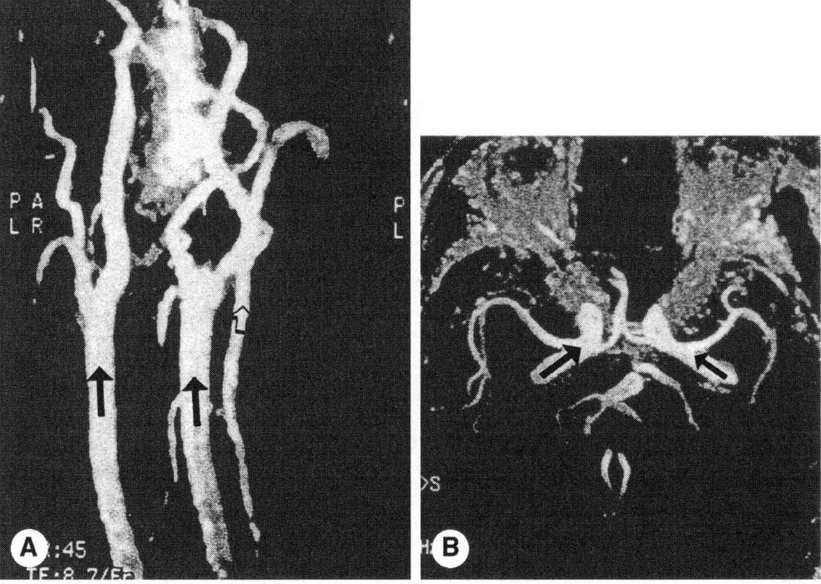

FIGURE 1.—(Case 1). Magnetic resonance angiography. **A**, Cervical region. Patent common carotid arteries are marked by solid arrows, and left vertebral artery by hollow arrow. Right vertebral artery is not visualized because of complete stenosis at point of origin. **B**, Circle of Willis. Large arrows indicate normal internal carotid arteries. Small arrow points to severely atrophic left posterior communicating artery. Right posterior communicating artery is not visualized in this axial view, nor in source images. (Courtesy of Welsh LW, Welsh JJ, Lewin B, et al: Vascular analysis of individuals with drop attacks. *Ann Otol Rhinol Laryngol* 113:245-251, 2004.)

bral and cervical vessels in vivo. MRA was conducted in 10 patients with drop attacks (6 men, 4 women; age range, 56-86 years; mean age, 72.8 years).

Results.—The majority of patients (6 of 10) showed evidence of multifocal vascular disease. Overall, multiple areas of occlusion, stenosis, or hypoplasia were visualized in the images of 8 of the 10 subjects. Specific anomalies of the vertebral and basilar arteries were observed in 4 patients, and in 8 patients there was evidence of nonvisualization of the posterior communicating arteries (Fig 1).

Conclusions.—The pathologic aberrations in the regional circulation of the hindbrain seen in these drop attack patients are supportive of the hypothesis that a transient hypovolemic episode may affect the neural activity involved in maintenance of muscular tone and postural stability.

▶ This report details intracranial MRA in 10 patients presenting with drop attacks. The authors found significant posterior circulation lesions in 8 of the 10 patients. They postulate that episodic hypotension leads to the drop attacks in these patients.

I am consulted about many patients with episodic dizziness. Most of these patients have orthostasis, typically due to their antihypertensive medication. The orthostasis is readily documented with positional blood pressure measurement. A small number of patients have true drop attacks. Until I read this report, I sent these patients for cardiac evaluation and told them I had nothing to offer. This article will change that practice. I will still look for arrythmias, but I will also obtain cerebral MRA to see if there are any lesions that are amenable to angioplasty. In the group of patients described in this article, 4 of the 8 patients had demonstrable lesions of the vertebral and basilar arteries, so perhaps 50% may be candidates for intervention.

J. M. Edwards, MD

Variations in Rates of Appropriate and Inappropriate Carotid Endarterectomy for Stroke Prevention in 4 Canadian Provinces

Kennedy J, Quan H, Ghali WA, et al (Univ of Calgary, Alta, Canada; Univ of Alberta, Edmonton, Canada)

CMAJ 171:455-459, 2004 12–17

Background.—Carotid endarterectomy (CE), when performed on appropriate patients, reduces the incidence of stroke, yet there are marked variations in rates of this procedure. We sought to determine reasons for the variation in CE rates in 4 Canadian provinces.

Methods.—We identified all CEs performed in 4 Canadian provinces between January 2000 and December 2001, inclusive. From chart review and expert assessment, we determined the proportion of these procedures that were appropriate, inappropriate or of uncertain appropriateness, using the RAND/UCLA Appropriateness Method. We sought to determine the varia-

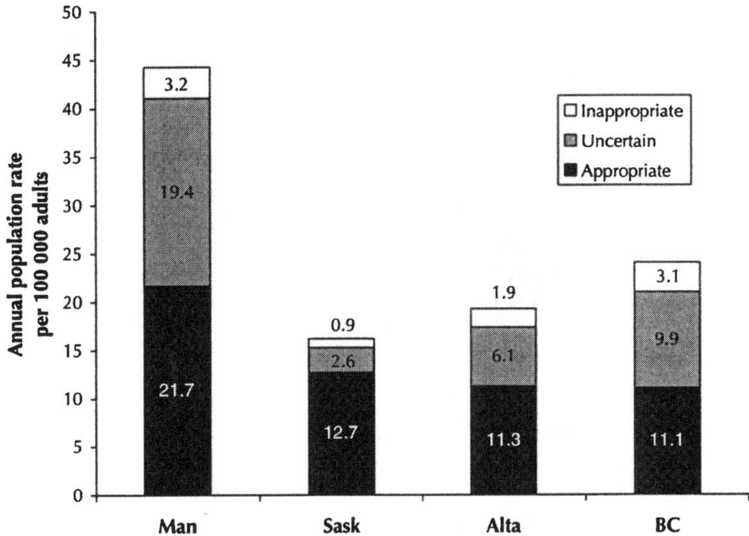

FIGURE 1.—Annual rates of appropriate, uncertain, and inappropriate carotid endarterectomy per 100 000 adults in 2000 and 2001, by province. *Abbreviations: Man*, Manitoba; *Sask*, Saskatchewan; *Alta*, Alberta; *BC*, British Columbia. (Courtesy of Kennedy J, Quan H, Ghali WA, et al: Variations in rates of appropriate and inappropriate carotid endarterectomy for stroke prevention in 4 Canadian provinces. *CMAJ* 171:455-459, 2004. Copyright 2004 Canadian Medical Association.)

tion in rates by province and whether the variation was due to differences in type of hospital, surgical specialty or surgical volume.

Results.—Overall, 1656 (52.3%) of the 3167 CEs studied were performed for appropriate indications. The proportions of appropriate procedures were 78.2% (176/225) in Saskatchewan, 58.7% (481/819) in Alberta, 49.1% (350/713) in Manitoba and 46.0% (649/1410) in British Columbia ($p < 0.001$ across provinces). Rates of appropriate procedures per 100 000 population ranged from 44.3 in Manitoba to 16.2 in Saskatchewan ($p < 0.001$ across provinces). CEs were more likely to be appropriate when performed by a neurosurgeon compared with all other surgeons (74.4% v. 49.4% were appropriate; $p < 0.001$), when performed by surgeons doing fewer than 31 procedures over 2 years compared with surgeons doing more than 31 (70.1% v. 49.5% were appropriate; $p < 0.001$) and when performed in hospitals doing fewer than 135 procedures per year compared with hospitals doing more than 135 (63.4% v. 49.1% were appropriate; $p < 0.001$). Overall, 10.3% of procedures were done for inappropriate reasons.

Interpretation.—Our findings suggest some overuse (for inappropriate or uncertain indications) but also some underuse (low population rates in some regions). High rates of CE are associated with lower rates of appropriateness for both surgeons and hospitals. That 1 in 10 CEs is done inappropriately suggests the need for preoperative assessment of appropriateness (Fig 1).

▶ There is a complex relationship between uncertainty, overuse, and underuse in the performance of any surgical procedure. It is clearly possible to have both over- and underuse of a procedure. It is, however, somewhat disconcerting to note that the appropriateness of carotid endarterectomy in this study was inversely related to surgery and hospital volume. This suggests that surgeons and hospitals performing high volumes of carotid surgery may do so because of a higher volume of inappropriate operations.

G. L. Moneta, MD

Patient Risk Perceptions for Carotid Endarterectomy: Which Patients Are Strongly Averse to Surgery?

Bosworth HB, Stechuchak KM, Grambow SC, et al (Durham Veterans Affairs Med Ctr, NC; Duke Univ, Durham, NC)
J Vasc Surg 40:86-91, 2004 12–18

Background and Purpose.—Patient risk perception for surgery may be central to their willingness to undergo surgery. This study examined potential factors associated with patient aversion of surgery.

Methods.—This is a secondary data analysis of a prospective cohort study that examined patients referred for evaluation of carotid artery stenosis at five Veterans Affairs Medical Centers. The study collected demographic, clinical, and psychosocial information related to surgery. This analysis focused on patient response to a question assessing their aversion to surgery.

Results.—Among the 1065 individuals, at the time of evaluation for carotid endarterectomy (CEA), 66% of patients had no symptoms, 16% had a transient ischemic attack, and 18% had stroke. Twelve percent of patients referred for CEA evaluation were averse to surgery. In adjusted analyses, increased age, black race, no previous surgery, lower level of chance locus of control, less trust of physicians, and less social support were significantly related to greater likelihood of surgery aversion among individuals referred for CEA evaluation. Patient degree of medical comorbidity and a validated measure of preoperative risk score were not associated with increased aversion to surgery.

Conclusions.—In previous work, aversion to CEA was associated with lack of receipt of CEA even after accounting for patient clinical appropriateness for surgery. We identified important patient characteristics associated with aversion to CEA. Interventions designed to assist patient decision making should focus on these more complex factors related to CEA aversion rather than the simple explanation of clinical usefulness.

▶ The authors identified a number of factors that were statistically associated with an aversion to surgery, including increased age, black ethnicity, no previous surgery, less trust of physicians, and less social support. The authors point out physicians typically think the major barriers to obtaining consent for surgery are a lack of understanding of the clinical utility of the surgery.

I admit I have never given a great deal of thought as to why some patients choose to have surgery and others refuse. Several of these factors are intuitive—previous surgery and loss of control. I have also seen studies describing issues of race and interactions with the medical system, but I was unaware that increased age and lack of social support had a relationship with a lower likelihood of consenting to surgery. I plan to change how I talk with patients as a result of this article. I will try to better assess their social support and their feelings about loss of control associated with surgery before asking their consent for a surgical procedure.

J. M. Edwards, MD

Octogenarians With Contralateral Carotid Artery Occlusion: A Cohort at Higher Risk for Carotid Endarterectomy?

Ballotta E, Renon L, Da Giau G, et al (Univ of Padua, Italy)

J Vasc Surg 39:1003-1008, 2004 12–19

Purpose.—Carotid angioplasty and stenting has been proposed as a treatment option for carotid occlusive disease in patients at high risk, including those 80 years of age or older or with contralateral carotid occlusion. We analyzed 30-day mortality and stroke risk rates of carotid endarterectomy (CEA) in patients aged 80 years or older with concurrent carotid occlusive disease.

Methods.—From a retrospective review of 1000 patients undergoing 1150 CEA procedures to treat symptomatic and asymptomatic carotid lesions over 13 years, we identified 54 patients (5.4%) aged 80 years or older with concurrent contralateral carotid occlusion. These patients were compared with 38 patients (3.8%) aged 80 years or older with normal or diseased patent contralateral carotid artery and 81 patients (8.1%) younger than 80 years with contralateral carotid occlusion. All CEA procedures involved either standard CEA with patching or eversion CEA, and were performed by the same surgeon, with the patients under deep general anesthesia and cerebral protection involving continuous perioperative electroencephalographic monitoring for selective shunting. Shunting criteria were based exclusively on electroencephalographic abnormalities consistent with cerebral ischemia.

Results.—The 30-day mortality and stroke rate in patients aged 80 years or older with concurrent contralateral carotid occlusion was zero.

Conclusions.—The concept of high-risk CEA needs to be revisited. Patients with two of the criteria considered high risk in the medical literature, that is, age 80 years or older and contralateral carotid occlusion, can undergo CEA with no greater risks or complications. Until prospective randomized trials designed to evaluate the role of carotid angioplasty and stenting have been completed, CEA should remain the standard treatment in such patients.

▶ This article reinforces my bias that CEA remains the standard therapy in elderly patients requiring intervention for carotid stenosis and that contralateral carotid occlusion is only a minor risk factor for periprocedural stroke. These opinions are based on this article along with other articles demonstrating a higher risk of stroke with carotid artery stenting in patients older than 80 years. This study clearly demonstrates that carotid surgery in an aged population with contralateral carotid occlusion can be carried out with minimal risk of death and stroke.

Until there is information from a randomized trial of CEA versus carotid artery stenting that demonstrates stenting is as good or better than surgery in older patients, I will continue to recommend surgery to the appropriate 80+-year-old patient. This is not a trivial issue, since, at least in the United States, octogenarians are the fastest-growing segment of the population.

J. M. Edwards, MD

Carotid Endarterectomy in Patients With Chronic Renal Insufficiency: A Recent Series of 184 Cases

Ascher E, Marks NA, Schutzer RW, et al (Maimonides Med Ctr, Brooklyn, NY)

J Vasc Surg 41:24-29, 2005 12–20

Background.—The published results of carotid endarterectomy (CEA) in chronic renal insufficiency (CRI) patients are contradictory, mostly because of the relatively small number of patients in these studies. To better assess the neurologic complications and mortality, we reviewed a recent and substantially larger series of CRI patients who underwent CEAs.

Methods.—From March 2000 to March 2003, 675 consecutive primary CEAs were performed in 609 patients (346 men, 57%) under general anesthesia. Asymptomatic carotid artery stenosis accounted for 71% of cases. CRI (serum creatinine level ≥ 1.5 mg/dL) was detected in 166 patients (27%) who underwent 184 CEAs. The remaining 443 patients (73%) had 491 CEAs.

Results.—Patients with CRI were different in age (76 ± 8 years vs 72 ± 9 years, $P < .001$), male gender (73% vs 51%, $P < .001$), coronary artery disease (50% vs 28%, $P < .001$), and diabetes mellitus incidence (38% vs 27%, $P < .02$). No significant difference in stroke rates was observed between the CRI patients and the control group (1.2% vs 0.5%). The mortality rate for CRI patients was 3%, whereas it was 0% for the control group ($P < .002$). The 143 CRI patients with serum creatinine levels from 1.5 to 2.9 mg/dL had a 0.7% mortality rate, whereas it was 17% for 23 patients with serum creatinine levels of 3 mg/dL or more ($P < .001$). The stroke rate for the former group was 0.7% and 4.3% for the latter group (NS). Asymptomatic (16) and symptomatic (7) patients with serum creatinine levels of 3 mg/dL or more had mortality rates of 13% and 28%, respectively, with $P = .6$.

Conclusion.—The high mortality rate observed in patients with serum creatinine levels of 3 mg/dL or more after CEA calls for a nonoperative approach in the management of asymptomatic patients.

▶ I commend the authors for their openness in publishing these data. I would have been tempted to shirk from publishing a subgroup analysis with a stroke and death rate of 17%. I admit to being very conservative about carotid surgery in the patients with creatinines in the 2.5 to 3.0 mg/dL range, but this is more to prevent dialysis-dependent renal failure than because I recognized that there was an extraordinary stroke and death rate; perhaps, this is a case of "being right for the wrong reason." Another take-home message from this article is that to benefit asymptomatic carotid patients with intervention, there has to be both an extremely low rate of periprocedural complications and a reasonable life expectancy—2 things that are not seen in patients with significantly elevated creatinine levels.

J. M. Edwards, MD

Local Versus General Anaesthetic for Carotid Endarterectomy

Rerkasem K, Bond R, Rothwell PM (Chiang Mai Univ, Thailand; Univ of Oxford, England)

Stroke 36:169-170, 2005 12–21

Background.—Carotid endarterectomy (CEA) has been shown to significantly reduce the risk of stroke in persons with recently symptomatic 70% to 99% carotid artery stenosis and to a lesser extent in persons with 50% to 69% stenosis. However, the benefit of CEA is dependent on maintenance of a low operative risk, which may in turn depend to some extent on the type of anesthesia used. Nonrandomized comparisons have suggested that CEA performed with the patient under local anesthesia is associated with a lower operative risk of stroke and death than CEA with general anesthesia. The operative risks of CEA with local anesthesia compared with CEA with general anesthesia were assessed.

Methods.—MEDLINE, EMBASE, and the Index to Scientific and Technical Proceedings were searched for pertinent studies by 2 independent reviewers. In addition, the Stroke Group trials register was searched, and hand searches were conducted of 13 relevant journals and the reference lists of articles identified. Finally, an advertisement of the review was placed in an issue of *Vascular News*.

Results.—Seven randomized trials involving 554 operations and 41 nonrandomized studies involving 25,622 patients were included in this study. However, the methodological quality of many of the nonrandomized trials was questionable. In 9 nonrandomized studies, the number of arteries as opposed to the number of patients, was unclear. Meta-analysis of the nonrandomized studies showed that the use of local anesthetic was associated with significant reductions in the odds of death (35 studies), stroke (31 studies), stroke or death (26 studies), myocardial infarction (22 studies), and pulmonary complications (7 studies) within 30 days of the operation. A meta-analysis of 7 randomized studies showed a nonsignificant trend toward reduced mortality within 30 days of the operation with local anesthesia. However, local anesthesia was associated with a more convincing reduction in local postoperative hemorrhage within 30 days of the operation. There was no evidence of a difference in the odds of operative stroke.

Conclusions.—There is insufficient evidence to allow reliable conclusions regarding the performance of CEA with local anesthesia versus general anesthesia. The findings of nonrandomized studies suggested that there may be potential benefits in the use of local anesthesia, but these studies may be biased.

► There is obvious potential for bias in nonrandomized trials. Overall, one must agree with the Cochrane reviewers. There is no scientifically valid evidence to support one form of anesthesia over another in the performance of carotid endarterectomy.

G. L. Moneta, MD

Prevention of Disabling and Fatal Strokes by Successful Carotid Endarterectomy in Patients Without Recent Neurological Symptoms: Randomised Controlled Trial

Halliday A, for the MRC Asymptomatic Carotid Surgery Trial (ACST) Collaborative Group (St George's Hosp, London; et al)

Lancet 363:1491-1502, 2004 12–22

Background.—Among patients with substantial carotid artery narrowing but no recent neurological symptom (stroke or transient ischaemia), the balance of surgical risks and long-term benefits from carotid endarterectomy (CEA) was unclear.

Methods.—During 1993-2003, 3120 asymptomatic patients with substantial carotid narrowing were randomised equally between immediate CEA (half got CEA by 1 month, 88% by 1 year) and indefinite deferral of any CEA (only 4% per year got CEA) and were followed for up to 5 years (mean 3.4 years). Kaplan-Meier analyses of 5-year risks are by allocated treatment.

Findings.—The risk of stroke or death within 30 days of CEA was 3.1% (95% CI 2.3-4.1). Comparing all patients allocated immediate CEA versus all allocated deferral, but excluding such perioperative events, the 5-year stroke risks were 3.8% versus 11% (gain 7.2% [95% CI 5.0-9.4], p<0.0001). This gain chiefly involved carotid territory ischaemic strokes (2.7% vs 9.5%; gain 6.8% [4.8-8.8], p<0.0001), of which half were disabling or fatal (1.6% vs 5.3%; gain 3.7% [2.1-5.2], p<0.0001), as were half the perioperative strokes. Combining the perioperative events and the non-perioperative strokes, net 5-year risks were 6.4% versus 11.8% for all strokes (net gain 5.4% [3.0-7.8], p<0.0001), 3.5% versus 6.1% for fatal or disabling strokes (net gain 2.5% [0.8-4.3], p=0.004), and 2.1% versus 4.2% just for fatal strokes (net gain 2.1% [0.6-3.6], p=0.006). Subgroup-specific analyses found no significant heterogeneity in the perioperative hazards or (apart from the importance of cholesterol) in the long-term postoperative benefits. These benefits were separately significant for males and females; for those with about 70%, 80%, and 90% carotid artery narrowing on ultrasound; and for those younger than 65 and 65-74 years of age (though not for older patients, half of whom die within 5 years from unrelated causes). Full compliance with allocation to immediate CEA or deferral would, in expectation, have produced slightly bigger differences in the numbers operated on, and hence in the net 5-year benefits. The 10-year benefits are not yet known.

Interpretation.—In asymptomatic patients younger than 75 years of age with carotid diameter reduction about 70% or more on ultrasound (many of whom were on aspirin, antihypertensive, and, in recent years, statin therapy), immediate CEA halved the net 5-year stroke risk from about 12% to about 6% (including the 3% perioperative hazard). Half this 5-year benefit involved disabling or fatal strokes. But, outside trials, inappropriate selection of patients or poor surgery could obviate such benefits.

► This is a later and larger variant of the Asymptomatic Carotid Atherosclerosis Study (ACAS). The study indicates benefit for patients with asymptomatic carotid stenosis who undergo prophylactic CEA. However, the data also indicate that, with good medical care, patients with high-grade carotid stenosis have an annual stroke risk of only about 2% without CEA. In addition, the morbidity and mortality rates of CEA must be low for any benefit to be achieved. Like the ACAS, the authors found no stratification of benefit of CEA in patients stratified for increasing carotid stenosis. In contrast to the ACAS, this study found a benefit for CEA for high-grade asymptomatic carotid stenosis in females.

G. L. Moneta, MD

The Risk and Benefit of Endarterectomy in Women With Symptomatic Internal Carotid Artery Disease

Alamowitch S, for the ASA and Carotid Endarterectomy (ACE) Trial Groups (Tenon Hosp, Paris; et al)

Stroke 36:27-31, 2005 12–23

Background and Purpose.—Perioperative risk and long-term benefit of carotid endarterectomy (CE) are not detailed in women with symptomatic internal carotid artery (ICA) stenosis. Our aim was to compare the efficacy of CE versus medical therapy in women and men with symptomatic ICA stenosis.

Methods.—Data were taken from the North American Symptomatic Carotid Endarterectomy Trial (873 women, 2012 men) and the ASA and Carotid Endarterectomy trial (335 women, 813 men).

Results.—The 30-day perioperative risk of death was higher in women than in men (2.3% versus 0.8%, P=0.002). Higher perioperative risk of stroke and death was also observed (7.6% versus 5.9%) but not statistically significant. With ≥70% stenosis, the 5-year absolute risk reduction (ARR) in stroke from CE was similar between women (15.1%) and men (17.3%). With 50% to 69% stenosis, CE was not beneficial in women (ARR=3.0%, P=0.94), contrary to men (ARR=10.0%, P=0.02). Medically treated women had low risk for stroke. A stroke prognosis instrument (SPI-II) assigned points to 7 factors that identified higher risk for medically treated women: 3 points for hemispheric (not retinal) event, history of diabetes, previous stroke; 2 for age older than 70 years, stroke (not transient ischemic attack); 1 for severe hypertension, history of myocardial infarction. CE was beneficial only for 29.0% of women with 50% to 69% stenosis who had the highest total score of 8 to 15 (ARR=8.9%).

Conclusions.—Women and men with ≥70% symptomatic stenosis had similar long-term benefit from CE, although the perioperative risks were higher for women. CE was not beneficial for women with 50% to 69% stenosis without other risk factors for stroke.

▶ This is a post-hoc subgroup analysis combining data from 2 large studies of similar design but different predetermined goals. Nevertheless, the suggestion that women do more poorly than men with CEA, even for high-grade stenosis, is consistent with the analysis from the European Carotid Surgery Trial as well as the North American Symptomatic Carotid Endarterectomy Trial.

G. L. Moneta, MD

Carotid Endarterectomy Relieves Pulsatile Tinnitus Associated With Severe Ipsilateral Carotid Stenosis

Kirkby-Bott J, Gibbs HH (St Mary's Hosp, London; Princess Alexandra Hosp, Brisbane, Qld, Australia)

Eur J Vasc Endovasc Surg 27:651-653, 2004 12–24

Objectives.—Pulsatile tinnitus is a rare and often disabling condition. Pulsatile tinnitus sometimes occurs in patients with severe atherosclerotic carotid stenosis. It is uncertain whether carotid endarterectomy (CEA) relieves pulsatile tinnitus in patients with severe carotid stenosis.

Design, Materials, and Methods.—This is a retrospective study of 14 patients with pulsatile tinnitus who underwent CEA. Demographic and clinical features and pre-operative duplex results were recorded. Operative results in this group were assessed.

Results.—CEA relieved symptoms of pulsatile tinnitus in 10 out of 14 cases (70%). Of 10 patients that had lateralisable tinnitus and ipsilateral surgery, 9 (90%) reported symptomatic improvement.

Conclusions.—CEA is effective in improving pulsatile tinnitus in patients with unilateral symptoms and severe ipsilateral carotid stenosis.

▶ I have not had a patient in my practice who complained of disabling pusatile tinnitus, although I have had a few patients who have complained of being able to hear a "whooshing" noise in their ear(s) every time their heart beats. The authors of this article quote an incidence of pusatile tinnitus in 2.6% of patients undergoing CEA, which I guess is about what I see. They found that about 70% of their patients had relief of the pulsatile tinnitus after CEA, including 1 who had relief of symptoms contralateral to the operated side.

The utility of this article is small but real. On the rare occasion when I am asked by a patient "Will the whooshing noise in my ear go away after surgery?", instead of answering "I don't know, probably not," I can now say with some confidence "there are 2 of 3 chances that it will." Or, if the symptoms are on the side of the planned surgery, "there is a 90% chance the surgery will relieve the noise symptoms."

J. M. Edwards, MD

Anti-platelet Effect of Aspirin Is Substantially Reduced After Administration of Heparin During Carotid Endarterectomy

Webster SE, Payne DA, Jones CI, et al (Univ of Leicester, England)
J Vasc Surg 40:463-468, 2004 12–25

Objectives.—Aspirin therapy is usually continued throughout the perioperative period to reduce the risk for thromboembolic stroke and myocardial infarction after carotid endarterectomy (CEA). Aspirin irreversibly binds cyclooxygenase-1, thereby reducing platelet aggregation for the lifetime of each platelet. However, recent research from this unit has shown that aggregation in response to arachidonic acid increases significantly, but transiently, during CEA, which suggests that the anti-platelet effect of aspirin is temporarily reversed. The purpose of the current study was to determine when this phenomenon occurs and to identify the possible mechanisms involved.

Methods.—Platelet aggregation was measured in platelet-rich plasma from 41 patients undergoing CEA who were stabilized with 150 mg of aspirin daily. Blood was taken at 8 time points: before anesthesia, after anesthesia, before heparinization, 3 minutes after heparinization, 3 minutes after shunt insertion, 10 minutes after flow restoration, 4 hours postoperatively, and 24 hours postoperatively. Platelet aggregation was also measured at similar times in a group of 18 patients undergoing peripheral angioplasty without general anesthesia.

Results.—All patient platelets were effectively inhibited by aspirin at the start of the operation. There was a significant intraoperative increase in platelet response to arachidonic acid in both groups of patients, which occurred within 3 minutes of administration of unfractionated heparin (Fig 1). In the CEA group this resulted in a greater than 10-fold increase in mean aggregation, to 5 mmol/L of arachidonic acid (5 mmol/L), rising from 3.9% ± 2.2% preoperatively to 45.1% ± 29.3% after administration of heparin ($P < .0001$) This increased aggregation persisted into the early postoperative period, but by 24 hours post operation aggregation had returned to near preoperative values. Aggregation in response to other platelet agonists (adenosine diphosphate, thrombin receptor agonist peptide) showed only a small increase at the same time, which could be accounted for by a parallel increase in the level of spontaneous aggregation.

Conclusion.—Administration of heparin significantly increases platelet aggregation in response to arachidonic acid, despite adequate inhibition by aspirin administered preoperatively. This apparent reversal in anti-platelet

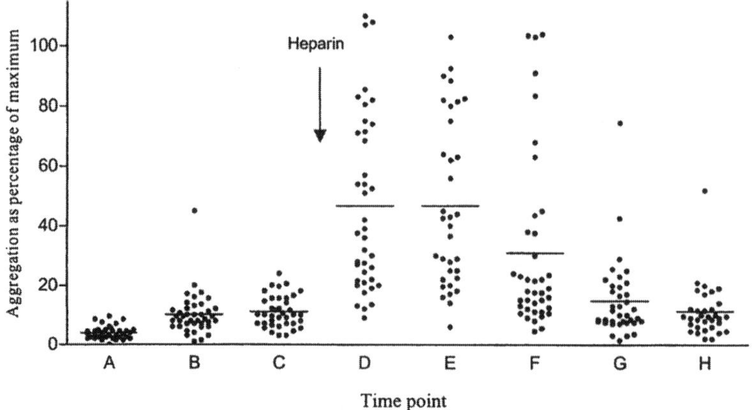

FIGURE 1.—Platelet aggregation in response to arachidonic acid (5 mmol/L) in patients undergoing carotid endarterectomy at time points *A*, pre-operative, at admission to hospital; *B*, After induction of anesthesia but before skin incision; *C*, after skin incision and soft tissue dissection but before heparinization; *D*, 3 minutes after heparin was administered, before insertion of shunt; *E*, 3 minutes after shunt opening; *F*, at the end of surgery, after flow restoration; *G*, 4 hours postoperatively; and *H*, 24 hours postoperatively but before the next dose of aspirin. (Reprinted by permission of the publisher from Webster SE, Payne DA, Jones CI, et al: Anti-platelet effect of aspirin is substantially reduced after administration of heparin during carotid endarterectomy. *J Vasc Surg* 40:463-468, 2004. Copyright 2004 by Elsevier.)

activity persisted into the immediate early postoperative period, and could explain why a small proportion of patients are at increased risk for acute cardiovascular events after major vascular surgery, despite aspirin therapy.

► The data show administration of heparin increases platelet aggregation in response to arachidonic acid. It does not demonstrate that the effect is clinically important. All my vascular surgical patients are on aspirin and all my patients with arterial reconstructions receive heparin intraoperatively. This report is not going to get me to change that practice.

G. L. Moneta, MD

► The authors found a significant increase in the platelet aggregation response to stimuli within minutes of exposure to heparin. This response did not occur in all patients, and it resolved in almost all patients by 4 hours after surgery. I am intrigued by this study. It has been my habit to treat all patients undergoing carotid surgery with low molecular weight dextran. My thought process was more for the thrombogenic surface of the endarterectomized artery than the possibility that the platelets may be activated by heparin, but now I wonder if this treatment may have had other unanticipated, but beneficial, effects.

I hope that this group continues their work and evaluates the effects of heparin on other antiplatelet agents, specifically clopidogrel. Until those data are available, I will treat most patients undergoing carotid surgery with clopidogrel, and I will continue to use dextran intraoperatively.

J. M. Edwards, MD

Beneficial Effects of Clopidogrel Combined With Aspirin in Reducing Cerebral Emboli in Patients Undergoing Carotid Endarterectomy

Payne DA, Jones CI, Thompson MM, et al (Univ of Leicester, England)

Circulation 109:1476-1481, 2004 12–26

Background.—Postoperative thromboembolic stroke affects 2% to 3% of patients undergoing carotid endarterectomy (CEA) and is preceded by 1 to 2 hours of increasing cerebral embolization. Previous work has demonstrated that high rates of postoperative embolization are associated with increased platelet reactivity to adenosine 5'-diphosphate (ADP). Our hypothesis was that preoperative administration of the platelet ADP antagonist clopidogrel could reduce postoperative embolization.

Methods and Results.—One hundred CEA patients on routine aspirin therapy (150 mg) were randomized to 75 mg clopidogrel (n=46) or placebo (n=54) the night before surgery. Platelet response to ADP was assessed by whole-blood flow cytometry. The number of emboli detected by transcranial Doppler within 3 hours of CEA was independently quantified. Time taken from flow restoration to skin closure was used as an indirect measure of the time to secure hemostasis. In comparison with placebo, clopidogrel produced a small (8.8%) but significant reduction in the platelet response to ADP ($P<0.05$) while conferring a 10-fold reduction in the relative risk of those patients having >20 emboli in the postoperative period (odds ratio, 10.23; 95% CI, 1.3 to 83.3; $P=0.01$, Fisher's exact test). However, in the clopidogrel-treated patients, the time from flow restoration to skin closure (an indirect marker of hemostasis) was significantly increased ($P=0.04$, Fisher's exact test), although there was no increase in bleeding complications or blood transfusions.

Conclusions.—This is the first study to show that a CEA patient's postoperative thromboembolic potential can be significantly reduced by targeted preoperative antiplatelet therapy without increasing the risk of bleeding complications.

▶ The data allow one to conclude that the use of clopidogrel as a perioperative antiplatelet agent results in increased time to hemostasis after restoration of flow during CEA. The data do not indicate that a reduction in postoperative embolization detected by transcranial Doppler translates into a reduction in clinical stroke. To determine whether perioperative use of clopidogrel will result in a decrease in stroke after CEA will require a very large, and perhaps not feasible, randomized trial. To determine clopidogrel results in an increase in pesky bleeding during CEA requires only operating on a few patients receiving clopidogrel in conjunction with their CEA. (See also comment to Abstract 12–25.)

G. L. Moneta, MD

Credentialing of Surgeons as Interventionalists for Carotid Artery Stenting: Experience From the Lead-In Phase of CREST

Hobson RW II, for the CREST Investigators (UMDNJ, Newark; et al)

J Vasc Surg 40:952-957, 2004 12–27

Background.—Credentialing of vascular surgeons to perform carotid artery stenting (CAS) continues to be a major issue confronting the specialty of Vascular Surgery. Cannulation of aortic arch branches, and placement of carotid antiembolic devices and stents constitute the major technical challenges to vascular surgeons becoming credentialed to perform CAS. The multicenter Carotid Revascularization Endarterectomy vs Stenting Trial (CREST), supported by the National Institute of Neurological Disorders and Stroke, National Institute of Health, reviews credentials of interventionalists, including surgeons, for the trial's "lead-in" phase of CAS to treat symptomatic (>50% stenosis) and asymptomatic (>70% stenosis).

Methods.—Vascular surgeons requesting participation in CREST must have achieved basic interventional credentialing criteria as recommended by the Society of Vascular Surgery. Each interventionalist is asked to submit notes and narrative summaries from a series of 10 to 30 CAS procedures for review by a multi-specialty review committee before being approved to participate in CREST. Thereafter, during the lead-in phase of CREST, each approved interventionalist is asked to perform CAS procedures using the study devices in as many as 20 patients. In this interim report from the CREST lead-phase, the association of specialty of operator (vascular surgeon, neurosurgeon, other specialist) and periprocedural stroke and death rate was examined in patients undergoing CAS. In addition, current enrollment volume in the lead-in phase by specialty of the principal investigator was examined.

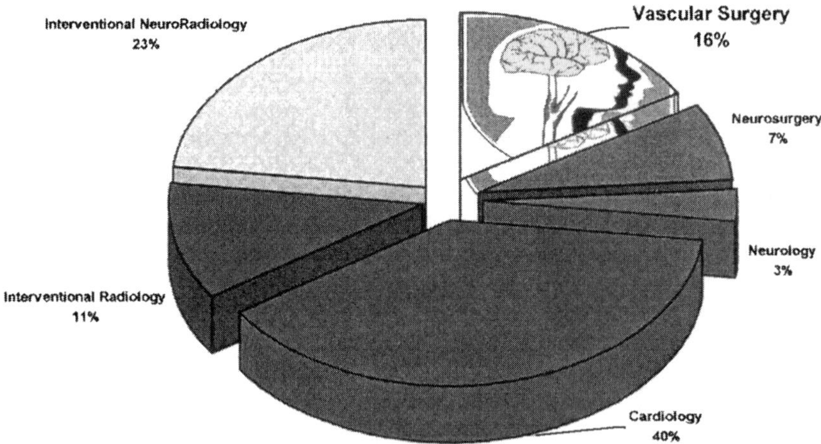

FIGURE 1.—Distribution of interventionalists credentialed by the Carotid Revascularization Endarterectomy vs Stenting Trial (n = 134). (Reprinted by permission of the publisher from Hobson RW II, for the CREST Investigators: Credentialing of surgeons as interventionalists for carotid artery stenting: Experience from the lead-in phase of CREST. *J Vasc Surg* 40:952-957, 2004. Copyright 2004 by Elsevier.)

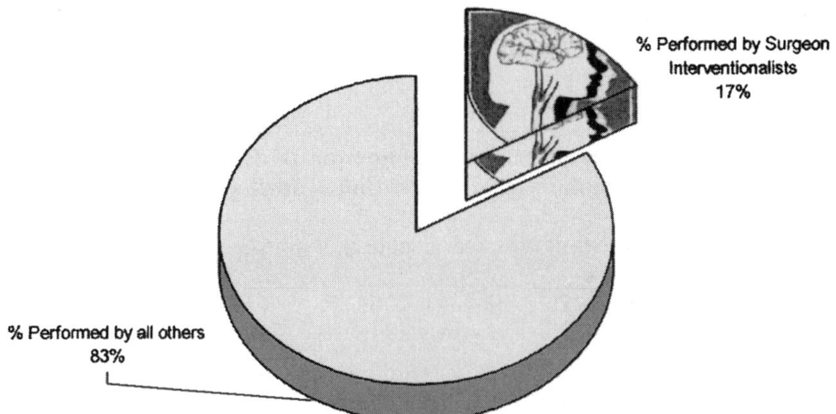

FIGURE 2.—Percentage of lead-in procedures performed by vascular surgeons and neurosurgeons vs all other interventionalists (n = 789). (Reprinted by permission of the publisher from Hobson RW II, for the CREST Investigators: Credentialing of surgeons as interventionalists for carotid artery stenting: Experience from the lead-in phase of CREST. *J Vasc Surg* 40:952-957, 2004. Copyright 2004 by Elsevier.)

Results.—Thirty-two of 134 (23.9%) CREST-credentialed interventionalists are vascular surgeons (n = 22; 16.4%) or neurosurgeons (n = 10; 7.5%). For events monitored through March 31, 2004, 789 patients had undergone CAS procedures performed by these 134 specialists. Thirty-day stroke and death rate was 4.6%, and myocardial infarction was observed in 1.1% of patients. Serious adverse events have not been clustered at individual institutions, and no significant differences have been observed between vascular surgeons or neurosurgeons and other credentialed specialists.

Conclusions.—Vascular surgeons with basic catheter and guide wire skills, particularly those who have incorporated diagnostic cerebral angiography into their practice, can be credentialed to perform CAS. Individuals or groups should devote a number of cases (n = 10-30 per surgeon) to CAS to accomplish this goal. Pending US Food and Drug Administration approval of devices and Center for Medicaid and Medicare Services reimbursement, institutional financial support for the performance of these procedures must be secured. The learning curve for CAS should not be considered so formidable as to discourage surgeons from adding these techniques of CAS to their procedural inventory (Figs 1 and 2).

► This article reviews the credentialing of surgeons, particular vascular surgeons, to be certified interventionalists in the multicenter CREST. The authors note several items of interest: first, that about 25% of the interventionalists in CREST are surgeons (about 16%, vascular surgeons), and second, that the surgeons tend to be quite productive. The authors also suggest, without supporting data, that previous experience with diagnostic cerebral arteriography is helpful in performing interventional cerebral procedures.

Although it appears as if it will be a while before the CREST is completed, it will be interesting to see if the final data breakdown in procedural complications will differ by specialty training. My gut feeling is that there will be no differences, but time will tell.

J. M. Edwards, MD

Training, Competency, and Credentialing Standards for Diagnostic Cervicocerebral Angiography, Carotid Stenting, and Cerebrovascular Intervention

Connors JJ III, for the NeuroVascular Coalition Writing Group (Cardiac and Vascular Inst, Miami, Fla; et al)

AJNR Am J Neuroradiol 25:1732-1741, 2004 12–28

Background.—Recent advances in noninvasive diagnostic neuroimaging have not replaced diagnostic cervicocerebral angiography, which remains the gold standard for evaluation and treatment of patients with cerebrovascular disease. In addition to a high level of technical expertise, the accurate performance and interpretation of diagnostic cervicocerebral angiography are dependent on in-depth cognitive knowledge of related neurological pathophysiology and neurovascular anatomy and pathology and an understanding of the many neurodiagnostic possibilities. The Accreditation Council for Graduate Medical Education (ACGME) has delineated the standards for competency in diagnostic cervicocerebral angiography and interventional procedures. The minimum training and experience necessary to provide adequate quality of patient care for extracranial cerebrovascular interventions, particularly carotid artery stenting, was defined.

Overview.—Stroke and permanent neurological deficit are significant risks associated with diagnostic cerebral angiography. In addition to the technical risk of cerebrovascular procedures, there is also a risk of misdiagnosis as a result of incorrect interpretation of the images. Endovascular interventions are associated with a higher risk than diagnostic angiography in all vascular beds. Potential benefit from "embolism protection" might make carotid stenting safer than is currently documented, but rates of procedural stroke and death still range from at least 2.8% in 1 registry to more than 6% at 30 days in other unpublished registries for both symptomatic and asymptomatic patients. Training guidelines for diagnostic arteriography and endovascular intervention are necessary for optimal and safe patient care. These guidelines have been formulated and published by numerous medical societies. Credentials committees at each hospital and institution must promote adequate standards of training and experience for initial accreditation in diagnostic cervicocerebral angiography that are uniform across all specialties, guarantee patient safety, and ensure continuous high quality of performance. It is expected that these credentials committees will guarantee that individual physicians diagnosing and treating cerebrovascular disease with endovascular procedures have enough formal training and experience in neuroscience and adequate training in the performance and interpretation of diagnostic cervicocerebral angiography and the implications of various findings to optimize the proper expected medical outcomes and ensure patient safety.

Conclusions.—Stringent credentialing criteria with formal neuroscience training as specified by published standards and as described in this document should be mandated for clinicians who perform carotid, vertebral, and intracranial cerebrovascular interventions, as is the case with coronary interventions.

▶ I find this self-serving document, at best, slightly insulting. While I have no issues with a group of societies issuing a joint statement on training, competency, and credentialing standards in the interest of patient safety, I have to wonder if that is the true purpose of this document. My reasoning for doubting the underlying purpose of this document is that somehow a year of specialized training for radiologists, neurologists, and neurosurgeons is enough to qualify as sufficient "cognitive" training but not for vascular surgeons. To totally ignore the fact that training in vascular surgery is additional training after general surgery and specifically includes diagnosis and treatment of cerebrovascular disease to me indicates that this document is more a turf-protecting document than a patient safety document.

It will only be a matter of time before some sharp plaintiff's attorney finds this document and uses it against a member of one of these societies who is performing carotid stenting but does not meet all the qualifications that the document has laid out. I know of at least one interventional radiologist in my city who does not have a certificate of added qualifications in diagnostic neuroradiology and who is performing carotid stenting. Does that mean both he and the hospital that has credentialed him are liable for bad outcomes?

J. M. Edwards, MD

Carotid Plaque Echolucency Increases the Risk of Stroke in Carotid Stenting: The Imaging in Carotid Angioplasty and Risk of Stroke (ICAROS) Study

Biasi GM, Froio A, Diethrich EB, et al (Univ of Milano-Bicocca, Milan, Italy; Gerardo Teaching Hosp, Milan, Italy; Arizona Heart Inst and Found, Phoenix; et al)

Circulation 110:756-762, 2004 12–29

Background.—Carotid artery stenting (CAS) has recently emerged as a potential alternative to carotid endarterectomy. Cerebral embolization is the most devastating complication of CAS, and the echogenicity of carotid plaque has been indicated as one of the risk factors involved. This is the first study to analyze the role of a computer-assisted highly reproducible index of echogenicity, namely the gray-scale median (GSM), on the risk of stroke during CAS.

Methods and Results.—The Imaging in Carotid Angioplasty and Risk of Stroke (ICAROS) registry included 418 cases of CAS collected from 11 international centers. An echographic evaluation of carotid plaque with GSM measurement was made preprocedurally. The onset of neurological deficits during the procedure and the postprocedural period was recorded. The overall rate of neurological complications was 3.6%: minor strokes, 2.2%, and major stroke, 1.4%. There were 11 of 155 strokes (7.1%) in patients with GSM ≤25 and 4 of 263 (1.5%) in patients with GSM >25 (P=0.005). Patients with severe stenosis (≥ 85%) had a higher rate of stroke (P=0.03). The effectiveness of brain protection devices was confirmed in those with GSM >25 (P=0.01) but not in those with GSM ≤25. Multivariate analysis revealed that GSM (OR, 7.11; P=0.002) and rate of stenosis (OR, 5.76; P=0.010) are independent predictors of stroke.

Conclusions.—Carotid plaque echolucency, as measured by GSM ≤25, increases the risk of stroke in CAS. The inclusion of echolucency measured as GSM in the planning of any endovascular procedure of carotid lesions allows stratification of patients at different risks of complications in CAS.

▶ The data indicate that patients with more echolucent plaques and higher degrees of internal carotid artery stenosis are at higher risk of neurologic complications with CAS. The embolic potential of soft (echolucent) plaques is obvious to all who have visualized such plaques at the time of carotid endarterectomy. The higher neurologic complication rate in patients with more severe stenosis may reflect a higher number of embolic particles resulting from crossing a tight lesion with an endovascular device.

G. L. Moneta, MD

Pro-CAS: A Prospective Registry of Carotid Angioplasty and Stenting

Theiss W, for the German Societies of Angiology and Radiology (Medizinische Klinik der Technischen Universität, Munich; et al)

Stroke 35:2134-2139, 2004 12–30

Background and Purpose.—The German Societies of Angiology and Radiology have instituted a prospective registry of carotid angioplasty and stenting (CAS) to limit uncontrolled use of CAS and to collect data about technique and results of CAS outside clinical trials.

Methods.—A total of 38 centers register their patients prospectively before CAS is performed. At discharge, technical details, periprocedural medication, and the clinical course are reported on a standardized form.

Results.—During the first 48 months, 3853 planned interventions were recorded, and CAS was actually attempted on 3267 patients of whom 1827 (56%) were symptomatic and 1433 (44%) were asymptomatic. In 3127 (98%) cases, stents were used, of which 2784 (89%) were of the self-expanding type. Other technical aspects such as the use of guiding catheters and protection devices varied widely among the centers. Periprocedural medication rather uniformly included aspirin and clopidogrel before and after CAS and high-dose heparin and atropin during CAS. CAS was successful in 3207 (98%) cases. There was a 0.6% (n=18) mortality rate, a 1.2%

(n=38) major stroke rate, and a 1.3% (n=41) minor stroke rate. The combined stroke and death rate was 2.8% (n=90).

Conclusions.—These prospective multicenter data are likely to give a realistic picture of the possibilities and limitations of CAS in the general community. They suggest that CAS may be performed with similar results in the general community as they have been reported by highly specialized centers and in clinical studies.

▶ There are ongoing trials evaluating efficacy of CAS versus carotid endarterectomy. These trials will determine the relative utility of the 2 procedures. In the meantime, articles such as this can be used to justify the randomized trials of carotid endarterectomy versus CAS. Because of all the limitations of a registry format, and the very short-term follow-up (in-hospital only) of patients in the registry, this article should not and cannot be used to justify performance of CAS in the community setting.

G. L. Moneta, MD

Routine Use of Cerebral Protection During Carotid Artery Stenting: Results of a Multicenter Registry of 753 Patients

Reimers B, Schlüter M, Castriota F, et al (Cardiology Dept, Mirano, Italy; Ctr for Cardiology and Vascular Intervention, Hamburg, Germany; Villa Maria Cecilia, Cotignola, Italy; et al)

Am J Med 116:217-222, 2004 12–31

Purpose.—To evaluate the short-term outcome of patients who underwent carotid stenting with the routine use of cerebral protection devices.

Methods.—In five centers, 808 successful stent procedures (of 815 attempted) were performed in 753 patients (557 [74%] men; mean [± SD] age, 70 ± 8 years). Cerebral protection involved distal filter devices (n=640), occlusive distal balloons (n=144), or proximal balloon protection (n=24).

Results.—The protection device was positioned successfully in 793 (98.2%) of the 808 attempted vessels. Neurologic complications occurred within 30 days after 46 procedures (5.6%), including seven major strokes, 17 minor strokes, and 22 transient ischemic attacks. There were four deaths (one following a major stroke). The 30-day incidence of stroke and death was 3.3% (27/815). The rate of stroke or death was 3.8% (8/213) for symptomatic lesions and 3.2% (19/602) for asymptomatic lesions ($P=0.87$), and 3.4% (25/729) in patients aged <80 years and 2% (2/86) in those aged ≥80 years ($P=0.81$). Protection device-related vascular complications, none of which led to neurologic symptoms, occurred after nine procedures (1.1%).

Conclusion.—In this uncontrolled study, routine cerebral protection during carotid artery stenting was technically feasible and clinically safe. The incidence of major neurologic complications in this study was lower than in

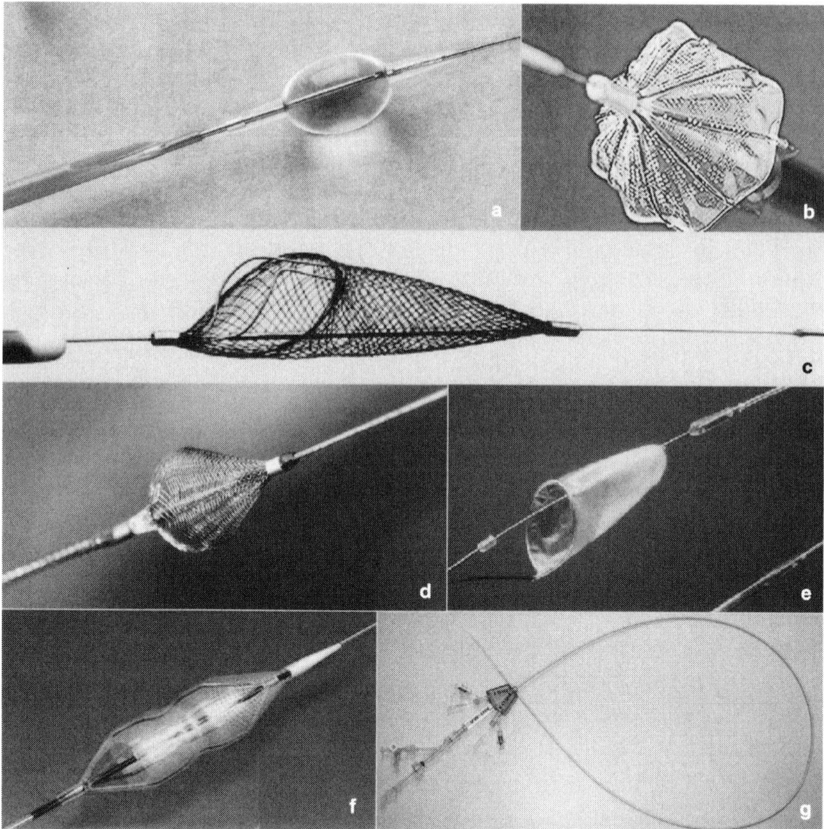

FIGURE.—Cerebral protection systems: (a) distal part of the PercuSurge distal balloon occlusion system (Medtronic, Santa Rosa, California); (b) the AngioGuard XP Filter with a porous polyurethane membrane (Cordis, Miami, Florida); (c) the Spider filter with nitinol basket (ev-3, Plymouth, Minnesota); (d) the Trap nitinol filter device (Microvena, White Bear Lake, Minnesota); (e) the FilterWire (porous polyurethane membrane) (Boston Scientific, Natick, Massachusetts); (f) the NeuroShield Filter (porous polyurethane membrane) (Abbott, Galway, Ireland); and (g) the Mo.Ma proximal balloon occlusion system (Invatec, Cenisio, Italy). (Reprinted from Reimers B, Schlüter M, Castriota F, et al: Routine use of cerebral protection during carotid artery stenting: Results of a multicenter registry of 753 patients. *Am J Med* 116:217-222, 2004. Copyright 2004, with permission from Elsevier Science.)

previous reports of carotid artery stenting without cerebral protection (Figure).

► These results come from a large prospectively maintained registry from 5 European centers. The incidence of major neurologic complications was lower than in previous reports of carotid stenting without cerebral protection. However, this was an uncontrolled study. Outcomes were not ascertained blindly, and no data were provided on long-term outcomes. One can only conclude routine use of cerebral protection devices is practical and may result in a lower rate of neurologic events associated with carotid artery stenting.

G. L. Moneta, MD

Protected Carotid-Artery Stenting Versus Endarterectomy in High-Risk Patients

Yadav JS, for the Stenting and Angioplasty With Protection in Patients at High Risk for Endarterectomy Investigators (Cleveland Clinic Found, Ohio; et al)
N Engl J Med 351:1493-1501, 2004 12–32

Background.—Carotid endarterectomy is more effective than medical management in the prevention of stroke in patients with severe symptomatic or asymptomatic atherosclerotic carotid-artery stenosis. Stenting with the use of an emboli-protection device is a less invasive revascularization strategy than endarterectomy in carotid-artery disease.

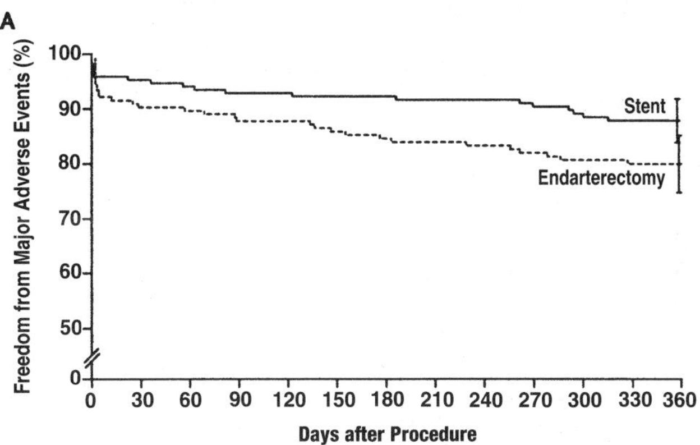

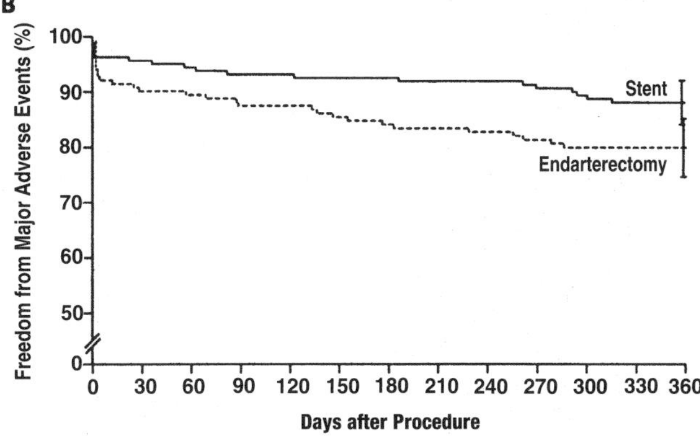

FIGURE 1.—Freedom from major adverse events at one year. In the intention-to-treat analysis (Panel A), the rate of event-free survival at one year was 87.8 percent among patients randomly assigned to carotid stenting, as compared with 79.9 percent among those randomly assigned to endarterectomy (P=0.053). In the actual-treatment analysis (Panel B), the rate of event-free survival at one year was 88.0 percent among patients who received a stent, as compared with 79.9 percent among those who underwent endarterectomy (P=0.048). I-bars represent 1.5 times the SE. (Reprinted by permission of *The New England Journal of Medicine* from Yadav JS, for the Stenting and Angioplasty With Protection in Patients at High Risk for Endarterectomy Investigators: Protected carotid-artery stenting versus endarterectomy in high-risk patients. *N Engl J Med* 351:1493-1501, 2004. Copyright 2004, Massachusetts Medical Society. All rights reserved.)

Methods.—We conducted a randomized trial comparing carotid-artery stenting with the use of an emboli-protection device to endarterectomy in 334 patients with coexisting conditions that potentially increased the risk posed by endarterectomy and who had either a symptomatic carotid-artery stenosis of at least 50 percent of the luminal diameter or an asymptomatic stenosis of at least 80 percent. The primary end point of the study was the cumulative incidence of a major cardiovascular event at 1 year—a composite of death, stroke, or myocardial infarction within 30 days after the intervention or death or ipsilateral stroke between 31 days and 1 year. The study was designed to test the hypothesis that the less invasive strategy, stenting, was not inferior to endarterectomy.

Results.—The primary end point occurred in 20 patients randomly assigned to undergo carotid-artery stenting with an emboli-protection device (cumulative incidence, 12.2 percent) and in 32 patients randomly assigned to undergo endarterectomy (cumulative incidence, 20.1 percent; absolute difference, −7.9 percentage points; 95 percent confidence interval, −16.4 to 0.7 percentage points; $P=0.004$ for noninferiority, and $P=0.053$ for superiority). At one year, carotid revascularization was repeated in fewer patients who had received stents than in those who had undergone endarterectomy (cumulative incidence, 0.6 percent vs. 4.3 percent; $P=0.04$).

Conclusions.—Among patients with severe carotid-artery stenosis and coexisting conditions, carotid stenting with the use of an emboli-protection device is not inferior to carotid endarterectomy (Fig 1).

▶ This study, first published in *USA Today*, has now appeared in *The New England Journal of Medicine*. The differences in the primary end points between the endarterectomy and stented group appear to be primarily driven by the higher number of myocardial infarctions, primarily non–Q-wave, in the endarterectomy group. Nearly three quarters of the patients were treated for asymptomatic stenosis. The applicability of the results of this trial for the overall care of carotid artery disease patients is very limited. Given the narrow therapeutic index of intervention for asymptomatic carotid stenosis, particularly recurrent carotid stenosis, it is likely that the large majority of patients entered into the trial would not have been, in many practices, suitable candidates for any carotid intervention, whether it be endarterectomy or stent. This was a bad trial that should never have been done and should never have been published.

G. L. Moneta, MD

Comparison of Angioplasty and Stenting With Cerebral Protection Versus Endarterectomy for Treatment of Internal Carotid Artery Stenosis in Elderly Patients

Kastrup A, Schulz JB, Raygrotzki S, et al (Univ of Tübingen, Germany; Univ of Jena, Germany)

J Vasc Surg 40:945-951, 2004 12–33

Purpose.—Carotid angioplasty and stenting (CAS) is being evaluated as an alternative to carotid endarterectomy (CEA) for treatment of severe carotid artery stenosis. Because CAS does not require general anesthesia and is less traumatic, it might be especially advantageous in older patients, but data comparing these 2 treatment methods in older patients are scarce.

Methods.—The periprocedural complication rates in 53 patients aged 75 years or older who had undergone protected CAS between June 2001 and April 2004 were compared with those in a group of 110 patients aged 75 years or older who had undergone CEA between January 1997 and December 2001, before widespread introduction of CAS procedures at our institution. All patients were evaluated by a neurologist both before and after surgery. According to the criteria set forth by the large trials the occurrence of minor, major, or fatal stroke, and myocardial infarction within 30 days was determined.

Results.—The demographic characteristics and indications for an intervention were similar in both treatment groups. Thirty patients (57%) in the CAS group had symptomatic carotid stenosis, compared with 69 patients (63%) in the CEA group. In neither group was there any fatal stroke or myocardial infarction. The 30-day stroke rate was significantly higher in the CAS group (4 minor, 2 major strokes; 11.3%) than in the CEA group (no minor, 2 major strokes; 1.8%; $P < .05$). Although the 30-day major stroke rate between CAS and CEA groups was comparable (3.8% vs 1.8%; $P = 0.6$), this effect was mainly attributable to a significantly higher rate of minor stroke in the CAS group (7.5% vs 0%; $P < .05$).

Conclusion.—Despite the use of cerebral protection devices, the neurologic complication rate in patients aged 75 years and older associated with CAS was significantly higher than with CEA performed by highly skilled surgeons at our academic institution. Although this finding is mainly based on a significantly higher rate of minor stroke in the CAS group, the common practice of preferentially submitting older patients to CAS is questionable, and should be abandoned until the results of further randomized trials are available.

▶ The authors reviewed their experience with 53 patients undergoing CAS with cerebral protection during a 3-year period and compared these results with 110 patients who had undergone carotid surgery in the period just before they began using CAS. The reason for the historic control patients was to attempt to prevent bias in treatment choice. This seems both rational and reasonable. Stroke rates in the surgery group were quite low (1.8%), and the overall complication rate in the surgery group was low. The same could not be said for the stenting group, where the stroke rate was 11.3% (major 3.8%, minor 7.5%). The authors note that the 2 patient groups were not selected randomly, but the demographics were very similar. An increased risk of stroke in elderly patients who undergo CAS has been previously noted.[1] No explanation is forthcoming why this group of patients is at increased risk of stroke or at what age the risk of stroke increases. I hope the Carotid Revascularization Endarterectomy versus Stent Trial (CREST) will shed some light on these very important questions, particularly the age cutoff.

J. M. Edwards, MD

Reference

1. Hobson RW II, Howard VJ, Roubin GS, et al: Carotid artery stenting is associated with increased complications in octogenarians: 30-day stroke and death rates in the CREST lead-in phase. *J Vasc Surg* 40:1106-1111, 2004.

Carotid Artery Stenting Is Associated With Increased Complications in Octogenarians: 30-Day Stroke and Death Rates in the CREST Lead-In Phase

Hobson RW II, for the CREST Investigators (Univ of Medicine and Dentistry of New Jersey, Newark; et al)

J Vasc Surg 40:1106-1111, 2004 12–34

Background.—A heightened risk of stroke and death among octogenarians undergoing carotid artery stenting (CAS) has been reported. The multicenter Carotid Revascularization Endarterectomy vs. Stent Trial (CREST) supported by the National Institute of Neurological Disorders, National Institutes of Health, compares the efficacy of carotid endarterectomy (CEA) and CAS in an ongoing clinical trial. This effort also includes a "lead-in" phase of symptomatic (>50% stenosis) and asymptomatic (>70% stenosis) patients. The protocol calls for patients to receive aspirin and clopidogrel before and 30-days after CAS and to be examined by a study neurologist preprocedure, at 24-hours, and at 30-day. The occurrence of stroke and death was reviewed by an independent clinical events committee.

Methods.—The association of age and periprocedural stroke and death was examined in 749 lead-in patients undergoing CAS (30.7% symptomatic, 69.3% asymptomatic). Patients were separated into four age categories: less than 60, 60 to 69, 70 to 79, and 80 years or older, and the proportion of patients with stroke and death during the 30-day periprocedural period was calculated for each category.

Results.—An increasing proportion of patients suffered stroke and death with increasing age (P = .0006); 2 (1.7%) of 120 patients under age 60, 3 (1.3%) of 229 aged 60 to 69, 16 (5.3%) of 301 aged 70 to 79, and 12 (12.1%) of 99 patients aged 80 years and older. These increasingly high complication rates at older ages were not mediated by adjustment for symptomatic status, use of antiembolic devices, gender, percentage of carotid stenosis, or the presence of distal arterial tortuosity.

Conclusions.—Interim results from the lead-in phase of CREST show that the periprocedural risk of stroke and death after CAS increases with age in the course of a credentialing registry. This effect is not mediated by potential confounding factors. Randomized trial data are needed to compare the CAS versus CEA periprocedural risk of stroke and death by age. Pending results from randomized studies, care should be taken when CAS is performed in older patient populations.

▶ The authors describe the early experience with the results during the lead-in phase of the multicenter CREST. During this phase, 749 patients were treated with carotid stenting. When divided into 4 age categories (<60 years, 60-69 years, 70-79 years, ≥80 years), the risk of stroke and death after carotid artery stenting was 1.7%, 1.3%, 5.3%, and 12.1% respectively. This report of an increased risk associated with carotid stenting in elderly patients is not an isolated report.[1] Kastrup et al (Abstract 12–33) found the same results in patients over the age of 75 even though cerebral protection with filter devices were used.

The reason for an increased stroke risk with stenting in the elderly population remains unclear to me. (A difficult arch anatomy may play a role.) The other issue that remains unclear is at what age the risk increases. Is it 70, 75, 80, or some age in between one of these ages? My hope is that the CREST study will answer this question.

J. M. Edwards, MD

Reference

1. Kastrup A, Schulz JB, Raygrotzki S, et al: Comparison of angioplasty and stenting with cerebral protection versus endarterectomy for treatment of internal carotid artery stenosis in elderly patients. *J Vasc Surg* 40:945-951, 2004.

Early Results of Carotid Stent Placement for Treatment of Extracranial Carotid Bifurcation Occlusive Disease

Powell RJ, Schermerhorn M, Nolan B, et al (Dartmouth-Hitchcock Med Ctr, Lebanon, NH; White River Junction Veterans Administration Hosp, Vt)

J Vasc Surg 39:1193-1199, 2004 12–35

Objective.—The purpose of this study was to review the initial results of carotid artery angioplasty with stenting (CAS) performed by vascular surgeons to treat bifurcation occlusive disease. Most patients were selected for CAS if they had indications for endarterectomy (CEA) but were considered at high risk for surgery.

Methods.—Since December 2000, 74 carotid arteries in 69 patients underwent CAS, with distal balloon embolization protection in 96%. Mean patient age was 72 years; 82% of patients were men. Indications for CAS included asymptomatic disease (62%), transient ischemic attack (TIA; 23%), and cerebrovascular accident (15%). Mean internal carotid artery diameter stenosis was 82%. CAS was chosen over CEA because of cardiac

(49%) or pulmonary (4%) comorbid conditions, hostile neck (25%), distal extent of disease (6%), and contralateral cranial nerve injury (1%). CAS was performed in 15% patients who were good surgical candidates, because of patient preference. Pathologic conditions were primary atherosclerosis (81%), recurrent carotid stenosis (18%), and dissection (1%). Procedures were transfemoral in 95% of cases and transcarotid in 5%. In 30% of cases the contralateral carotid artery had 80% or greater stenosis or was completely occluded.

Results.—Technical success was achieved in 96% of cases. There were no deaths, no major strokes, one minor stroke (National Institutes of Health Stroke Scale, 3), and one TIA (neurologic event rate, 2.6%). The single minor stroke resolved completely by 1 month. One patient (1.3%) had a perioperative myocardial infarction. Transient neurologic changes occurred in 8% of patients during the protection balloon inflation, and all resolved with deflation. Bradyarrhythmia requiring pharmacologic treatment occurred in 14% of patients. At mean follow-up of 6 months there have been two instances of recurrent stenosis greater than 50% as noted at duplex scanning. During the same period, 266 carotid CEAs were performed, with a neurologic event rate of 0.8% (major stroke, 0.4%; no minor strokes; TIA, 0.4%) and a myocardial infarction rate of 3%. Combined stroke and death rate was 1.3% in patients who underwent CAS and 0.5% in patients who underwent CEA.

Conclusion.—CAS with cerebral protection can be performed safely in patients at high surgical risk, with low perioperative morbidity and mortality. The durability of the procedure must be determined with longer follow-up.

► The authors reviewed their experience with carotid stent placement with cerebral protection in patients deemed high risk for either anatomical or medical reasons. All procedures were performed by surgeons with catheter skills.

In the 74 high-risk patients treated during a 5-year period, no deaths or major strokes occurred, and the complications were 1.3%, minor stroke; 1.3%, myocardial infarction; and 1.3%, TIA. The take-home message from this article is that well-performed procedures in carefully selected patients, even if they are high risk, will have excellent outcomes. A corollary is that vascular surgeons can be well trained to perform carotid stenting procedures.

J. M. Edwards, MD

Transcervical Carotid Stenting With Internal Carotid Artery Flow Reversal: Feasibility and Preliminary Results

Criado E, Doblas M, Fontcuberta J, et al (Stony Brook Univ, NY; Complejo Hospitalario de Toledo, Spain)

J Vasc Surg 40:476-483, 2004 12–36

Objective.—Transfemoral carotid artery stenting (CAS), with or without distal protection, is associated with risk for cerebral and peripheral embolism and access site complications. To establish cerebral protection before crossing the carotid lesion and to avert transfemoral access complications, the present study was undertaken to evaluate a transcervical approach for CAS with carotid flow reversal for cerebral protection.

Methods.—Fifty patients underwent CAS through a transcervical approach. All patients with symptoms had greater than 60% internal carotid artery (ICA) stenosis, and all patients without symptoms had greater than 80% ICA stenosis. Twenty-one patients (42%) had symptomatic disease or ipsilateral stroke, and 8 patients (16%) had contralateral stroke. Four patients (8%) had recurrent stenosis, 7 patients (14%) had contralateral ICA occlusion, and 1 patient (2%) had undergone previous neck radiation. Twenty-seven procedures (54%) were performed with local anesthesia, and 23 (46%) with general anesthesia. Using a cervical cutdown, flow was reversed in the ICA by occluding the common carotid artery and establishing a carotid-jugular vein fistula. Pre-dilation was selective, and 8-mm to 10-mm self-expanding stents were deployed and post-dilated with 5-mm to 6-mm balloons in all cases.

Results.—The procedure was technically successful in all patients, without significant residual stenoses. No strokes or deaths occurred. There was 1 wound complication (2%). All patients were discharged within 2 days of surgery. Mean flow reversal time was 21.4 minutes (range, 9-50 minutes). Carotid flow reversal was not tolerated in 2 patients (4%). Early in the experience, carotid flow reversal was not possible in 1 patient, and there were 1 major and 3 minor common carotid artery dissections, which resolved after stent placement. One intraoperative transient ischemic attack (2%) occurred in 1 patient in whom carotid flow was not reversed, and 1 patient with a contralateral ICA occlusion had a contralateral transient ischemic attack. At 1 to 12 months of follow-up, all patients remained asymptomatic, and all but 1 stent remained patent.

Conclusion.—Transcervical CAS with carotid flow reversal is feasible and safe. It can be done with the patient under local anesthesia, averts the complications of the transfemoral approach, and eliminates the increased complexity and cost of cerebral protection devices. Transcervical CAS is feasible when the transfemoral route is impossible or contraindicated, and may be the procedure of choice in a subset of patients in whom carotid stenting is indicated.

► While the debate over the relative benefit of CAS and carotid endarterectomy continues, the technique of CAS continues to evolve. One of the primary issues in CAS is distal emboli. The current state of the art appears to be a distal filter, although complications are associated with its use, and it does not prevent all emboli from passing. For this reason, several groups are working on CAS with flow reversal in the carotid system.

I think both flow reversal and distal filters can reduce distal emboli; it is not clear which is preferred. Part of this is due to the fact that some patients have a limited inflow, such as those with contralateral internal carotid artery occlusion, who may not tolerate flow reversal and who will be better off with a distal filter. Also, the technology of the filters will likely improve with time. If I had to guess, I would say that filters will win out because of the fact that they are simpler and do not require a surgeon, even if flow reversal in some ways makes "more sense."

J. M. Edwards, MD

Radiotherapy-induced Supra-aortic Trunk Disease: Early and Long-term Results of Surgical and Endovascular Reconstruction

Hassen-Khodja R, for the University Association for Research in Vascular Surgery (Univ Hosp of Nice, France; Petié-Salpêtriére Univ, Paris)

J Vasc Surg 40:254-261, 2004 12–37

Purpose.—Few articles have dealt specifically with management of radiotherapy-induced supra-aortic trunk disease. We investigated the results of surgical and endovascular treatment of these lesions, and present our findings in a large series of patients.

Methods.—The study was conducted at 11 centers. Over 10 years 64 patients with radiotherapy-induced supra-aortic trunk disease underwent surgical or endovascular treatment. Data were collected retrospectively in a consecutive cohort of patients, and were analyzed with the Kaplan-Meier method.

Results.—Mean patient age was 64.4 years. The indications for radiotherapy included breast cancer (30%), head and neck malignancies (50%), and lymphomas (19%). The mean interval between irradiation and arterial revascularization was 15.2 years. Thirteen of the 64 patients (20%) had asymptomatic disease, and 51 patients (80%) had symptomatic disease. Ninety-two stenotic or occlusive lesions were observed, which involved the common carotid artery (n = 62), the subclavian artery (n = 26), or the innominate artery (n = 4). Twenty-three patients (36%) had multiple supra-aortic trunk lesions, but only 8 patients underwent reconstruction of multiple supra-aortic trunks. Five patients (8%) underwent sternotomy for revascularization from the ascending aorta. Forty-seven patients required revascularization of a common carotid artery; procedures included bypass grafting (n = 30), angioplasty with stent placement (n = 13), carotid-carotid transposition (n = 2), and endarterectomy (n = 2). Fifteen patients underwent restoration of a subclavian artery. One patient died on postoperative day 5, of stroke after early occlusion of an intercarotid crossover bypass graft. Mean follow-up was 37 months (range, 2-120 months). Ten late deaths occurred during follow-up. The probability of survival at 4 years was 78.1% ± 8.6%. During follow-up, 6 patients had stroke, 4 bypass occlusions occurred and 3 stenoses occurred in the revascularized arteries. At 4 years the probability of freedom from stroke was 85% ± 8.8%. At 4 years the primary patency rate was 79.3% ± 8.5% and the secondary patency rate was 87.9% ± 7.2%.

Conclusions.—In light of the context, the results of arterial revascularization to treat radiation-induced arterial lesions of the supra-aortic trunk are satisfactory (Fig 1).

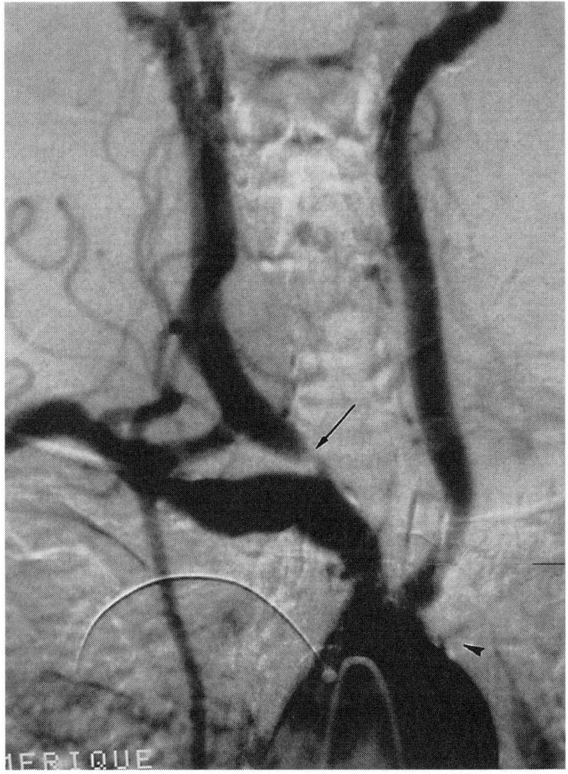

FIGURE 1.—Patient 3. Arteriogram reveals stenosis at the origin of the right common carotid artery (*arrow*) and occlusion of the left subclavian artery (*arrowhead*) in a patient who underwent radiotherapy to treat cancer of the right breast 16 years previously and cancer of the left breast 6 years previously. (Reprinted by permission of the publisher from Hassen-Khodja R, for the University Association for Research in Vascular Surgery: Radiotherapy-induced supra-aortic trunk disease: Early and long-term results of surgical and endovascular reconstruction. *J Vasc Surg* 40:254-261, 2004. Copyright 2004 by Elsevier.)

► This is nice compilation of a large number of patients with a relatively rare problem. I cannot say that I have any immediate use for this article, but I find it reassuring to know that it exists. The patients in this group are in many ways the ones I dread seeing in clinic. Because I work in a tertiary referral center, it is difficult to refer them elsewhere. Yet, although I do see patients like this every few years, I do not have great experience with them. Nothing in the article is really a surprise—angioplasty for short lesions, vein over prosthetic, and so forth.

J. M. Edwards, MD

Restenosis After Carotid Angioplasty, Stenting, or Endarterectomy in the Carotid and Vertebral Artery Transluminal Angioplasty Study (CAVATAS)

McCabe DJH, for the CAVATAS Investigators (Univ College London; et al)

Stroke 36:281-286, 2005 12–38

Background and Purpose.—Carotid and Vertebral Artery Transluminal Angioplasty Study (CAVATAS) patients with carotid stenosis were randomized between endovascular treatment and endarterectomy. The rates of residual severe stenosis and restenosis and their contribution to recurrent symptoms was unclear.

Methods.—Endovascular patients were treated by balloon angioplasty alone (88%) or stenting (22%). Patches were used in 63% of endarterectomy patients. Carotid stenosis was categorized as mild (0% to 49%), moderate (50% to 69%), severe (70% to 99%), or occluded, using standardized Doppler ultrasound criteria at the examination closest to 1 month (n=283) and 1 year (n=347) after treatment. Recurrent cerebrovascular symptoms during follow-up were analyzed.

Results.—More patients had ≥70% stenosis of the ipsilateral carotid artery 1 year after endovascular treatment than after endarterectomy (18.5% versus 5.2%, P=0.0001). Residual severe stenosis was present in 6.5% of patients at 1 month after endovascular treatment. Between 1 month and 1 year, restenosis to ≥70% stenosis occurred in 10.5% of the endovascular group. After endarterectomy, 1.7% had residual severe stenosis at 1 month, and 2.5% developed severe restenosis. The results were significantly better after stenting compared with angioplasty alone at 1 month (P<0.001) but not at 1 year. Recurrent ipsilateral symptoms were more common in endovascular patients with severe stenosis (5/32 [15.6%]) compared with lesser degrees of stenosis at 1 year (11/141 [7.8%], P=0.02), but most were transient ischemic attacks and none were disabling or fatal strokes. There were no recurrent symptoms in the 9 endarterectomy patients with ≥70% stenosis at 1 year.

Conclusions.—Carotid stenosis 1 year after endovascular treatment is partly explained by poor initial anatomical results and partly by restenosis. The majority of patients were treated by angioplasty without stenting. Further randomized studies are required to determine whether newer carotid stenting techniques are associated with a lower risk of restenosis. The low rate of recurrent stroke in both endovascular and endarterectomy patients suggests that treatment of restenosis should be limited to patients with recurrent symptoms, but long term follow up data are required.

► This article should have been dead upon arrival to the editorial office of *Stroke*. It has so little relevance to modern practice that one wonders why it was published. Problems with the CAVATAS study began with the poor initial clinical results with both endovascular and surgical treatment. The fact that stents were used in only a small minority of patients in this study makes the endovascular results irrelevant to modern practice. The duplex criteria for identification of high-grade stenosis used in this study are highly sensitive but, likely, have poor specificity. This may be especially so in the patients treated with stents. We need to hope the CREST investigators do a better job. The CAVATAS study does not help clarify the role of endovascular treatment in the management of carotid artery stenosis. It should sink beneath the waves.

G. L. Moneta, MD

In-Stent Recurrent Stenosis After Carotid Artery Stenting: Life Table Analysis and Clinical Relevance

Lal BK, Hobson RW II, Goldstein J, et al (UMDNJ-New Jersey Med School, Newark)

J Vasc Surg 38:1162-1169, 2003 12–39

Objectives.—Carotid artery stenting has been proposed as an alternative to carotid endarterectomy in cerebral revascularization. Although early results from several centers have been encouraging, concerns remain regarding long-term durability of carotid artery stenting. We report the incidence, characteristics, and management of in-stent recurrent stenosis after long-term follow-up of carotid artery stenting.

Methods.—Carotid artery stenting (n = 122) was performed in 118 patients between September 1996 and March 2003. Indications included recurrent stenosis after previous carotid endarterectomy (66%), primary lesions in patients at high-risk (29%), and previous ipsilateral cervical radiation therapy (5%). Fifty-five percent of patients had asymptomatic stenosis; 45% had symptomatic lesions. Each patient was followed up with serial duplex ultrasound scanning. Selective angiography and repeat intervention were performed when duplex ultrasound scans demonstrated 80% or greater in-stent recurrent stenosis. Data were prospectively recorded, and were statistically analyzed with the Kaplan-Meier method and log-rank test.

Results.—Carotid artery stenting was performed successfully in all cases, with the WallStent or Acculink carotid stent. Thirty-day stroke and death rate was 3.3%, attributable to retinal infarction (n = 1), hemispheric stroke (n = 1), and death (n = 2). Over follow-up of 1 to 74 months (mean, 18.8 months), 22 patients had in-stent recurrent stenosis (40%-59%, n = 11; 60%-79%, n = 6; ≥80%, n = 5), which occurred within 18 months of carotid artery stenting in 13 patients (60%). None of the patients with in-stent recurrent stenosis exhibited neurologic symptoms. Life table analysis and Kaplan-Meier curves predicted cumulative in-stent recurrent stenosis 80% or greater in 6.4% of patients at 60 months. Three of five in-stent recurrent stenoses occurred within 15 months of carotid artery stenting, and one each occurred at 20 and 47 months, respectively. Repeat angioplasty was performed once in 3 patients and three times in 1 patient, and repeat stenting in 1 patient, without complications. One of these patients demonstrated asymptomatic internal carotid artery occlusion 1 year after repeat intervention.

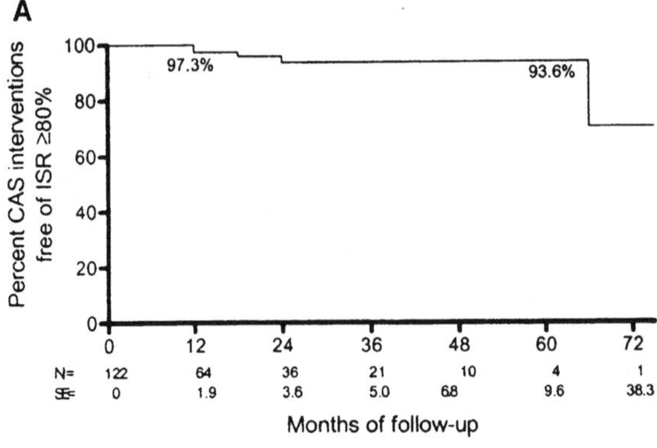

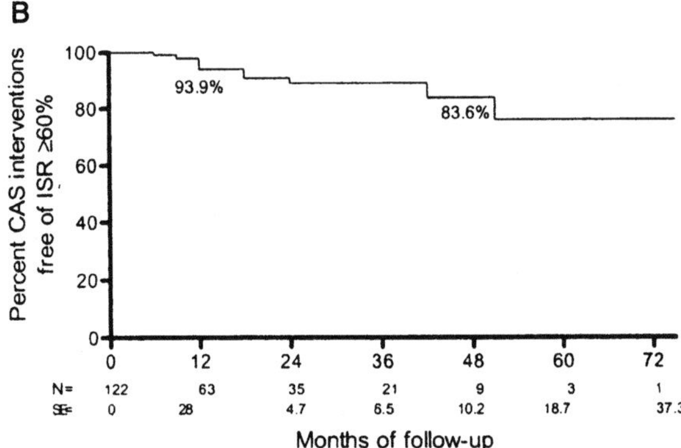

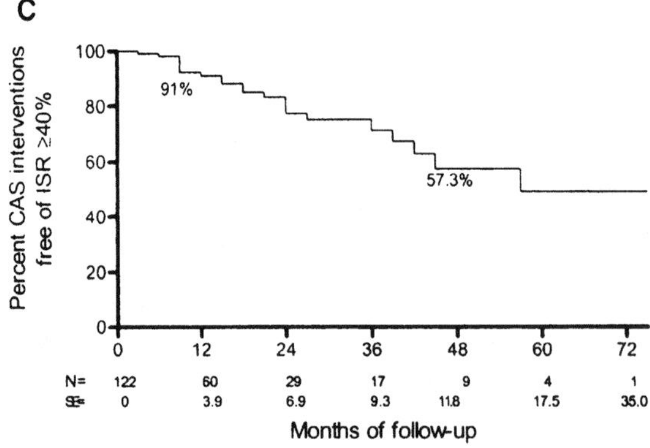

FIGURE 3.—Cumulative life table analysis. **A**, Projected recurrence rates for 1 and 5 years were 2.7% and 6.4%, respectively, for clinically significant disease (in-stent restenosis ≥80%). Cumulative rates of in-stent recurrent stenosis 60% or greater at 1 and 4 years were 6.2% and 16.4%, respectively (**B**), and of in-stent recurrent stenosis 40% or greater were 9.0% and 42.7%, respectively (**C**). (Reprinted by permission of the publisher from Lal BK, Hobson RW II, Goldstein J, et al: In-Stent recurrent stenosis after carotid artery stenting: Life table analysis and clinical relevance. *J Vasc Surg* 38:1162-1169, 2003. Copyright 2003 by Elsevier.)

Conclusions.—Carotid artery stenting can be performed with a low incidence of periprocedural complications. The cumulative incidence of clinically significant in-stent recurrent stenosis (≥80%) over 5 years is low (6.4%). In-stent restenosis was not associated with neurologic symptoms in the 5 patients noted in this cohort. Most instances of in-stent recurrent stenosis occur early after carotid artery stenting, and can be managed successfully with endovascular techniques (Fig 3).

► My major concern about the long-term outcome of carotid stenting has been the risk of in-stent restenosis. To date, there have been few good studies concerning the frequency of this phenomenon. In our local community, I have rarely seen it, and it is not clear to me whether it is more or less common than restenosis is after carotid endarterectomy.

My interpretation of these data is that in a group of patients thought to be at high risk for restenosis, the restenosis rate after stenting is relatively low.

On the basis of this article and other data in the literature, it appears there is not much difference in long-term risk of restenosis between carotid endarterectomy and carotid stenting. I await the outcome of the multicenter Carotid Revascularization Endarterectomy versus Stent Trial (CREST) and other trials to see if this is really true.

J. M. Edwards, MD

Ultrasound-Enhanced Systemic Thrombolysis for Acute Ischemic Stroke

Alexandrov AV, for the CLOTBUST Investigators (Univ of Texas, Houston; et al)

N Engl J Med 351:2170-2178, 2004 12–40

Background.—Transcranial Doppler ultrasonography that is aimed at residual obstructive intracranial blood flow may help expose thrombi to tissue plasminogen activator (t-PA). Our objective was to determine whether ultrasonography can safely enhance the thrombolytic activity of t-PA.

Methods.—We treated all patients who had acute ischemic stroke due to occlusion of the middle cerebral artery with intravenous t-PA within three hours after the onset of symptoms. The patients were randomly assigned to receive continuous 2-MHz transcranial Doppler ultrasonography (the target group) or placebo (the control group). The primary combined end point was complete recanalization as assessed by transcranial Doppler ultrasonography or dramatic clinical recovery. Secondary end points included recovery at 24 hours, a favorable outcome at three months, and death at three months.

Results.—A total of 126 patients were randomly assigned to receive continuous ultrasonography (63 patients) or placebo (63 patients). Symptomatic intracerebral hemorrhage occurred in three patients in the target group and in three in the control group. Complete recanalization or dramatic clinical recovery within two hours after the administration of a t-PA bolus occurred in 31 patients in the target group (49 percent), as compared with 19 patients in the control group (30 percent; P=0.03). Twenty-four hours after

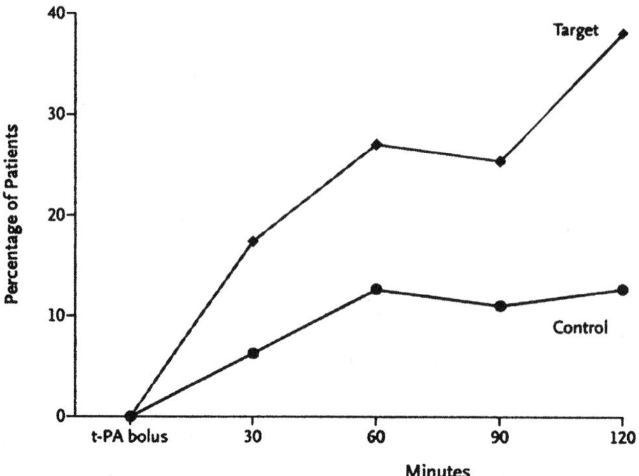

FIGURE 2.—Rate of sustained complete recanalization within two hours after administration of a t-PA bolus. A trend toward the achievement of complete recanalization was observed over time with active treatment with the use of transcranial Doppler ultrasonography. Complete recanalization had occurred at 30 minutes after the t-PA bolus in 4 patients in the control group (6 percent; 95 percent confidence interval, 1.8 to 15.5) and in 11 patients in the target group (18 percent; 95 percent confidence interval, 9.0 to 29.1). At 60 minutes, 8 patients in the control group (13 percent; 95 percent confidence interval, 5.6 to 23.5) and 17 in the target group (27 percent; 95 percent confidence interval, 16.6. to 39.7) had complete recanalization. At 90 minutes, 7 patients in the control group (11 percent; 95 percent confidence interval, 4.6 to 21.6) and 16 in the target group (25 percent; 95% confidence interval, 15.3 to 27.9) had complete recanalization. At 120 minutes, 8 patients in the control group (13 percent; 95% confidence interval, 5.6 to 23.5) and 24 in the target group (38 percent; 95 percent confidence interval, 26.1 to 51.2) had complete recanalization. All 63 patients per group were accounted for at each time point. (Reprinted by permission of *The New England Journal of Medicine* from Alexandrov AV, for the CLOTBUST Investigators: Ultrasound-enhanced systemic thrombolysis for acute ischemic stroke. *N Engl J Med* 351:2170-2178, 2004. Copyright 2004, Massachusetts Medical Society. All rights reserved.)

treatment of the patients eligible for follow-up, 24 in the target group (44 percent) and 21 in the control group (40 percent) had dramatic clinical recovery (P=0.7). At three months, 22 of 53 patients in the target group who were eligible for follow-up analysis (42 percent) and 14 of 49 in the control group (29 percent) had favorable outcomes (as indicated by a score of 0 to 1 on the modified Rankin scale) (P=0.20).

Conclusions.—In patients with acute ischemic stroke, continuous transcranial Doppler augments t-PA-induced arterial recanalization, with a nonsignificant trend toward an increased rate of recovery from stroke, as compared with placebo (Fig 2).

▶ This study indicates enhancement of t-PA therapy with transcranial Doppler in patients with acute ischemic stroke can be achieved safely and may improve the efficacy of systemic therapy with t-PA in cases of acute ischemic stroke. The mechanism of US enhancement of thrombolysis is unclear and may relate to US-induced cavitation effects, resulting in increased permeability of the thrombus to t-PA. The vascular laboratory may someday have a therapeutic role in the treatment of patients with acute ischemic stroke.

G. L. Moneta, MD

Analysis of the Safety and Efficacy of Intra-arterial Thrombolytic Therapy in Ischemic Stroke

Lisboa RC, Jovanovic BD, Alberts MJ (Northwestern Univ, Chicago)

Stroke 33:2866-2871, 2002 12–41

Background and Purpose.—Intra-arterial thrombolytic therapy (IAT) may be a treatment option for patients with ischemic stroke. We analyzed the safety and efficacy of IAT on the basis of published data.

Methods.—We searched computerized databases for studies using IAT in ≥10 patients with ischemic stroke. Some studies had control patients for comparison. Data were collected on age, stroke territory, time to treatment, medication, site of arterial occlusion and recanalization on angiogram, outcomes, and symptomatic intracranial hemorrhage (SICH).

Results.—The analysis included 27 studies with 852 patients who received IAT and 100 control subjects. There were more favorable outcomes in the IAT than in the control group (41.5% versus 23%, P=0.002), with a lower mortality rate for IAT (IAT, 27.2%; control group, 40%, P=0.004). The IAT group had an odds ratio of 2.4 (95% CI, 1.45 to 3.85) for favorable outcome. SICH was more frequent in the IAT group compared with the control group (9.5% versus 3%, P=0.046). The subgroup of patients receiving a combination of intravenous thrombolytic therapy and IAT had more favorable outcomes than the IAT alone subgroup, but this trend did not reach statistical significance (53.6% versus 41.5%, P=0.1). Among the patients treated with IAT, those who had supratentorial strokes were more likely to have favorable outcomes than those with infratentorial strokes (42.2% versus 25.6%; P=0.001; odds ratio, 2.0; 95% CI, 1.33 to 3.0).

Conclusions.—IAT for ischemic stroke appears efficacious but carries an increased risk of SICH. Further prospective studies are needed to prove the safety and efficacy of IAT in stroke.

► This study will not affect my practice patterns. Most of the patients I see with acute stroke have contraindications to thrombolysis. I am on occasion called to the emergency department to see 1 of our vascular clinic patients who has had an acute stroke, but typically the stroke team has also been called. In the rare case where I am going to make the treatment decision, I do not think the data presented in this article are strong enough for me to select intra-arterial thrombolytic therapy over IV thrombolytic therapy.

J. M. Edwards, MD

Frequency of Thrombolytic Therapy in Patients With Acute Ischemic Stroke and the Risk of In-Hospital Mortality: The German Stroke Registers Study Group

Heuschmann PU, for the German Stroke Registers Study Group and for the Competence Net Stroke (Univ of Muenster, Germany; et al)

Stroke 34:1106-1113, 2003 12–42

Background and Purpose.—There is little information about early outcome after intravenous application of tissue-type plasminogen activator (tPA) for stroke patients treated in community-based settings. We investigated the association between tPA therapy and in-hospital mortality in a pooled analysis of German stroke registers.

Methods.—Ischemic stroke patients admitted to hospitals cooperating within the German Stroke Registers Study Group (ADSR) between January 1, 2000, and December 31, 2000, were analyzed. The ADSR is a network of regional stroke registers, combining data from 104 academic and community hospitals throughout Germany. Patients treated with tPA were matched to patients not receiving tPA on the basis of propensity scores and were analyzed with conditional logistic regression. Analyses were stratified for hospital experience with the administration of tPA.

Results.—A total of 13,440 ischemic stroke patients were included. Of these, 384 patients (3%) were treated with tPA. In-hospital mortality was significantly higher for patients treated with tPA compared with patients not receiving tPA (11.7% versus 4.5%, respectively; $P<0.0001$). After matching for propensity score, overall risk of inpatient death was still increased for patients treated with tPA (odds ratio [OR], 1.7; 95% CI, 1.0 to 2.8). Patients receiving tPA in hospitals that administered ≤5 thrombolytic therapies in 2000 had an increased risk of in-hospital mortality (OR, 3.3; 95% CI, 1.1 to 9.9). No significant influence of tPA use for risk of inpatient death was found in hospitals administering >5 thrombolytic treatments per year (OR, 1.3; 95% CI, 0.8 to 2.4).

Conclusions.—In-hospital mortality of ischemic stroke patients after tPA use varied between hospitals with different experience in tPA treatment in routine clinical practice. Our study suggested that thrombolytic therapy in hospitals with limited experience in its application increase the risk of in-hospital mortality.

▶ This study demonstrates 2 issues in the translation of clinical studies to the real world. One is the reluctance of physicians to use drugs with life-threatening side effects unless they are comfortable with them, and the second is that the use of life-threatening drugs or procedures should be done in higher-volume centers. I admit to being a bit surprised that the volume cutoff for tPA is as low as 5 uses per year. I am not surprised that the use of tPA is low. Even in our center, with a dedicated stroke team, the use of tPA is far from universal, and in a center without a dedicated team, I would expect a very low rate.

The higher mortality rate is part of what I see as the trade-off of treatment of stroke with thrombolytics. Some patients will have clot lysis with improvement in flow and resolution of symptoms, but others will suffer intracranial or other hemorrhage and will die. I would expect a slightly higher mortality rate and a higher recovery rate.

J. M. Edwards, MD

13 Vascular Trauma

Blunt Carotid Artery Injury: The Futility of Aggressive Screening and Diagnosis

Mayberry JC, Brown CV, Mullins RJ, et al (Oregon Health & Science Univ, Portland; Los Angeles County/Univ of Southern Calif)

Arch Surg 139:609-613, 2004 13–1

Background.—Blunt carotid artery injury (BCI) remains a rare but potentially lethal condition. Recent studies recommend that aggressive screening based on broad criteria (hyperextension-hyperflexion mechanism of injury, basilar skull fracture, cervical spine injury, midface fracture, mandibular fracture, diffuse axonal brain injury, and neck seat-belt sign) increases the rate of diagnosis of BCI by 9-fold. If this recommendation becomes a standard of care, it will require a major consumption of resources and may give rise to liability claims. The benefits of aggressive screening are unclear because the natural history of asymptomatic BCI is unknown and the existing treatments are controversial.

Hypothesis.—The lack of an aggressive angiographic screening protocol does not result in delayed BCI diagnosis or BCI-related neurologic deficits.

Methods.—A 10-year medical record review of patients with BCI was undertaken in 2 level I academic trauma centers. In both centers, urgent screening for BCI was performed in patients with focal neurologic signs or neurologic symptoms unexplainable by results of computed tomography of the brain as well as in selected patients undergoing angiography for another reason.

Results.—Of 35,212 blunt trauma admissions, 17 patients (0.05%) were diagnosed as having BCI. Six showed no evidence of BCI-related neurologic symptoms during hospitalization or prior to death as a result of associated injuries. Eleven sustained a BCI-related stroke, 9 of whom had it within 2 hours of injury. The remaining 2 had a delayed diagnosis (9 and 12 hours after injury) and received only anticoagulation because the lesions were surgically inaccessible. Just 1 of these 2 patients met the criteria for BCI screening and could have been offered earlier treatment, of uncertain benefit, if we had adopted an aggressive screening policy.

Conclusions.—Of the few patients with BCI, most remain asymptomatic or develop neurologic deficits shortly after injury. Although a widely applied, resource-consuming screening program may increase the rate of early diagnosis of BCI, an improvement in outcome is uncertain. A cost-effectiveness analysis should be done before trauma surgeons accept an aggressive screening protocol as the standard of care.

► Nonselective screening for BCI by angiography or the vascular laboratory is not practical. However, I see no reason why essentially routine CT scans of the head and abdomen in bluntly injured patients cannot be extended to the neck routinely.

G. L. Moneta, MD

Anticoagulation Is the Gold Standard Therapy for Blunt Carotid Injuries to Reduce Stroke Rate

Cothren CC, Moore EE, Biffl WL, et al (Univ of Colorado, Denver; Brown Med School, Providence, RI)

Arch Surg 139:540-546, 2004 13–2

Hypothesis.—Aggressive screening, early angiographic diagnosis, and prompt anticoagulation for blunt carotid artery injuries (CAIs) improves neurologic outcome.

Design.—From January 1, 1996, through December 31, 2002, there were 13,280 blunt trauma admissions to our level I center, of which 643 underwent screening angiography for blunt CAI on the basis of a protocol including injury patterns and symptoms. Patients without contraindications underwent anticoagulation immediately for documented lesions.

Setting.—A state-designated, level I urban trauma center.

Patients.—Of the 643 patients undergoing screening angiography, 114 (18%) had confirmed CAI.

Intervention.—Early angiographic diagnosis and prompt anticoagulation.

Main Outcome Measures.—Diagnosis, stroke rate, and complications stratified by method of intervention.

Results.—A CAI was identified in 114 patients during the 7-year study period; the majority were men (71%), with a mean ± SD age of 34 ± 1.3 years and a mean ± SD Injury Severity Score of 29 ± 1.5. Seventy-three patients underwent anticoagulation after diagnosis (heparin in 54, low-molecular-weight heparin in 2, antiplatelet agents in 17); none had a stroke. Of the 41 patients who did not receive anticoagulation (because of a contraindication in 27, symptoms before diagnosis in 9, and carotid coil or stent in 5), 19 patients (46%) developed neurologic ischemia. Ischemic neurologic events occurred in 100% of patients who presented with symptoms before angiographic diagnosis and those receiving a carotid coil or stent without anticoagulation.

Conclusions.—Our prospective evaluation of blunt CAIs suggests that early diagnosis and prompt anticoagulation reduce ischemic neurologic events and their disability. The optimal anticoagulation regimen, however, remains to be established.

► This report raises 2 principal issues. The first is screening. The aggressive screening program in this article utilized standard catheter-based angiography. That won't work in most places. I think with modern CT scanners, many injuries could be discovered as part of a CT scan performed as a routine assessment of the multiply injured patient (see Abstract 13–1). Once an injury is discovered, anticoagulation appears effective. A stent can be used if the patient can be anticoagulated. Stenting without anticoagulation leads to thrombotic complications. Therefore, significant injuries in patients who cannot be anticoagulated probably should be repaired surgically, even though this is exactly the group of patients in which it would be nice to avoid operation.

G. L. Moneta, MD

Vascular Injuries in Knee Dislocations: The Role of Physical Examination in Determining the Need for Arteriography

Stannard JP, Sheils TM, Lopez-Ben RR, et al (Univ of Alabama at Birmingham)

J Bone Joint Surg Am 86-A:910-915, 2004 13–3

Background.—Popliteal artery injury is frequently associated with knee dislocation following blunt trauma, an injury that is being seen with increasing frequency. The primary purpose of the present study was to evaluate the use of physical examination to determine the need for arteriography in a large series of patients with knee dislocation. The secondary purpose was to evaluate the correlation between physical examination findings and clinically important vascular injury in the subgroup of patients who underwent arteriography.

Methods.—One hundred and thirty consecutive patients (138 knees) who had sustained an acute multiligamentous knee injury were evaluated at our level-1 trauma center between August 1996 and May 2002 and were included in a prospective outcome study. Four patients (four knees) were lost to follow-up, leaving 126 patients (134 knees) available for inclusion in the study. The results of the physical examination of the vascular status of the extremities were used to determine the need for arteriography. The mean duration of follow-up was nineteen months (range, eight to forty-eight months). Physical examination findings, magnetic resonance imaging findings, and surgical findings were combined to determine the extent of ligamentous damage.

Results.—Nine patients had flow-limiting popliteal artery damage, for an overall prevalence of 7%. Ten patients had abnormal findings on physical examination, with one patient having a false-positive result and nine having a true-positive result. The knee dislocations in the nine patients with popliteal artery damage were classified, according to the Wascher modification of the Schenck system, as KD-III (one knee), KD-IV (seven knees), and KD-V (one knee).

Conclusions.—Selective arteriography based on serial physical examinations is a safe and prudent policy following knee dislocation. There is a strong correlation between the results of physical examination and the need for arteriography. Increased vigilance may be justified in the case of a patient with a KD-IV dislocation, for whom serial examinations should continue for at least forty-eight hours.

▶ This series adds to 6 previous retrospective series, involving a total of 283 knee dislocations, that used arteriography selectively to evaluate for vascular injury. While physical examination is clearly effective in screening for popliteal artery injury associated with knee dislocation, it is subjective. The use of the ankle-brachial index (ABI), as proposed by Lynch and Johansen,[1] is preferred and provides objective data. Arteriography can be justified in traumatized limbs with an ABI of less than 0.9.

G. L. Moneta, MD

Reference

1. Lynch K, Johansen K: Can Doppler pressure measurement replace "exclusion" arteriography in the diagnosis of occult extremity arterial trauma? *Ann Surg* 214:737-741, 1991.

Iatrogenic Arterial Injury Is an Increasingly Important Cause of Arterial Trauma

Giswold ME, Landry GJ, Taylor LM, et al (Oregon Health and Sciences Univ, Portland)

Am J Surg 187:590-593, 2004 13–4

Background.—Iatrogenic arterial injuries (IAI) may result from any invasive diagnostic or therapeutic procedure. The relative occurrence and severity of IAI compared with those of penetrating and blunt vascular trauma is unknown. A review of arterial trauma at a university hospital level 1 trauma center, with a focus on iatrogenic injury, forms the basis of this report.

Methods.—Patients treated for arterial trauma from January 1994 through October 2002 were identified from prospectively maintained registries. Record review included injury etiology, type of repair, 30-day all-cause mortality, and permanent morbidity. Permanent morbidity was defined as amputation or loss of extremity function.

Results.—In all, 252 patients required treatment, 85 (33.7%) from IAI, 86 (34.1 %) from penetrating trauma, and 81 (32.1%) from blunt trauma. During the study period, the number of IAIs per year increased (Fig 1). Femoral artery injury from percutaneous intervention (50, 58.8%) was the most frequent IAI; intraoperative injury (including 14 tumor resections and 5 orthopedic procedures) was next most frequent (23, 27.1%). Three patients (3.5%) with IAI had permanent morbidity. The 30-day all-cause mortality was 7.1% (6) for patients with IAI.

Conclusions.—Iatrogenic arterial injury is increasingly frequent and caused one third of the arterial trauma at our level 1 trauma center. These data suggest education and training regarding IAI deserves equal priority with the study of penetrating vascular trauma.

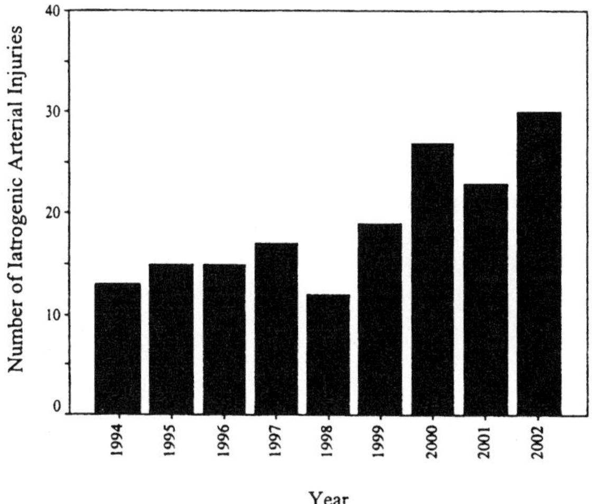

FIGURE 1.—Number of iatrogenic arterial injuries per year from 1994 through 2002. (Reprinted from Giswold ME, Landry GJ, Taylor LM, et al: Iatrogenic arterial injury is an increasingly important cause of arterial trauma. *Am J Surg* 187:590-593, 2004. Copyright 2004, with permission from Excerpta Medica Inc.)

▶ The study points out vascular injury is not just a problem of our major urban war zone trauma centers. As more and more people with various levels of training stick holes in arteries, the number of IAIs can only be expected to increase.

G. L. Moneta, MD

The Role of Clinical Examination in Excluding Vascular Injury in Haemodynamically Stable Patients With Gunshot Wounds to the Neck. A Prospective Study of 59 Patients

Mohammaed GS, Pillay WR, Barker P, et al (Univ of Natal, Durban, South Africa)

Eur J Vasc Endovasc Surg 28:425-430, 2004 13–5

Objective.—To prospectively evaluate the safety and accuracy of physical examination in determining the management of stable patients with gunshot wounds to the neck.

Design.—Prospective study of 59 patients with gunshot wounds to the neck.

Patients and Methods.—Fifty-nine stable patients with gunshot wounds to the neck managed between December 2001 and August 2003. All patients had a physical examination and routine angiography according to a written protocol approved by the research ethics committee. The sensitivity, specificity, and predictive values of physical examination were assessed and compared with the angiographic findings.

Results.—Thirteen patients with positive findings on physical examination (history of bleeding, haematoma, minimal bleeding, thrill, bruit and pulse deficit) and 10 patients without clinical signs of vascular injury had vascular injury. A sensitivity of 57%, specificity 53%, positive predictive value 43% and negative predictive value of 67% were calculated for physical examination alone in detecting vascular injury.

Conclusion.—Findings on physical examination are not good predictors of vascular injury in stable patients with gunshot wounds to the neck. Our findings question the validity of physical examination alone, as a safe and accurate assessment of patients with gunshot wounds to the neck. Arteriography or ultrasonography is needed to identify vascular injuries.

▶ Two previous articles suggested physical examination was an important component in ruling out vascular injury in the neck after penetrating trauma.[1,2] This was not the case in this series. Thirty-four percent of the vascular injuries in the neck after gunshot wounds were missed by physical examination. This article argues strongly for continued use of objective imaging studies in the assessment of penetrating injuries to the neck.

G. L. Moneta, MD

References

1. Sekharan J, Dennis JW, Veldenz HC, et al: Continued experience with physical examination alone for evaluation and management of penetrating zone 2 neck injuries: Results of 145 cases. *J Vasc Surg* 32:483-489, 2000.
2. Gasparri MG, Lorelli DR, Kralovich KA, et al: Physical examination plus chest radiography in penetrating periclavicular trauma: The appropriate trigger for angiography. *J Trauma* 49:1029-1033, 2000.

Vascular Injury During Anterior Lumbar Surgery

Brau SA, Delamarter RB, Schiffman ML, et al (Spine Access Surgery Associates, Los Angeles; Univ of California, Los Angeles; Occupational Care Centers of Los Angeles; et al)

Spine J 4:409-412, 2004 13–6

Background Context.—With the number of anterior lumbar procedures expected to increase significantly over the next few years, it is important for spine surgeons to have a good understanding about the incidence of vascular complications during these operations.

Purpose.—To determine the incidence of vascular injury in 1,315 consecutive cases undergoing anterior lumbar surgery at various levels from L2 to S1.

Study Design/Setting.—Patients undergoing anterior lumbar surgery were studied.

Patient Sample.—A total of 1,310 consecutive patients undergoing 1,315 anterior lumbar procedures between August 1997 and December 2002 were included in the study.

Outcome Measures.—All patients were evaluated for incidence of vascular injury during and immediately after surgery.

Method.—A concurrent database was maintained on all these cases. All the patients had distal pulse evaluation preoperatively. Patients with venous injuries were further analyzed to determine location and extent of injury, amount of blood loss, completion of the procedure and postoperative sequelae. Patients with pulse deficits or evidence of ischemia during or immediately after surgery were further analyzed in particular in relation to demographic, preoperative variables and management.

Results.—Six patients were identified as having left iliac artery thrombosis (0.45%), and 19 had major vein lacerations (1.4%).

Conclusion.—This study shows that the incidence of vascular injury is relatively low (25 in 1,315 or 1.9%). Because only five of these patients experienced significant sequelae from the approach, it appears that anterior lumbar surgery is quite safe, although it must be carried out with utmost respect for the vessels to avoid possible catastrophic outcomes.

▶ Anterior exposure of the lumbar spine results in a small incidence of injuries to the iliac arteries and veins and, occasionally, to the vena cava at the level of the iliac bifurcation. These injuries can be very difficult to manage intraoperatively, and deep venous thrombosis and ischemic limbs can result. This can be a major surprise to a patient, and the result is often a lawsuit. If one is going to participate in these operations, it is worthwhile to spend some time becoming familiar with the techniques involved. Just because you operate in the retroperitoneum does not mean you are familiar with the extensive mobilization of the vessels that can be required in these cases. Books are not just for doorstops.

G. L. Moneta, MD

An Analysis of 124 Surgically Managed Brachial Artery Injuries

Zellweger R, Hess F, Nicol A, et al (Univ of Cape Town, South Africa)

Am J Surg 188:240-245, 2004 13–7

Background.—A 3-year review of surgically managed brachial artery injuries is presented.

Methods.—The medical records were analyzed for demographic data, mechanism of injury, associated injuries, treatment, and outcome.

Results.—There were 113 males and 11 females with a mean age of 28.7 years. The majority of the injuries were caused by stab and gunshot wounds in 57.3% and 29%, respectively. Primary anastomosis was possible in 47 patients, whereas 73 patients required vein interposition grafting. Lower arm fasciotomy was performed in 15 patients (12.1%) (Fig 1). Associated injuries included peripheral nerve lesions in 77 (62.1%), nonpaired brachial vein injuries in 17 (13.7%), and concomitant humerus fracture in 12 (9.7%) patients. Thirty-nine patients (31.5%) had remote injuries.

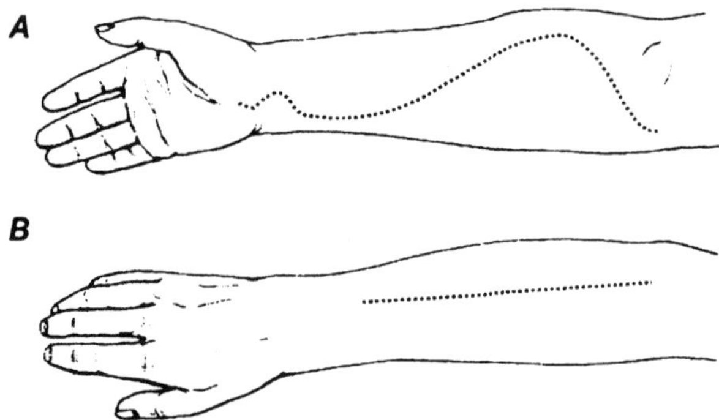

FIGURE 1.—(A) Thompson and (B) Henry approach to the compartments of the forearm. (Reprinted from Zellweger R, Hess F, Nicol A, et al: An analysis of 124 surgically managed brachial artery injuries. *Am J Surg* 188:240-245, 2004. Copyright 2004, with permission from Excerpta Medica Inc.)

Conclusions.—The primary repair of penetrating brachial artery injuries was possible in approximately one third of the patients. Approximately two thirds of the patients had associated nerve lesions. Critical limb ischemia rarely occurred.

► The article highlights the fact that associated nerve injuries are common with brachial artery injury. Primary repair of the brachial artery is possible in only a minority of patients. Be prepared to use a vein graft.

G. L. Moneta, MD

14 Nonatherosclerotic Conditions

Clinical Review of Patients Treated for Atypical Claudication: A 28-Year Experience

Turnipseed WD (Univ of Wisconsin, Madison)

J Vasc Surg 40:79-85, 2004 14–1

Purpose.—This article describes patient demographic data, as well as diagnosis and treatment of symptomatic lower extremity claudication that has no apparent vascular or orthopedic cause.

Methods.—A retrospective review was performed of records for 843 patients who received surgical treatment between 1975 and 2003. All patients had a detailed history, and underwent physical examination and selected noninvasive vascular testing. Noninvasive popliteal entrapment screening tests and compartment pressure measurements for isolated superficial muscle pain were routine. Duplex scanning or arteriography were used only when arteriovenous disease or popliteal entrapment syndrome was suspected.

Results.—The study population included 549 female patients (65%) and 294 male patients (35%). Their mean age was 29 years (range, 12-71 years). The most common symptoms were isolated lower extremity muscle cramping (100%), foot paresthesia (20%), and medial tibial bone pain (1%). Causes of symptoms included chronic compartment syndrome (796 patients, 94%), functional popliteal entrapment syndrome (33 patients, 4%), and medial tibial syndrome (14 patients, 2%). Pathologic findings included overuse injury (756 patients, 89%), blunt limb trauma (60 patients, 7%), or gait anomaly (34 patients, 4%). Surgery for compartment release included fasciotomy (100 patients, 12%) or fasciectomy (696 patients, 88%). Surgery for functional popliteal entrapment included excision of the plantaris muscle and soleal band (33 patients). Medial tibial release included soleal and transverse fasciectomy, with periosteal cautery of the tibial insertions. Complete symptomatic relief was achieved in 92% of compartment release procedures, 100% of popliteal entrapment release procedures, and 80% of medial tibial release procedures.

Conclusion.—Atypical claudication represents a collection of syndromes that can be permanently and effectively treated with surgical intervention.

► Patients with atypical claudication are vexing problems for the vascular surgeon. No one has more experience in dealing with these patients than Dr Turnipseed. This is one of those articles that should be kept handy for periodic reference as needed. The workup and treatment suggested make sense and result in favorable outcomes of properly selected patients.

G. L. Moneta, MD

Management of Arteriovenous Malformations: A Multidisciplinary Approach

Lee B-B, Do YS, Yakes W, et al (Sungkyunkwan Univ, Seoul, Korea)

J Vasc Surg 39:590-600, 2004 14–2

Background.—Management of arteriovenous malformations (AVMs) remains challenging because of their unpredictable behavior and high recurrence rate. A multidisciplinary approach based on a new classification scheme and improved diagnostic techniques may improve their management. The purpose of this study was to review our experience with combined embolotherapy, sclerotherapy (embolo/sclerotherapy), and surgical procedures to manage AVMs.

Methods.—A total of 797 patients with congenital vascular malformations (January 1995 through December 2001) was investigated with noninvasive studies. Once an AVM was diagnosed, all underwent angiographic confirmation as a roadmap for treatment. Embolo/sclerotherapy and surgical procedures were instituted by the multidisciplinary team with periodic follow-up per protocol. Seventy-six patients with AVMs were reviewed retrospectively to assess the diagnosis and management by a multidisciplinary approach.

Results.—Seventy-six (9.5% of all CVM) patients had AVMs (Fig 1), mostly infiltrating, extratruncular form (61/76). Embolo/sclerotherapy with various combinations of absolute ethanol, *N*-butyl cyanoacrylate (NBCA), contour particles, and coils were used in 48 patients. Sixteen patients with surgically accessible localized lesions completed preoperative embolism and sclerotherapy through 24 sessions, with subsequent surgical excision with minimal morbidity. Interim results were excellent, with no evidence of recurrence in all 16 patients with a mean follow-up of 24 months. Thirty-two patients with surgically inaccessible lesions (infiltrating) were treated with embolism and sclerotherapy alone. There were nine failures in a total of 171 sessions. Interim results with a mean of 19 months' follow-up of embolism and sclerotherapy alone were excellent in the majority (25/32) and good to fair among the rest (7/32). However, 31 complications, mostly minor (27/31), occurred in 30 sessions. Four major complications occurred, including facial nerve palsy, pulmonary embolism, deep vein thrombosis, and massive necrosis of an ear cartilage.

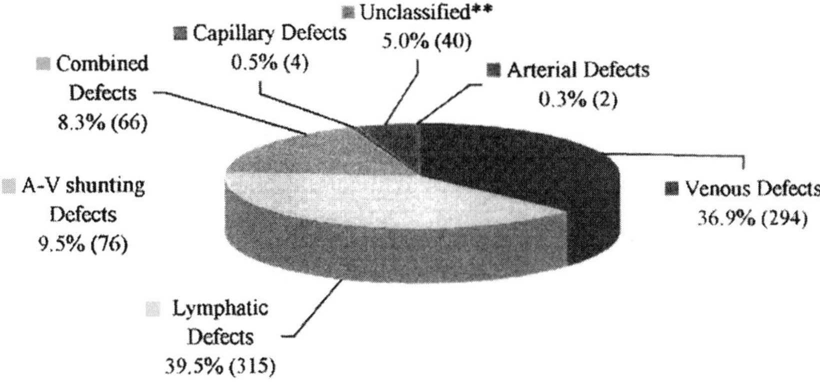

FIGURE 1.—Congenital vascular malformation based on the Hamburg classification for 797 patients registered at CVM Clinic, Vascular Center, Samsung Medical Center (January 1995 through December 2001): 446 females and 351 males; mean age 22.1 years (range, 14 days to 81 years). **Due to various factors including young age, final diagnosis was temporarily deferred until conclusive diagnostic procedures could be included. Unclassified malformations are, however, mostly venous malformations clinically and subsequently confirmed as venous malformations after lymphatic malformations, etc, were properly ruled out. In addition to these deferred diagnostic cases, there were truly unclassifiable malformations from hemangioma as well as capillary malformations clinically and/or histopathologically. (Reprinted by permission of the publisher from Lee B-B, Do YS, Yakes W, et al: Management of arteriovenous malformations: A multidisciplinary approach. *J Vasc Surg* 39:590-600, 2004. Copyright 2004 by Elsevier.)

Conclusions.—Diagnosis and management of AVMs by a multidisciplinary approach that integrates surgical therapy with embolism and sclerotherapy appears to improve the results and management with limited morbidity and no recurrence during early follow-up.

▶ The best results with any therapy will only occur when the therapy is applied to the disease process to which it is most suited. Classification and treatment of congenital vascular malformations is a black box to most vascular surgeons. This article illustrates how a better understanding of the variants of congenital vascular malformations can lead to a logical treatment strategy and potentially improved results. Nevertheless, the strategy outlined is daunting and fraught with significant potential complications. This is one vascular disorder where evaluation and treatment should take place in specialized centers by ongoing multidisciplinary teams. These are not small community hospital procedures.

G. L. Moneta, MD

Vascular Anomalies in Alagille Syndrome: A Significant Cause of Morbidity and Mortality

Kamath BM, Spinner NB, Emerick KM, et al (Univ of Pennsylvania, Philadelphia; Northwestern Univ, Chicago; Univ of Manitoba, Winnipeg, Canada; et al)
Circulation 109:1354-1358, 2004 14–3

Background.—Alagille syndrome (AGS) is a dominantly inherited multisystem disorder involving the liver, heart, eyes, face, and skeleton, caused by mutations in *Jagged1*. Intracranial bleeding is a recognized complication and cause of mortality in AGS. There are multiple case reports of intracranial vessel abnormalities and other vascular anomalies in AGS. The objective of this study was to characterize the nature and spectrum of vascular anomalies in AGS.

Method and Results.—Retrospective chart review of 268 individuals with AGS was performed. Twenty-five patients (9%) had noncardiac vascular anomalies or events. Sixteen patients had documented structural vascular abnormalities. Two had basilar artery aneurysms, 7 had internal carotid artery anomalies, and another had a middle cerebral artery aneurysm. Moyamoya disease was described in 1 patient. Three of the 16 patients had aortic aneurysms, and 2 had aortic coarctations. One of the patients with a basilar artery aneurysm also had coarctation of the aorta. One of the individuals with an internal carotid artery anomaly also had renal artery stenosis. Nine more patients had intracranial events without documented vessel abnormalities. Vascular accidents accounted for 34% of the mortality in this cohort.

Conclusions.—The vascular anomalies described in our cohort of AGS individuals identify an underrecognized and potentially devastating complication of this disorder. It is a major cause of morbidity and mortality in this population, accounting for 34% of the mortality. We have also reviewed the body of evidence supporting a role for *Jagged1* and the Notch signaling pathway in vascular development.

▶ I had not heard of this syndrome before. Most of the vascular anomalies associated with AGS are intercranial, but a few involve the aorta and visceral or peripheral arteries. The article is also interesting in that it suggests a particular mechanistic abnormality in vascular development (Notch signaling pathway, which I also had never heard of) as an etiology for developmental vascular anomalies.

G. L. Moneta, MD

Compelling Nature of Arterial Manifestations in Behçet Disease

Iscan ZH, Vural KM, Bayazit M (Turkiye Yuksek Ihtisas Hosp, Sihhiye-Ankara, Turkey)

J Vasc Surg 41:53-58, 2005 14–4

Introduction.—We present our experience with surgical treatment of arterial complications in Behçet disease (vasculo-Behcet disease), and the long-term results and pitfalls of surgical treatment.

Material and Methods.—Between January 1990 and January 2003, 20 consecutive patients underwent surgery to treat vasculo-Behcet disease. Most patients (17 of 20) were men, with mean age of 38.4 years.

Results.—Thirty-four operations were performed in 20 patients. The operative mortality rate was 5.8% (2 patients). There were 17 emergency operations, 6 because of ruptured primary abdominal aneurysms. There were

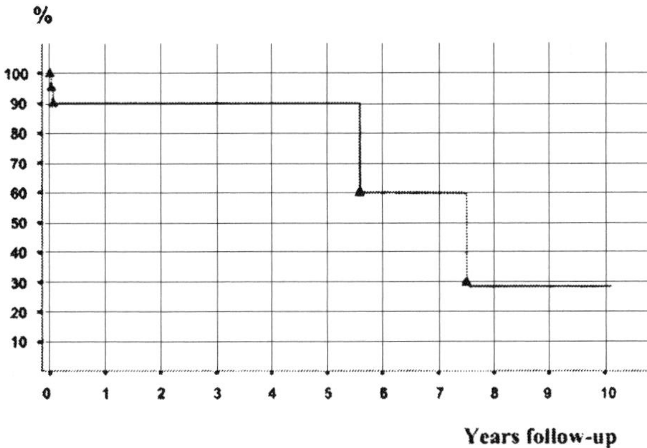

FIGURE 3.—Survival after vascular manifestation, including early hospital mortality. (Reprinted by permission of the publisher from Iscan ZH, Vural KM, Bayazit M: Compelling nature of arterial manifestations in Behçet disease. *J Vasc Surg* 41:53-58, 2005. Copyright 2005 by Elsevier.)

five others with critical limb ischemia, resulting in 3 amputations. All patients were followed up postoperatively on average for 44 months (range, 6 months-14 years). Two additional patients were lost to follow-up. After the initial operation 10-year survival rate was 30% (Fig 3), 10-year complication-free survival rate was 13% (Fig 4), and 5-year repeat operation-free survival rate was 26%.

Conclusion.—Although surgical intervention should be postponed until active inflammation has subsided, often this is not possible, because of the emergent nature of these problems. Most arterial complications of vasculo-Behcet disease present with a pseudoaneurysm rupture or with impending

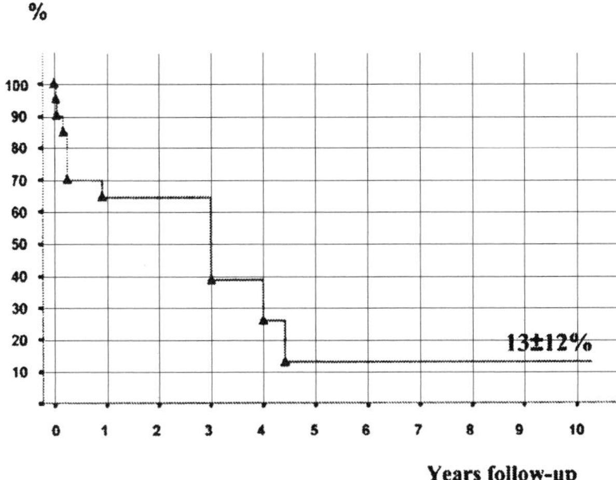

FIGURE 4.—Major arterial complication-free survival. (Reprinted by permission of the publisher from Iscan ZH, Vural KM, Bayazit M: Compelling nature of arterial manifestations in Behçet disease. *J Vasc Surg* 41:53-58, 2005. Copyright 2005 by Elsevier.)

rupture. An aggressive surgical approach can be life-saving in such instances, and should be undertaken regardless of long-term complications, which are more common when the operation is performed in the presence of active inflammation. Early and late results can be improved by individualizing, selecting a disease-free area for reconstruction, and eliminating use of autologous graft material.

▶ Behçet disease is rare. Vascular involvement occurs in only a minority, and involvement of a major artery in only 1% to 2%. Nevertheless, it will get your attention if a Behçet patient with arterial involvement washes up on your beach. The take-home message is to use prosthetic material to repair the arterial complications of Behçet disease, even if they involve an infrainguinal artery. Also try to avoid operating during an acute inflammatory episode.

G. L. Moneta, MD

Prevalence and Associations of an Abnormal Ankle-Brachial Index in Systemic Lupus Erythematosus: A Pilot Study

Theodoridou A, Bento L, D'Cruz DP, et al (St Thomas' Hosp, London)

Ann Rheum Dis 62:1199-1203, 2003 14–5

Background.—Accelerated atheroma is a well recognised complication of systemic lupus erythematosus (SLE). Its aetiology is multifactorial and several methods may be used to detect early signs of atheroma.

Methods.—Patients aged ≤55 years were screened using the ankle-brachial index (ABI). Ninety one patients aged ≤55 years and fulfilling the revised American College of Rheumatology criteria for SLE were studied. The ABI was measured using a contour wrapped 12 cm cuff attached to a mercury sphygmomanometer and an 8 MHz Doppler probe in the arms and legs; a ratio of <1 was considered abnormal.

Results.—The mean (SD) age of the patients was 39.0 (9.2) years. Of the 91 patients studied, 34 (37%) had an abnormal ABI. Only one patient was mildly symptomatic. Abnormal ABI correlated with age but not with disease duration, cumulative steroid dosage, ECLAM score, or any other traditional risk factors for atherosclerosis. In comparison with population studies, the prevalence of an ABI <1 in the patients with SLE with a mean age of 39 years was similar to that in adults aged over 80.

Conclusion.—In this pilot study, patients with SLE with a mean age of 39 years had a high prevalence of an abnormal ABI. The ABI is a simple non-invasive tool for the early detection of accelerated atheroma in SLE.

▶ Since atherosclerosis is at least in part an inflammatory disease and SLE has an inflammatory component, it makes some sense, in a superficial sort of way, that patients with SLE have evidence of premature atherosclerosis as assessed by ABI. I wonder if patients with SLE will benefit in the same manner from aspirin, β-blockers, and statin therapy as patients with peripheral vascular disease associated with traditional cardiovascular risk factors? This article has not answered the question of whether traditional risk modifications should be used in the SLE patient.

G. L. Moneta, MD

Combination Treatment of Venous Thoracic Outlet Syndrome: Open Surgical Decompression and Intraoperative Angioplasty

Schneider DB, Dimuzio PJ, Martin ND, et al (Univ of California, San Francisco; Thomas Jefferson Univ, Philadelphia)

J Vasc Surg 40:599-603, 2004 14–6

Objective.—Residual subclavian vein stenosis after thoracic outlet decompression in patients with venous thoracic outlet syndrome is often treated with postoperative percutaneous angioplasty (PTA). However, interval recurrent thrombosis before postoperative angioplasty is performed can be a vexing problem. Therefore we initiated a prospective trial at 2 referral institutions to evaluate the safety and efficacy of combined thoracic outlet decompression with intraoperative PTA performed in 1 stage.

Methods.—Over 3 years 25 consecutive patients (16 women, 9 men; median age, 30 years) underwent treatment for venous thoracic outlet syndrome with a standard protocol at 2 institutions. Twenty-one patients (84%) underwent preoperative thrombolysis to treat axillosubclavian vein thrombosis. First-rib resection was performed through combined supraclavicular and infraclavicular incisions. Intraoperative venography and subclavian vein PTA were performed through a percutaneous basilic vein approach. Postoperative anticoagulation therapy was not used routinely. Venous duplex ultrasound scanning was performed postoperatively and at 1, 6, and 12 months.

Results.—Intraoperative venography enabled identification of residual subclavian vein stenosis in 16 patients (64%), and all underwent intraoperative PTA with 100% technical success (Fig 2). Postoperative duplex scans documented subclavian vein patency in 23 patients (92%). Complications included subclavian vein recurrent thrombosis in 2 patients (8%), and both underwent percutaneous mechanical thrombectomy, with restoration of patency in 1 patient. One-year primary and secondary patency rates were 92% and 96%, respectively, at life-table analysis.

Conclusions.—Residual subclavian vein stenosis after operative thoracic outlet decompression is common in patients with venous thoracic outlet syndrome. Combination treatment with surgical thoracic outlet decompression and intraoperative PTA is a safe and effective means for identifying and treating residual subclavian vein stenosis. Moreover, intraoperative PTA may reduce the incidence of postoperative recurrent thrombosis and eliminate the need for venous stent placement or open venous repair.

► This approach is reasonable if somehow one knows which patients with venous thoracic outlet syndrome require operation. It is, however, very clear that not all patients with primary upper extremity venous thrombosis require op-

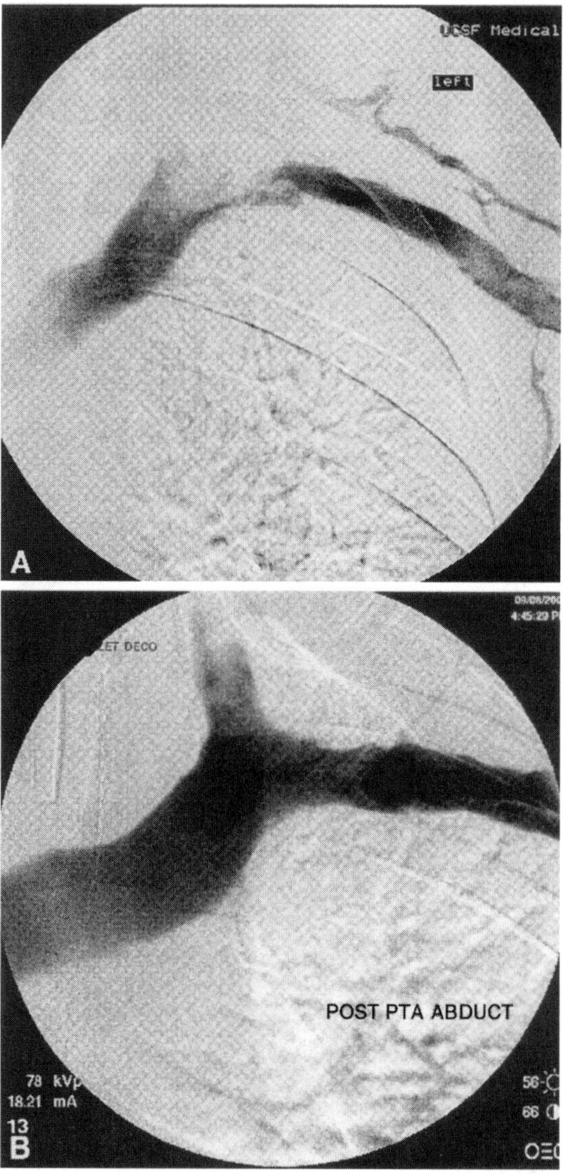

FIGURE 2.—Left upper extremity venograms. **A**, Preoperative venogram after successful thrombolysis demonstrates subclavian vein stenosis within the costoclavicular space. **B**, Completion venogram after percutaneous transluminal angioplasty (PTA) with 14-mm balloon demonstrates widely patent subclavian vein with the arm abducted. (Reprinted by permission of the publisher from Schneider DB, Dimuzio PJ, Martin ND, et al: Combination treatment of venous thoracic outlet syndrome: Open surgical decompression and intraoperative angioplasty: *J Vasc Surg* 40:599-603, 2004. Copyright 2004 by Elsevier.)

eration. It is important to keep in mind that the goal is a patient who does well, not just a patent vein.

We have had the same problems with postoperative hematomas in patients treated with surgical decompression and angioplasty. A take-home point from this article would seem to be to avoid postoperative anticoagulation in these patients unless the initial primary upper extremity venous thrombosis was extensive.

G. L. Moneta, MD

Portal Vein Thrombosis in Children and Adolescents: The Low Prevalence of Hereditary Thrombophilic Disorders

Pinto RB, Silveira TR, Bandinelli E, et al (Hosp de Clínicas de Porto Alegre, Brazil; Universidade Federal do Rio Grande do Sul, Porto Alegre, Brazil)

J Pediatr Surg 39:1356-1361, 2004 14–7

Purpose.—The aim of this study was to determine the frequency of thrombophilic disorders in children and adolescents with portal vein thrombosis (PVT) as well as assessing the hereditary character of this disorder.

Methods.—A 2-year prospective study was carried out in pediatric PVT patients (n = 14), their parents (n = 25), and an age-matched control group free of liver disease (n = 28). The presence of PVT was assessed by means of Doppler ultrasound scan or angiography. None of the PVT patients presented biochemical or histologic signs of liver disease.

Results.—The frequency in PVT patients of protein C (PC), protein S (PS) and antithrombin (AT) deficiency was 42.9% ($P < .05$ *v* controls), 21.4% ($P > .05$) and 7.1% ($P > .05$), respectively. None of the controls or parents of PVT patients presented hereditary PC, PS, or AT deficiency. One PVT patient and one control ($P = .999$) presented prothrombin G20210A mutation. Homozygous methylenetetrahydrofolate reductase C677T genotype was observed in 3 of 14 (21.4%) PVT patients and in 5 of 28 (17.9%; $P = .356$) controls. None of these patients presented factor V G1691A mutation.

Conclusions.—PC deficiency was frequent in pediatric PVT patients and does not seem to be an inherited condition. The hereditary prothrombotic disorders do not seem to play a vital role in thrombosis in children and adolescents with PVT.

► Hypercoagulable states are common in children with PVT; however, they do not appear to be inherited and therefore must be considered acquired or a mutation. The data do not argue for genetic testing or hypercoagulable screening of siblings of children with PVT but do suggest pediatric patients with portal vein thrombosis undergo thrombophilia screening.

G. L. Moneta, MD

Acute Mesenteric Venous Thrombosis: A Better Outcome Achieved Through Improved Imaging Techniques and a Changed Policy of Clinical Management

Zhang J, Duan ZQ, Song QB, et al (China Med Univ, Shenyang)

Eur J Vasc Endovasc Surg 28:329-334, 2004 14–8

Objective.—To analyse and compare the results obtained from acute mesenteric venous thrombosis (MVT) patients before and after the change of the clinical management principle, to assess the factors responsible for the recent better outcome and determine the best management for this disease.

Materials and Methods.—We retrospectively reviewed 41 patients treated for acute MVT admitted in our hospital between 1978 and 2003. Before 1995 (Group I), our policy was to perform surgery in patients with suspected acute MVT. After 1995 (Group II), we changed our policy to a medical approach when achievable. Each patient in this study was assessed for diagnosis, initial management (operative or non-operative), mortality, duration of hospitalisation, and outcome.

Results.—There were 13 in Group I, 28 in Group II. The mean duration of diagnoses made after admission was 7.3 S.D. 2.6 days for patients in Group I, and 1.5 S.D. 1.2 days for those in Group II ($p < 0.01$, Student's t-test). Eleven patients underwent operations and two patients received non-operative treatment initially in group I, the mortality was 39%; while nine patients underwent operations and 19 patients received non-operative management in group II, the mortality was 11% ($p < 0.05$). No death occurred in the patients with initial non-operative management. The mean duration of hospitalisation was 26 S.D. 6.8 days in Group I and 12.6 S.D. 4.6 days in

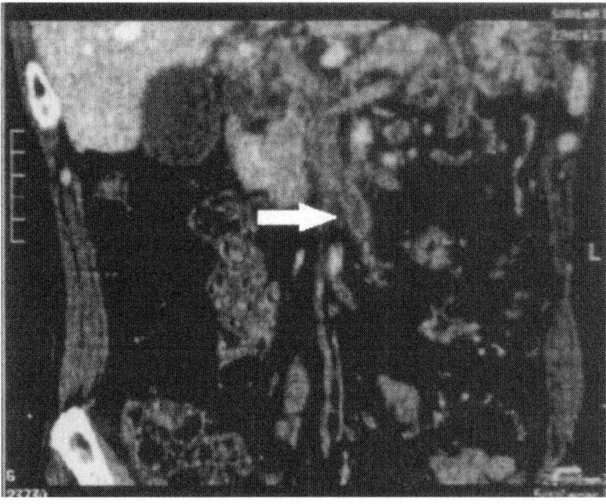

FIGURE 2.—Coronal reformation of three-dimensional helical CT angiography shows a filling defect in the superior mesenteric vein (*arrow*). (Reprinted from Zhang J, Duan ZQ, Song QB, et al: Acute mesenteric venous thrombosis: A better outcome achieved through improved imaging techniques and a changed policy of clinical management. *Eur J Vasc Endovasc Surg* 28:329-334, 2004. Copyright 2004 by permission of the publisher.)

Group II ($p < 0.01$, Student's *t*-test). No significant difference in 2-year survival rate between the two groups.

Conclusion.—Recent improvements in imaging techniques and better understanding of the aetiology have led to a dramatic change in the principle and policy of clinical management for acute MVT, which leads to a more favourable outcome of acute MVT (Fig 2).

▶ It is difficult to draw any real conclusions from this article. The authors describe their recent improved results with MVT to a greater willingness to anticoagulate patients even after an operation and/or bowel resection. Clearly, anticoagulation initially and postoperatively makes sense in patients with MVT; it is usually easier to deal with bleeding than more dead intestine.

G. L. Moneta, MD

Mesenteric Venous Thrombosis With Transmural Intestinal Infarction: A Population-Based Study

Acosta S, Ögren M, Sternby N-H, et al (Malmö Univ, Sweden; Uppsala Univ, Sweden)

J Vasc Surg 41:59-63, 2005 14–9

Objective.—To determine the cause-specific mortality from and incidence of transmural intestinal infarction caused by mesenteric venous thrombosis (MVT) in a population-based study and to evaluate the findings at autopsy by evaluating autopsies and surgical procedures.

Methods.—All clinical (n = 23,446) and forensic (n = 7569) autopsies performed in the city of Malmö between 1970 and 1982 (population 264,000 to 230,000) were evaluated. The autopsy rate was 87%. The surgical procedures were performed in 1970, 1976, and 1982. Autopsy protocols coded for intestinal ischemia or mesenteric vessel occlusion, or both, were identified in a database. In all, 997 of 23,446 clinical and 9 of 7,569 forensic autopsy protocols were analyzed. A 3-year sample of the surgical procedures, comprising 21.3% (11,985 of 56,251) of all operations performed during the entire study period, was chosen to capture trends of diagnostic and surgical activity. In a nested case-control study within the clinical autopsy cohort, four MVT-free controls, matched for gender, age at death, and year of death were identified for each fatal MVT case to evaluate the clinical autopsy findings.

Results.—Four forensic and 23 clinical autopsies demonstrated MVT with intestinal infarction (Fig 1). Seven patients were operated on, of whom six survived. The cause-specific mortality ratio was 0.9:1000 autopsies. The incidence was 1.8/100,000 person years. At autopsy, portal vein thrombosis and systemic venous thromboembolism occurred in 2 of 3 and 1 of 2 of the cases, respectively. Obesity was an independent risk factor for fatal MVT ($P = .021$).

Conclusions.—The estimated incidence of MVT with transmural intestinal infarction was 1.8/100,000 person years. Portal vein thrombosis, sys-

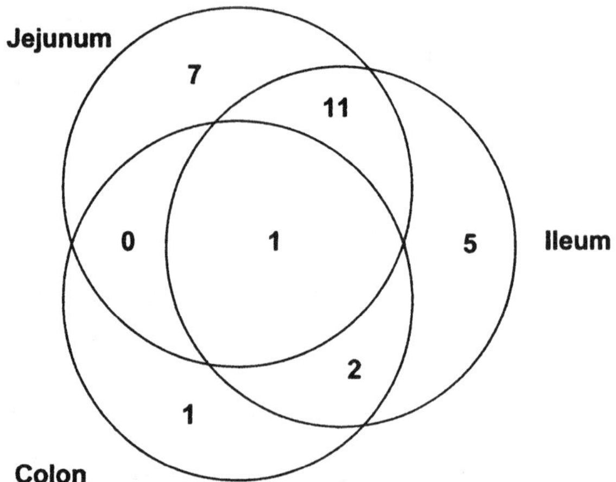

FIGURE 1.—Venn diagram showing the extent of intestinal infarction in 27 patients with mesenteric venous thrombosis and transmural intestinal infarction. (Reprinted by permission of the publisher from Acosta S, Ögren M, Sternby N-H, et al: Mesenteric venous thrombosis with transmural intestinal infarction: A population-based study. *J Vasc Surg* 41:59-63, 2005. Copyright 2005 by Elsevier.)

temic venous thromboembolism and obesity were associated with fatal MVT.

► Many, perhaps most, cases of MVT can be managed nonoperatively. It is likely the prevalence of MVT is underestimated. The study does point out that MVT can result in large lengths of infarcted intestine. The association of obesity with MVT is a finding I was previously unaware of. Perhaps the increased intra-abdominal pressure associated with obesity leads to relative intra-abdominal venous stasis and increased risk of MVT.

G. L. Moneta, MD

15 Venous Thrombosis and Pulmonary Embolization

Estrogen Plus Progestin and Risk of Venous Thrombosis

Cushman M, for the Women's Health Initiative Investigators (Univ of Vermont, Burlington; et al)

JAMA 292:1573-1580, 2004 15–1

Context.—Postmenopausal hormone therapy increases the risk of venous thrombosis. It is not known whether other factors influencing thrombosis add to this risk.

Objective.—To report final data on incidence of venous thrombosis in the Women's Health Initiative Estrogen Plus Progestin clinical trial and the association of hormone therapy with venous thrombosis in the setting of other thrombosis risk factors.

Design, Setting, and Participants.—Double-blind randomized controlled trial of 16,608 postmenopausal women between the ages of 50 and 79 years, who were enrolled in 1993 through 1998 at 40 US clinical centers with 5.6 years of follow up; and a nested case-control study. Baseline gene variants related to thrombosis risk were measured in the first 147 women who developed thrombosis and in 513 controls.

Intervention.—Random assignment to 0.625 mg/d of conjugated equine estrogen plus 2.5 mg/d of medroxyprogesterone acetate, or placebo.

Main Outcome Measures.—Centrally validated deep vein thrombosis and pulmonary embolus.

Results.—Venous thrombosis occurred in 167 women taking estrogen plus progestin (3.5 per 1000 person-years) and in 76 taking placebo (1.7 per 1000 person-years); hazard ratio (HR), 2.06 (95% confidence interval [CI], 1.57-2.70). Compared with women between the ages of 50 and 59 years who were taking placebo, the risk associated with hormone therapy was higher with age: HR of 4.28 (95% CI, 2.38-7.72) for women aged 60 to 69 years and 7.46 (95% CI, 4.32-14.38) for women aged 70 to 79 years. Compared with women who were of normal weight and taking placebo, the risk associated with taking estrogen plus progestin was increased among overweight and obese women: HR of 3.80 (95% CI, 2.08-6.94) and 5.61 (95% CI, 3.12-10.11), respectively. Factor V Leiden enhanced the hormone-associated risk of thrombosis with a 6.69-fold increased risk compared with women in the placebo group without the mutation (95% CI, 3.09-14.49). Other genetic variants (prothrombin 20210A, methylenetetrahydrofolate reductase C677T, factor XIII Val34Leu, PAI-1 4G/5G, and factor V HR2) did not modify the association of hormone therapy with venous thrombosis.

Conclusions.—Estrogen plus progestin was associated with doubling the risk of venous thrombosis. Estrogen plus progestin therapy increased the risks associated with age, overweight or obesity, and factor V Leiden.

▶ There are immense implications here with respect to use of equine-derived postmenopausal hormone therapy for treatment of menopausal symptoms. It appears women undergoing postmenopausal hormone therapy with equine-derived estrogens are at increased risk of venous thromboembolic events. Certain categories of patients are at prohibitive risk.

G. L. Moneta, MD

Esterified Estrogens and Conjugated Equine Estrogens and the Risk of Venous Thrombosis

Smith NL, Heckbert SR, Lemaitre RN, et al (Univ of Washington, Seattle; Group Health Cooperative, Seattle; Univ Med Ctr, Leiden, The Netherlands)

JAMA 292:1581-1587, 2004 15–2

Context.—Clinical trial evidence indicates that estrogen therapy with or without progestins increases venous thrombotic risk. The findings from these trials, which used oral conjugated equine estrogens, may not be generalizable to other estrogen compounds.

Objective.—To compare risk of venous thrombosis among esterified estrogen users, conjugated equine estrogen users, and nonusers.

Design, Setting, and Participants.—This population-based, case-control study was conducted at a large health maintenance organization in Washington State. Cases were perimenopausal and postmenopausal women aged 30 to 89 years who sustained a first venous thrombosis between January 1995 and December 2001 and controls were matched on age, hypertension status, and calendar year.

Main Outcome Measure.—Risk of first venous thrombosis in relation to current use of esterified or conjugated equine estrogens, with or without concomitant progestin. Current use was defined as use at thrombotic event for cases and a comparable reference date for controls.

Results.—Five hundred eighty-six incident venous thrombosis cases and 2268 controls were identified. Compared with women not currently using hormones, current users of esterified estrogen had no increase in venous thrombotic risk (odds ratio [OR], 0.92; 95% confidence interval [CI], 0.69-1.22). In contrast, women currently taking conjugated equine estrogen had an elevated risk (OR, 1.65; 95% CI, 1.24-2.19). When analyses were restricted to estrogen users, current users of conjugated equine estrogen had a higher risk than current users of esterified estrogen (OR, 1.78; 95% CI, 1.11-2.84). Among conjugated equine estrogen users, increasing daily dose was associated with increased risk (trend *P* value = .02). Among all estrogen users, concomitant progestin use was associated with increased risk compared with use of estrogen alone (OR, 1.60; 95% CI, 1.13-2.26).

Conclusion.—Our finding that conjugated equine estrogen but not esterified estrogen was associated with venous thrombotic risk needs to be replicated and may have implications for the choice of hormones in perimenopausal and postmenopausal women.

▶ Just as all quarterbacks and surgeons are not equal, estrogens when used in perimenopausal and postmenopausal women are also not the same. The reported findings have significant implications for potential selection of perimenopausal and postmenopausal hormone therapy. Perhaps the increased venous thromboembolic risk associated with equine-derived estrogens reported by the Women's Health Initiative (see Abstract 15–1) can be avoided or lowered by using an alternative estrogen preparation.

G. L. Moneta, MD

Factor V Leiden and the Risk of Venous Thromboembolism in the Adult Danish Population

Juul K, Tybjaerg-Hansen A, Schnohr P, et al (Herlev Univ, Denmark; Copenhagen Univ; Bispebjerg Univ, Copenhagen)

Ann Intern Med 140:330-337, 2004 15–3

Background.—Odds ratios for venous thromboembolism (deep venous thrombosis and pulmonary embolism) derived from case-control studies range from 3 to 16 for heterozygotes compared with noncarriers and up to 79 for homozygotes compared with noncarriers.

Objective.—To estimate risks for venous thromboembolism in the adult Danish population according to factor V Leiden genotype.

Design.—Cohort study with 23 years of follow-up.

Setting.—Adult Danish population.

Participants.—9253 randomly selected individuals.

Measurements.—Hospitalization and death from venous thromboembolism, factor V Leiden genotype, and additional thromboembolic risk factors.

Results.—Adjusted hazard ratios in heterozygotes and homozygotes compared with noncarriers were 2.7 (95% CI, 1.8 to 3.8) and 18 (CI, 4.1 to 41) for venous thromboembolism overall, 2.4 (CI, 1.3 to 3.8) and 22 (CI, 0 to 60) for deep venous thrombosis, and 3.0 (CI, 1.7 to 4.9) and 11 (CI, 0 to 33) for pulmonary embolism. The lowest absolute 10-year risks for venous thromboembolism in factor V Leiden heterozygotes and homozygotes—0.7% (CI, 0.5% to 1.0%) and 3% (CI, 1% to 8%)—were found in nonsmokers younger than 40 years of age with a body mass index below 25 kg/m^2; the corresponding highest risks—10% (CI, 7% to 14%) and 51% (CI,

13% to 100%)—were found in smokers older than 60 years of age with a body mass index above 30 kg/m² (Fig 2).

Conclusions.—Hazard ratios for venous thromboembolism in factor V Leiden heterozygotes and homozygotes compared with noncarriers in the adult Danish population were approximately 3 and 18, respectively. The simultaneous presence of smoking, obesity, and old age resulted in absolute

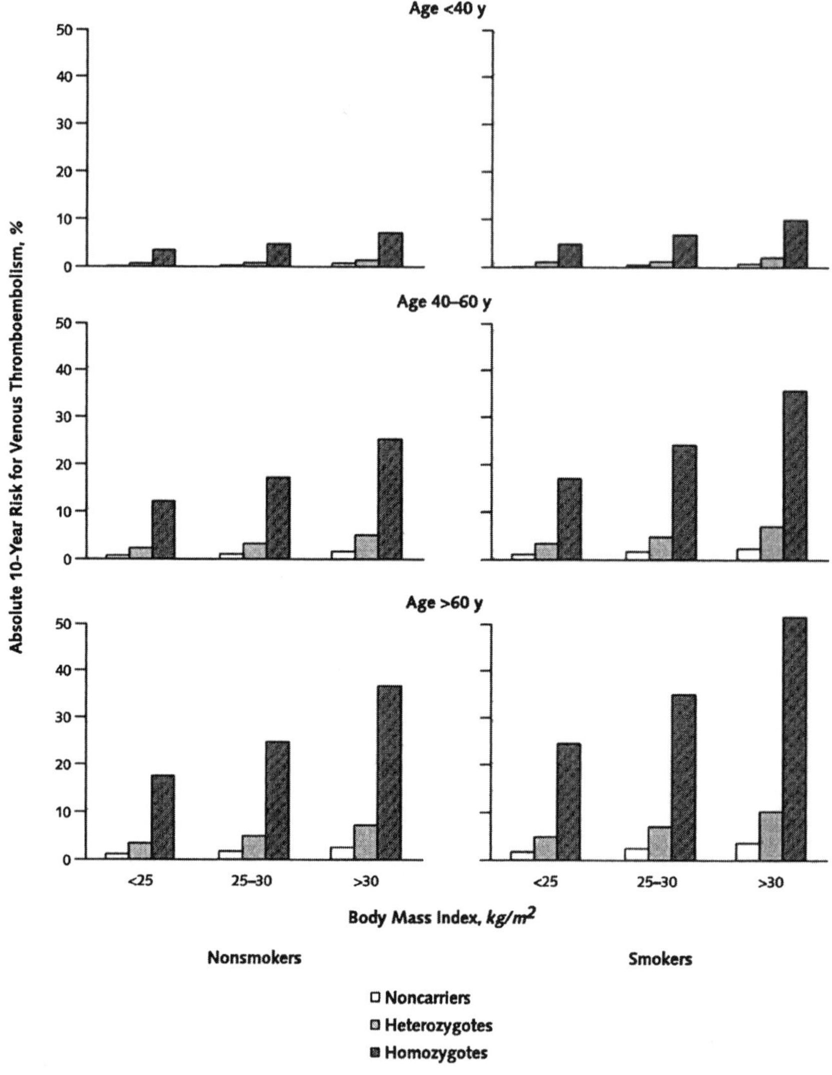

FIGURE 2.—Absolute 10-year risk for venous thromboembolism (deep venous thrombosis and pulmonary embolism combined) according to age, smoking, body mass index, and factor V Leiden genotype. (Courtesy of Juul K, Tybjaerg-Hansen A, Schnohr P, et al: Factor V Leiden and the risk of venous thromboembolism in the adult Danish population. *Ann Intern Med* 140:330-337, 2004.)

10-year thromboembolic risks of 10% in heterozygotes and 51% in homozygotes.

▶ The article reinforces the fact risk factors for venous thromboembolism (VTE) are not linearly additive. Risk is basically exponential. Individual risk factors for VTE somehow act in synergy. The overall risk in a patient with multiple risk factors for VTE is considerably higher than that predicted by the individual contributions of each risk factor.

G. L. Moneta, MD

Inhibition of Annexin V Binding to Cardiolipin and Thrombin Generation in an Unselected Population With Venous Thrombosis

Hanly JG, Smith SA, Anderson D (Dalhousie Univ, Halifax, NS, Canada)

J Rheumatol 30:1990-1993, 2003 15–4

Objective.—To examine the effect on annexin V binding to cardiolipin (CL) and *in vitro* thrombin generation by plasma samples from an unselected population of patients with confirmed venous thrombosis and matched controls. The prevalence of autoimmune antiphospholipid antibodies (aPL) was also determined.

Methods.—A total of 111 patients who presented to a single emergency room with symptoms suggestive of venous thromboembolic (VTE) disease were studied. In 34 patients the diagnosis of lower limb deep venous thrombosis (DVT) and/or pulmonary embolus (PE) was confirmed (VTE+ group). In the remaining 77 patients the diagnostic workup was negative (VTE− group). Plasma samples were collected prior to the initiation of anticoagulation and examined for IgG anticardiolipin (aCL), IgG anti-β_2-glycoprotein I (GPI), and IgG anti-prothrombin (aPT antibodies) by ELISA. In addition, the effect of individual patient and control plasma samples on annexin V binding to CL and on *in vitro* thrombin generation was determined by a competitive ELISA and a chromogenic assay, respectively.

Results.—The prevalence and levels of IgG aCL, anti-β_2-GPI, and aPT antibodies were similar in the VTE+ and VTE− groups. However, plasma samples from the VTE+ group caused a significant inhibition of in vitro thrombin generation (mean ± SD Z score: −0.66 ± 0.97 vs 0.26 ± 1.46; $p < 0.001$) and a concurrent but less impressive inhibition of annexin V binding to CL (mean ± SD Z score: −2.53 ± 1.44 vs −2.05 ± 1.61; $p = 0.123$). Upon analyzing a panel of clinical and laboratory variables, only age and inhibition of thrombin generation were significantly associated with VTE disease.

Conclusion.—Our findings suggest that subtle abnormalities in annexin V physiology may contribute to the procoagulant state in patients with idiopathic venous thrombosis.

▶ Despite improvement in detection of hypercoagulable states, many patients with unprovoked VTE have no identifiable hypercoagulable abnormality. The study suggests that annexin V abnormalities may result in a minor hypercoagulable state. It is unclear if annexin V abnormalities can act in isolation to produce venous thrombosis.

G. L. Moneta, MD

Excess Risk of Cancer in Patients With Primary Venous Thromboembolism: A National, Population-based Cohort Study

Murchison JT, Wylie L, Stockton DL (Royal Infirmary of Edinburgh-Little, France; NHS Scotland, Edinburgh)

Br J Cancer 91:92-95, 2004 15–5

Background.—The association between thrombotic phenomena and cancer was observed as long ago as 1865. In the intervening years, many studies have documented the increased risk of cancer patients for the development of deep venous thrombosis (DVT) and pulmonary embolism (PE). In more recent years, an association has been noted between the initial diagnosis of venous thromboembolism (VTE) and a subsequent increased risk of cancer. This association has been investigated in several studies, but conclusions have ranged from a no-excess risk to a definitely increased risk. Whether the incidence of cancer was increased in a large population-based cohort of Scottish patients with a new diagnosis of VTE was determined. In addition, the excess risk of cancer in relation to the time since diagnosis of VTE and the patient age at diagnosis were assessed. Those cancers that were particularly associated with previous VTE in this population were identified.

Methods.—A nationwide retrospective cohort study was conducted in Scotland to assess the risk of cancer in patients diagnosed with VTE from 1982 to 2000. Patients who were presumed to be visitors to Scotland at the time of diagnosis were excluded, as were pregnant women and patients who had undergone surgery in the 6 weeks before VTE diagnosis. Patients with a

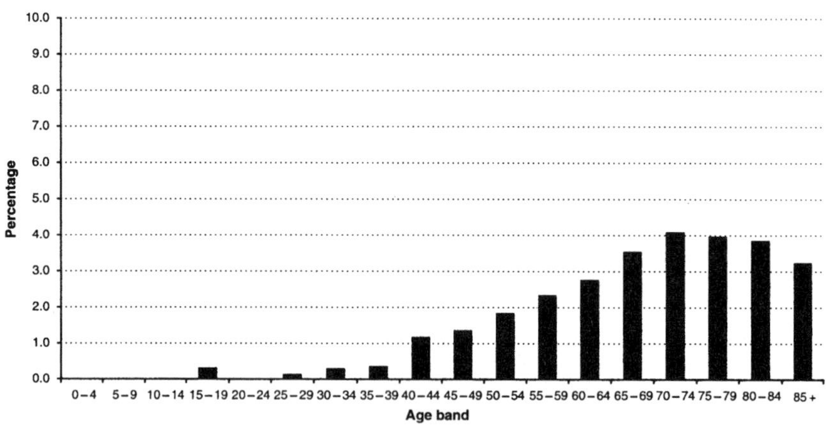

FIGURE 1.—Percentage of patients who developed cancer within 1–12 months after the first episode of VTE in relation to the total number of VTE patients, by age at VTE diagnosis. (Courtesy of Murchison JT, Wylie L, Stockton DL: Excess risk of cancer in patients with primary venous thromboembolism: A national, population-based cohort study. *Br J Cancer* 91:92-95, 2004. Reprinted by Nature Publishing.)

previous primary malignant cancer and those with cancer diagnosed within 1 month of the diagnosis of VTE were also excluded.

Results.—A total of 77,572 patients were identified with DVT/PE or both between 1981 and 2000. After application of the exclusion criteria, the study cohort comprised 59,334 patients (55% female, 45% male). The median duration of follow-up was 32 months. During the 19 years included in the study, 7.5% of patients were diagnosed with a first primary cancer at least 1 month after the diagnosis of VTE. The standardized incidence rate (SIR) for all cancers was 1.28 compared with the expected incidence, as calculated from the incidence of first malignancies in Scotland. A high excess risk of being diagnosed with cancer within 1 to 6 months after diagnosis of VTE was noted, with a slowly declining but still-significant excess risk for each 6-month follow-up for up to 2 years (Fig 1).

Conclusions.—In this Scottish population, significantly increased risks of cancer were sustained for 2 years after VTE diagnosis, particularly in patients with ovarian tumors and lymphomas. Younger patients also were at an increased relative risk from this association.

▶ Another bit of evidence suggesting undetected malignancy may be the underlying cause of some venous VTEs. This study does not answer the question of whether the patients with idiopathic VTE should be screened for malignancy. In addition, we do not know whether malignancies diagnosed after VTE have an improved prognosis. Some data suggest cancer diagnosed after VTE is often advanced and has a poor prognosis.[1]

G. L. Moneta, MD

Reference

1. Sorensen H, Mellemkjaer L, Olsen J, et al: Prognosis of cancers associated with venous thromboembolism. *N Engl J Med* 343:1846-1850, 2000.

The Risk of Recurrent Venous Thromboembolism in Men and Women

Kyrle PA, Minar E, Bialonczyk C, et al (Univ of Vienna; Wilhelminenspital, Vienna; Hanusch Krankenhaus, Vienna)

N Engl J Med 350:2558-2563, 2004 15–6

Background.—Whether a patient's sex is associated with the risk of recurrent venous thromboembolism is unknown.

Methods.—We studied 826 patients for an average of 36 months after a first episode of spontaneous venous thromboembolism and the withdrawal of oral anticoagulants. We excluded pregnant patients and patients with a deficiency of antithrombin, protein C, or protein S; the lupus anticoagulant; cancer; or a requirement for potentially long-term antithrombotic treatment. The end point was objective evidence of a recurrence of symptomatic venous thromboembolism.

Results.—Venous thromboembolism recurred in 74 of the 373 men, as compared with 28 of the 453 women (20 percent vs. 6 percent; relative risk

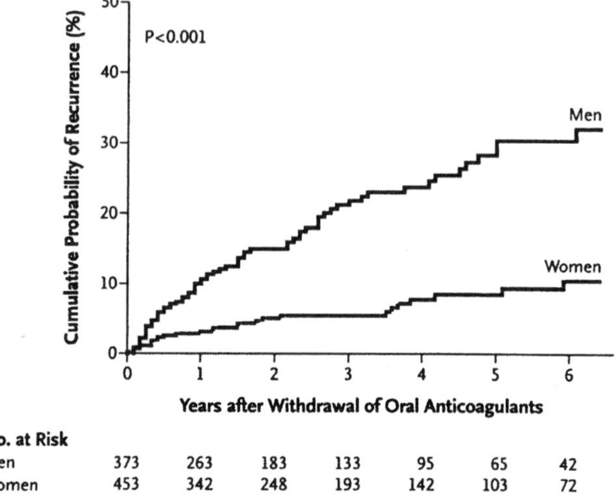

FIGURE 1.—Kaplan–Meier estimates of the likelihood of recurrent venous thromboembolism according to sex. The cumulative probability of recurrent venous thromboembolism was greater among men than women (P<0.001 by the log-rank test). (Reprinted by permission of *The New England Journal of Medicine* from Kyrle PA, Minar E, Bialonczyk C, et al: The risk of recurrent venous thromboembolism in men and women. *N Engl Med J* 350:2558-2563, 2004. Copyright 2004, Massachusetts Medical Society. All rights reserved.)

of recurrence, 3.6; 95 percent confidence interval, 2.3 to 5.5; P<0.001). The risk remained unchanged after adjustment for age, the duration of anticoagulation, and the presence or absence of a first symptomatic pulmonary embolism, factor V Leiden, factor II G20210A, or an elevated level of factor VIII or IX. At five years, the likelihood of recurrence was 30.7 percent among men, as compared with 8.5 percent among women (P<0.001). The relative risk of recurrence was similar among women who had had their first thrombosis during oral-contraceptive use or hormone-replacement therapy and women in the same age group in whom the first event was idiopathic.

Conclusions.—The risk of recurrent venous thromboembolism is higher among men than women (Fig 1).

▶ There have been previous studies evaluating the risk of recurrent venous thromboembolism (VTE).[1,2] These studies did not specifically look at sex as a risk of recurrent VTE. It seems unlikely, however, that it would have been overlooked. This study therefore represents the first major study implicating male sex as a risk factor for recurrent VTE. There are getting to be fewer and fewer reasons to be male!

G. L. Moneta, MD

References

1. Prandoni P, Lensing AW, Cogo A, et al: The long-term clinical course of acute deep venous thrombosis. *Ann Intern Med* 125:1-17, 1996.

2. Baglin T, Luddington R, Brown K, et al: Incidence of recurrent venous thromboembolism in relation to clinical and thrombophilic risk factors: Prospective cohort study. *Lancet* 362:523-526, 2003.

Predictive Value of D-Dimer Test for Recurrent Venous Thromboembolism After Anticoagulation Withdrawal in Subjects With a Previous Idiopathic Event and in Carriers of Congenital Thrombophilia

Palareti G, Legnani C, Cosmi B, et al (Univ Hosp S Orsola-Malpighi, Bologna, Italy; Univ of Ferrara, Italy)

Circulation 108:313-318, 2003 15–7

Background.—We have shown that normal D-dimer levels obtained after the discontinuation of oral anticoagulant treatment (OAT) has a high negative predictive value for recurrent venous thromboembolism (VTE). The aim of the present study was to assess the predictive value of D-dimer for recurrent VTE in subjects with a previous unprovoked event who are either carriers of inherited thrombophilia or not.

Method and Results.—We prospectively evaluated 599 patients (301 males) with a previous VTE episode. They were repeatedly examined for D-dimer levels after OAT withdrawal and were screened for inherited thrombophilic alterations. Alterations were detected in 130 patients (21.7%), factor V Leiden (70 patients; 2 of whom were homozygotes) and prothrombin mutation (38 patients) were the most prevalent ones. Recurrent events were recorded in 58 subjects (9.7%) during a follow-up of 870.7 patient-years. Altered D-dimer levels at 1 month after OAT withdrawal were associated with a higher rate of subsequent recurrence in all subjects investigated, especially in those with an unprovoked qualifying VTE event (hazard ratio, 2.43; 95% confidence interval, 1.18 to 4.61) and in those with thrombophilia (hazard ratio, 8.34; 95% confidence interval, 2.72 to 17.43). The higher relative risk for recurrence of altered D-dimer was confirmed by multivariate analysis after adjustment for other risk factors. The negative predictive value of D-dimer was 92.9% and 95.8% in subjects with an unprovoked qualifying event or with thrombophilia, respectively.

Conclusions.—D-dimer levels measured 1 month after OAT withdrawal have a high negative predictive value for recurrence in subjects with unprovoked VTE who are either carriers or not carriers of congenital thrombophilia.

▶ Recent studies have suggested prolonged anticoagulation after idiopathic VTE results in lower rates of recurrence.[1] Perhaps a selective approach to prolonged anticoagulation after venous thrombosis can be based on D-dimer testing? This could potentially spare some patients with deep vein thrombosis prolonged anticoagulation.

G. L. Moneta, MD

Reference

1. Ridker PM, Goldhaber SZ, Danielson E, et al: Long-term, low-intensity warfarin therapy for the prevention of recurrent venous thromboembolism. *N Engl J Med* 348:1425-1434, 2003.

Negative D-Dimer Result to Exclude Recurrent Deep Venous Thrombosis: A Management Trial

Rathbun SW, Whitsett TL, Raskob GE (Univ of Oklahoma, Oklahoma City)
Ann Intern Med 141:839-845, 2004 15–8

Background.—All of the available diagnostic tests for deep venous thrombosis (DVT) have limitations for excluding acute recurrent DVT. Measurement of plasma D-dimer by using an automated quantitative assay may be useful as a rapid exclusion test in patients with suspected recurrent DVT.

Objective.—To test the safety of withholding additional diagnostic testing and heparin treatment in patients who have a negative D-dimer result at presentation (using the automated quantitative assay STA-Liatest D-di), regardless of their symptoms.

Design.—Prospective cohort study.

Setting.—Academic medical center in the United States.

Patients.—300 consecutive patients with suspected recurrent DVT.

Intervention.—Patients underwent D-dimer testing at presentation. In patients with negative D-dimer results, heparin therapy was withheld, and no further diagnostic testing for DVT was done as part of the initial evaluation. Patients with positive D-dimer results underwent compression ultrasonography.

Measurements.—The primary outcome measure was a diagnosis of new symptomatic venous thromboembolism confirmed by diagnostic testing during the 3-month follow-up period.

Results.—Of the 300 study patients, the D-dimer result was negative at presentation in 134 patients (45%; negative cohort) and positive at presentation in 166 patients. Of the 166 patients, compression ultrasonography documented new DVT in 54 patients. Compression ultrasonography findings were normal in 79 patients and were inconclusive in 33 patients. After 3 months of follow-up, 1 of 134 patients in the negative cohort had confirmed venous thromboembolism (0.75% [95% CI, 0.02% to 4.09%]). Venous thromboembolism on follow-up could not be definitively excluded in 5 patients with recurrent leg symptoms and in 1 patient who died. If these patients are considered to have venous thromboembolism, the incidence during the 3-month follow-up period would be 6.0% (CI, 2.6% to 11.4%) (8 of 134 patients).

Limitations.—There is no accepted diagnostic reference standard for recurrent DVT. The precision of the estimate of the incidence of venous thromboembolism on follow-up and the generalizability to settings other than an academic health center should be evaluated.

Conclusions.—Measurement of plasma D-dimer by using the automated quantitative assay STA-Liatest D-di seems to provide a simple method for excluding acute recurrent DVT in symptomatic patients.

► Diagnosis of recurrent DVT is often difficult in the setting of the presence of old residual thrombus. Studies suggest a negative D-dimer in patients with suspected recurrent DVT may safely allow withholding heparin therapy. There are, however, a number of limitations to this study. Many of the patients in this study were on warfarin therapy, and we don't know the effects of warfarin on D-dimer testing. In addition, patients could have had recurrent DVT that was unable to be diagnosed by available diagnostic techniques. However, it does appear safe to withhold heparin in patients with possible recurrent DVT who have a negative D-dimer test.

G. L. Moneta, MD

Incidence of Deep Vein Thrombosis After Varicose Vein Surgery

van Rij AM, Chai J, Hill GB, et al (Univ of Otago, Dunedin, New Zealand)

Br J Surg 91:1582-1585, 2004 15–9

Background.—Varicose vein surgery is generally considered to have little risk of postoperative deep vein thrombosis (DVT). This prospective study examined the incidence of DVT in patients undergoing varicose vein surgery.

Methods.—Lower leg veins were assessed before operation by duplex ultrasonography in 377 patients, and reassessed 2–4 weeks after surgery, and again at 6 and 12 months. Patients were instructed to contact a physician if symptoms consistent with DVT occurred before the scheduled follow-up appointment. Preoperative prophylaxis (a single dose of subcutaneous heparin) was left to the discretion of the vascular surgeon.

Results.—DVT was detected in 20 (5.3 per cent) of the 377 patients. Of these, only eight were symptomatic and no patient developed symptoms consistent with pulmonary embolus. Eighteen of the 20 DVTs were confined to the calf veins. Subcutaneous heparin did not alter the outcome. No propagation of thrombus was observed and half of the DVTs had resolved without deep venous reflux at 1 year.

Conclusion.—The incidence of DVT following varicose vein surgery was higher than previously thought, but these DVTs had minimal short- or long-term clinical significance (Table 1).

► Prophylaxis for venous thrombosis in patients undergoing varicose vein surgery is controversial. Based on the results of this study, the current guidelines suggested by the American College of Chest Physicians and the Scottish Guideline Network to limit DVT prophylaxis in varicose vein surgery to those patients with DVT risk factors are appropriate. Patients with multiple risk factors perhaps should be considered for extended prophylaxis.

G. L. Moneta, MD

TABLE 1.—Risk Factors for, and Incidence of, Deep Vein Thrombosis After Varicose Vein Surgery

	DVT (n = 20)	No DVT (n = 357)	P*
Age (years)			
< 40	0 (0)	56	0·055†
40-55	9 (5·7)	150	
55-70	8 (6·4)	117	
> 70	3 (8)	34	
Disease type			0·106
Primary	7 (3·5)	191	
Recurrent	13 (7·3)	166	
Severity (CEAP)			
1-2	7 (3·9)	173	
3-4	6 (4·4)	129	
5-6	7 (11)	55	0·021‡
Thromboprophylaxis			0·612
Perioperative	6 (4·5)	127	
None	14 (5·7)	230	
Previous DVT			0·361
Clinical and/or confirmed	4 (8)	46	
None	16 (4·9)	311	
Family history			0·006
Yes	4 (19)	17	
No	16 (4·5)	339	
Obesity			0·591
Obese	2 (4)	51	
Not obese	18 (5·6)	306	
Oral contraceptive or HRT use			0·247
Yes	1 (7)	5	
No	18 (5·6)	306	

Values in parentheses are percentages. CEAP, clinical, etiology, anatomy, pathology (classification); DVT, deep vein thrombosis; HRT, hormone replacement therapy.

*χ^2 test.

†Less than 40 years *versus* 40 years and older;

‡ severe disease (CEAP class 5 and 6) *versus* less severe disease (CEAP classes 1-4).

(Courtesy of van Rij AM, Chai J, Hill GB, et al: Incidence of Deep Vein Thrombosis After Varicose Vein Surgery. *Br J Surg* 91:1582-1585, 2004. Reprinted by permission of Blackwell Publishing.)

Electronic Alerts to Prevent Venous Thromboembolism Among Hospitalized Patients

Kucher N, Koo S, Quiroz R, et al (Harvard Med School, Boston; Univ of Pennsylvania, Philadelphia; Partners HealthCare System, Wellesley, Mass)
N Engl J Med 352:969-977, 2005 15–10

Background.—Prophylaxis against deep-vein thrombosis in hospitalized patients remains underused. We hypothesized that the use of a computer-alert program to encourage prophylaxis might reduce the frequency of deep-vein thrombosis among high-risk hospitalized patients.

Methods.—We developed a computer program linked to the patient database to identify consecutive hospitalized patients at risk for deep-vein thrombosis in the absence of prophylaxis. The program used medical-record numbers to randomly assign 1255 eligible patients to an intervention group,

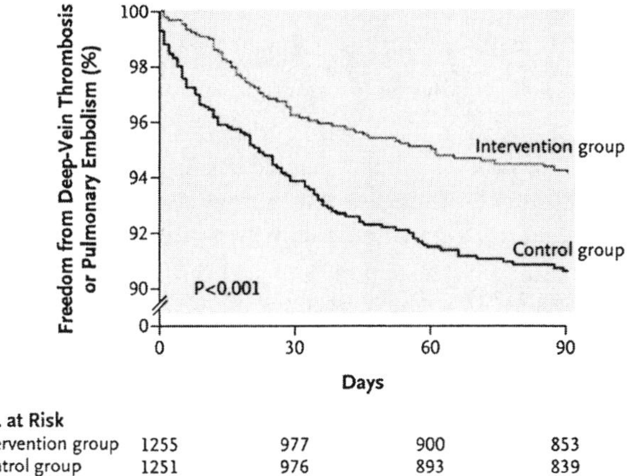

FIGURE 1.—Kaplan–Meier estimates of the absence of deep-vein thrombosis or pulmonary embolism in the intervention group and the control group. P<0.001 by the log-rank test for the comparison of the outcome between groups at 90 days. (Reprinted by permission of *The New England Journal of Medicine* from Kucher N, Koo S, Quiroz R, et al: Electronic alerts to prevent venous thromboembolism among hospitalized patients. *N Engl J Med* 352:969-977, 2005.)

in which the responsible physician was alerted to a patient's risk of deep-vein thrombosis, and 1251 patients to a control group, in which no alert was issued. The physician was required to acknowledge the alert and could then withhold or order prophylaxis, including graduated compression stockings, pneumatic compression boots, unfractionated heparin, low-molecular-weight heparin, or warfarin. The primary end point was clinically diagnosed, objectively confirmed deep-vein thrombosis or pulmonary embolism at 90 days.

Results.—More patients in the intervention group than in the control group received mechanical prophylaxis (10.0 percent vs. 1.5 percent, P<0.001) or pharmacologic prophylaxis (23.6 percent vs. 13.0 percent, P<0.001). The primary end point occurred in 61 patients (4.9 percent) in the intervention group, as compared with 103 (8.2 percent) in the control group; the Kaplan-Meier estimates of the likelihood of freedom from deep-vein thrombosis or pulmonary embolism at 90 days were 94.1 percent (95 percent confidence interval, 92.5 to 95.4 percent) and 90.6 percent (95 percent confidence interval, 88.7 to 92.2 percent), respectively (P<0.001) (Fig 1). The computer alert reduced the risk of deep-vein thrombosis or pulmonary embolism at 90 days by 41 percent (hazard ratio, 0.59; 95 percent confidence interval, 0.43 to 0.81; P=0.001).

Conclusions.—The institution of a computer-alert program increased physicians' use of prophylaxis and markedly reduced the rates of deep-vein thrombosis and pulmonary embolism among hospitalized patients at risk.

▶ The necessity of venous thromboembolism (VTE) prophylaxis in hospitalized patients is widely acknowledged. Yet prophylaxis is underutilized. VTE prophylaxis can be increased and clinically evident VTE decreased through use of a physician alert system that notifies physicians as to the patient's VTE risk.

Despite this, only 33.5% of patients in the intervention group receive prophylaxis. Additional measures will be required to maximize VTE prophylaxis in hospitalized patients.

G. L. Moneta, MD

Randomized Clinical Trial of Low Molecular Weight Heparin With Thigh-Length or Knee-Length Antiembolism Stockings for Patients Undergoing Surgery

Howard A, Zaccagnini D, Ellis M, et al (Imperial College of Science, Technology, and Medicine, London)

Br J Surg 91:842-847, 2004 15–11

Background.—This was a randomized clinical trial to determine the efficacy and safety of a 'blanket' protocol of low molecular weight heparin (LMWH) and the best length of antiembolism stocking, for every patient requiring surgery under general anaesthesia.

Methods.—Of 426 patients interviewed, 376 agreed to be randomized to receive one of three types of stocking: thigh-length Medi thrombexin® climax™ (Medi UK, Hereford, UK), knee-length thrombexin® climax™ and thigh-length Kendall T.E.D.™ (Tyco Healthcare UK, Redruth, UK). All patients received LMWH thromboprophylaxis. Duplex ultrasonography was used to assess the incidence of postoperative deep vein thrombosis (DVT).

Results.—No postoperative DVT occurred in 85 patients at low or moderate risk. Nineteen DVTs occurred, all in the 291 high-risk patients: two with the Medi thigh-length stockings, 11 with the Medi knee-length stockings (odds ratio 0.18 (95 per cent confidence interval 0.04 to 0.82); P = 0.026) and six with the Kendall T.E.D.™ thigh-length stockings. No patient developed a pulmonary embolism. Stocking groups were similar for age, sex, thromboembolic risk, type of operation and compliance. One significant bleeding complication occurred.

Conclusion.—A single protocol comprising LMWH and thigh-length stockings abolished DVT in low- and moderate-risk patients, and reduced the rate of DVT to 2 per cent in high-risk patients.

▶ The authors' simple protocol of a good-quality thigh-length stocking and LMWH has produced excellent prophylaxis against DVT in both high-risk and moderate- and low-risk patients. The protocol is simple and appears safe to use. This study is limited by relatively short follow-up with assessment of postoperative venous thrombosis being performed only on postoperative days 5 and 7.

G. L. Moneta, MD

Superiority of Fondaparinux Over Enoxaparin in Preventing Venous Thromboembolism in Major Orthopedic Surgery Using Different Efficacy End Points

Turpie AGG, Bauer KA, Eriksson BI, et al (Hamilton Health Sciences-Gen Hosp, Ont, Canada; VA Boston Healthcare System; Sahlgrenska Univ, Göteborg, Sweden; et al)

Chest 126:501-508, 2004 15–12

Study Objectives.—To assess the relevance of various efficacy end points established for thromboprophylaxis trials, we compared the results of the fondaparinux phase III program in major orthopedic surgery using the original primary efficacy end point with those obtained when the efficacy end points recently suggested by the American College of Chest Physicians (ACCP) Consensus Conference on Antithrombotic Therapy and the European Committee for Proprietary Medicinal Products (CPMP) were used.

Setting and Patients.—Fondaparinux was compared with enoxaparin in four multicenter, randomized, double-blind trials of major orthopedic surgery. The original primary efficacy end point consisted of a composite of deep-vein thrombosis detected by mandatory bilateral venography, documented symptomatic deep-vein thrombosis, or pulmonary embolism up to day 11. The efficacy end point established by the ACCP Consensus Conference on Antithrombotic Therapy comprises any proximal deep-vein thrombosis, symptomatic proven deep-vein thrombosis or pulmonary embolism, or fatal pulmonary embolism, and that established by the European CPMP comprises any proximal deep-vein thrombosis, symptomatic proven pulmonary embolism, or death from any cause.

Interventions.—Patients were randomized to receive either subcutaneous fondaparinux (2.5 mg once daily) starting postoperatively or approved enoxaparin regimens.

Results.—Using the original end point of the fondaparinux studies, the incidence of venous thromboembolism was 13.7% (371 of 2,703 patients) in the enoxaparin group compared with 6.8% (182 of 2,682 patients) in the fondaparinux group, with a common odds reduction of 55.2% ($p = 10^{-17}$); 95% confidence interval, 45.8% to 63.1%) in favor of fondaparinux. The respective incidences of efficacy end points with enoxaparin and fondaparinux were 3.3% and 1.7%, respectively, according to the ACCP definition, and 3.9% and 2.1%, respectively, according to the CPMP definition. The common odds reduction in favor of fondaparinux was 49.6% ($p < 0.001$) and 48.0% ($p < 0.001$), respectively.

Conclusions.—Fondaparinux was consistently more effective than enoxaparin in preventing venous thromboembolism in patients undergoing major orthopedic surgery, irrespective of the established composite outcomes used.

► This is basically a rehash of the 4 major trials evaluating the efficacy of fondaparinux when compared with enoxaparin in preventing venous thromboembolism in patients undergoing major hip and knee surgery. The major difference here was to eliminate asymptomatic calf vein thrombi as an end point. Indeed, asymptomatic calf vein thrombosis was by far the most frequent end point in the fondaparinux trials. The results of the current analysis still favor fondaparinux, but the absolute differences are not that great and the drug is still not that well accepted. I don't know whether this is a tribute to the marketing prowess of those who make low molecular weight heparin, the savvy of practicing physicians, or both.

G. L. Moneta, MD

Evaluation of D-Dimer in the Diagnosis of Suspected Deep-Vein Thrombosis

Wells PS, Anderson DR, Rodger M, et al (Univ of Ottawa, Ont, Canada; Dalhousie Univ, Halifax, NS, Canada; Univ of Western Ontario, London, Canada; et al)

N Engl J Med 349:1227-1235, 2003 15–13

Background.—Several diagnostic strategies using ultrasound imaging, measurement of D-dimer, and assessment of clinical probability of disease have proved safe in patients with suspected deep-vein thrombosis, but they have not been compared in randomized trials.

Methods.—Outpatients presenting with suspected lower-extremity deep-vein thrombosis were potentially eligible. Using a clinical model, physicians evaluated the patients and categorized them as likely or unlikely to have deep-vein thrombosis. The patients were then randomly assigned to undergo ultrasound imaging alone (control group) or to undergo D-dimer testing (D-dimer group) followed by ultrasound imaging unless the D-dimer test was negative and the patient was considered clinically unlikely to have deep-vein thrombosis, in which case ultrasound imaging was not performed.

Results.—Five hundred thirty patients were randomly assigned to the control group, and 566 to the D-dimer group. The overall prevalence of deep-vein thrombosis or pulmonary embolism was 15.7 percent. Among patients for whom deep-vein thrombosis had been ruled out by the initial diagnostic strategy, there were two confirmed venous thromboembolic events in the D-dimer group (0.4 percent; 95 percent confidence interval, 0.05 to 1.5 percent) and six events in the control group (1.4 percent; 95 percent confidence interval, 0.5 to 2.9 percent; P=0.16) during three months of follow-up. The use of D-dimer testing resulted in a significant reduction in the use of ultrasonography, from a mean of 1.34 tests per patient in the control group to 0.78 in the D-dimer group (P=0.008). Two hundred eighteen patients (39 percent) in the D-dimer group did not require ultrasound imaging.

Conclusions.—Deep-vein thrombosis can be ruled out in a patient who is judged clinically unlikely to have deep-vein thrombosis and who has a negative D-dimer test. Ultrasound testing can be safely omitted in such patients.

► The study indicates it is possible to safely omit venous US studies in highly selected patients with a low probability of deep venous thrombosis. Implementation of this protocol may allow vascular laboratories to reduce after-hours venous duplex studies and improve working conditions and retention of vascular technologists.

G. L. Moneta, MD

Withholding Anticoagulation After a Negative Result on Duplex Ultrasonography for Suspected Symptomatic Deep Venous Thrombosis

Stevens SM, Elliott CG, Chan KJ, et al (Univ of Utah, Salt Lake City; Franklin Square Hosp Center, Baltimore, Md)

Ann Intern Med 140:985-991, 2004 15–14

Background.—Negative results on simplified compression ultrasonography cannot rule out symptomatic deep venous thrombosis (DVT) without further testing, such as repeated ultrasonography several days later. Repeated testing is costly and inconvenient, and patients are sometimes less likely to return for follow-up tests.

Objective.—To determine the rate of venous thromboembolism when anticoagulation is withheld in patients with symptoms of DVT of the leg after negative results on a single examination with comprehensive duplex ultrasonography.

Design.—Prospective clinical cohort study.

Setting.—Peripheral vascular laboratory of a tertiary care academic hospital.

Patients.—445 consecutive patients in whom a first episode of symptomatic DVT was suspected.

Intervention.—The researchers examined the entire leg with comprehensive duplex ultrasonography, using compression and Doppler techniques. Anticoagulation was withheld from the group with negative results. Patients were observed for thromboembolic events for 3 months.

Measurements.—All patients who had new or progressive symptoms or signs of venous thromboembolism during follow-up underwent objective testing.

Results.—Comprehensive duplex ultrasonography yielded normal results in 384 patients (86.3%) and showed DVT in 61 patients (13.7%). Nineteen cases of DVT (31.1%) were isolated to the deep veins of the calf. Nine patients in the negative cohort (2.3%) were excluded from analysis because they received anticoagulation for reasons unrelated to venous thromboembolism. Three of 375 patients (0.80% [95% CI, 0.16% to 2.33%]) in the normal cohort had symptomatic venous thrombosis during the 3-month follow-up. All 384 patients in the negative cohort completed follow-up.

Limitations.—The study was conducted at a single tertiary care center by a peripheral vascular staff with substantial experience in duplex ultrasonography, which may limit the applicability of the results to other institutions. Pregnant patients were excluded.

Conclusions.—It is safe to withhold anticoagulation after negative results on comprehensive duplex ultrasonography in nonpregnant patients with a suspected first episode of symptomatic DVT of the leg. New or progressive symptoms should prompt further testing.

► Results of this study compare favorably with previous studies utilizing serial normal compression US examinations limited to the proximal leg veins. The data here confirm the clinical impression that a complete duplex examination of the lower extremities detects clinically important DVT at all levels. A single negative complete duplex examination for DVT should replace repeated testing of proximal veins. A single negative, technically adequate, complete duplex study allows withholding anticoagulation in patients suspected of DVT provided there are no new or increasing symptoms suggestive of DVT.

G. L. Moneta, MD

Does Repeat Duplex Ultrasound for Lower Extremity Deep Vein Thrombosis Influence Patient Management?

Ascher E, DePippo PS, Hingorani A, et al (Maimonides Med Ctr, Brooklyn, NY)

Vasc Endovasc Surg 38:525-531, 2004 15–15

Introduction.—The clinical significance of lower extremity deep vein thrombus (DVT) propagation in the setting of anticoagulation therapy remains unclear. The purpose of this study is to compare results of thrombus outcome found with repeat duplex ultrasonography to the incidence of pulmonary embolism and mortality. During a recent 18-month period, 457 patients were diagnosed with lower extremity DVT with duplex ultrasonography and their data were retrospectively analyzed. Repeat examinations were available for review in 118 patients (51 men, 67 women). Results of repeat duplex exams were divided into 4 groups: resolved, improved, unchanged, or extended proximally. All patients received heparin and warfarin therapy. Ventilation-perfusion ($\dot{V}/\dot{Q}$) scans were obtained only for signs and symptoms of pulmonary embolism (n=30). Mortality, the prevalence of high-probability $\dot{V}/\dot{Q}$ scans, frequency of intracaval filter insertion, gender, mean age, mean prothrombin time (PT), mean partial thromboplastin time (PTT), mean number of repeat ultrasounds per patient, and mean time over which the repeat ultrasounds took place were compared among the 4 groups. Patients who had proximal extension of DVT (19%) on repeat duplex ultrasound had an increased prevalence of pulmonary embolism ($p<0.05$). Also, patients whose DVT resolved were younger ($p<0.05$). There was no difference among the 4 groups in mortality, placement of Greenfield filters, mean PT, mean PTT, mean number of ultrasound exams per patient, or mean follow-up time over which the exams took place. Proximal extension of DVT documented by repeat duplex ultrasound is a significant risk factor for pulmonary embolism. Repeat duplex ultrasound can identify a group of patients who may benefit from insertion of an intracaval filter device.

► There are almost as many reasons to "justify" placement of venae cavae filters as there are patients with DVT. We already know from multiple previous studies that DVT is very active and often propagates somewhat even with anticoagulation. I don't think this is a reason to place a filter unless it can be demonstrated that such a policy prevents death from pulmonary embolism. This study did not demonstrate that death from pulmonary embolism was decreased by using DVT progression under anticoagulation as an indicator for filter placement. I think we are getting very close to treating the doctor and his or her wallet rather than treating the patient.

G. L. Moneta, MD

Extended Lower Limb Venous Ultrasound for the Diagnosis of Proximal and Distal Vein Thrombosis in Asymptomatic Patients After Total Hip Replacement

Elias A, Cadène A, Elias M, et al (Rangueil Univ, Toulouse, France; Hospices Civils de Lyon, Lyons, France)

Eur J Vasc Endovasc Surg 27:438-444, 2004 15–16

Objective.—To assess the performance of extended lower limb venous ultrasound (US) for the diagnosis of asymptomatic deep vein thrombosis (DVT) and to estimate a 3-month DVT incidence on repeated US after total hip replacement.

Design.—Diagnostic performance study and prospective cohort study.

Materials and Methods.—US was compared to phlebography in 70 consecutive patients and interobserver agreement was assessed in the last 48 patients at day 8. US was repeated in these 48 patients at day 13 and day 90.

Results.—Phlebography demonstrated a DVT in 18/70 (26%) patients, with five proximal and 13 distal and US in 23/70 (33%) patients, with eight proximal and 15 distal. Sensitivity and specificity of US with 95% CI were 94% (73–100) and 89% (76–96), respectively. Sensitivity in isolated distal vein thrombosis was 92% (67–99). The Kappa coefficient for agreement between observers was 0.84 (0.66–1.00). Follow-up showed a DVT in 15/48 (31%) patients on day 8, in 20/48 patients (42%) on day 13. DVT recurred in two patients during follow-up.

Conclusions.—The incidence of asymptomatic DVT is still significant despite prophylaxis but most DVTs remain distal and occur in the first 2 weeks. Extended US could replace phlebography for systematic screening in clinical trials using surrogate endpoints in view of its high accuracy and reliability.

► This study helps dispel the widespread belief that US is poor for detecting asymptomatic calf vein thrombus. With modern equipment it can be basically as good as venography. I do not think venography is still necessary to evaluate venous thromboembolism end points in trials for detection of asymptomatic DVT.

G. L. Moneta, MD

Fondaparinux or Enoxaparin for the Initial Treatment of Symptomatic Deep Venous Thrombosis: A Randomized Trial

Büller HR, for the Matisse Investigators (Univ of Amsterdam; et al)

Ann Intern Med 140:867-873, 2004 15–17

Background.—The current standard initial therapies for deep venous thrombosis are low-molecular-weight heparin and unfractionated heparin. In a dose-ranging study of patients with symptomatic deep venous thrombosis, fondaparinux had efficacy and a safety profile similar to those of low-molecular-weight heparin (dalteparin).

Objective.—To evaluate whether fondaparinux has efficacy and safety similar to those of enoxaparin in patients with deep venous thrombosis.

Design.—Randomized, double-blind study.

Setting.—154 centers worldwide.

Patients.—2205 patients with acute symptomatic deep venous thrombosis.

Intervention.—Fondaparinux, 7.5 mg (5.0 mg in patients weighing <50 kg and 10.0 mg in patients weighing >100 kg) subcutaneously once daily, or enoxaparin, 1 mg/kg of body weight, subcutaneously twice daily for at least 5 days and until vitamin K antagonists induced an international normalized ratio greater than 2.0.

Measurements.—The primary efficacy outcome was the 3-month incidence of symptomatic recurrent venous thromboembolic complications. The main safety outcomes were major bleeding during initial treatment and death. An independent, blinded committee adjudicated all outcomes.

Results.—43 (3.9%) of 1098 patients randomly assigned to fondaparinux had recurrent thromboembolic events compared with 45 (4.1%) of 1107 patients randomly assigned to enoxaparin (absolute difference, −0.15 percentage point [95% CI, −1.8 to 1.5 percentage points]). Major bleeding occurred in 1.1% of patients receiving fondaparinux and 1.2% of patients receiving enoxaparin. Mortality rates were 3.8% and 3.0%, respectively.

Limitations.—Follow-up was incomplete in 0.4% of fondaparinux-treated patients and 1.0% of enoxaparin-treated patients.

Conclusions.—Once-daily subcutaneous fondaparinux was at least as effective (not inferior) and safe as twice-daily, body weight-adjusted enoxaparin in the initial treatment of patients with symptomatic deep venous thrombosis.

▶ The fondaparinux guys keep trying and the doctors are still not buying. Despite the attractiveness of fondaparinux the market is relegating it to a boutique status drug (see also Abstract 15–12).

G. L. Moneta, MD

Combined Regional Thrombolysis and Surgical Thrombectomy for Treatment of Iliofemoral Vein Thrombosis

Blättler W, Heller G, Largiadèr J, et al (Angio Bellaria Centre for Vascular Diseases, Zurich, Switzerland; Inselspital Bern, Switzerland)

J Vasc Surg 40:620-625, 2004 15–18

Objective.—In at least half of patients with iliofemoral deep vein thrombosis post-thrombotic syndrome develops when only anticoagulant therapy is given. We combined thrombolysis, applied under ischemic conditions, with surgical thrombectomy to restore patency and valve function. The technique and the short-term and long-term results in 2 patient series are reported.

Methods.—A catheter was inserted into a foot vein of the thrombosed leg, and the limb was excluded from the circulation with a pneumatic cuff placed on the thigh with the patient under general anesthesia. Urokinase (0.5 million–3 million IU) and heparin were infused and allowed to act for 30 minutes while the pelvic axis was cleared with a Fogarty catheter through an inguinal venotomy. The external iliac vein was then clamped and the cuff removed. Thrombi that detached from the wall were flushed out with reactive hyperemia and squeezed out with manual leg compression (Fig 2). The blood was retrieved, washed, and transfused back into the patient. Various additional procedures were performed to secure outflow. Two patient series are reported: 1 with 12 consecutive patients and 1 with 21 patients who were successfully treated 6 to 10 years previously. Follow-up data were obtained for all patients after 1 year and for 18 of 21 patients after 6 to 10 years. Patency and valve function were assessed with duplex scanning or venography. Studies of blood coagulation and the kinetics of urokinase were performed in 5 additional patients.

Results.—Vein patency and valve function were restored in all consecutive patients. At 1 year none of the 33 patients had had recurrence, and none

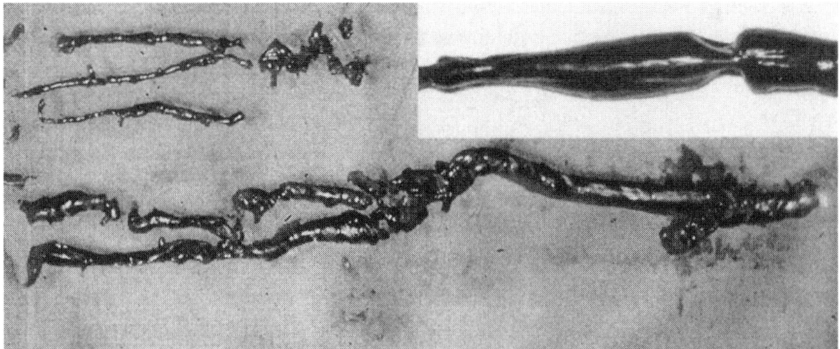

FIGURE 2.—Usually, the thrombi appearing in the operating field are only partly degraded. Here, they are assembled to demonstrate the completeness of the thrombectomy. The impressions of the valves are depicted in the insert. (Reprinted by permission of the publisher from Blättler W, Heller G, Largiadèr J, et al: Combined regional thrombolysis and surgical thrombectomy for treatment of iliofemoral vein thrombosis. *J Vasc Surg* 40:620-625, 2004. Copyright 2004 by Elsevier.)

showed clinical signs of post-thrombotic syndrome. At 6 to 10 years 3 of 18 patients had experienced another venous thromboembolism, but none in the treated leg. Sixteen legs were asymptomatic without compression therapy, and 2 had venous claudication. Coagulation studies showed a trace concentration of urokinase and a mild decrease in fibrinogen in the systemic circulation. The concentration of urokinase in blood collected from the treated leg was only 1% of that infused.

Conclusion.—Regional thrombolysis combined with surgical thrombectomy is relatively easy to perform and seems safe. Vein patency and valve function were restored, and post-thrombotic syndrome was prevented. Additional procedures to overcome pelvic vein obstructions were required in 11 of 33 patients (33%). The procedure should be tested against standard anticoagulation therapy in patients with acute iliofemoral thrombosis.

► The authors have shown they can safely combine thrombolysis with open thrombectomy in patients with iliofemoral deep venous thrombosis. How much the lytic agent itself really adds to the procedure is unclear as there is no control group. This is basically a "how I do it" report. There is no real science here. (See also Abstract 15–19.)

G. L. Moneta, MD

Surgical Thrombectomy Followed by Intraoperative Endovascular Reconstruction for Symptomatic Ilio-Femoral Venous Thrombosis

Schwarzbach MHM, Schumacher H, Böckler D, et al (Univ of Heidelberg, Germany)

Eur J Vasc Endovasc Surg 29:58-66, 2005 15–19

Objectives.—To evaluate the efficacy of surgical thrombectomy combined with endovascular reconstruction for acute ilio-femoral/caval venous thrombosis.

Methods.—Twenty consecutive patients with acute, symptomatic ilio-femoral/-caval thrombosis underwent valve-preserving thrombectomy with immediate endovascular repair between October 1996 and October 2003 (Fig 3). Thrombectomy was classified by intraoperative venography as: TYPE I = complete, TYPE II = partial, TYPE III = complete with stenosis other than thrombus, TYPE IV = permanent occlusion. TYPEs I and IV were excluded from this analysis because endovascular repair was not performed.

Results.—Left-sided venous thrombosis predominated (90%). Lesions were located in the common iliac vein (85%), the external iliac vein (10%), and the inferior vena cava (5%). Three TYPE II lesions and 17 TYPE III lesions (11 spurs, one hypoplasia, one fibrosis, one haematoma, and three others) were diagnosed. Catheter-directed recanalisation (thrombectomy/thrombolysis) resolved TYPE II lesions in three patients. Balloon angioplasty (one patient), iliac stenting (15 patients [two with thrombolysis]), and caval stenting (one patient) were employed in TYPE III stenoses. No

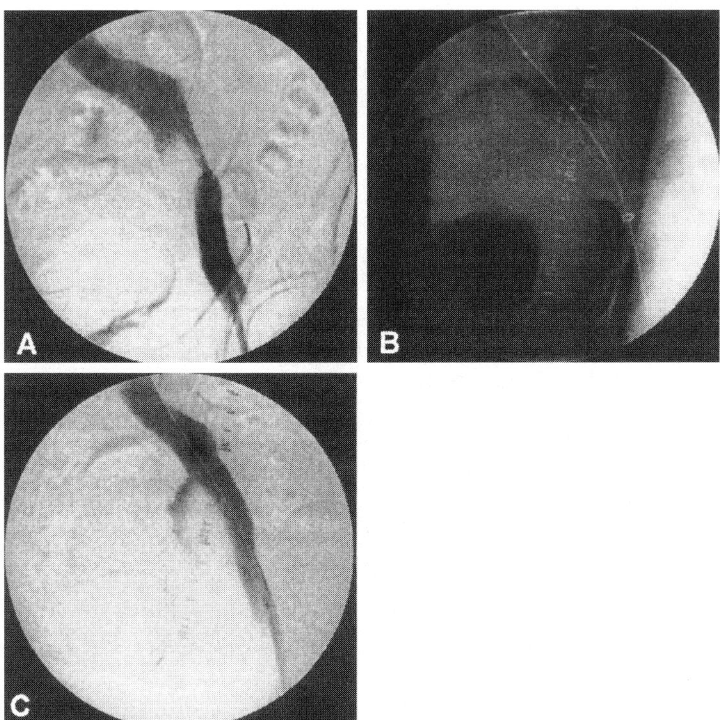

FIGURE 3.—A 62-year-old man underwent transfemoral thrombectomy with subsequent ascending venography. The venous angiogram shows a stenosis of the external iliac vein (TYPE III thrombectomy) (**A**). The stenosis was treated by deployment of a Palmaz XXL stent (**B**) and the reconstruction was patent on completion phlebography (**C**). Fifteen months after treatment the reconstruction was patent and the patient was free of swelling and pain. (Courtesy of Schwarzbach MHM, Schumacher H, Böckler D, et al: Surgical thrombectomy followed by intraoperative endovascular reconstruction for symptomatic ilio-femoral venous thrombosis. *Eur J Vasc Endovasc Surg* 29:58-66, 2005. Copyright 2005, by permission of the publisher.)

serious complication or death occurred. Mean follow-up was 21 months. Of 20 patients clinical results were excellent in 18 patients who maintained patency of their reconstructed iliac veins. Primary and secondary patency rates were 80 and 90%, respectively.

Conclusions.—Ilio-caval venous obstructions detected intraoperatively can be reconstructed in a one-stage combined procedure. The specific endovascular approach depends on the type of residual venous obstruction. Excellent mid-term results indicate that the proposed thrombectomy classification (TYPE I–IV) and treatment algorithm optimises the results in selected patients with symptomatic venous thrombosis.

► Modern technology and pharmacology are being used to tweak the old operation of venous thrombectomy (see also Abstract 15–18). It will be interesting to see if these new adjuncts will add enough to the old operation of venous thrombectomy that the procedure becomes more widely performed. As vascular surgeons place more filters and stents, I think more and more surgeons will be giving venous thrombectomy a new look.

G. L. Moneta, MD

C-Reactive Protein and Red Cell Aggregation Correlate With Late Venous Function After Acute Deep Venous Thrombosis

Krieger E, van Der Loo B, Amann-Vesti BR, et al (Univ Hosp Zurich, Switzerland; Univ of Zurich, Switzerland)

J Vasc Surg 40:644-649, 2004 15–20

Objective.—Risk factors leading to development and subsequent progression of chronic venous insufficiency after acute deep venous thrombosis (DVT) are only partially identified. Inflammation and rheologic abnormalities might have a causative role. The purpose of this study was to investigate C-reactive protein (CRP), D-dimer, and blood rheologic parameters in patients after acute DVT in relation to clinical outcome.

Subjects and Methods.—Patients with a history of acute proved DVT underwent clinical examination and duplex ultrasound scanning of the veins, and Venous Clinical Severity Score (VCSS) and Venous Segmental Disease Score (VSDS) were calculated. Further, CRP, D-dimer, and several rheologic parameters were determined and related to outcome as assessed with venous scores.

Results.—Forty-three patients were examined 28 (median) months after the index event. Patients had higher CRP ($P < .001$), D-dimer ($P < .001$), red blood cell aggregation ($P < .01$), fibrinogen concentration ($P < .01$), and leukocyte count ($P < .05$) than did healthy control subjects. CRP and red blood cell aggregation were positively correlated with VCSS ($r = 0.42$ and $P < .01$, and $r = 0.30$ and $P < 0.05$, respectively) (Fig 1). Multivariate regression analysis showed that the relation between CRP and VCSS was independent of

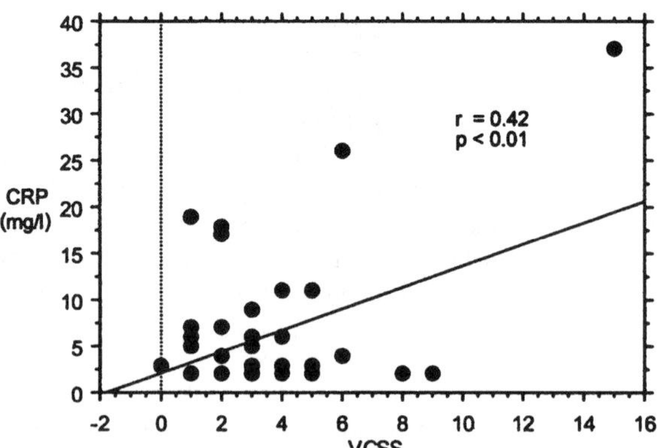

FIGURE 1.—Correlation between C-reactive protein and Venous Clinical Severity Score (*VCSS*). (Reprinted by permission of the publisher from Krieger E, van Der Loo B, Amann-Vesti BR, et al: C-Reactive protein and red cell aggregation correlate with late venous function after acute deep venous thrombosis. *J Vasc Surg* 40:644-649, 2004. Copyright 2004 by Elsevier.)

other laboratory and rheologic parameters and of age, total thrombus load, duration of compression therapy after the index event, recurrence, recanalization, and presence of comorbid conditions ($P < .05$).

Conclusions.—CRP is independently related to the severity of venous dysfunction in patients after acute DVT. Chronic inflammation as well as changes in blood rheologic parameters may be causally involved in the development of chronic venous insufficiency occurring in the medium-term and long-term course after acute DVT.

► Dr. Wakefield and his colleagues at the University of Michigan have convinced us inflammation is associated with acute DVT. Now we have the suggestion that inflammatory markers may also be predictive of late venous function after DVT. It is always nice to see observations in patients parallel observations in the laboratory. The cause-effect relationship between CRP levels and late venous function still remains to be established.

G. L. Moneta, MD

Iliac Compression Syndrome and Recanalization of Femoropopliteal and Iliac Venous Thrombosis: A Prospective Study With Magnetic Resonance Venography

Fraser DGW, Moody AR, Morgan PS, et al (Queen Elizabeth Hosp, Birmingham, England; Sunnybrook and Women's College Health Science Centre, Toronto; Univ Hosp, Nottingham, England)

J Vasc Surg 40:612-619, 2004 15–21

Objectives.—Poor iliac vein recanalization has been associated with compression of the left common iliac vein by the right common iliac artery (RCIA/LCIV compression); however, this finding has been difficult to confirm. In a baseline study, RCIA/LCIV compression was detected with magnetic resonance imaging in patients with deep venous thrombosis. We compared recanalization of left femoropopliteal and iliac thrombosis with and without RCIA/LCIV compression.

Methods.—This was a prospective blinded study carried out in a 1355-bed university hospital. Thirty-one patients were recruited from consecutive cohorts of patients with iliofemoral and femoropopliteal DVT who underwent direct thrombus magnetic resonance imaging, venous enhanced peak arterial magnetic resonance venography, and magnetic resonance arteriography as part of the baseline study relating RCIA/LCIV compression to extent of thrombosis. Magnetic resonance venography was performed 6 weeks, 6 months, and 1 year after diagnosis of deep venous thrombosis. Femoropopliteal and iliac venous segments that were occluded at diagnosis were classified as occluded, partially occluded, or patent on follow-up scans.

Results.—At 6-week follow-up, recanalization of all segments was incomplete. At both 6-month and 1-year follow-up, recanalization of left iliac segments associated with RCIA/LCIV compression was poorer compared with recanalization of left iliac segments not associated with compression (6 of 6

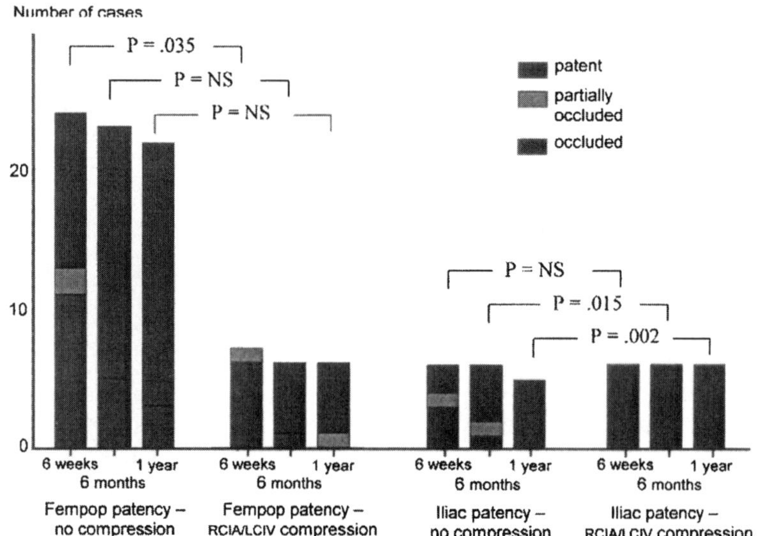

FIGURE 2.—Patency of femoropopliteal and iliac veins during follow-up divided according to the presence of compression of the left common iliac vein by the right common iliac artery (*RCIA/LCIV compression*). Recanalization of femoropopliteal and iliac segments not associated with RCIA/LCIV compression remained occluded. Failure of femoropopliteal vein recanalization associated with RCIA/LCIV compression at 6 weeks may have been related to more extensive thrombosis at presentation and persistent occlusion of adjacent iliac veins. *Fempop,* femoropopliteal; *NS,* nonsignificant. (Reprinted by permission of the publisher from Fraser DGW, Moody AR, Morgan PS, et al: Iliac compression syndrome and recanalization of femoropopliteal and iliac venous thrombosis: A prospective study with magnetic resonance venography. *J Vasc Surg* 40:612-619, 2004. Copyright 2004 by Elsevier.)

occluded vs 1 of 6 occluded and 1 of 6 partially occluded at 6 months, P=.015; 6 of 6 occluded vs 5 of 5 patent at 1 year, P=.002). This was due to complete failure of recanalization of left common iliac veins associated with RCIA/LCIV compression in 6 of 6 cases. All other iliac and femoropopliteal segments including left external iliac veins associated with RCIA/LCIV compression had high rates of recanalization at both 6 months and 1 year (Fig 2).

Conclusion.—RCIA/LCIV compression is associated with persistent occlusion of the left common iliac vein. The recanalization rate for all other femoropopliteal and iliac segments was high.

► This is modern technology to confirm a 40-year-old observation.[1]

G. L. Moneta, MD

Reference

1. Cockett FB, Thomas ML: The iliac compression syndrome. *Br J Surg* 52:816-821, 1965.

Below-Knee Elastic Compression Stockings to Prevent the Post-Thrombotic Syndrome: A Randomized, Controlled Trial

Prandoni P, Lensing AWA, Prins MH, et al (Univ Hosp of Padua, Italy; Academic Med Ctr, Amsterdam; Academic Hosp, Maastricht, The Netherlands)
Ann Intern Med 141:249-256, 2004 15–22

Background.—Because only limited evidence suggests that elastic stockings prevent the post-thrombotic syndrome in patients with symptomatic deep venous thrombosis (DVT), these stockings are not widely used.

Objective.—To evaluate the efficacy of compression elastic stockings for prevention of the post-thrombotic syndrome in patients with proximal DVT.

Design.—Randomized, controlled clinical trial.

Setting.—University hospital.

Patients.—180 consecutive patients with a first episode of symptomatic proximal DVT who received conventional anticoagulant treatment.

Interventions.—Before discharge, patients were randomly assigned to wear or not wear below-knee compression elastic stockings (30 to 40 mm Hg at the ankle) for 2 years. Follow-up was performed for up to 5 years.

Measurements.—The presence and severity of the post-thrombotic syndrome were scored by using a standardized scale.

Results.—Post-thrombotic sequelae developed in 44 of 90 controls (severe in 10) and in 23 of 90 patients wearing elastic stockings (severe in 3). All but 1 event developed in the first 2 years. The cumulative incidence of the post-thrombotic syndrome in the control group versus the elastic stockings group was 40.0% (95% CI, 29.9% to 50.1%) versus 21.1% (CI, 12.7% to 29.5%) after 6 months, 46.7% (CI, 36.4% to 57.0%) versus 22.2% (CI, 13.8% to 30.7%) after 1 year, and 49.1% (CI, 38.7% to 59.4%) versus

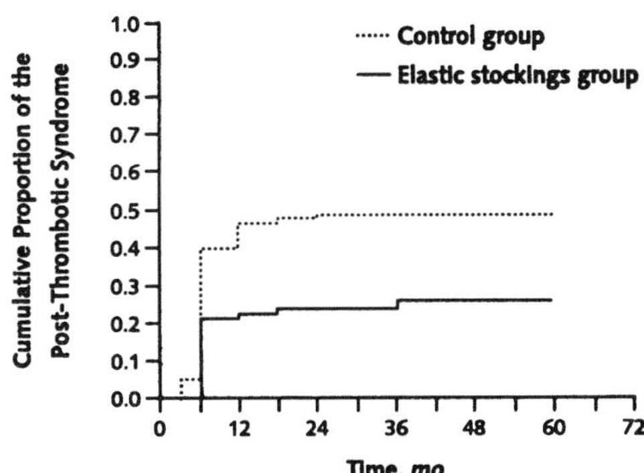

Patients at risk, *n*

Control group	90	54	47	43	41	40	40	33	26	20	16
Elastic stockings group	90	71	69	66	64	63	62	59	48	31	24

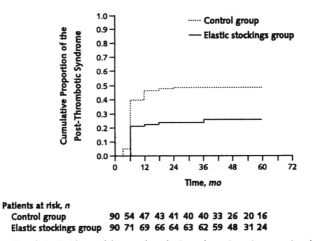

FIGURE 2.—Cumulative incidence of the post-thrombotic syndrome in patients wearing elastic stockings and those in the control group. (Courtesy of Prandoni P, Lensing AWA, Prins MH, et al: Below-knee elastic compression stockings to prevent the post-thrombotic syndrome: A randomized, controlled trial. *Ann Intern Med* 141:249-256, 2004.)

24.5% (CI, 15.6% to 33.4%) after 2 years (Fig 2). After adjustment for baseline characteristics, the hazard ratio for the post-thrombotic syndrome in the elastic stockings group compared with controls was 0.49 (CI, 0.29 to 0.84; $P = 0.011$).

Limitations.—This study lacked a double-blind design.

Conclusions.—Post-thrombotic sequelae develop in almost half of patients with proximal DVT. Below-knee compression elastic stockings reduce this rate by approximately 50%.

► This study, along with a previous study by Brandjes et al,[1] indicate a beneficial effect of prophylactic compression stockings for preventing postthrombotic syndrome in patients with symptomatic proximal DVT. Patients with proximal DVT should be treated with elastic compression stockings to reduce the symptoms of postthrombotic syndrome.

G. L. Moneta, MD

Reference

1. Brandjes DP, Büller HR, Heijboer H, et al: Randomised trial of effect of compression stockings in patients with symptomatic proximal-vein thrombosis. *Lancet* 349:759-762, 1997.

Preservation of Venous Valve Function After Catheter-Directed and Systemic Thrombolysis for Deep Venous Thrombosis

Laiho MK, Oinonen A, Sugano N, et al (Helsinki Univ)

Eur J Vasc Endovasc Surg 28:391-396, 2004 15–23

Objectives.—The aim of the study was to assess venous reflux and the obstruction pattern after catheter-directed and systemic thrombolysis of deep iliofemoral venous thrombosis.

Patients.—Thirty-two patients treated either with systemic (16) or catheter-directed local thrombolysis (16) for massive iliofemoral thrombosis were identified from the hospital registry.

Methods.—Clinical evaluation at follow up was based on the CEAP classification and disability score. Reflux was assessed by colour duplex ultrasonography and standardised reflux testing. A vascular surgeon blinded to treatment established the clinical status of the lower limb following the previous DVT.

Results.—Valvular competence was preserved in 44% of patients treated with catheter-directed thrombolysis compared with 13% of those treated with systemic thrombolysis ($p = 0.049$, Chi squared). Reflux in any deep vein was present in 44% of patients treated by catheter-directed lysis compared with 81% of patients receiving systemic thrombolysis ($p = 0.03$, Chi squared). Reflux in any superficial vein was observed in 25% vs. 63% of the patients, respectively ($p = 0.03$, Chi squared). There were significantly more patients with venous insufficiency of classes C0-1 in the group treated with catheter-directed thrombolysis.

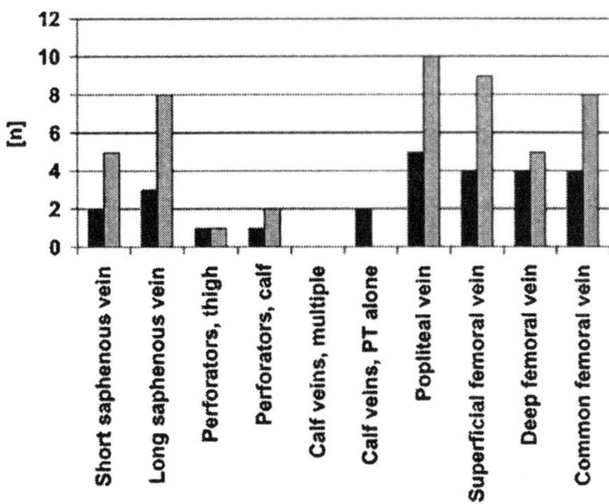

FIGURE 1.—Anatomical distribution of incompetent venous segments after deep vein thrombosis in patients treated with catheter-directed thrombolysis (black column) and systemic thrombolysis (light grey column). (Courtesy of Laiho MK, Oinonen A, Sugano N, et al: Preservation of venous valve function after catheter-directed and systemic thrombolysis for deep venous thrombosis. *Eur J Vasc Endovasc Surg* 28:391-396, 2004. Copyright 2004, by permission of the publisher.)

Conclusion.—In this clinical series venous valvular function was better preserved after iliofemoral DVT when treated with catheter-directed thrombolysis (Fig 1).

▶ In this retrospective study, systemic thrombolysis did not work to preserve valve function after DVT. Catheter-directed thrombolysis did not work well either. Without controls this study adds nothing to the already incomprehensible literature on lytic therapy to preserve late valve function after DVT.

G. L. Moneta, MD

Role of a Quantitative D-Dimer Assay in Determining the Need for CT Angiography of Acute Pulmonary Embolism

Abcarian PW, Sweet JD, Watabe JT, et al (Kaiser Found Hosp, Honolulu, Hawaii)

AJR 182:1377-1381, 2004 15–24

Objective.—Our goal was to use the results of a quantitative D-dimer assay to determine the need for pulmonary CT angiography in patients suspected of having acute pulmonary embolism.

Materials and Methods.—From July 2001 to December 2002, 755 patients underwent pulmonary CT angiography for the evaluation of acute pulmonary embolism. A rapid, fully automated quantitative D-dimer assay was obtained in more than half the patients. The electronic medical records of the patients were subsequently reviewed to analyze the negative predictive value of the D-dimer assay in the diagnostic workup of acute pulmonary embolism and to determine the outcome of the patients who had negative findings on both D-dimer assay and pulmonary CT angiography at 3-month follow-up.

Results.—Of the 755 patients who underwent pulmonary CT angiography, 666 (88.2%) had negative findings, 73 (9.7%) had positive findings, and 16 (2.1%) were indeterminate. A total of 426 patients underwent both pulmonary CT angiography and D-dimer level evaluation, and 84 of these had negative findings (< 0.4 µg/mL) on D-dimer assay. Eighty-two of the 84 patients with negative findings on D-dimer assay had negative findings on pulmonary CT angiography; two were indeterminate and both subsequently had low-probability ventilation-perfusion studies. Among patients with positive D-dimer assays, no one with a level between 0.4 and 1.0 µg/mL had pulmonary CT angiography with findings positive for pulmonary embolism.

Conclusion.—A quantitative D-dimer assay was effective in excluding the need for pulmonary CT angiography and had high negative predictive value when the D-dimer level was less than 1.0 µg/mL.

▶ There is now enough literature out there to support use of D-dimer testing in evaluation of patients with suspected venous thromboembolism (VTE). I think physicians are on pretty solid ground withholding anticoagulation and other diagnostic studies for VTE in patients suspected of VTE but in whom D-dimer levels are very low.

G. L. Moneta, MD

Upper-Extremity Deep Vein Thrombosis: A Prospective Registry of 592 Patients

Joffe HV, for the Deep Vein Thrombosis (DVT) FREE Steering Committee (Harvard Med School, Boston; Duke Univ, Durham, NC)

Circulation 110:1605-1611, 2004 15–25

Background.—Upper-extremity deep vein thrombosis (UEDVT) occurs spontaneously or sometimes develops as a complication of pacemaker use, long-term use of a central venous catheter (CVC), or cancer.

Method and Results.—To improve our understanding of UEDVT, we compared the demographics, symptoms, risk factors, prophylaxis, and initial management of 324 (6%) patients with central venous catheter (CVC)–associated UEDVT, 268 (5%) patients with non–CVC-associated UEDVT, and 4796 (89%) patients with lower-extremity DVT from a prospective US multicenter DVT registry. The non–CVC-associated UEDVT patients were younger (59.218.2 versus 64.216.9 years old; P<0.0001), less often white (65% versus 73%; P<0.01), leaner (body mass index [BMI] 26.87.1 versus 28.57.3 kg/m^2; P<0.001), and more likely to smoke (19% versus 13%; P=0.02) than the lower-extremity DVT patients. By way of propensity analysis and multivariable logistic regression analysis, we determined that an indwelling CVC was the strongest independent predictor of UEDVT (odds ratio [OR], 7.3; 95% confidence interval [CI], 5.8 to 9.2). An age of <67 years, a BMI of <25 kg/m^2, and hospitalization were the independent predictors of non–CVC-associated UEDVT. Most (68%) UEDVT patients were evaluated while they were inpatients. Only 20% of the 378 UEDVT patients who did not have an obvious contraindication to anticoagulation received prophylaxis at the time of diagnosis.

Conclusions.—UEDVT risk factors differ from the conventional risk factors for lower-extremity DVT. Our findings identify deficiencies in our current understanding and the prophylaxis of UEDVT and generate hypotheses for future research efforts.

► In addition to the obvious risk factor of a CVC for production of UEDVT, the authors point out differences between the risk factors for UEDVT and lower extremity DVT. Younger age and mean body weight as well as inpatient status independently predicted UEDVT. The data suggest possible underlying differences in the pathophysiology of UEDVT versus lower extremity DVT.

G. L. Moneta, MD

Characterization and Probability of Upper Extremity Deep Venous Thrombosis

Schmittling ZC, McLafferty RB, Bohannon WT, et al (Illinois Univ, Springfield)
Ann Vasc Surg 18:552-557, 2004 15–26

Introduction.—The objective of this study was to characterize patient demographics, risk factors, and anatomic distribution of upper extremity deep venous thrombosis (UEDVT) to develop a probability model for diagnosis. A retrospective review of all patients who underwent color-flow duplex scanning (CDS) for clinically suspected acute UEDVT over a 5-year period was performed. Patient risk factors and clinical symptoms were evaluated as predictors. Technically adequate complete CDS of 177 upper extremities (UEs) of arms were reviewed. CDS scanning identified acute UE venous thrombosis in 53 (30%) of the arms examined with deep system involvement in 40 (23%). Of the UEs affected, the subclavian was involved in 64%, the axillary in 25%, the internal jugular in 32%, the brachial in 36%, the cephalic in 32%, and the basilic in 47%. Multivariate analysis identified limb tenderness (odds ratio 9.3), history of central venous catheterization (odds ratio 7.0), and malignancy (odds ratio 2.9) as positive predictors for UEDVT (Table 4). Erythema (odds ratio 0.12) and suspected pulmonary embolism (odds ration 0.06) were identified as negative predictors. A predictive model was designed from these variables. The anatomic distribution of UEDVT obtained from this study is consistent with previous reviews. Potential positive and negative risk factors can be identified from which a predictive model can be designed. Use of this model can help focus clinical suspicion, improve color-flow duplex utilization, and provide timely treatment with anticoagulation.

TABLE 4.—Multivariate Analysis of Clinical Variables and Risk Factors

Clinical Variable	Odds Ratio	95% CI
Tenderness	9.3	2.4-35.5
Central venous catherization	7	2.9-17
Malignancy	2.9	1.3-6.7
Suspicion of PE	0.12	0.02-0.62
Erythema	0.06	0.01-0.68

(Courtesy of Schmittling ZC, McLafferty RB, Bohannon WT, et al: Characterization and probability of upper extremity deep venous thrombosis. *Ann Vasc Surg* 18:552-557, 2004.)

▶ This study parallels previous studies in lower extremities using clinical findings as predictors of venous thrombosis. As with clinical findings in the lower extremities, no findings in the upper extremity are sufficiently sensitive or specific in themselves to determine the need for duplex sonography. The next step will be to evaluate the use of D-dimer testing in patients with possible UEDVT.

G. L. Moneta, MD

Risk Factors and Recurrence Rate of Primary Deep Vein Thrombosis of the Upper Extremities

Martinelli I, Battaglioli T, Bucciarelli P, et al (Univ of Milano, Italy)

Circulation 110:566-570, 2004 15–27

Background.—One third of cases of upper-extremity deep vein thrombosis (DVT) are primary, ie, they occur in the absence of central venous catheters or cancer. Risk factors for primary upper-extremity DVT are not well established, and the recurrence rate is unknown.

Method and Results.—We studied 115 primary upper-extremity DVT patients and 797 healthy controls for the presence of thrombophilia due to factor V Leiden, prothrombin G20210A, antithrombin, protein C, protein S deficiency, and hyperhomocysteinemia. Transient risk factors for venous thromboembolism were recorded. Recurrent upper-extremity DVT was evaluated prospectively over a median of 5.1 years of follow-up. The adjusted odds ratio for upper-extremity DVT was 6.2 (95% CI 2.5 to 15.7) for factor V Leiden, 5.0 (95% CI 2.0 to 12.2) for prothrombin G20210A, and 4.9 (95% CI 1.1 to 22.0) for the anticoagulant protein deficiencies. Hyperhomocysteinemia and oral contraceptives were not associated with upper-extremity DVT. However, in women with factor V Leiden or prothrombin G20210A who were taking oral contraceptives, the odds ratio for upper-extremity DVT was increased up to 13.6 (95% CI 2.7 to 67.3). The recurrence rate was 4.4% patient-years in patients with thrombophilia and 1.6% patient-years in those without thrombophilia. The hazard ratio for recurrent upper-extremity DVT in patients with thrombophilia compared with those without was 2.7 (95% CI 0.7 to 9.8).

Conclusions.—Inherited thrombophilia is associated with an increased risk of upper-extremity DVT. Oral contraceptives increase the risk only when combined with inherited thrombophilia. The recurrence rate of primary upper-extremity DVT is low but tends to be higher in patients with thrombophilia than in those without.

► Patients with primary upper extremity DVT (UEDVT) can be considered for investigation of inherited thrombophilia. The relatively low risk of upper UEDVT recurrence even in patients with thrombophilia, however, does not support prolonged or lifelong anticoagulation of all patients with UEDVT. This is regardless of thrombophilia status. Nevertheless, knowledge of thrombophilia status may be important when the patient undergoes future surgical procedures or develops additional risk factors for DVT.

G. L. Moneta, MD

Elevated Plasma Factor VIII and D-Dimer Levels as Predictors of Poor Outcomes of Thrombosis in Children

Goldenberg NA, for the Mountain States Regional Thrombophilia Group (Univ of Colorado, Denver; et al)
N Engl J Med 351:1081-1088, 2004 15–28

Background.—Elevated levels of plasma factor VIII and D-dimer predict recurrent venous thromboembolism in adults. We sought to determine whether an elevation of factor VIII, D-dimer, or both at diagnosis and persistence of the laboratory abnormality after three to six months of anticoagulant therapy correlate with poor outcomes of thrombosis in children.

Methods.—We evaluated levels of factor VIII and D-dimer and additional components of an extensive laboratory thrombophilia (i.e., hypercoagulability) panel at the time of diagnosis in 144 children with a radiologically confirmed acute thrombotic event. All patients were treated initially with heparin and then with either warfarin or low-molecular-weight heparin for at least three to six months, according to the current standard of care. Patients were examined at follow-up visits 3, 6, and 12 months after diagnosis and then annually, at which times testing was repeated in children with previously abnormal factor VIII and D-dimer test results and a uniform evaluation for the post-thrombotic syndrome was performed.

Results.—Among 82 children for whom complete data were available regarding laboratory test results at diagnosis and thrombotic outcomes during follow-up, 67 percent had factor VIII levels above the cutoff value of 150 IU per deciliter, D-dimer levels above 500 ng per milliliter, or both at diagnosis, and at least one of the two laboratory values was persistently elevated in 43 percent of the 75 patients in whom testing was performed after three to six months of anticoagulant therapy. Fifty-one percent of the 82 patients had a poor outcome (i.e., a lack of thrombus resolution, recurrent thrombosis, or the post-thrombotic syndrome) during a median follow-up of 12 months (range, 3 months to 5 years). Elevated levels of factor VIII, D-dimer, or both at diagnosis were highly predictive of a poor outcome (odds ratio, 6.1; P=0.008), as was the persistence of at least one laboratory abnormality at three to six months (odds ratio, 4.7; P=0.002). The combination of a factor VIII level above 150 IU per deciliter and a D-dimer level above 500 ng per milliliter at diagnosis was 91 percent specific for a poor outcome, and after three to six months of standard anticoagulation, the combination was 88 percent specific.

Conclusions.—Elevated levels of plasma factor VIII, D-dimer, or both at diagnosis and a persistent elevation of at least one of these factors after standard-duration anticoagulant therapy predict a poor outcome in children with thrombosis.

▶ Children with thrombosis should not be considered just small adults. Children have lower concentrations of physiologic inhibitors of the coagulation system and a more limited fibrinolytic capacity than do adults. These differences in the coagulation system between adults and children are particularly prominent in the first year of life and at the time of puberty and adolescence.[1] This study's stratification of specific levels of factor VIII and D-dimer in children with thrombosis should help guide anticoagulation therapy in children.

G. L. Moneta, MD

Reference

1. Andrew M: Developmental hemostasis: Relevance to thromboembolic complications in pediatric patients. *Thromb Haemost* 74:415-425, 1995.

16 Chronic Venous and Lymphatic Disease

Correlation of Duplex Ultrasound Scanning-derived Valve Closure Time and Clinical Classification in Patients With Small Saphenous Vein Reflux: Is Lesser Saphenous Vein Truly Lesser?

Lin JC, Iafrati MD, O'Donnell TF Jr, et al (Tufts–New England Med Ctr, Boston)

J Vasc Surg 39:1053-1058, 2004 16–1

Objective.—We recently identified small saphenous vein (SSV) reflux as a significant risk factor for ulcer recurrence in patients with severe chronic venous insufficiency (CVI) undergoing perforator vein ligation. In this study we examined the role of SSV reflux in patients across the spectrum of CVI.

Methods.—From March 15, 1997, to December 24, 2002, clinical and duplex ultrasound (US) scanning data from all valve closure time studies performed in our vascular laboratory were prospectively recorded. Valve closure time in the deep and superficial leg veins was assessed with the rapid cuff deflation technique; reflux time greater than 0.5 seconds was considered abnormal. SSV reflux was correlated with the CEAP classification system and eventual surgical procedure. Data were analyzed with Pearson χ^2 analysis.

Results.—We analyzed 722 limbs in 422 patients, 265 (63%) female patients and 157 (37%) male patients, with a mean age of 48 ± 12.8 years (range, 16-85 years). In the entire cohort the cause was congenital (Ec) in 5 patients, primary (Ep) in 606 patients, and secondary (Es) in 112 patients. SSV reflux was present in 206 limbs (28.5%) evaluated. Among limbs with SSV reflux, Ec = 4 (2%), Ep = 162 (79%), and Es = 40 (19%). SSV reflux did not correlate with gender, side, or age. The prevalence of SSV reflux increases with increasing severity of clinical class: C1-C3, 25.8% versus C4-C6, 36.1% ($P = .006$). SSV reflux is highly associated with deep venous reflux, 35.2% of femoral vein reflux ($P = .015$), 35.8% of femoral vein plus popliteal vein reflux ($P = .001$), and 40.5% of isolated popliteal vein reflux ($P < .001$). Great saphenous vein (GSV) reflux was identified in 483 (67%) limbs studied with valve closure time, whereas SSV reflux was present in 206 (28%) limbs. In this cohort, 127 GSV or SSV surgical procedures were performed subsequent to valve closure time examination. Among these operations 107 (84%) were GSV procedures, and only 20 (16%) were SSV procedures.

Conclusion.—SSV reflux is most common in patients demonstrating severe sequelae of CVI, such as lipodermatosclerosis or ulceration. The increasing prevalence of SSV reflux in more severe clinical classes and the strong association of SSV reflux and deep venous reflux suggest that SSV may have a significant role in CVI. Our data further show that, in our institution, a GSV with reflux is more than twice as likely to be surgically corrected as an SSV with reflux. It is time for the SSV to assume greater importance in the treatment of lower extremity venous disease. Future improvements in surgical techniques for access and visualization of the SSV may facilitate this method.

▶ The Tufts–New England Medical Center group continues their investigations of SSV incompetence in primary and secondary venous disease. There is an association with deep vein reflux and advanced stages of chronic venous disease suggesting an important role of SSV reflux in CVI, justifying surgical treatment of incompetent SSVs. It is unclear, though, whether perhaps benefits of such treatment overweight the risks of complications. This awaits demonstration of SSV treatment outcomes in patients with different clinical and anatomic patterns of chronic venous disease.

F. Lurie, MD, PhD

Prevalence, Anatomic Patterns, Valvular Competence, and Clinical Significance of the Giacomini Vein

Delis KT, Knaggs AL, Khodabakhsh P (Imperial College, London; Mayo Clinic, Rochester, Minn)

J Vasc Surg 40:1174-1183, 2004 16–2

Objective.—Coursing the posterior thigh as a tributary or trunk projection of the small saphenous vein (SSV), the Giacomini vein's clinical significance in chronic venous disease (CVD) remains undetermined. This cross-sectional controlled study examined the prevalence, anatomy, competency status, and clinical significance of the Giacomini vein across the clinical spectrum of CVD in relation to the SSV termination.

Methods.—One hundred eighty-nine consecutive subjects (301 limbs) with suspected CVD (109 men, 80 women; age, 18-87 years [median, 61

FIGURE 1.—Schematic representation of thigh extension (Giacomini vein) of small saphenous vein (*SSV*) in limbs with a typical saphenopopliteal junction (**A**) and in limbs with a high or a very high SSV termination (**B**). See Methods for definitions. Epitomized are the single or multiple endings (see Table III) of Giacomini vein. Percentage attached to named veins represents cumulative occurrence in limbs with (**A**) a typical saphenopopliteal junction alone (236 of 301; great saphenous vein, 33% [78 of 236]; posterior thigh muscle veins, 17% [40 of 236]; femoral vein, 8% [19 of 236]; popliteal vein, 100% [236 of 236]) and (**B**) with a high or a very high SSV termination alone (65 of 301; great saphenous vein, 42% [27 of 65]; profunda femoral vein, 11% [7 of 65]; posterior thigh muscle veins, 27% [18 of 65]; femoral vein, 14% [9 of 65]). Differences in cumulative proportions not statistically significant. *Abbreviation: Giac V,* Giacomini vein. (Reprinted by permission of the publisher from Delis KT, Knaggs AL, Khodabakhsh P: Prevalence, anatomic patterns, valvular competence, and clinical significance of the Giacomini vein. *J Vasc Surg* 40:1174-1183, 2004. Copyright 2004 by Elsevier.)

FIGURE 1

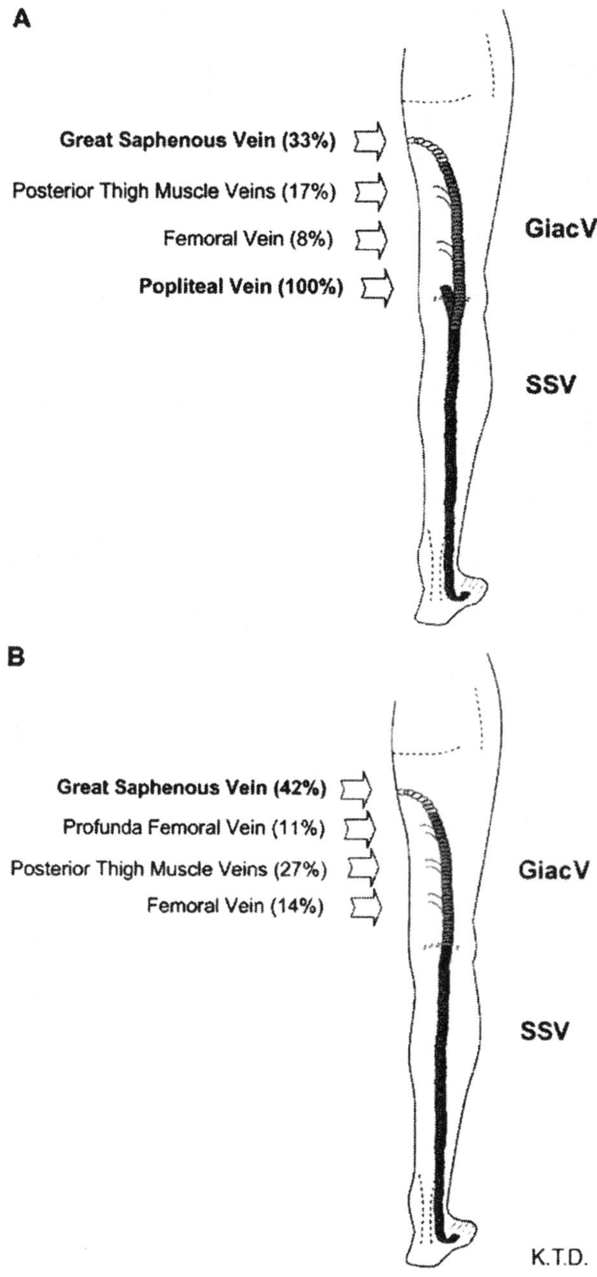
A
Great Saphenous Vein (33%)
Posterior Thigh Muscle Veins (17%)
Femoral Vein (8%)
Popliteal Vein (100%)
GiacV
SSV
B
Great Saphenous Vein (42%)
Profunda Femoral Vein (11%)
Posterior Thigh Muscle Veins (27%)
Femoral Vein (14%)
GiacV
SSV
K.T.D.

years]) underwent examination, clinical class (CEAP) stratification, and duplex ultrasound determination of the sites and extent of reflux >0.5 sec) and Giacomini vein's anatomy (Fig 1).

Results.—A Giacomini vein was found in 70.4% of limbs (212 of 301; 95% confidence interval, 65%-75.6%). Extent, pattern, and sites of reflux in all named superficial and deep veins were evenly distributed in limbs with and without a Giacomini vein; perforator vein incompetence in thigh and calf was also balanced (all, $P > .2$). Giacomini vein had no effect ($P > .2$) on SSV termination anatomy, displaying a similar prevalence in classes C(0-6). In 212 limbs, either as a tributary or trunk projection of the SSV, the Giacomini vein ascended subfascially (n = 210) to the lower (8%; n = 17), middle (47.6%; n = 101), or upper (44.3%; n = 94) thigh, and terminated at the deep system (45.3%; n = 96) and/or perforated the fascia (64.2%; n = 136), to join the superficial system. Giacomini vein morphology was not affected by the SSV termination anatomy and CEAP clinical class. Incompetence was detected less often ($P < .001$) in the Giacomini vein (4.7%; n = 10 of 212) than in the saphenous trunks cumulatively (53.3%; n = 113 of 212). Yet the odds ratio of Giacomini incompetence was 11.94 (7 of 33 over 3 of 169) in the presence of SSV reflux, and 11.67 (6 of 23 over 4 of 179) when both the great saphenous vein (proximal, proximal plus distal) and SSV were incompetent.

Conclusion.—Found in more than two thirds of limbs, the Giacomini vein has a complex anatomy that is linked vastly to the deep or superficial veins of the posteromedial thigh, but is unaffected by the anatomy of SSV termination and CEAP clinical class. Its presence proved insignificant to the extent, pattern, sites, and clinical severity of venous incompetence, yet the Giacomini vein was far less often susceptible to reflux than the saphenous trunks were. Routine Giacomini vein investigation is not justified in view of these findings. Investigation could be considered selectively in limbs with SSV incompetence, with or without great saphenous vein incompetence, supported by the high odds of concomitant Giacomini vein reflux.

▶ Using duplex US, the authors confirmed earlier anatomic studies indicating the presence of a Giacomini vein in more than 70% of extremities with CVD. In addition, this report provides interesting information that, when present, Giacomini veins have valvular insufficiency in less than 5% of extremities. They are incompetent when the great saphenous vein, SSV, or both, are incompetent. The indication for treatment of incompetent Giacomini veins is still not clear. It will be interesting to learn what happens to Giacomini vein reflux after successful treatment of saphenous incompetence.

F. Lurie, MD, PhD

Iliac Vein Compression in an Asymptomatic Patient Population
Kibbe MR, Ujiki M, Goodwin AL, et al (Northwestern Univ, Chicago)
J Vasc Surg 39:937-943, 2004 16–3

Objective.—May-Thurner syndrome is a well-recognized anatomic variant that is associated with the development of symptomatic acute venous thrombosis of the left iliac vein. However, the natural frequency of compression of the left iliac vein and its clinical significance in asymptomatic disease has not been established. Therefore the purpose of this descriptive anatomic study was to determine the incidence of left common iliac vein compression in an asymptomatic population.

Methods.—A retrospective analysis of medical records and helical abdominal computed tomography scans was conducted in 50 consecutive patients evaluated in the emergency department because of abdominal pain. Medical records were reviewed for symptoms and risk factors for deep venous thrombosis, and data were collected and reported according to the Joint Society Reporting Standards for acute lower extremity venous thrombosis. All computed tomography was performed with intravenous contrast medium, and 2-mm to 5-mm axial images were obtained. The minor diameter of the common iliac arteries and veins was measured. The technique of transverse image measurement was validated with multiplanar reconstructions and orthogonal diameter measurements in a subset of subjects. Statistical analysis was performed with the Student *t* test or Spearman rank correlation.

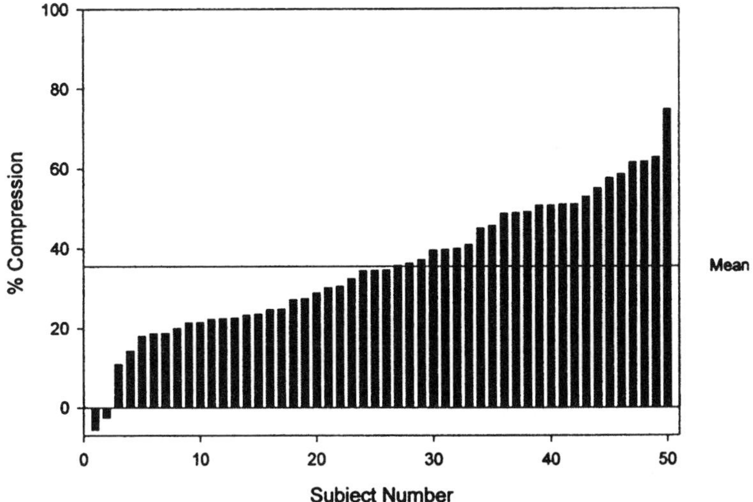

FIGURE 1.—Individual results of percent compression of the left iliac vein as measured on axial CT images with transverse linear measurements. (Reprinted by permission of the publisher from Kibbe MR, Ujiki M, Goodwin AL, et al: Iliac vein compression in an asymptomatic patient population. *J Vasc Surg* 39:937-943, 2004. Copyright 2004 by Elsevier.)

Results.—Mean age of subjects without symptoms was 40 years (range, 19-85 years), and 60% (n = 30) were female patients. The mean acute lower extremity venous thrombosis risk factor score was 1.16 ± 0.23 (range, 0-6; maximum possible score, 28). It was surprising that 24% (n = 12) of patients had greater than 50% compression and 66% (n = 33) had greater than 25% compression (Fig 1). Mean compression of the left common iliac vein was 35.5% (range, −5.6%-74.8%). The structure most often compressing the left common iliac vein against the vertebral body was the right common iliac artery (84%). There was no strong correlation between patient age or common iliac artery size and compression of the left common iliac vein. However, women had greater mean compression of the left common iliac vein (women, 41.2% ± 3.1%; men, 27.0% ± 3.0%; P =.003).

Conclusion.—Hemodynamically significant left common iliac vein compression is a frequent anatomic variant in asymptomatic individuals. Therefore compression of the left iliac vein may represent a normal anatomic pattern that has thus far been thought of as a pathologic condition.

▶ This report confirms earlier anatomic data that left iliac vein compression is widely present in asymptomatic individuals. Although patients were studied in the horizontal position and CT scans were obtained during the arterial phase, the magnitude of prevalence of left iliac vein compression is astonishing: two thirds of all patients had at least 25% compression, and in one fourth it was 50% or greater. One can conclude that perhaps a noncompressed left iliac vein is relatively rare. This publication suggests a careful reexamination of the relationship between left iliac vein compression and acute and chronic venous disease.

F. Lurie, MD, PhD

Compression Stockings Reduce Occupational Leg Swelling

Partsch H, Winiger J, Lun B (Univ of Vienna; Ganzoni Management AG, Winterthur, Switzerland; Research Dept of Ganzoni Group, St Just, France)

Dermatol Surg 30:737-743, 2004 16–4

Background.—Evening edema of the legs is a physiologic phenomenon occurring after sitting and standing.

Objective.—The objective of this study was to investigate which compression pressure is necessary to prevent leg swelling.

Methods.—In 12 volunteers, the volume of both lower legs was measured in the morning and 7 h later, the difference being defined as evening edema (mL). The procedure was carried out for 4 days, in which the subjects wore below-knee stockings of different compression levels alternatively on one leg only in a random order. Compression pressure was assessed using the HATRA device.

Results.—The average evening edema of the noncompressed legs was 62.4 mL on the left side and 94.4 mL on the right side (n.s.). Evening edema was significantly reduced to 40.3 mL by light support stockings, to −34.1

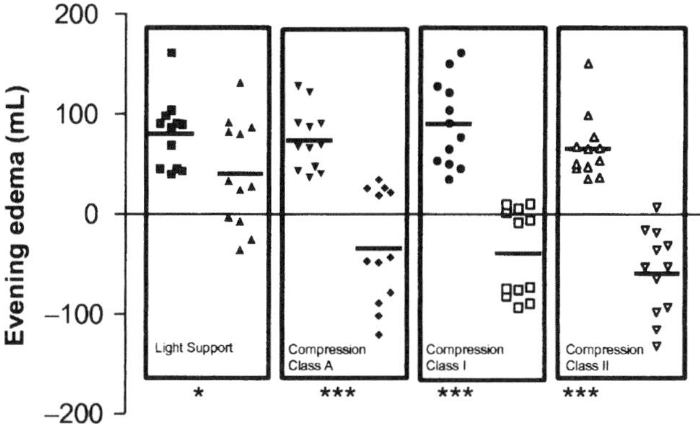

FIGURE 4.—Reduction of evening edema with light support stockings (*p<0.05), prevention with compression stockings between classs A and class II (***p<0.0001). The *shapes on the left side in each box* represent the values without stockings ("evening edema"); the *shapes on the right side* represent the values after different stockings on the same leg. (Courtesy of Partsch H, Winiger J, Lun B: Compression stockings reduce occupational leg swelling. *Dermatol Surg* 30:737-743, 2004. Copyright 2004 by the American Society for Dermatologic Surgery, Inc. Published by Blackwell Publishing.)

mL by compression class A, to −39.6 by compression class I, and to −59.1 mL by compression class II (Fig 4). Mainly stockings exerting a pressure above 10 mmHg improved subjective symptoms.

Conclusion.—Calf-length compression stockings with a pressure range between 11 and 21 mmHg are able to reduce or totally prevent evening edema and may therefore be recommended for people with a profession connected with long periods of sitting or standing.

► This is perhaps the first investigation accounting for all major factors influencing outcomes of elastic compression. It includes direct measurement of applied pressures and has demonstrated a significant reduction of occupational edema by wearing compression stockings. Demonstrated benefits of low-pressure stockings suggest tissue pressure may be much lower than theoretic hydrostatic pressure. The importance of this finding is that some patients may get the same benefit from wearing class I, or class A stockings versus the much less "patient friendly" class II stockings.

F. Lurie, MD, PhD

Effectiveness and Safety of Calcium Dobesilate in Treating Chronic Venous Insufficiency: Randomized, Double-blind, Placebo-controlled Trial

Labs K-H, for the CVI Study Group (Univ of Basel, Switzerland; et al)

Phlebology 19:123-130, 2004 16–5

Background.—Chronic venous insufficiency (CVI) is a common problem with significant medical and socioeconomic effects. A need exists for effective conservative treatment of CVI. The efficacy of calcium dobesilate (CaD) for reducing CVI-related peripheral edema was determined.

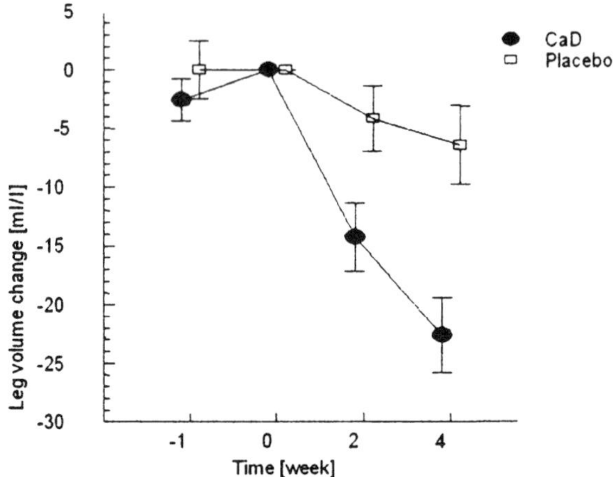

FIGURE 3.—Change in leg volume during the treatment period, in a subset of patients with previous therapy (SSS = 1) or with CEAP C4 or with CVI duration > 12 years (median ± MADN/$\sqrt{n}$). *Abbreviations: SSS*, Previous treatment with compression stockings, sclerotherapy or venous stripping; *MADN*, median absolute deviation normalized; *CaD*, calcium dobesilate; *CVI*, chronic venous insufficiency. (Courtesy of Labs K-H, for the CVI Study Group: Effectiveness and safety of calcium dobesilate in treating chronic venous insufficiency: Randomized, double-blind, placebo-controlled trial. *Phlebology* 19:123-130, 2004.)

Methods.—A randomized, double-blind, parallel group trial was conducted in centers in Switzerland and France. Study participants were enrolled in a 1-week screening period followed by a 4-week treatment phase with review at day 14 and a 2-week follow-up phase with no treatment. Patients were randomly assigned to receive 500 mg of CaD 3 times per day or matching placebo. The primary end point was the change of the lower leg volume (LV) of the more diseased leg between baseline and week 4. LV was calculated on the basis of a truncated cone model. Secondary end points included change of leg perimeters, evaluation of the patient's subjective symptomatology on a 10-cm visual analog scale, and assessment on a 7-point scale of the overall efficacy of the study drug by the patient and investigator at the conclusion of the study.

Results.—Patients in the CaD group showed a median reduction of leg volume of 25.5 ± 33.6 mL/L tissue. The difference in the median change of the leg volume between the treatment groups at week 4 was −12.2 mL/L tissue (Fig 3). The effects of CaD were independent of the duration of CVI (in contrast with findings in the placebo group) and were more pronounced in the more severely diseased patients. No significant differences were seen in safety variables between groups.

Conclusions.—These findings were in agreement with those of previous trials and supportive of the effectiveness and tolerability of CaD for the treatment of CVI.

► An unusually high magnitude of placebo effect, especially in the patients with a short history of venous disease, emphasizes the need for double-blind studies. Assuming the majority of patients had primary disease with saphenous reflux, their symptoms could be controlled by stripping or endovenous treatment. Using drug treatment gave them very little benefit. The maximal differences between the placebo and treatment groups were 1.32 mm in ankle circumference and 1.5 mm in calf circumference. The clinical significance of such small changes is questionable. Despite the authors' optimism, drug treatment appears suboptimal in patients who can be effectively managed by surgery.

F. Lurie, MD, PhD

Sodium Tetradecyl Sulfate for Sclerotherapy Treatment of Veins: Is Compounding Pharmacy Solution Safe?

Goldman MP (Dermatology/Cosmetic Laser Associates of La Jolla, Inc, Calif)

Dermatol Surg 30:1454-1456, 2004 16–6

Objective.—The objective was to determine the composition of three available solutions of sodium tetradecyl sulfate from compounding pharmacies in comparison to pharmaceutical-grade sodium tetradecyl sulfate, Fibrovein (STD Pharmaceuticals, Ltd.).

Methods.—Solutions of 3% sodium tetradecyl sulfate were obtained from three compounding pharmacies. An analysis of their composition was performed.

Results.—All samples of 3% sodium tetradecyl sulfate obtained had a different concentration of sodium tetradecyl sulfate than that stated on the bottle (range, 2.59%-3.39%). Significant concentrations of the contaminant carbitol were present in samples from all three sources (0.33%-4.18%).

Conclusion.—The production of 3% sodium tetradecyl sulfate by these three compounding pharmacies appears to occur by simple dilution of a 27% industrial detergent solution that is not manufactured for use in humans. Physicians need to be aware that the stated concentration may not be correct and that along with sodium tetradecyl sulfate, potentially harmful contaminants may be present in the solution.

► Physicians and surgeons who use compounding pharmacies as a source of IV solutions should be aware of the results of this study. Concentrations of carbitol as high as 4.18% may present potential risk, especially when large volumes of sclerosant are injected. It is unclear how much the variability in pH and concentration of sodium tetradecyl in these solutions contributes to treatment outcomes.

F. Lurie, MD, PhD

Microfoam Ultrasound-guided Sclerotherapy of Varicose Veins in 100 Legs

Barrett JM, Allen B, Ockelford A, et al (Palm Clinic, Auckland, New Zealand; Dermatology/Cosmetic Laser Associates of La Jolla, Inc, Calif)

Dermatol Surg 30:6-12, 2004 16–7

Background.—Microfoam ultrasound-guided sclerotherapy (UGS) has been shown to be effective for closure of the saphenous trunks for treatment of varicose veins. The effectiveness of UGS treatment from both clinical and patient quality-of-life perspectives was determined retrospectively.

Methods.—This retrospective analysis was conducted among 100 randomly selected legs, including 55 left and 45 right legs. The greater saphenous vein was treated in 89 legs, and the short saphenous vein was treated in 23 legs. Both the greater and short saphenous veins were treated in 12 patients. Patients were asked to complete a quality-of-life survey and were evaluated clinically, with the use of visual assessment and duplex scanning. All of the patients had been treated for varicose veins of the leg with UGS with a mean of 22.5 months of follow-up. The end point of treatment was closure of incompetent saphenous trunks, incompetent branch veins, and all associated varicosities. Follow-up treatment was provided at 3 months, if required, which occurred in 31% of legs. The success of UGS therapy was measured on the basis of clinical assessment and patient satisfaction.

Results.—The average number of USG treatments required to close incompetent varicose veins was 2.1, using an average of 8.7 mL of foam scle-

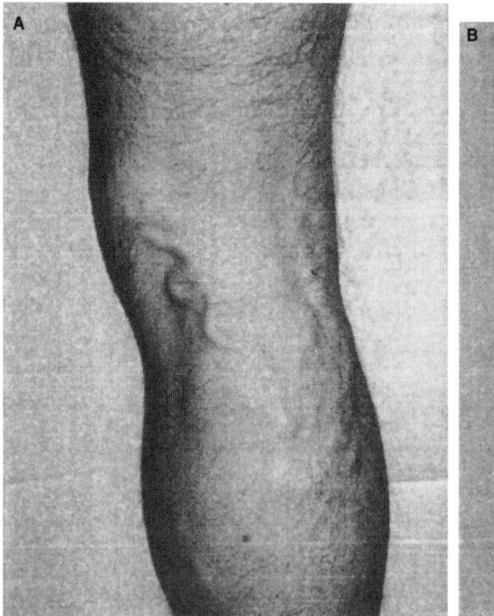

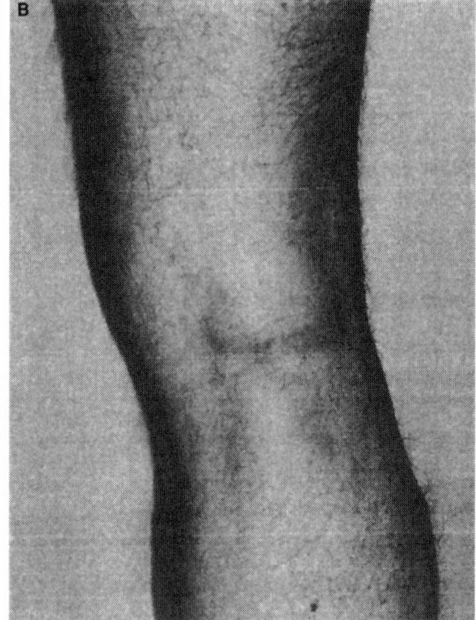

FIGURE 10.—(A) Before UGS. (B) One week after UGS. (Courtesy of Barrett JM, Allen B, Ockelford A, et al: Microfoam ultrasound-guided sclerotherapy of varicose veins in 100 legs. *Dermatol Surg* 30:6-12, 2004. Reprinted by permission of Blackwell Publishing.)

rosing solution. Patient satisfaction was high—100% of patients believed that their legs were successfully treated; resolution of all symptoms were seen by 85% of patients, and resolution of all varicose veins by 92% of patients (Fig 10).

Conclusions.—USG foam sclerotherapy is a safe and effective treatment for all varicose veins, providing high patient satisfaction with outcomes and improvement in the patients' quality of life.

▶ This study has demonstrated high patient satisfaction with microfoam sclerotherapy in 100 symptomatic and asymptomatic patients who underwent microfoam sclerotherapy of saphenous veins. This was despite the fact that 31 patients needed retreatment at 3 months. The authors used a variety of concentrations and doses of polidocanol and sodium tetradecyl sulphate. This variability of treatment techniques indicates modern sclerotherapy is still more a form of art than science. Neurologic complications, deep vein thrombosis, and local phlebitis can occur after foam sclerotherapy, but the incidence is low. US follow-up indicated that, unlike after radiofrequency obliteration or endovenous laser therapy, saphenous veins remain visible 2 years after foam sclerotherapy. This raises the concern of late recanalization.

F. Lurie, MD, PhD

Prospective Randomised Study of Endovenous Radiofrequency Obliteration (Closure) Versus Ligation and Vein Stripping (EVOLVeS): Two-Year Follow-up

Lurie F, Creton D, Eklof B, et al (Univ of Hawaii, Honolulu; Clinique Ambroise Pare, Nancy, France; Vein Inst of New Jersey, Morristown; et al)

Eur J Vasc Endovasc Surg 29:67-73, 2005 16–8

Purpose.—To study intermediate clinical outcomes, rates of recurrent varicosities and neovascularisation, ultrasound changes of the GSV, and the quality of life changes in patients from EVOLVeS trial.

Methods.—Forty five patients were re-examined 1 year and 65 two years after treatment. Follow-up visits included clinical examination with CEAP classification and calculation of venous clinical severity score (VCSS), ultrasound examination, and a quality of life questionnaire.

Results.—The clinical course of the disease (CEAP, VCSS) was similar in the two treatment groups. 51% of the GSV trunks occluded by RFO underwent progressive shrinkage with the external diameter decreased from 6.3 SD 1.4 mm at 72 h after treatment to 2.9 SD 1.5 mm at 2 years. An additional 41% of the GSV became undetectable by ultrasound at 2-year follow up. In two patients we observed re-opening of an initially closed GSV lumen. Neovascularisation was found in one RFO case and in four S and L cases. Cumulative rates of recurrent varicose veins at combined 1 and 2 years follow-up were 14% for RFO and 21% for S and L (NS). The difference in global QOL score in favour of RFO re-appeared at 1 year and remained significant at 2 years after treatment.

Conclusion.—The 2-year clinical results of radiofrequency obliteration are at least equal to those after high ligation and stripping of the GSV. In the vast majority of RFO patients the GSV remained permanently closed, and underwent progressive shrinkage to eventual sonographic disappearance. Recurrence and neovascularisation rates were similar in the two groups although limited patient numbers prevent reliable statistical analysis. Improved quality of life scores persisted through the 2-year observations in the RFO group compared to the S and L group.

▶ Another piece of evidence suggesting that, at least in the short-term, catheter-based interventions for obliteration of the greater saphenous vein (GSV) are at least as effective as traditional ligation and stripping procedures. There are still details to be worked out regarding catheter-based obliteration of the GSV, such as the long-term effects of preservation of the proximal GSV branches, and when, and if, to combine stab phlebectomy or sclerotherapy with catheter-based treatment of the GSV.

G. L. Moneta, MD

Deep Venous Thrombosis After Radiofrequency Ablation of Greater Saphenous Vein: A Word of Caution

Hingorani AP, Ascher E, Markevich N, et al (Maimonides Med Ctr, Brooklyn, NY)

J Vasc Surg 40:500-504, 2004 16–9

Purpose.—Radiofrequency ablation (RFA) of the greater saphenous vein (GSV; "closure") is a relatively new option for treatment of venous reflux. However, our initial enthusiasm for this minimally invasive technique has been tempered by our preliminary experience with its potentially lethal complication, deep venous thrombosis (DVT).

Methods.—Seventy-three lower extremities were treated in 66 patients with GSV reflux, between April 2003 and February 2004. There were 48 (73%) female patients and 18 (27%) male patients, with ages ranging from 26 to 88 years (mean, 62 ± 14 years). RFA was combined with stab avulsion of varicosities in 55 (75%) patients and subfascial ligation of perforator veins in 6 (8%) patients. An ATL HDI 5000 scanner with linear 7-4 MHz probe and the SonoCT feature was used for GSV mapping and procedure guidance in all procedures. GSV diameter determined the size of the RFA catheter used. Veins less than 8 mm in diameter were treated with a 6F catheter (n = 54); an 8F catheter was used for veins greater than 8 mm in diameter (n = 19). The GSV was cannulated at the knee level. The tip of the catheter was positioned within 1 cm of the origin of the inferior epigastric vein (first GSV tributary). All procedures were carried out according to manufacturer guidelines.

Results.—All patients underwent venous duplex ultrasound scanning 2 to 30 days (mean, 10 ± 6 days) after the procedure. The duplex scans documented occlusion of the GSV in 70 limbs (96%). In addition, DVT was found in 12 limbs (16%). Eleven patients (92%) had an extension of the occlusive clot filling the treated proximal GSV segment, with a floating tail beyond the patent inferior epigastric vein into the common femoral vein (Figure). Another patient developed acute occlusive clots in the calf muscle (gastrocnemius) veins. Eight patients were readmitted and received anticoagulation therapy. Four patients were treated with enoxaparin on an ambulatory basis. None of these patients had pulmonary embolism. Initially 3 patients with floating common femoral vein clots underwent inferior vena cava filter placement. Of the 19 limbs treated with the 8F RFA catheter, GSV clot extension developed in 5 (26%), compared with 7 of 54 (13%) limbs treated with the 6F RFA catheter (P = .3). No difference was found between the occurrence of DVT in patients who underwent the combined procedure (RFA and varicose vein excision) compared with patients who underwent GSV RFA alone (P =.7). No statistically significant differences were found in age or gender of patients with or without postoperative DVT (P = NS).

Conclusion.—Patients who underwent combined GSV RFA and varicose vein excision did not demonstrate a higher occurrence of postoperative DVT compared with patients who underwent RFA alone. Early postoperative du-

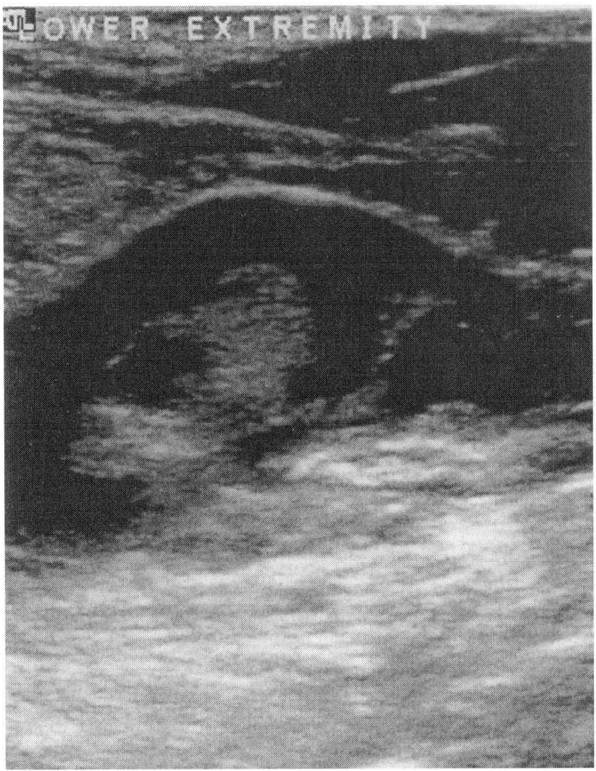

FIGURE.—Free-floating common femoral vein thrombus. (Reprinted by permission of the publisher from Hingorani AP, Ascher E, Markevich N, et al: Deep venous thrombosis after radiofrequency ablation of greater saphenous vein: A word of caution. *J Vasc Surg* 40:500-504, 2004. Copyright 2004 by Elsevier.)

plex scans are essential, and should be mandatory in all patients undergoing RFA of the GSV.

▶ This is a lot of DVT following RFA. The 16% incidence of DVT after RFA of the GSV in this series far exceeds multiple previous reports suggesting a DVT incidence of less than 1%. Eleven of 12 observed DVTs originated from the proximal-treated GSV segment and extended into the common femoral vein and thus were directly related to treatment. Preserving flow from the epigastric vein into the common femoral vein during endovenous ablation is thought to be an intraoperative protective measure against DVT. Another intriguing bit of information is that all proximal DVTs underwent complete lysis within 3 to 14 days of anticoagulation therapy. The take-home message is that patients after RFA should be monitored with duplex US a day after the procedure.

F. Lurie, MD, PhD

The Effect of Long Saphenous Vein Stripping on Deep Venous Reflux

MacKenzie RK, Allan PL, Ruckley CV, et al (Royal Infirmary, Edinburgh, Scotland; Heartlands Hosp, Birmingham, England)

Eur J Vasc Endovasc Surg 28:104-107, 2004 16–10

Background.—The addition of long saphenous vein (LSV) stripping to sapheno-femoral junction (SFJ) disconnection and multiple stab avulsions (MSAs) in the course of varicose vein (VV) surgery is associated with a significant reduction in recurrence, and a significant improvement in quality of life. It is hypothesised that these benefits relate, at least in part, to a favourable effect of stripping on deep venous reflux.

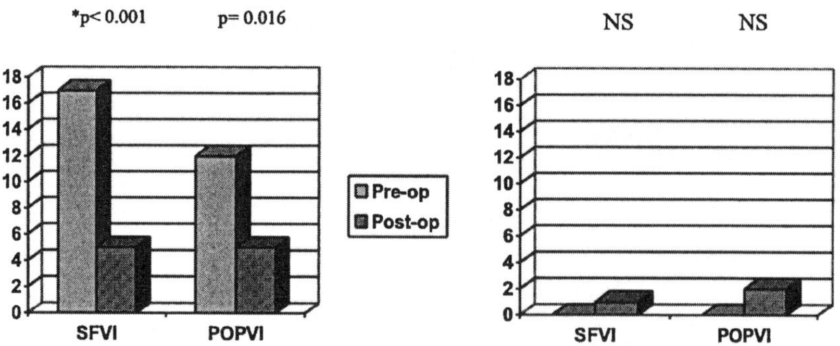

FIGURE 1.—Presence of deep venous incompetence pre- and post-operatively in patients with complete stripping of the long saphenous vein in the thigh. *Asterisk*, McNemars test comparing pre-operative and 2 year post-operative prevalence of reflux. *Abbreviations: DVR*, Deep venous reflux (popliteal and superficial femoral vein); *SFVI*, superficial femoral vein incompetence; *POPVI*, popliteal vein incompetence. (Reprinted from MacKenzie RK, Allan PL, Ruckley CV, et al: The effect of long saphenous vein stripping on deep venous reflux. *Eur J Vasc Endovasc Surg* 28:104-107, 2004. Copyright 2004, by permission of the publisher.)

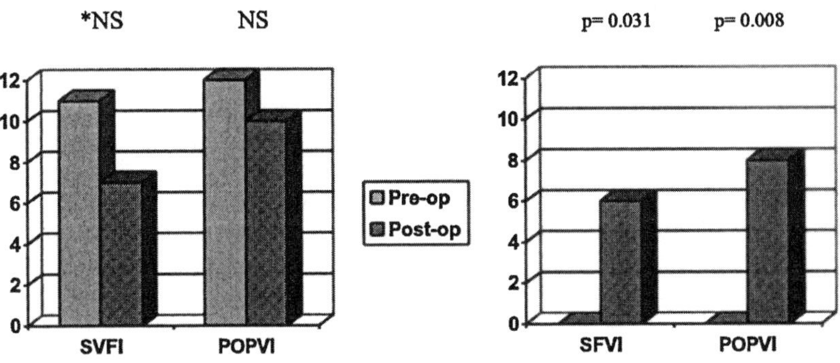

FIGURE 2.—Presence of deep venous incompetence pre- and post-operatively in patients with incomplete stripping of the long saphenous vein in the thigh. *Asterisk*, McNemars test comparing pre-operative and 2 year post-operative prevalence of reflux. *Abbreviations: DVR*, Deep venous reflux (popliteal and superficial femoral vein); *SFVI*, superficial femoral vein incompetence; *POPVI*, popliteal vein incompetence. (Reprinted from MacKenzie RK, Allan PL, Ruckley CV, et al: The effect of long saphenous vein stripping on deep venous reflux. *Eur J Vasc Endovasc Surg* 28:104-107, 2004. Copyright 2004, by permission of the publisher.)

Objective.—To examine the effect of long saphenous vein (LSV) stripping on deep venous reflux (DVR).

Methods.—This was prospective study of 62 consecutive patients (77 limbs) CEAP class 2-6, undergoing SFJ disconnection and MSAs, with and without successful stripping of the LSV to the knee. A duplex ultrasound examination was performed pre-operatively and at a median (IQR) of 24 (23-25) months post-operatively. Completely stripped limbs were defined as those in whom complete stripping of the LSV to the knee was confirmed on post-operative duplex. Reflux ≥0.5 s. was considered pathological.

Results.—Pre-operatively, 32 (42%) limbs had deep venous reflux (DVR). Post-operative duplex at 24 months revealed that the LSV had been completely stripped in 29 (38%) limbs. In patients with pre-operative DVR, complete stripping was associated with a significant reduction in the prevalence of superficial femoral vein (SFV) ($p < 0.001$) and popliteal vein (PV) reflux ($p = 0.016$), McNemar test) on post-operative duplex (Fig 1). By contrast, in patients without pre-operative DVR, incomplete stripping was associated with the development of SFV ($p = 0.031$) and PV ($p = 0.008$) reflux (Fig 2).

Conclusions.—Complete LSV stripping abolishes DVR in a significant proportion of limbs, whereas failure to strip is frequently associated with the development of new DVR. These data support for routine stripping and suggest that the benefits of stripping may relate, at least in part, to a favourable impact on deep venous function.

▶ The data suggest that successful stripping of a refluxing greater saphenous vein (GSV) may improve reflux in the femoral and popliteal veins. An incomplete stripping may lead to the development of new DVR in the femoral and popliteal veins. This study reaffirms the growing realization that DVR may derive from the presence of superficial venous reflux (see 2005 YEAR BOOK OF VASCULAR SURGERY, pp 360-362). Patients with a combination of DVR and superficial venous reflux may benefit from stripping of a refluxing GSV and, in fact, may be harmed by leaving a refluxing GSV in situ.

G. L. Moneta, MD

Fate of Great Saphenous Vein After Radio-Frequency Ablation: Detailed Ultrasound Imaging

Salles-Cunha SX, Rajasinghe H, Dosick SM, et al (Jobst Vascular Ctr, Toledo, Ohio)

Vasc Endovasc Surg 38:339-344, 2004 16–11

Introduction.—Radio-frequency ablation (RFA) of the great saphenous vein (GSV) is an endovascular alternative to stripping. To determine long-term effectiveness, the fate of GSV treated for valvular insufficiency with RFA was evaluated in detail with ultrasound imaging (US). One hundred lower extremities were examined with high-resolution color flow US, an average of 8 months after RFA treatment of an incompetent GSV. For every cm of the RFA-treated segment, the US observation was classified as follows: absent, occluded, or recanalized. Lengths of vein segments in each class were added and percentages of absent, occluded, or recanalized segments were calculated. Five groups were identified. Group I (n = 15): segment of treated GSV was absent. Group II (n = 4): segment of treated GSV was visualized and occluded (these vein segments had no flow and were shrunk and "fibrotic" or thrombosed without clear evidence of significant shrinkage). Group III (n = 1): segment of treated GSV was recanalized. Group IV (n = 27): segment of treated GSV was obstructed (absent or occluded). Group V (n = 53): segment of treated GSV was partially recanalized, on average being 53% absent, 32% occluded, and 15% recanalized. Maximum recanalization was 50% of treated segment. RFA was successful in obliterating all of the GSV treated segment in 46% of veins (groups I, 15%, plus II, 4%, plus IV, 27%) and obliterated more than half of the treated vein segment in 53% of the cases (group V). A dynamic process of recanalization and thrombosis warrants further evaluation to determine if and how a collateral network may develop.

▶ This report provides detailed information on US images of the GSV between 4 and 14 months after RFA. It confirmed previous reports that the GSV after RFA undergoes progressive shrinkage and eventually disappears either entirely or segment by segment. Recanalization was rare in this study. The association of untreated branches that provide inflow and outflow to recanalized segments suggests that incompetent tributaries and perforators should be treated at the time of RFA.

F. Lurie, MD, PhD

Neovascularization and Recurrent Varicose Veins: More Histologic and Ultrasound Evidence

van Rij AM, Jones GT, Hill GB, et al (Univ of Otago, Dunedin, New Zealand)

J Vasc Surg 40:296-302, 2004 16–12

Background.—The recurrence of varicose veins is a common and costly consequence of varicose vein surgery. Despite the long history and vast experience of varicose vein surgery, the exact cause of recurrence is still unknown. This study aims to investigate the cause of recurrence further by correlating findings from duplex ultrasound scans, resin casts, and histologic investigation at the recurrence of the saphenofemoral junction. In particular, frequency and neovascularization are evaluated.

Method.—Forty-nine saphenofemoral junctions (SFJs) from 42 patients who presented for re-operation on their varicose veins were examined with duplex ultrasound and physiologic air plethysmography tests before surgery. All patients had reflux at the groin for which surgery was carried out. Specimens taken during surgery were sectioned and stained for conventional histology and immunohistology, and 5 specimens were infused with resin to form a cast of the venous vasculature (Fig 5).

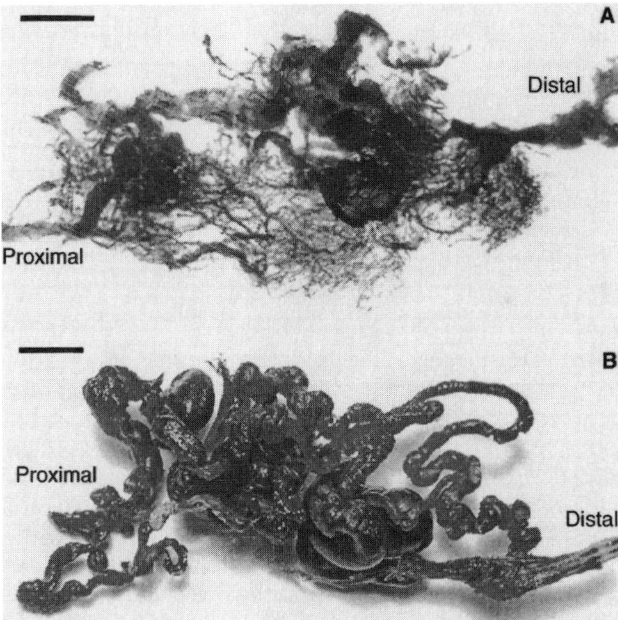

FIGURE 5.—Vascular casts of recurrent refluxing saphenofemoral junction specimens. Casts injected from the saphenofemoral junction show resin present in the connecting network of vessels. Notice the variation in the size of the abundant tortuous vessels in both specimens. **A**, Though several channels are larger, there are more than 100 channels running in a similar proximal distal direction. **B**, Three large-diameter tortuous channels dominate the cast; however, there are also many small channels present in continuity. Note the injecting cannula (distal). Scale bars: **A**, 5 mm; **B**, 10 mm. (Reprinted by permission of the publisher from van Rij AM, Jones GT, Hill GB, et al: Neovascularization and recurrent varicose veins: more histologic and ultrasound evidence. *J Vasc Surg* 40:296-302, 2004. Copyright 2004 by Elsevier.)

Results.—All but 3 re-operation specimens (94%) showed multiple vessels at the stump site of the previous SFJ ligation. Neovascular channels of variable size, number, and tortuosity accounted for the ultrasound appearances and reflux to recurrent varicosities in the vast majority of specimens. These new vessels connected to the common femoral vein at the site of the previous SFJ. In 2 incompetent junctions without femoral vein involvement, while small vessels were seen surrounding the femoral stump scar, ultrasound and histology confirmed both neovascular and residual (enlarged collateral) connections from epigastric and pudendal vessels into the thigh.

Conclusion.—Neovascularisation is the major cause for ultrasound-confirmed recurrence of reflux in the groin following varicose vein surgery.

▶ Increasing attention to the genesis of recurrent varicose veins, especially in the groin, has been recently fueled by discussion of endovenous treatment of the great saphenous vein (GSV) that leaves the SFJ and proximal GSV tributaries open. According to this study, neovascularization occurs in every extremity with previously ligated SFJ stumps. Ligated GSVs recanalize or form new channels within the tract of the stripped GSV. Small sample size, selected population of groin recurrences, and unknown time from the initial surgery limit the generalization of these findings. Thus, how often neovascularization truly happens after surgery remains unknown. The anatomic pattern of reconnection suggests that neovascularization is likely associated with surgical trauma and less so with remaining proximal tributaries.

F. Lurie, MD, PhD

Saphenofemoral Venous Channels Associated With Recurrent Varicose Veins Are Not Neovascular

El Wajeh Y, Giannoukas AD, Guilliford CJ, et al (Sheffield Vascular Inst, England; Northern Gen Hosp, Sheffield, England)

Eur J Vasc Endovasc Surg 28:590-594, 2004 16–13

Background.—Recurrence of varicose veins after apparently adequate surgery is common. Neovascularisation, the formation of new vascular channels between a venous surgery site and new varicosities, is thought to be an important cause of recurrence. The aim of this study was to provide histological evidence of the 'neovascularisation' process.

Method.—Tissue samples from the region of the previously ligated saphenofemoral junction (SFJ) were taken from 14 limbs with recurrent varicose veins and from nine control limbs. Tissue samples were analysed histologically for overall vascularity, and the presence of intimal circular fibrosis, intimal eccentric fibrosis, medial thickened elastosis, and thrombosis in the microscopic thin walled vessels within the tissue. The same samples were analysed immunohistoligically for S100, a neural marker, and Ki-67 (Mib 1), a marker of endothelial proliferation. Absent S100 and positive Ki-67 were considered as evidence of new vessels.

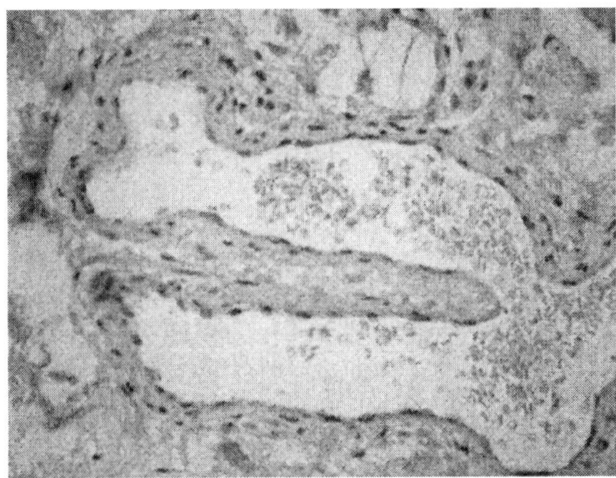

FIGURE 2.—Vascular endothelial cells are negative for Mib-1 antibody staining (original magnification ×400). (Reprinted from El Wajeh Y, Giannoukas AD, Guilliford CJ, et al: Saphenofemoral venous channels associated with recurrent varicose veins are not neovascular. *Eur J Vasc Endovasc Surg* 28:590-594, 2004. Copyright 2004, by permission of the publisher.)

Result.—No significant difference was found between the venous recurrence and control groups in respect to histological features. S100 positive nerve fibrils were seen associated with dilated venous channels in the majority of both redo and control groups ($p=1$, Fisher's exact test). Only one section stained positively with Ki-67 (Mib1) in a single vascular channel for a few endothelial cells. The remaining control and redo cases were negative for Mib 1 ($p=1$, Fisher's exact test) (Fig 2).

Conclusion.—We found little evidence of neovascularisation associated with recurrent varicose veins in the saphenofemoral region. The venous channels that develop at the previously ligated SFJ may represent adaptive dilatation of pre-existing venous channels (vascular remodelling), probably in response to abnormal haemodynamic forces.

▶ Comparison of tissue samples from 14 limbs with recurrent varicose veins and 9 control limbs showed no difference in immunohistochemical identification of perivascular nerves and proliferative markers. The authors conclude that neovascular vessels are no more common in saphenofemoral recurrent varicose veins than in other postsurgical scar tissue.

Aside from an obvious lack of statistical power, these findings raise an important question of the natural history of venous insufficiency and the dynamics of postsurgical tissue changes. If neovascularization is stimulated by surgical trauma, it should occur early after treatment. If this is the case, the incidence of recurrent varicose veins may be lowered by minimizing surgical trauma. If these reconnecting vessels (either preexisting or new) develop in the course of the natural history of venous disease, proliferative changes should be more likely to happen later after surgery. (See also Abstract 16–12.)

F. Lurie, MD, PhD

Treatment of Venous Leg Ulcers With Dermagraft

Omar AA, Mavor AID, Jones AM, et al (Faculty of Medicine, Shebinel-Kom, Egypt; General Infirmary, Leeds, England; Univ of York, England)
Eur J Vasc Endovasc Surg 27:666-672, 2004 16–14

Background.—A number of different treatment approaches have been recommended for the treatment of venous ulceration, including local ulcer treatment, compression and drug therapy. Recent advances in tissue engineering have resulted in living tissues being developed for cutaneous wound repair and skin replacement. The aim of this pilot study was to compare the rate of healing of venous ulcers in patients treated with Dermagraft (a human fibroblast-derived dermal replacement) and compression therapy or compression therapy alone.

Methods.—A total of 18 patients with venous ulceration of the leg were recruited into the pilot study. Ten patients were treated with Dermagraft and compression therapy, and eight patients were treated with compression therapy alone. Healing was assessed by ulcer tracing and computerised planimetry. Skin perfusion was measured by laser Doppler.

Results.—Five (50%) of the patients treated with Dermagraft and one (12.5%) control patient had healed by the end of the 12-week study period (NS). The total ulcer area rate of healing and linear rate of healing was significantly improved in patients treated with Dermagraft ($P = 0.001$ and $P = 0.006$, respectively, Mann-Whitney U-test) (Fig 2). The number of capillaries increased in both the treatment and control group. Peri-ulcer skin perfusion increased by 20% in patients treated with Dermagraft, compared with 4.9% in the control group.

Conclusion.—The data from this small pilot study suggests that Dermagraft is associated with improved healing of venous ulceration. Following this pilot study, further clinical studies are needed to confirm the validity of these results in 'hard to heal' venous leg ulcers.

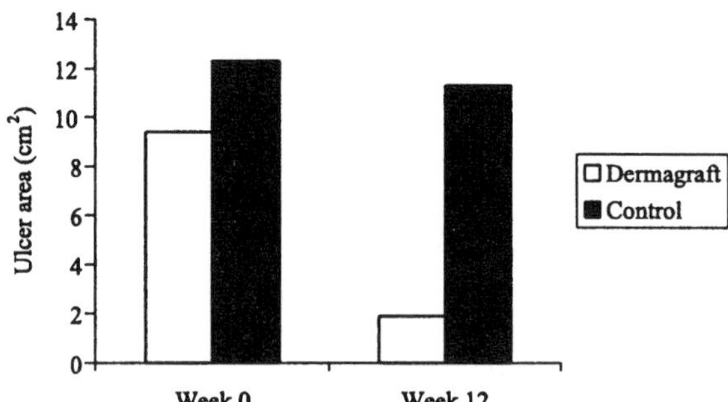

FIGURE 2.—Mean ulcer area before treatment and at week 12. (Reprinted from Omar AA, Mavor AID, Jones AM, et al: Treatment of venous leg ulcers with Dermagraft. *Eur J Vasc Endovasc Surg* 27:666-672, 2004. Copyright 2004, by permission of the publisher.)

► This study is too small to draw any definitive conclusion regarding the utility of this product in healing venous ulcers. We have used it on a few patients in our clinic. Anecdotally, it seemed to have helped on occasion. Clearly, however, there is no definitive evidence that Dermagraft offers any advantage over traditional compressive therapy in the healing of venous ulcers.

G. L. Moneta, MD

Randomized Clinical Trial of Four-Layer and Short-Stretch Compression Bandages for Venous Leg Ulcers (VenUS I)

Nelson EA, for the VenUS I Collaborators (Univ of York, England)

Br J Surg 91:1292-1299, 2004 16–15

Background.—A randomized clinical trial was undertaken to determine the relative effectiveness of four-layer and short-stretch bandaging for venous ulceration.

Methods.—A total of 387 adults with a venous ulcer, who were receiving leg ulcer treatment either in primary care or as a hospital outpatient, were recruited to this parallel-group open study and randomized to either four-layer or short-stretch bandages. Follow-up continued until the patient's reference leg was ulcer free or for a minimum of 12 months. The primary endpoint was time to complete healing of all ulcers on the reference leg. Secondary outcomes included proportion of ulcers healed, health-related quality of life, withdrawals and adverse events. Analysis was by intention to treat.

Results.—Unadjusted analysis identified no statistically significant difference in median time to healing: 92 days for four-layer and 126 days for short-stretch bandages. However, when prognostic factors were included in a Cox proportional hazards regression model, ulcers treated with the short-stretch bandage had a lower probability of healing than those treated with the four-layer bandage: hazard ratio 0.72 (95 per cent confidence interval 0.57 to 0.91). More adverse events and withdrawals were reported with the short-stretch bandage.

Conclusion.—Venous leg ulcers treated using a four-layer bandage healed more quickly than those treated with a short-stretch bandage.

► This randomized study confirms the effectiveness of elastic compression in ulcer healing. It provides information on healing time of ulcers—3 months with the 4-layer compression and 4 months with short-stretch bandages. Although the difference between the 2 techniques was statistically significant, interpretation of the data is impeded by uncontrolled and unknown pressure applied by the bandages to each individual leg. It would be interesting to know how many of the 387 patients had surgically correctible disease. In primary disease, for example, surgical treatment may provide faster healing and better long-term results. An important finding was that nearly one third of the enrolled patients withdrew from the study because they could not tolerate compression or their condition deteriorated. Elastic bandaging can be effective, but it is not for every patient. The choice of bandages, and perhaps the optimal pressure applied by bandages, is still to be defined by further studies.

F. Lurie, MD, PhD

Proliferative Capacity of Venous Ulcer Wound Fibroblasts in the Presence of Platelet-Derived Growth Factor

Vasquez R, Marien BJ, Gram C, et al (Boston Univ; Wyoming Valley Surgical Associates, Wilkes-Barre, Pa)

Vasc Endovasc Surg 38:355-360, 2004 16–16

Introduction.—Growth factors have been demonstrated to increase the proliferation of wound fibroblasts. Platelet-derived growth factor (PDGF) is a potent cell mitogen. However, the role of PDGF in chronic venous ulcers is inconclusive. This study investigated whether PDGF stimulates venous ulcer fibroblasts to proliferate. Fibroblasts (fb) were isolated from 8 venous ulcers wounds (w-fb) and normal skin (n-fb) of the ipsilateral thigh via punch biopsies. Fibroblasts were plated at 1,500 cells/dish in Dulbecco's Modified Eagle Medium + 10% calf serum (CM) and treated with/without PDGF-αβ (10 ng/mL) for 15 days. Growth rates were calculated. Western blotting and immunocytochemistry staining determined basal levels for PDGF-α and -β receptors, respectively. Growth rates were significantly lower in w-fb than in n-fb (1,579 ±546 vs 13,782 ±5,882 cells/day, $p=0.019$). PDGF-αβ treatment caused n-fb to increase their proliferative capacity relative to complete media (20,393 ±6,572 vs 13,782 ±5,882 cells/day, $p=0.005$). However, PDGF-αβ had no significant effect on w-fb proliferation over CM (1,030 ±264 and 1,579 ±546 cells/day, $p=0.15$). In the presence of PDGF-αβ, w-fb had a significantly attenuated growth rate over n-fb (1,030 ±264 vs 20,393 ±6,572 cells/day, $p=0.019$). Western blot and immunocytochemistry analysis revealed diminished basal levels of PDGF-α and -β receptors, respectively, in ulcer fibroblasts. Venous ulcer fibroblasts had decreased proliferation. PDGF-αβ had no effect on the growth rate of venous ulcer fibroblasts. In venous ulcers, decreased basal levels of fibroblast PDGF-α and -β receptors may explain reduced proliferation. Further clinical studies are needed to elucidate the role growth factors may play in venous ulcers.

► This study demonstrates basic biological differences between venous ulcers and other chronic wounds. Fibroblasts cultured from venous ulcers have deficient levels of PDGF receptors, and this perhaps explains, in part, their inability to respond to usual proliferative stimuli. Based on this report, PDGF-based treatment for venous ulcers should not work. As any good scientific study, this one leaves us with more questions than answers. How reversible are these changes in fibroblasts, and how are the changes connected to venous hypertension?

F. Lurie, MD, PhD

Surgical Disobliteration of Postthrombotic Deep Veins—Endophlebectomy—Is Feasible

Puggioni A, Kistner KL, Eklof B, et al (Univ of Hawaii, Honolulu)

J Vasc Surg 39:1048-1052, 2004 16–17

Objective.—Partial obstruction of postthrombotic veins is caused by endovenous scar tissue, which creates synechiae and septae that narrow and sometimes block the lumen. We have performed surgical disobliteration, or endophlebectomy, of chronically obstructed venous segments during various kinds of deep venous reconstructions to increase the flow through previously obstructed segments. In this article we describe the endophlebectomy technique, and report the availability of this procedure as an adjunct to deep venous reconstructions for the treatment of postthrombotic chronic venous insufficiency.

Patients and Methods.—Between July 1996 and February 2003, surgical disobstruction of 23 deep venous segments was performed in 13 patients in association with 14 deep venous reconstructions to treat advanced postthrombotic chronic venous insufficiency. Postthrombotic veins were surgically exposed, and a longitudinal venotomy was carried out at a variable length. The synechiae and masses attached to the intimal layer were carefully excised (Figure). Mean duplex scanning follow-up was 10.8 ± 8.2 months (median, 8 months; range, 1-28 months).

Results.—In 10 patients (77%) the treated segments remained primarily patent at median follow-up of 8 months (range, 1-28 months). Early thrombosis near the endophlebectomy site occurred in 3 patients, at 2, 5, and 12 days, respectively, after surgery. In 2 patients with early thrombosis further interventions were carried out with success. In a third patient with early postoperative thrombosis the final outcome was recanalization and reflux.

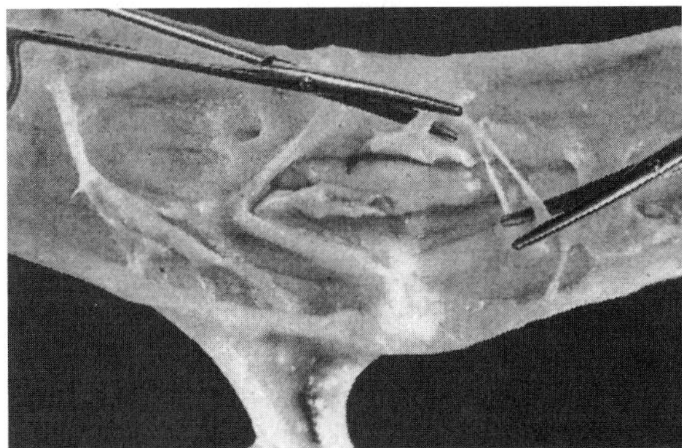

FIGURE.—On opening the vein the synechiae attached to the intimal layer are placed on tension and carefully removed with scissors by snipping their attachments to the intimal surface of the vein. (Reprinted by permission of the publisher from Puggioni A, Kistner KL, Eklof B, et al: Surgical disobliteration of postthrombotic deep veins—endophlebectomy—is feasible. *J Vasc Surg* 39:1048-1052, 2004. Copyright 2004 by Elsevier.)

These results yielded an overall secondary patency rate of 93%. No perioperative pulmonary embolism was observed.

Conclusion.—This series demonstrates that surgical disobliteration of postthrombotic deep veins is technically feasible, and led to patency of the segments for the duration of follow-up for up to 28 months (mean, 10.8 ± 8.2 months). We used this technique with the objective of disobstructing postthrombotic veins, to increase flow through a previously narrowed lumen. Postoperative thrombosis at the site of endophlebectomy occurred in 23% of patients. Although this early experience is encouraging, further studies and longer follow-up are necessary to assess the durability of the procedure.

▶ Two aspects of this article are important to me as a coauthor. First is the description of pathologic changes inside the postthrombotic vein. Synechiae that could not always be detected by venography or US not only obstruct the flow, but also restrict venous wall movement in reaction to physiologic changes in blood flow. Second, success of the procedure requires not only meticulous surgical technique, but also must have adequate inflow to, and outflow from, the treated segment.

F. Lurie, MD, PhD

Second-Generation Percutaneous Bioprosthetic Valve: A Short-term Study in Sheep

Pavenik D, Kaufman J, Uchida B, et al (Oregon Health & Science Univ, Portland)

J Vasc Surg 40:1223-1227, 2004 16–18

Objectives.—To eliminate occasional tilting of the original bioprosthetic venous valve (BVV) a second-generation BVV has been developed. This study was performed to evaluate deployment, stability, and short-term function of the second-generation BVV in an animal model.

Methods.—A second-generation percutaneously placed BVV consisting of a square stent and lyophilized small intestinal submucosa attached to a second square stent (DS BVV) or Z-stent (ZS BVV) was tested (Fig 1). DS BVVs (n = 32) were constructed with a nitinol (n = 28) or stainless steel double stent (n = 4), and ZS BVVs (n = 16) were made of nitinol (n = 8) or stainless steel (n = 4). BVVs were implanted percutaneously through a femoral vein approach into the jugular vein in 24 female sheep with an over-the-wire 13F or 10F delivery system. All BVVs were placed across the natural valve of the proximal jugular vein. Deployment, stability, and function of BVVs were studied at immediate venography with contrast medium injections peripheral and central to the BVVs. Animals underwent follow-up venography and were sacrificed at 6 weeks (n = 24). Gross pathologic examination was performed.

Results.—Jugular vein diameter ranged from 9.8 to 14.4 mm (mean, 12.1 ± 1.2 mm) in 24 sheep. The 10-mm to 12-mm valve was deployed in 27 jugu-

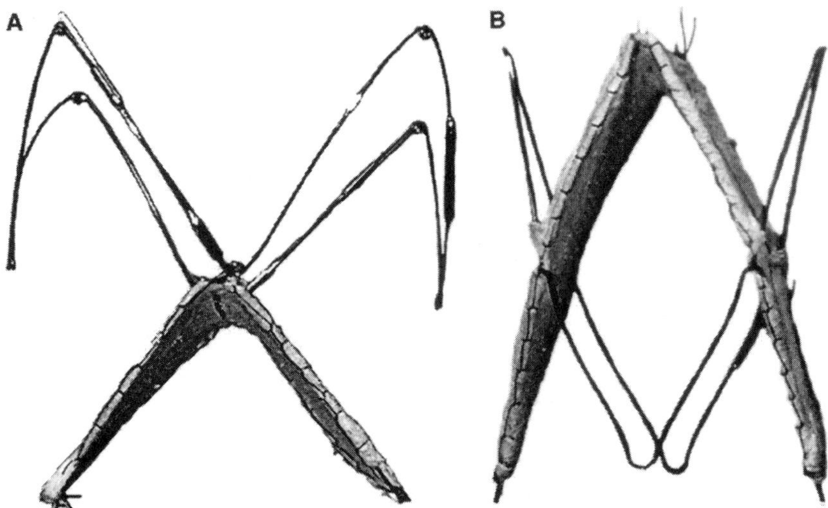

FIGURE 1.—Second-generation bioprosthetic venous valve. A, Stainless steel Z-stent is attached to apex of original square stent valve. Z-stent has barbs at its upper bends. B, Nonrestrained nitinol double-stent bioprosthetic venous valve with 4 barbs for maximal vein diameter of 12 to 14 mm. (Reprinted by permission of the publisher from Pavenik D, Kaufman J, Uchida B, et al: Second-generation percutaneous bioprosthetic valve: a short-term study in sheep. *J Vasc Surg* 40:1223-1227, 2004. Copyright 2004 by Elsevier.)

lar veins, and the 12-mm to 14-mm valve was deployed in 21 jugular veins. No tilting was seen at placement of 48 BVVs into the jugular veins, and all valves exhibited good function on immediate venograms. Angiographic competency for the nitinol and stainless steel ZS BVV (100%) was similar to that for the nitinol DS BVV (92.3%; P = .488) but was significantly better than for the stainless steel DS BVV at 6 weeks (50%; P = .03). Dysfunction of 4 valves was caused by either nitinol DS BVV oversizing (n = 2) or intimal hyperplasia with the stainless steel DS BVV (n = 2).

Conclusion.—Placement without tilting appears essential for proper valve function. The second-generation BVV enables placement without tilting. Exact matching of valve size with vein diameter is necessary for good valve function.

► This group in Portland, working together with Cook Inc, gives us hope that someday clinical use of an implantable venous valve will be a reality. Animal testing demonstrates nonthrombogenicity and function for up to 1 year. Importantly, this report identifies a number of technical problems that can be solved by further improvements in valve construction. One of the major problems in both the animal studies and the limited experience in patients was stent sizing and selection of placement site. Exactly where implantable valves should be placed to gain a desirable clinical outcome remains unknown.

F. Lurie, MD, PhD

Incidence of Chronic Thromboembolic Pulmonary Hypertension After Pulmonary Embolism

Pengo V, for the Thromboembolic Pulmonary Hypertension Study Group (Univ Hosp of Padua, Italy; et al)

N Engl J Med 350:2257-2264, 2004 16–19

Background.—Chronic thromboembolic pulmonary hypertension (CTPH) is associated with considerable morbidity and mortality. Its incidence after pulmonary embolism and associated risk factors are not well documented.

Methods.—We conducted a prospective, long-term, follow-up study to assess the incidence of symptomatic CTPH in consecutive patients with an acute episode of pulmonary embolism but without prior venous thromboembolism. Patients with unexplained persistent dyspnea during follow-up underwent transthoracic echocardiography and, if supportive findings were present, ventilation-perfusion lung scanning and pulmonary angiography. CTPH was considered to be present if systolic and mean pulmonary-artery pressures exceeded 40 mm Hg and 25 mm Hg, respectively; pulmonary-capillary wedge pressure was normal; and there was angiographic evidence of disease.

Results.—The cumulative incidence of symptomatic CTPH was 1.0 percent (95 percent confidence interval, 0.0 to 2.4) at six months, 3.1 percent (95 percent confidence interval, 0.7 to 5.5) at one year, and 3.8 percent (95 percent confidence interval, 1.1 to 6.5) at two years. No cases occurred after two years among the patients with more than two years of follow-up data. The following increased the risk of CTPH: a previous pulmonary embolism (odds ratio, 19.0), younger age (odds ratio, 1.79 per decade), a larger perfusion defect (odds ratio, 2.22 per decile decrement in perfusion), and idiopathic pulmonary embolism at presentation (odds ratio, 5.70).

Conclusions.—CTPH is a relatively common, serious complication of pulmonary embolism. Diagnostic and therapeutic strategies for the early identification and prevention of CTPH are needed.

► CTPH is apparently much more common than previously suspected. Previous articles suggested an incidence of 0.1% to 0.5% after acute nonfatal pulmonary embolism.[1] The disease, however, is not inevitably associated with symptomatic venous thromboembolism[2] and does not share the usual systemic and coagulation risk factors with venous thromboembolism. The whitish yellow, fibrotic organized thrombosis in a patient with CTPH strongly resembles chronic venous thrombosis of the extremities. The key to CTPH may lie in improving resolution of the thrombotic process.

G. L. Moneta, MD

References

1. Fedullo PF, Auger WR, Kerr KM, et al: Chronic thromboembolic pulmonary hypertension. *N Engl J Med* 345:1465-1472, 2001.

2. Lang IM: Chronic thromboembolic pulmonary hypertension—Not so rare after all. *N Engl J Med* 350:2236-2238, 2004.

Klippel-Trénaunay Syndrome: The Importance of "Geographic Stains" in Identifying Lymphatic Disease and Risk of Complications

Maari C, Frieden IJ (Univ of Montreal; Univ of California, San Francisco)

J Am Acad Dermatol 51:391-398, 2004 16–20

Background.—Klippel-Trénaunay syndrome (KTS) is a rare congenital anomaly classically defined as the triad of vascular stain, soft tissue and/or bony hypertrophy, and venous varicosities.

Objective.—To determine whether the morphologic characteristics of the associated vascular stains in KTS are predictive of the presence of lymphatic involvement and/or complications.

Setting.—Outpatient dermatology practice, tertiary care medical center.

Methods.—We retrospectively reviewed all cases of KTS identified between January 1989 and September 2001 at the University of California San Francisco (UCSF) Department of Dermatology. Forty patients were identified. We further classified them by type of cutaneous vascular stain, either "geographic" or "blotchy/segmental" (Fig 4). Patients were further classified as having definite, probable, possible, or no evidence of lymphatic disease. We also reviewed the charts for other possibly associated manifestations and complications of KTS.

Results.—Of those with sharply demarcated geographic stains (n=22), 21 had definite or probable evidence of lymphatic disease. Of those with blotchy port-wine stains (n=17), 16 had possible or no evidence of lymphatic disease ($P < .001$). Determination of the type of stain had 95% sensitivity and 94% specificity in differentiating the definite or probable presence of definite or probable lymphatic disease from possible or no evidence of lymphatic disease. Complications occurred in 19 (86%) of 22 patients with a geographic stain vs 7 of 17 (41%) with a blotchy/segmental stain ($P < .003$).

Conclusion.—This study demonstrates that the presence of a geographic vascular stain is a predictor of the risk of both associated lymphatic malformation and complications in patients with KTS. Since these stains are present at birth, this clinical observation can help in identifying individuals with KTS at greatest risk for complications and in need of closer observation.

▶ Congenital vascular malformations are difficult to study. Each report of a clinical series adds to our knowledge. This retrospective series brings another dimension to the complexity of KTS by demonstrating that 56% of these patients have a definite or probable lymphatic component. It also demonstrates a probable association between the geographic pattern of cutaneous staining and the presence of lymphatic disease. Since the cutaneous stains are often

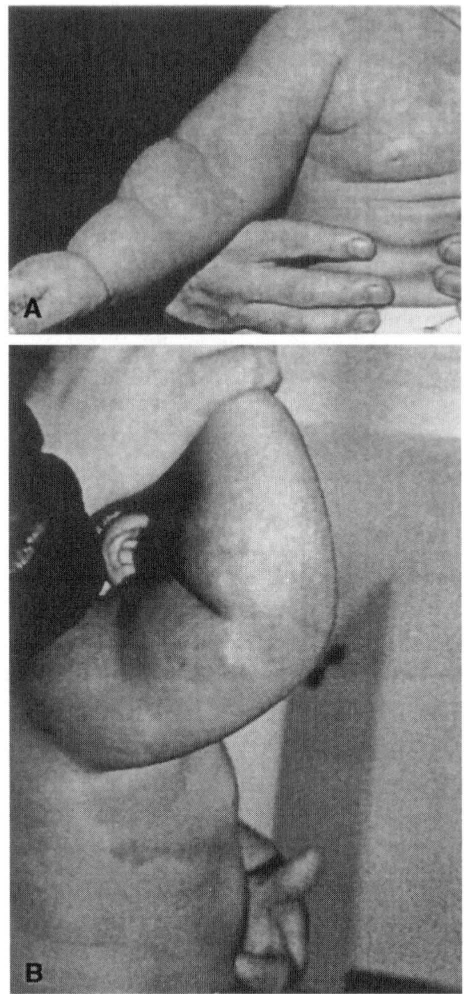

FIGURE 4.—A, Blotchy/Segmental stain on the arm of a young infant; front view. B, Blotchy/Segmental stain on the arm of same infant; side view. (Reprinted by permission of the publisher from Maari C, Frieden IJ: Klippel-Trénaunay syndrome: The importance of "geographic stains" in identifying lymphatic disease and risk of complications. *J Am Acad Dermatol* 51:391-398, 2004. Copyright 2004 by Elsevier.)

apparent at birth, possible associations can be investigated prospectively. Hopefully, careful monitoring of patients with geographic stains can lead to the diagnosis of lymphatic disease at earlier stages when treatment may be more effective.

F. Lurie, MD, PhD

Microsurgical Techniques for Lymphedema Treatment: Derivative Lymphatic-Venous Microsurgery

Campisi C, Boccardo F (Univ of Genoa, Italy)

World J Surg 28:609-613, 2004 16–21

Introduction.—We analyzed clinicopathologic and imaging features of chronic peripheral lymphedema to identify imaging findings indicative of its exact etiopathogenesis and to establish the optimal treatment strategy. One of the main problems of microsurgery for lymphedema is the discrepancy between the excellent technical possibilities and the subsequently insufficient reduction of the lymphedematous tissue fibrosis and sclerosis. Appropriate treatment based on pathologic studies and surgical outcome have not been adequately documented. Over the past 25 years, 676 patients with peripheral lymphedema have been treated with microsurgical lymphatic-venous anastomoses. Of these patients, 447 (66%) were available for long-term follow-up study. Objective assessment was undertaken by water volumetry and lymphoscintigraphy. Objectively, volume changes showed a significant improvement in 561 patients (83%), with an average reduction of 67% of the excess volume. Of the 447 patients followed, 380 (85%) have been able to discontinue the use of conservative measures, with an average follow-up of more than 7 years and average reduction in excess volume of 69%. There was an 87% reduction in the incidence of cellulitis after microsurgery. Microsurgical lymphatic-venous anastomoses have a place in the treatment of peripheral lymphedema and should be the therapy of choice in patients who are not sufficiently responsive to nonsurgical treatment. Improved results can be expected with operations performed early, during the first stages of lymphedema.

▶ This article presents 25 years of experience performing microsurgical lympho-venous anastomoses in 676 patients with chronic lymphedema. As perhaps the largest series and the most successful report on this subject, it deserves attention. Initial successes of microsurgical lympho-venous anastomoses were reported in the late 1960s by Capozza Armenio (Italy) and by Politowski (Poland). Long-term results have been disappointing. Careful patient selection and surgical technique likely contribute to the superb results reported in this article. However, these results must be reproduced in other centers.

F. Lurie, MD, PhD

17 Technical Notes

Management of Juxtarenal Aortic Aneurysms and Occlusive Disease With Preferential Suprarenal Clamping Via a Midline Transperitoneal Incision: Technique and Results

Ryan SV, Calligaro KD, McAffee-Bennett S, et al (Pennsylvania Hosp, Philadelphia; VA Med Ctr, Philadelphia)

Vasc Endovasc Surg 38:417-422, 4 17–1

Introduction.—Surgical management of juxtarenal aortic (JR-Ao) aneurysms and occlusive disease may include supraceliac aortic clamping, a retroperitoneal approach, or medial visceral rotation. The authors report their results using preferential direct suprarenal aortic clamping via a midline transperitoneal incision. Between July 1, 1992, and July 31, 2001, they treated 58 patients with JR-Ao disease (44 aneurysmal, 14 occlusive) via a midline incision without medial visceral rotation. Preferential suprarenal aortic clamping was used in 53 cases (42 proximal to both renal arteries, 11 proximal to the left renal artery only) and supraceliac or supramesenteric clamping in 5 cases when there was insufficient space for an aortic clamp between the superior mesenteric artery and renal arteries. This strategy avoided mesenteric ischemia associated with supraceliac clamping in the majority of cases and afforded better exposure of the right renal artery than obtainable with a left retroperitoneal approach or medial visceral rotation. Eleven patients underwent concomitant renal revascularization. Critical adjuncts included the following: (1) selective left renal vein (LRV) division if the vein stump pressure was < 35 mm Hg (suggesting sufficient renal venous collaterals existed), (2) bilateral renal artery occlusion during aortic clamping to prevent thromboembolism, (3) flushing of aortic debris before restoring renal perfusion, and (4) routine administration of perioperative intravenous mannitol and renal-dose dopamine. Patients with type IV thoracoabdominal aneurysms, ruptured aneurysms, or JR-Ao disease approached via a retroperitoneal incision (severely obese patients, re-do aortic surgery) were excluded. No patients died or required dialysis during their hospital stay. The LRV was divided in 12 (21%) cases and reanastomosed in 2 cases (elevated stump pressures). The average suprarenal clamp time was 26 minutes (range, 10-60). Postoperative serum creatinine remained > 0.5 ng/dL above baseline in 3 (5%) patients. These results support suprarenal aortic clamping with a midline transperitoneal incision as the optimal strategy for treating juxtarenal aortic aneurysms and occlusive disease. The authors believe that selective left renal vein division enhances juxtarenal aortic exposure, and routine administration of renal protective agents, along with occlusion of both renal arteries during suprarenal aortic clamping, are critical adjuncts in performing these operations.

▶ Surgeons should be familiar with both the retroperitoneal and transperitoneal approach to the juxtarenal and visceral aorta. Both have advantages and disadvantages. The retroperitoneal approach with the left kidney mobilized up, however, will allow one to avoid dividing the LRV. A supraceliac clamp also is not usually required with a retroperitoneal kidney up approach for juxtarenal surgery. In our practice, the transperitoneal approach to the aorta is largely limited to patients with large right iliac aneurysms. I cannot remember the last time I divided a LRV in conjunction with JR-Ao surgery.

G. L. Moneta, MD

Total Laparoscopic Abdominal Aortic Aneurysm Repair With Reimplantation of the Inferior Mesenteric Artery

Javerliat I, Coggia M, Di Centa I, et al (Ambroise Paré Univ, Boulogne-Billancourt, France; Versailles Saint Quentin en Yvelines Univ, France)

J Vasc Surg 39:1115-1117, 2004 17–2

Background.—The development of laparoscopic aortic surgery for the treatment of aortic aneurysms has presented the vascular surgeon with the need to revascularize the inferior mesenteric artery (IMA) to prevent ischemic colitis. The first case of a total laparoscopic abdominal aortic aneurysm (AAA) repair with reimplantation of the IMA was described.

Case Report.—Man, 70, with body weight of 92 kg, was a smoker with chronic obstructive pulmonary disease and was referred to the authors for treatment of an infrarenal AAA. A CT scan showed an aneurysm 55 mm in diameter, with mural thrombus, and a moderately calcified aorta. The patient was scheduled for total laparoscopic endoaneurysmorrhaphy with aortoaortic bypass. Doppler US scans after the procedure showed that vascular flow to the left colon was compromised. In addition, reverse bleeding from the IMA was poor, and the colon was gray, without peristalsis. Colon viability was not ensured; therefore, it was decided to reimplant the IMA on the prosthesis. Extubation was performed on the same day. The postoperative course was uneventful, and the patient made an excellent recovery, with minimal pain and return to a general diet on the fifth day. A control angiogram showed a patent IMA without morphologic abnormalities on the tube graft. The patient's recovery was complete with no clinical symptoms at a 2 months' follow-up. Additional follow-up US and CT scans showed no hemodynamic or morphologic anomalies (Figure).

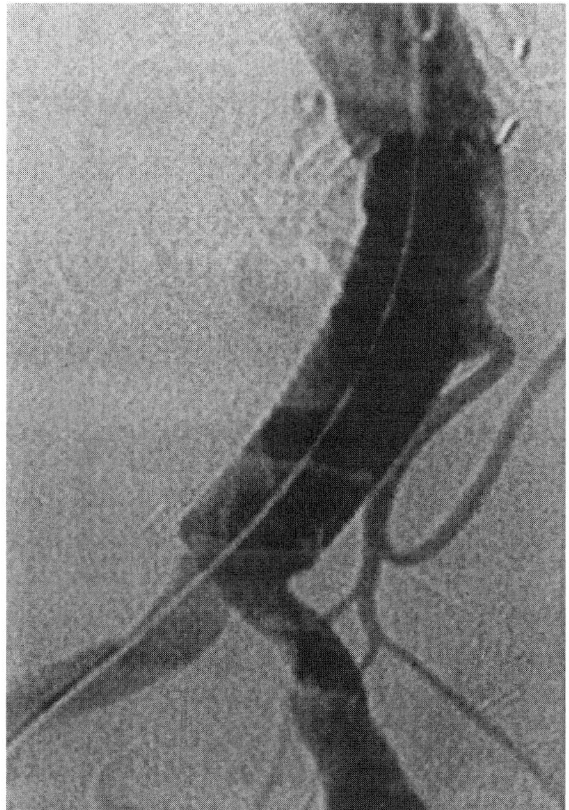

FIGURE.—Postoperative angiogram shows aortoaortic bypass graft with inferior mesenteric artery reimplantation. (Reprinted by permission of the publisher from Javerliat I, Coggia M, Di Centa I, et al: Total laparoscopic abdominal aortic aneurysm repair with reimplantation of the inferior mesenteric artery. *J Vasc Surg* 39:1115-1117, 2004. Copyright 2004 by Elsevier.)

Conclusions.—The first reported case of total laparoscopic AAA repair with reimplantation of the IMA had a successful outcome.

► You have to admire the persistence of this group from France. They have clearly become extremely good at a technique for which there is very little interest elsewhere. With endovascular aneurysm repair becoming applicable to more and more aneurysms, it is very difficult to imagine why anyone would want to take the time and energy to become expert in the laparoscopic repair of abdominal aortic aneurysms. (See also Abstract 7–3.)

G. L. Moneta, MD

Robotically Assisted Aorto-Femoral Bypass Grafting: Lessons Learned From Our Initial Experience

Desgranges P, Bourriez A, Javerliat I, et al (Henri Mondor Hosp, Creteil, France)

Eur J Vasc Endovasc Surg 27:507-511, 2004 17–3

Objective.—The da Vinci Surgical System (Intuitive Surgical Inc., Sunnyvale, CA) is a computer-enhanced telemanipulator that may help to overcome some limitations of traditional laparoscopic instruments. This prospective study was performed to assess the safety and feasibility of robotically assisted aorto-femoral bypass grafting (AF).

Methods.—Five patients undergoing elective AF were enrolled in this study. In three patients, a laparotomy of 6 cm was first performed, the aorta being exposed using an Omnitract° retractor. In two patients, aortic dissection was performed with laparoscopy, with the patient in a modified right lateral decubitus position. In all patients, the proximal anastomosis was attempted with the da Vinci system by a remote surgeon. The role of the assistant at the patient's side was limited to exposure, haemostasis and maintaining traction on the running sutures performed by the robot. Six weeks after the operation, all patients underwent a duplex scan of the graft.

Results.—Mean operative time was 188 min. Robotically assisted aortic anastomoses were successfully completed in four out of five patients. In these four patients, adequate blood flow was observed within the graft with no need for conversion for haemostasis. In the fifth patient, despite an adequate laparoscopic aortic dissection, the anastomosis was impossible to perform

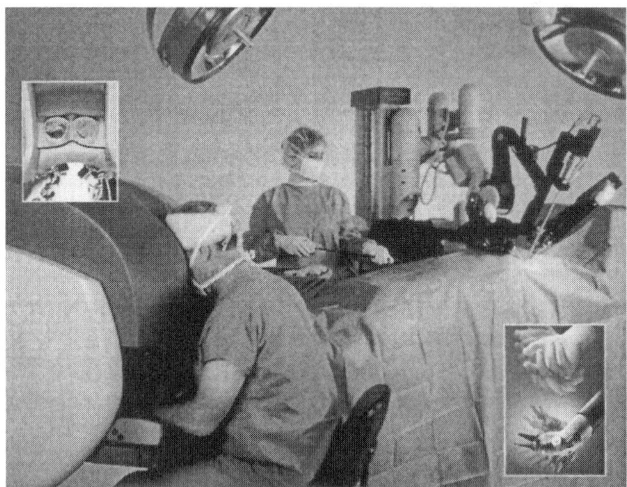

FIGURE 2.—General view of the da Vinci surgical system with the surgeon console and the surgical cart. *Left insert*, magnified 3D display of the operative field; *right insert*, EndoWrist technology gives a total of seven degrees of freedom at the tip of instruments mimicking the up-down and side-to-side flexibility of the human wrist. (Reprinted from Desgranges P, Bourriez A, Javerliat I, et al: Robotically assisted aorto-femoral bypass grafting: Lessons learned from our initial experience. *Eur J Vasc Endovasc Surg* 27:507-511, 2004. Reprinted by permission of the publisher.)

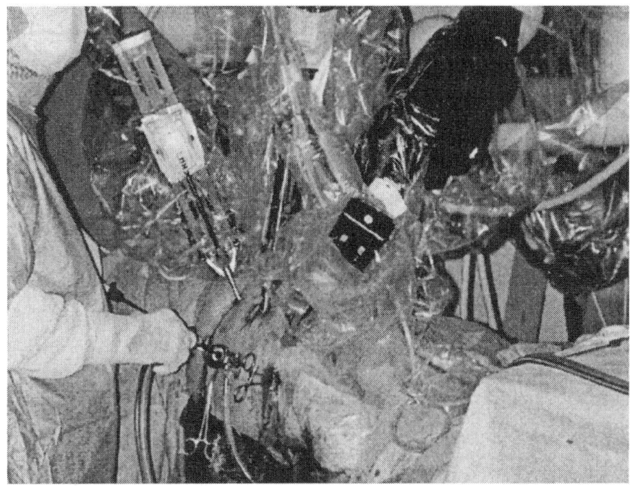

FIGURE 3.—View of the surgical cart with the da Vinci right and left arms and camera in action with the help of the assistant surgeon. (Reprinted from Desgranges P, Bourriez A, Javerliat I, et al: Robotically assisted aorto-femoral bypass grafting: Lessons learned from our initial experience. *Eur J Vasc Endovasc Surg* 27:507-511, 2004. Reprinted by permission of the publisher.)

due to external conflicts between the robotic arms. A conversion using conventional suture was successfully performed. No robot-related complications were noted. Six weeks after the operation, the duplex scans demonstrated a graft patency of 100%.

Conclusion.—Robotically assisted anastomoses are possible by their unique ability to combine conventional laparoscopic surgery with stereoscopic 3D magnification and ultra-precise suturing techniques due to the flexibility of the robotic-wristed instruments using different motion scaling of surgeon hand movements. In addition, prior training in laparoscopic aortic surgery is not necessary for surgeons to obtain the level required for suturing. Further clinical trials are needed to explore the clinical potential and value of robotically assisted AF (Figs 2 and 3).

► The da Vinci robotic system appears to be generating a great deal of interest in some circles. It may eventually have an application in vascular surgery, but I doubt it will be for abdominal aortic surgery. The same basic points from the previous abstract (Abstract 17–2) also apply here.

G. L. Moneta, MD

Protruding Aortic Arch Thrombus: Treatment With Minimally Invasive Surgical Approach

Schneiderman J, Feinberg MS, Schwammenthal E, et al (Sheba Med Ctr, Tel Hashomer, Israel; Tel Aviv Univ, Israel)

J Vasc Surg 40:1083-1088, 2004 17–4

Background.—Protruding aortic arch thrombus is associated clinically with life-threatening emboli. Definitive treatment for aortic arch thrombus removal has demanded complicated vascular surgical procedures, with high morbidity and mortality.

Method and Results.—Transesophageal echocardiography (TEE) enabled diagnosis of a protruding thrombus at the aortic arch in 5 patients, and a simultaneous lesion in the descending aorta in 1 patient. Four patients had visceral emboli, coinciding with peripheral emboli in 2 patients, and the fifth patient had peripheral and cerebral emboli. One patient had had ischemic stroke and femoral emboli a few months previously. Mean patient age was 51 years. None had clinical evidence of coronary or peripheral atherosclerotic occlusive disease. Risk factors included hypertension (n = 2), smoking (n = 4), and preexisting thrombophilia (n = 4). Five patients underwent TEE-guided aortic balloon thrombectomy from the arch with a 34-mm occluding balloon catheter. One patient also underwent balloon thrombectomy from the descending aorta with a 14F Foley catheter. Access into the

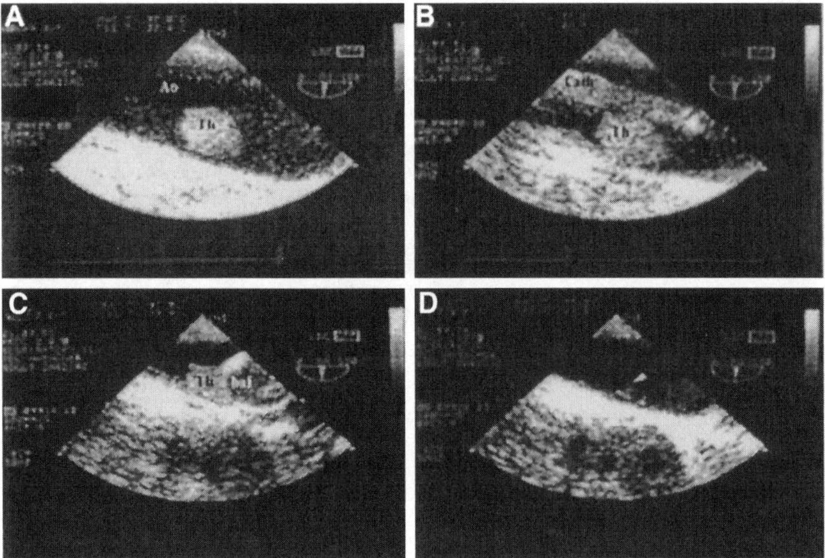

FIGURE 2.—A, Intraoperative transesophageal echocardiograms of the descending aorta (*Ao*), distal third, longitudinal view, with a pedunculated protruding thrombus (*Th*). B-D, Sequence of balloon extraction. B, Foley catheter (*Cath*) is introduced beyond thrombus. C, Balloon inflation (*bal*) and thrombus withdrawal. D, Remnant thrombus (*arrowhead*). (Reprinted by permission of the publisher from Schneiderman J, Feinberg MS, Schwammenthal E, et al: Protruding aortic arch thrombus: Treatment with minimally invasive surgical approach. *J Vasc Surg* 40:1083-1088, 2004. Copyright 2004 by Elsevier.)

aorta was obtained through the iliac artery (n = 4) during laparotomy because of visceral ischemia or through the transfemoral approach (n = 2). Previous procedures included superior mesenteric embolectomy (n = 3), segmental bowel resection (n = 1), splenectomy (n = 1), and peripheral arterial embolectomy n = 3). Real-time intraoperative TEE enabled visualization of the protruding thrombus and assisted with maneuvering of the balloon catheter. At completion peripheral thrombectomy thrombus material was retrieved in 4 patients. Postoperatively there were no clinically proved new procedure-related visceral emboli, and all patients received anticoagulant therapy thereafter. Follow-up TEE within 2 weeks and up to 7 years revealed no recurrent aortic arch thrombus.

Conclusions.—TEE-guided aortic balloon thrombectomy used in 6 procedures was effectively completed without visceral or peripheral ischemic complications. It enabled removal of the life-threatening source of emboli from the proximal aorta, thereby averting the need of major aortic surgery (Fig 2).

▶ Thrombectomy of the thoracic aorta with TEE guidance is an interesting idea. One obviously worries about embolization to the visceral arteries. Induction of the catheter through an iliac artery to allow visceral inspection seems prudent. However, until more cases are reported, we really won't know if visceral embolization will be a problem with this approach. Clearly, the authors' patients were well served by this procedure.

G. L. Moneta, MD

Surgical Treatment of Persistent Type 2 Endoleaks With Increase of the Aneurysm Sac: Indications and Technical Notes

Ferrari M, Sardella SG, Berchiolli R, et al (Azienda Ospedaliera Pisa (AOP), Italy; Univ of Pisa, Italy; Vascular Surgery IDI IRCCS Rome)

Eur J Vasc Endovasc Surg 29:43-46, 2005 17–5

Objective.—Unsolved type 2 endoleaks and aneurysmal sac increasing after endovascular aneurysm repair (EVAR) can be fixed with surgical sacotomy, ligation of the patent backbleeding vessels and preservation of the endograft. The aim of the paper is to highlight the technique as a feasible procedure in alternative to the removal of the graft.

Materials and Methods.—Four male patients whose aneurysm sac maximum transverse diameter had increased by 5 mm or more, without evidence of endoleak, migration or structural alteration of the endografts. The surgical access was by medial laparotomy in one case, flank incision in two cases and mini-laparotomy with laparoscopic assistance in the fourth case. Patients were followed with spiral CT and duplex ultrasound at discharge and at 6-12 months.

Results.—All procedures were carried out, without complication. Two patients required intensive care unit (ICU) admission and the average postoperative hospital stay was 10 days (range 6-13). All patients are currently alive with a functioning endograft, at an average follow-up of 14.7 months.

Conclusions.—Sacotomy, leaving the endograft in place, appears to be a feasible therapeutic option, less invasive than conversion to open repair. This technique merits further study.

► The aneurysm sac after EVAR can clearly be opened without disrupting the endograft repair. The authors left some aneurysm sacs open after repair of the endoleak site. I am not sure there is any advantage to leaving the sac open and would suggest reclosure of the sac if possible.

G. L. Moneta, MD

Infrascrotal, Perineal, Femorofemoral Bypass for Arterial Graft Infection at the Groin

Illuminati G, Caliò FG, D'Urso A, et al (Univ of Rome "La Sapienza,"; Sant'Anna Hosp, Catanzaro, Italy)

Arch Surg 139:1314-1319, 2004 17–6

Hypothesis.—Infrascrotal, perineal, femorofemoral bypass is an acceptable procedure for treating infection of a prosthetic arterial graft limited to a unilateral groin.

Design.—A consecutive sample clinical study with a mean follow-up of 29 months.

Setting.—The surgical department of an academic tertiary care center and an affiliated secondary care center.

Patients.—Nineteen patients with a mean age of 68 years with prosthetic graft infection at the outflow anastomosis on a femoral artery at the Scarpa triangle underwent an infrascrotal, perineal, femorofemoral bypass, with excision of the graft material limited at the groin. The recipient artery was the profunda femoris artery in 12 cases, the superficial femoral in 5, and the distal common femoral artery in 2.

Main Outcome Measures.—Cumulative survival, recurrence of sepsis, primary graft patency, and limb salvage rates expressed by standard life-table analysis.

Results.—Postoperative mortality rate was 5%. Cumulative (SE) survival rate was 65% (11.6%) at 3 years. Cumulative (SE) rate of freedom from recurrent sepsis was 88% (8.6%) at 3 years. Cumulative (SE) primary patency and limb salvage rates were 86% (9.4%) and 91% (7.9%), respectively, at 3 years.

Conclusion.—Femorofemoral bypass with an infrascrotal perineal approach is a valuable procedure for the treatment of femoral arterial graft infection limited at a unilateral groin.

► Vascular surgeons should be familiar with the infrascrotal route for a femorofemoral bypass. The authors use saphenous vein for some of their bypasses. I don't think the long-term patency of saphenous vein femorofemoral bypasses is that good and would try to avoid them. When faced with groin infection requiring femorofemoral bypass, our group is now preferentially using a femoral vein as the conduit. The infrascrotal technique described here should not be necessary if an autogenous conduit is used to treat arterial graft infection in the groin and the anastomoses covered with local muscle flaps. (See Abstracts 4–11 and 17–7.)

G. L. Moneta, MD

Rotational Muscle Flap Closure for Acute Groin Wound Infections Following Vascular Surgery

Illig KA, Alkon JE, Smith A, et al (Univ of Rochester, NY)

Ann Vasc Surg 18:661-668, 2004 17–7

Introduction.—Since 1996, 41 patients have presented to our institution with deep but localized groin infection following bypass (30) or isolated femoral artery surgery (11). These patients were treated with antibiotics, debridement, and rotational muscle flap coverage either immediately or within a few days. Patients had one of three patterns: serous leak from a groin incision within a few days of operation (Acute, $n = 10$), early serous leak that later became grossly infected (Acute-observed, $n = 8$), or obvious purulent drainage following an initially normal, healed wound (Delayed, $n = 23$). Patients with early leak had nearly uniformly polymicrobial infections with a preponderance of gram-negative organisms, whereas most of those with late purulence had monobacterial infection with *Staphylococcus aureus*. At exploration, 26 of 41 suture lines were exposed. Rectus femoris flaps were used in 35 patients (85% of cases) for coverage, and graft preservation was at-

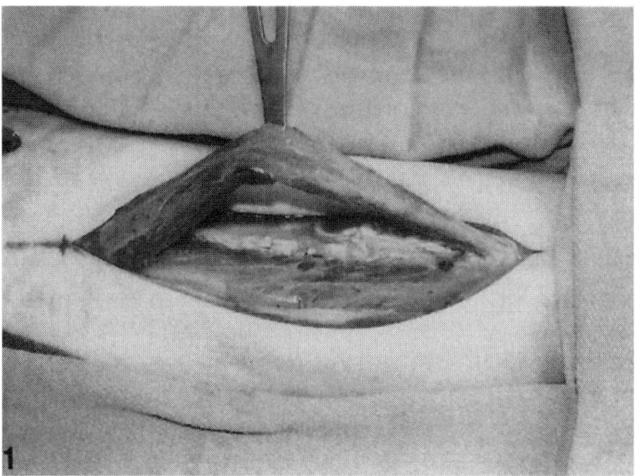

FIGURE 1.—Dissection and elevation of rectus femoris. Its blood supply is derived from the protunda femoris and enters the muscle via a proximal pedicle, thus it remains well perfused when its contribution to the quadriceps tendon is divided distally. The groin is to the left, and the knee to the right. (Courtesy of Illig KA, Alkon JE, Smith A, et al: Rotational muscle flap closure for acute groin wound infections following vascular surgery. *Ann Vasc Surg* 18:661-668, 2004.)

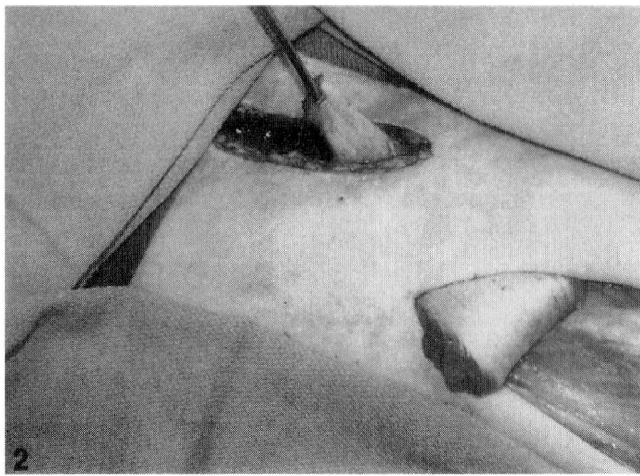

FIGURE 2.—Rectus femoris being mobilized to groin wound through a skin tunnel. Note the more than adequate length available. (Courtesy of Illig KA, Alkon JE, Smith A, et al: Rotational muscle flap closure for acute groin wound infections following vascular surgery. *Ann Vasc Surg* 18:661-668, 2004.)

tempted in all 8 vein grafts and 16 of 23 prosthetic grafts. Only one flap failed and there were no instances of anastomotic bleeding. There were no deaths directly attributable to reexploration and flap coverage, although 10 patients died during the index hospitalization. Durable coverage with no long-term evidence of infection was achieved in 24 patients with mean follow-up of 23 (range 10-66) months and another 12 had no evidence of local problems despite shorter follow-up; only 5 patients (12%) overall had evidence of persistent graft infection or unexplained bacteremia. In patients with attempted graft salvage, limb salvage was 97% at 6 months and 85% at 1 year. Although early mortality is high, deaths are not related to the flap procedure itself, local outcome is excellent, and graft and limb salvage are

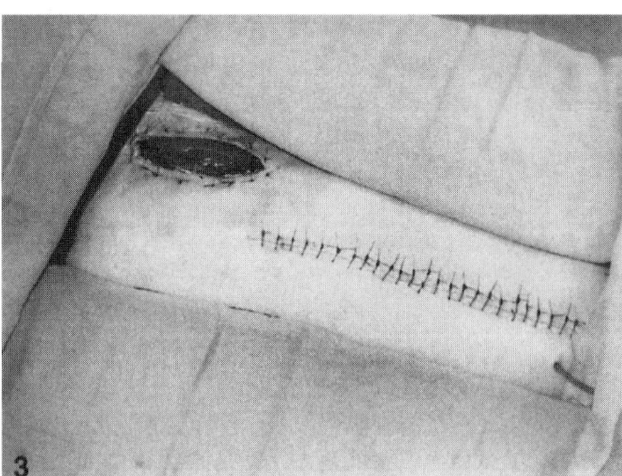

FIGURE 3.—The nearly finished result, awaiting a skin graft. (Courtesy of Illig KA, Alkon JE, Smith A, et al: Rotational muscle flap closure for acute groin wound infections following vascular surgery. *Ann Vasc Surg* 18:661-668, 2004.)

good; results are much worse if an initially draining wound is treated too late. Local rotational muscle flap closure is an excellent solution for acute infections involving the groin following vascular procedures (Figs 1-3).

▶ Muscle flap coverage of exposed vascular grafts in the groin has turned out to work remarkably well. The rectus femoris flap appears to be the muscle of choice for many and is probably more reliable than a sartorius flap. It is important to note that the rectus muscle receives its blood supply from the profunda femoris artery. It may be wise to consider alternative flaps in patients with occluded or highly diseased profunda femoris arteries.

G. L. Moneta, MD

Let It Be: Salvage of Exposed Hemodialysis Grafts With Fasciocutaneous Island Flaps

Isenberg JS (Univ of Oklahoma, Norman)

Microsurgery 24:134-138, 2004 17–8

Background.—Vascular access is a vital component in both acute and chronic settings. Gore-Tex grafts are durable and easily implanted; however, a risk of infection can still be present with these prosthetics. Once infection occurs, it is standard procedure to remove the prosthetic. Few reconstructive options are available for wound closure on the volar forearm. The radial artery island fasciocutaneous flap is a legitimate but underused option for wound closure and hemodialysis graft salvage. The outcomes of a series of hemodialysis grafts salvaged with island fasciocutaneous flaps were reported.

Methods.—A prospective review was performed of all patients presenting in a 4-year period with infected and/or contaminated hemodialysis grafts.

Results.—Of the 17 patients presenting for repair of exposed hemodialysis grafts, 5 patients were identified who underwent attempted graft salvage with fasciocutaneous island flaps. All the patients (3 women, 2 men; mean age, 58 years) had at least 2 concurrent medical conditions in addition to renal failure (Fig 1). Of the 5 patients, 4 had a history of heavy tobacco use. Reconstructive procedures in all patients were based on the radial artery and included 3 arterial fasciocutaneous flaps and 2 septocutaneous perforator flaps. Healing of 2 skin grafts at donor sites was delayed for an overall complication rate of 60%, with an overall graft salvage rate of 80%. At 6 months, no patient demonstrated vascular insufficiency in the reconstructed limb.

Conclusions.—Graft removal has been the traditional management for exposed dialysis grafts. The outcomes of a series of patients with renal failure and exposed forearm hemodialysis grafts were discussed. All of the wounds were closed satisfactorily with arterial fasciocutaneous and septocutaneous flaps. In 4 of 5 cases, the graft was salvaged at 6 months.

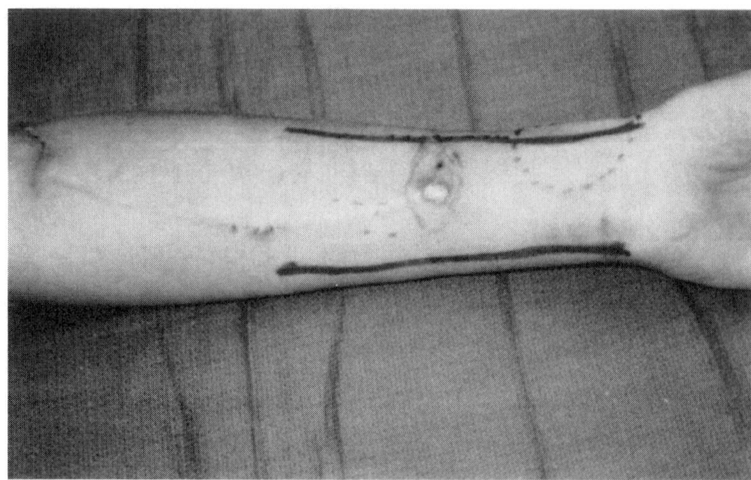

FIGURE 1.—A 45-year-old right-hand-dominant woman with end-stage renal failure and an exposed Gore-Tex hemodialysis graft in distal right forearm. Graft was patent and still being accessed at time of presentation. Patient showed no evidence of infection, and did not have an elevated white blood cell count. (Courtesy of Isenberg JS: Let it be: Salvage of exposed hemodialysis grafts with fasciocutaneous island flaps. *Microsurgery* 24:134-138, 2004. Copyright 2004 Wiley-Liss, Inc. Reprinted by permission of John Wiley & Sons, Inc.)

► It is important to know about these sorts of flaps. But most cases of exposed small areas of prosthetic dialysis access grafts can be more simply treated by rerouting the graft around the exposed part and excising the contaminated piece of graft.

G. L. Moneta, MD

Vacuum-assisted Conservative Treatment for the Management and Salvage of Exposed Prosthetic Hemodialysis Access

Vallet C, Saucy F, Haller C, et al (Univ Hosp, Lausanne, Switzerland)

Eur J Vasc Endovasc Surg 28:397-399, 2004 17–9

Background.—Several reports have described complications associated with expanded polytetrafluoroethylene (ePTFE) graft placement for hemodialysis vascular access. Recurrent puncture of prosthetic dialysis accesses may cause erosion and ulcer formation in the skin over the prosthetic material, and contamination of the wound may lead to infection of the graft. Once a graft is infected, standard treatment is to remove the graft. A vacuum-assisted closure device (VAC) can be used for the management of complicated wounds. The use of a vacuum dressing combined with IV antibiotics after wound debridement to allow salvage of ePTFE grafts is described.

Methods.—The study group was composed of 3 men and 1 woman with a median age of 66.2 years. All of the patients had wound dehiscence over

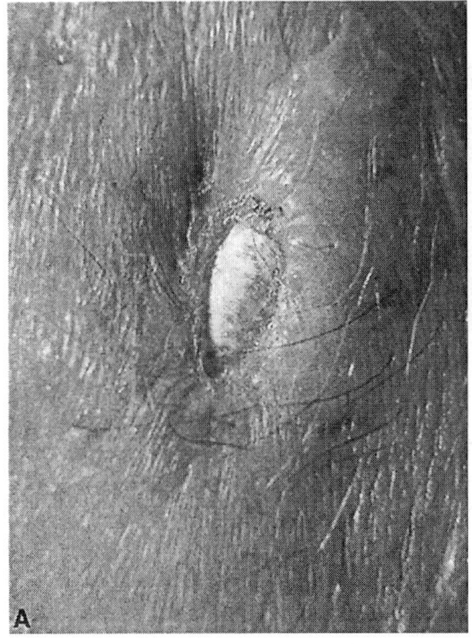

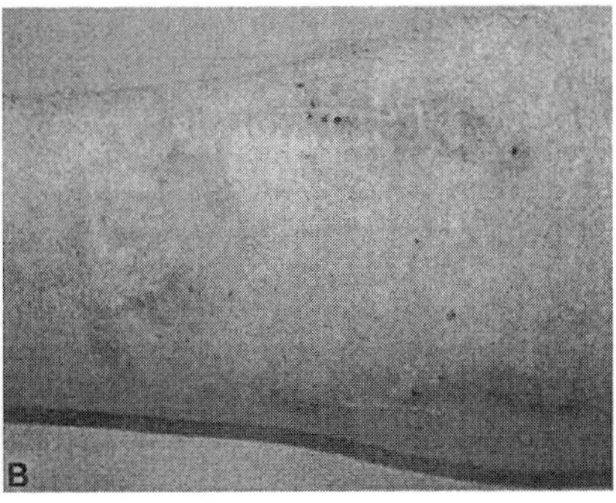

FIGURE 2.—Result after local skin flap. (Reprinted from Vallet C, Saucy F, Haller C, et al: Vacuum-assisted conservative treatment for the management and salvage of exposed prosthetic hemodialysis access. *Eur J Vasc Endovasc Surg* 28:397-399, 2004. Copyright 2004 by permission of the publisher.)

ePTFE grafts for hemodialysis access. Treatment consisted of wound débridement and application of a vacuum dressing, combined with IV antibiotics. A VAC device was used on all of the wounds.

Results.—Wound dehiscence over the graft developed in 2 patients after repeated skin puncture. A third patient had a wound dehiscence after surgery after a small infected hematoma was evacuated over the prosthetic material. A voluminous hematoma developed in the fourth patient at the anterior aspect of the elbow after puncture. Retraction of the wound over the ePTFE graft was obtained in 3 patients, with development of granulation tissue on two thirds of the graft's circumference. In these patients, coverage of the prosthetic material was obtained by a local skin flap under local anesthesia (Fig 2). In all patients, the combination of debridement, IV antibiotics, and negative-pressure therapy allowed salvage of the prosthesis without discontinuation of hemodialysis. The wounds have been stable from 7 to 9 months.

Conclusions.—Salvage of exposed prosthetic hemodialysis access was accomplished in 4 patients with the surgeons using a combination of aggressive local care, vacuum-assisted therapy, and systemic antibiotics.

▶ Another use of the wound VAC. However, the same comment applies to this article as to the previous abstract.

G. L. Moneta, MD

The Surgically Created Arteriovenous Fistula: A Forgotten Alternative to Venous Access

Carsten CG III, Taylor SM, Cull DL, et al (Greenville Hosp System, SC)

Ann Vasc Surg 18:635-639, 2004 17–10

Introduction.—The care of patients requiring lifelong intravenous access was revolutionized with the development of tunneled catheters and implantable ports. These devices are not without complications, however, and selected patients may benefit from alternative modalities to maintain access for such therapies as parenteral nutrition, phlebotomy, or chemotherapy. Use of surgically created arteriovenous (AV) fistulae as an alternative to central venous access has been described. This report reviews our experience using AV access for central venous access. An AV access database of more than 800 active patients was reviewed and all patients who had autogenous or synthetic AV fistulae created exclusively for central venous access between July 1, 2001, and December 31, 2003, were identified. Outcomes were assessed. A total of 853 new accesses were placed during the time period. Six fistulae in six patients (0.7%) were placed for central access. All patients (5 males, 1 female, mean age, 42.8 years) required access for intermittent parenteral nutrition or intravenous fluids secondary to short-gut syndrome (n = 5) or gastroparesis (n = 1). All patients had failed at least two prior catheter-based accesses before access placement was considered. Procedures were all brachial artery based and included autogenous brachiobasilic vein fistulae with elevation or transposition (n = 3), autogenous brachiocephalic fistula (n = 1), autogenous brachiobasilic graft with transposed greater saphenous vein (n = 1), and a prosthetic brachiobasilic graft with ePTFE (n = 1). There was one perioperative autogenous fistula thrombosis treated with thrombectomy and revision. A total of seven late revisions (thrombectomy, thrombectomy with venous outflow revision, fistula elevation, and 4 percutaneous angioplasties) in four patients were required. All fistulae were patent and functional at the end of the review period (mean follow-up, = 393 days; range, 35-757 days). Daily access was performed by family members (n = 2) or nurses (n = 4). One patient received small bowel transplantation and no longer required use of his patent fistula. One patient died of liver failure 382 days after fistula placement with a patent fistula. These results show that, while often forgotten and infrequently used, AV access can be a durable alternative to catheter-based venous access.

► AV fistulas can be used for long-term central access. They were more frequently used before the development of modern tunneled catheters and have little use today. One advantage is the lack of need for a permanent indwelling device. An AV fistula for central access should be considered in the patient who requires permanent central access and is prone to catheter infection. The usual complications of AV fistula, however, are still to be expected.

G. L. Moneta, MD

Long-term Results of Through-Knee Amputation With Dorsal Musculocutaneous Flap in Patients With End-Stage Arterial Occlusive Disease

Kock H-J, Friederichs J, Ouchmaev A, et al (Univ of Heidelberg, Germany; Technical Univ Munich)

World J Surg 28:801-806, 2004 17–11

Introduction.—A modified technique of knee joint disarticulation using a dorsal musculocutaneous flap of the gastrocnemius muscle was first described in 1985. The operative results in 66 patients (33 women, 33 men; mean age 66.7 ± 11.3 years, range 42-93 years) with gangrene due to peripheral vascular disease with 69 knee disarticulations are reported. After a mean survival period of 35.2 months (0-116 months), 88% ($n = 58$) of the patients had died owing to cardiopulmonary reasons. The in-hospital 48-day mortality was 9%. Nine patients (14%) underwent reamputation at the above-knee level, and five patients underwent operative revision of the soft tissue. After discharge from the hospital, 35 of 60 patients (58%) were able to walk with the aid of a prosthesis. We conclude that knee disarticulation with the use of a myocutaneous gastrocnemius flap is a safe, functionally acceptable operative method in high risk vascular patients (Fig 2).

▶ Patients who cannot have a below-knee amputation but may be ambulatory with a prosthesis probably do a little better with through-knee versus transfemoral amputations. This is a nice technique for performing a through-knee amputation. I think it will be infrequently needed. The technique described is for those patients who cannot have a functional below-knee amputation but still have enough of a posterior flap to cover the through-knee site and may be ambulatory with a prosthesis.

G. L. Moneta, MD

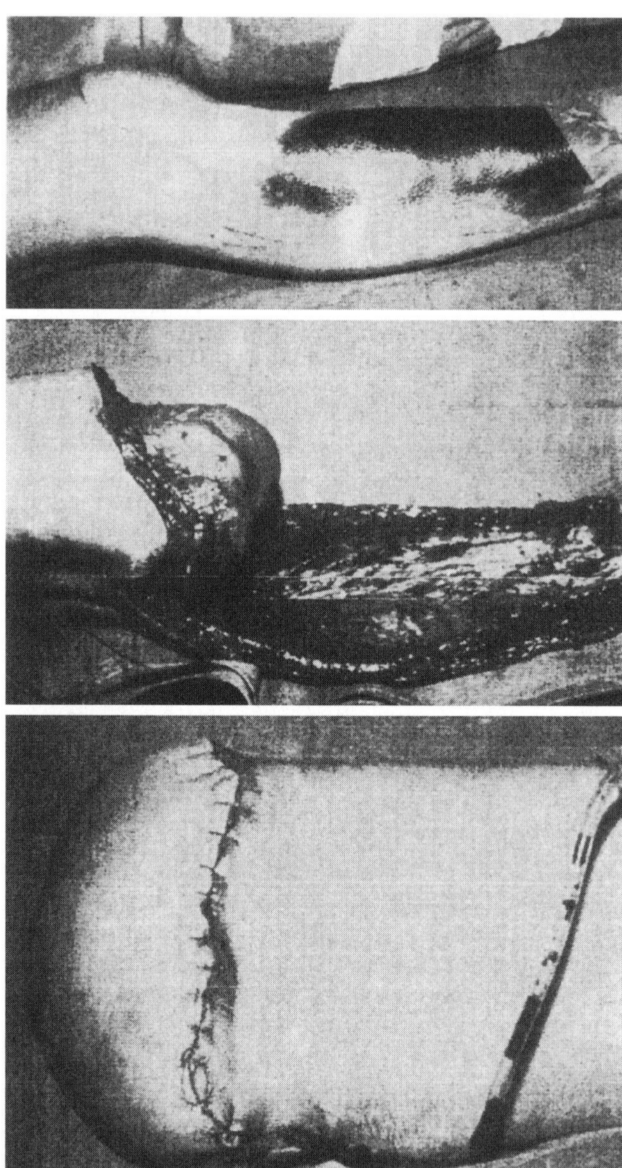

FIGURE 2.—Original through-knee operation technique using a dorsal musculocutaneous flap of the gastrocnemius muscle. (From Klaes and Eigler, with permission.) (Courtesy of Kock H-J, Friederichs J, Ouchmaev A, et al: Long-term results of through-knee amputation with dorsal musculocutaneous flap in patients with end-stage arterial occlusive disease. *World J Surg* 28:801-806, 2004. Copyright Springer-Verlag.)

To Clot or Not to Clot? That Is the Question in Central Venous Catheters

Cadman A, Lawrance JAL, Fitzsimmons L, et al (Univ of Manchester, England; Christie Hosp, Manchester, England)

Clin Radiol 59:349-355, 2004 17–12

Introduction.—AIM: To establish the relationship between the tip position of tunnelled central venous catheters (CVC) and the incidence of venous thrombosis.

Materials and Methods.—A randomly sampled, retrospective review of 428 CVC inserted into 334 patients was performed. The chest radiograph obtained post-catheter insertion, as well as follow-up radiographs, linograms, venograms and Doppler ultrasounds (US), were reviewed.

Results.—The median follow-up was 72 days (range 1-720 days), with a total follow-up of 23,040 line days. Venous thrombosis occurred in five out of 191 (2.6%) CVC in a distal position (distal third of the superior vena cava (SVC) or right atrium (RA)), five of 95 (5.3%) in an intermediate position (middle third of the SVC) and 20 of 48 (41.7%) in a proximal position (proximal third SVC or thoracic inlet veins). There was a significant difference in thrombosis rate between lines sited with the tip in a distal compared with a proximal position ($p<0.0005$). CVC with tips in a proximal position were 16 times more likely to thrombose than those in a distal position. None of the 58 CVC with the tip located in the RA thrombosed or caused complications.

Conclusion.—Distal placement of tunnelled CVC, either in the distal third of the SVC or proximal RA is optimal (Fig 3).

▶ The recommendation for a more distal position of a CVC tip to prevent catheter-associated venous thrombosis is not new, but deserves emphasis. The study has a number of potential limitations. No follow-up was recorded in

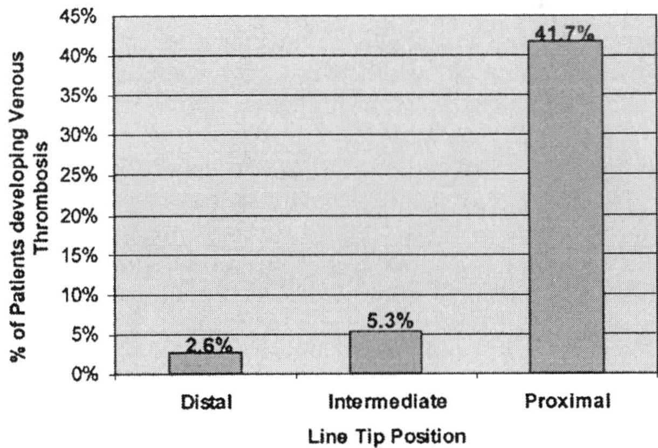

FIGURE 3.—The incidence of radiologically proven venous thrombosis correlated with line tip position. (Reprinted by permission of the publisher from Cadman A, Lawrance JAL, Fitzsimmons L, et al: To clot or not to clot? That is the question in central venous catheters. *Clin Radiol* 59:349-355, 2004. Copyright 2004 by Elsevier Science Inc.)

one third of the patients, patient follow-up notes were not reviewed, and cases of clinically suspected venous thrombosis that were not imaged were not included. Nevertheless, the authors' recommendation for more distal positioning of venous catheter tips to avoid CVC-associated venous thrombosis remains valid.

G. L. Moneta, MD

A New Type of Magnification System in Vascular Surgery—An Evaluation Study

Hofmann WJ, Walter J, Czerny M, et al (St John's Hosp, Salzburg, Austria; Univ of Vienna)

Eur J Vasc Endovasc Surg 27:676-678, 2004 17–13

Background.—Loupe magnification is a commonly used technique in vascular surgery. The magnification of available loupe systems is up to 8×. However, the depth of field and the field of view decrease with every increase in magnification. Thus, when surgeons use standard high-magnification loupes with a narrow depth of field, they must either adjust their posture or adjust the position of the operating table to be in accordance with the working distance of the magnifying system. An experience with a new type of magnification system to overcome the limitations of standard surgical loupes—the Varioscope® AF 3—was described. This system was developed in close cooperation with a surgical department.

Overview.—The Varioscope AF 3 system is composed of a dynamic Keplerian telescope mounted on a headset (Fig 1). The cost of the system ranges from 14,000 to 16,000 Euro, depending on the features included. This system can provide an infinitely variable range of magnification from 3.6× to 7.2×, and the working distance ranges from 300 to 600 mm. In addition to the zoom function, the Varioscope has a focus function that is activated automatically or on demand. The Varioscope was used in 221 procedures from June 2000 to May 2002. No technical failures occurred, and no intraoperative adverse events were attributable to the optical system. A comparison was conducted of the results and operating times of 98 carotid endarterectomies and 123 infrainguinal revascularizations performed using the Varioscope (group A) with the same number of operations performed using conventional loupe systems (group B). The operating times of carotid endarterectomies and tibial and pedal reconstructions were significantly shorter in the group in which the Varioscope was used. Early primary patency rates of peripheral vascular reconstructions showed no significant differences between the groups (98.3% of patients in group A vs. 95.1% of patients in group B). No significant difference also in the perioperative major complication rate was noted between the groups (4.5% for group A vs. 4.1% for group B).

Conclusions.—The Varioscope can allow vascular surgeons to refocus the system at any time, enabling them to maintain the most efficient and ergonomic working position at all times.

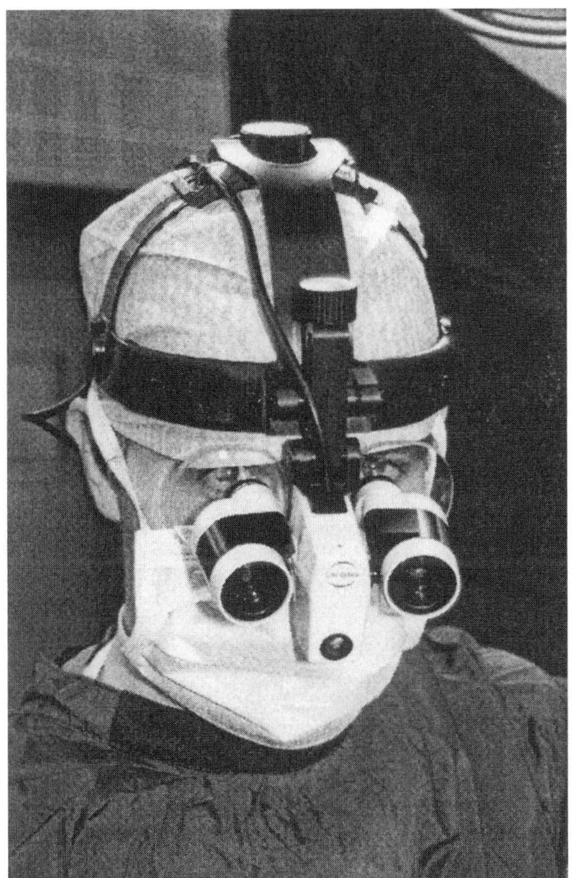

FIGURE 1.—The Varioscope® AF 3 mounted on the head set. (Reprinted from Hofmann WJ, Walter J, Czerny M, et al: A new type of magnification system in vascular surgery—an evaluation study. *Eur J Vasc Endovasc Surg* 27:676-678, 2004. Copyright 2004 by permission of the publisher.)

▶ This device looks interesting. The ability to vary magnification and focal lengths without changing loupes or looking "around" the telescopes would seem to be an advantage over traditional surgical telescopes. However, I think it will need to be less expensive and more compact and lighter before it will gain widespread use.

G. L. Moneta, MD

Subject Index

A

B

C

D

E

F

G

H

I

K

L

M

N

O

P

Q

R

S

T

U

V

W

Author Index

A

B

C

I

J

K

L

M

N

O

P

Q

R

S

T

U

V

W

X

Y

Z